SYSTEM OF OPHTHALMOLOGY

The proposed scheme for the "System of Ophthalmology" is as follows, but its division into different volumes is liable to alteration.

SYSTEM OF OPHTHALMOLOGY

EDITED BY

SIR STEWART DUKE-ELDER

VOL. XI

DISEASES OF THE LENS AND VITREOUS; GLAUCOMA AND HYPOTONY

WITH 686 ILLUSTRATIONS AND 9 COLOURED PLATES

LONDON

HENRY KIMPTON

1969

Reprinted 1971

Standard Book Number 85313 755 2

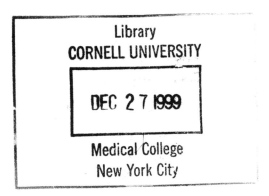
MADE AND PRINTED IN GREAT BRITAIN

Published in London by
Henry Kimpton
205 Great Portland Street, W.1

CONTRIBUTORS

The Sections on DISEASES OF THE LENS and DISEASES
OF THE VITREOUS were written by

Sir Stewart Duke-Elder
G.C.V.O., F.R.S.

The Section on GLAUCOMA AND HYPOTONY was written by

Sir Stewart Duke-Elder

and

Barrie Jay
M.D., F.R.C.S.

**(Consultant Surgeon, Moorfields Eye Hospital
Consultant Ophthalmic Surgeon, The London Hospital)**

PREFACE

THIS Volume completes the series of this *System* dealing with diseases of the eye itself and therefore includes three subjects which to some extent are unrelated.

During the last thirty years there has been no striking revolution in our ideas on the diseases of the lens apart from the great improvement in the several surgical techniques now available for their treatment. Cataract, the most important of these, has certainly received much attention but, despite the immense amount of research which has been devoted to the elucidation of its ætiology, our knowledge of the biochemistry of the normal or pathological lens has not yet reached the stage when the rapidly accumulating but somewhat disconnected data can be integrated into a coherent story. We still must be content with the vague statement that it is a senile degeneration wherein the essential determinant is anoxia because the necessary enzymes lose their efficiency—perhaps a definition of senescence itself.

Diseases of the vitreous body are usually secondary degenerations and although we know more about the minutiæ of their various clinical manifestations, recent advances are again mainly surgical in nature, for it may be said that an operative attack on some of the worst consequences of these has now been inaugurated.

While the ætiology of simple glaucoma still remains obscure, although the site of the obstruction of the aqueous is now known with more certainty than in the past and the progress of the disease can now be more accurately assessed, our ideas on closed-angle glaucoma have undergone a complete revolution. Largely through the introduction of gonioscopy as a popular method of examination, the immediate origin of this condition is now clear and our understanding of the mechanism of pupillary blockage and closure of the drainage angle has made the operation for its prophylaxis and cure in the early stages one of the safest and most satisfactory procedures in the whole of surgery. In many cases the cause of the condition is thus completely explained, but in others it may be that recent stress on the simple mechanics of the local condition in the eye has tended to obscure our appreciation of the part the general constitution of the patient may play in the basic ætiology of the disease, for in many cases the eye shares in the fortunes of the entire body of which it is a part. At the present moment it may be that ophthalmologists are sometimes acting as myopic carpenters rather than good physicians; but this tendency will doubtless be corrected in time.

STEWART DUKE-ELDER.

INSTITUTE OF OPHTHALMOLOGY,
UNIVERSITY OF LONDON,
1969

ACKNOWLEDGEMENTS

IN the first place I must thank Mr. James R. Hudson for assistance in writing the section on modern techniques in the surgical extraction of cataract; he has also helped me in compiling the references in the literature on diseases of the lens. Mr. John H. Dobree assisted me with the references in the section on diseases of the vitreous. To both of them I am indebted.

As in the previous Volumes, I have been provided with illustrations from a large number of authors, all of whom have showed great kindness in this respect. Without their help the value of this book would have been considerably lowered. These are all acknowledged in the appropriate legends to the figures. Among them, however, I am more than happy to make especial note of Professor Norman Ashton of the Institute of Ophthalmology and Dr. L. E. Zimmerman of the Armed Forces Institute of Pathology in Washington, D.C. Again, for the many illustrations I have obtained from the Medical Illustration Department of the Institute of Ophthalmology, from Dr. Peter Hansell and his staff, I am extremely grateful. Finally, Dr. F. N. L. Poynter has helped me with historical portraits from the Wellcome Institute of the History of Medicine.

As in the previous Volumes of this *System*, I must thank Miss Mina H. T. Yuille of the Library of the Institute of Ophthalmology and Mr. A. J. B. Goldsmith for helping me by reading the proofs, and Miss Rosamund E. Soley for her usual invaluable help in preparing the manuscript, reading the proofs, arranging the illustrations, verifying the bibliographies and writing the Index. Mr. George and Mr. Ronald Deed have again proved to be the most sympathetic and understanding of publishers.

STEWART DUKE-ELDER.

CONTENTS

SECTION I
DISEASES OF THE LENS

Chapter I
General Considerations

Chapter II
The Capsule and Subcapsular Epithelium

Chapter III
Cataract

CONTENTS

CHAPTER IV

DISPLACEMENTS OF THE LENS

SECTION II

DISEASES OF THE VITREOUS BODY

CHAPTER V

DISEASES OF THE VITREOUS BODY

SECTION III

GLAUCOMA AND HYPOTONY

Chapter VI

Introduction

Chapter VII

Simple Glaucoma

CHAPTER X

OCULAR HYPOTONY

SECTION I

DISEASES OF THE LENS

BY

Sɪʀ Sᴛᴇᴡᴀʀᴛ Dᴜᴋᴇ-Eʟᴅᴇʀ

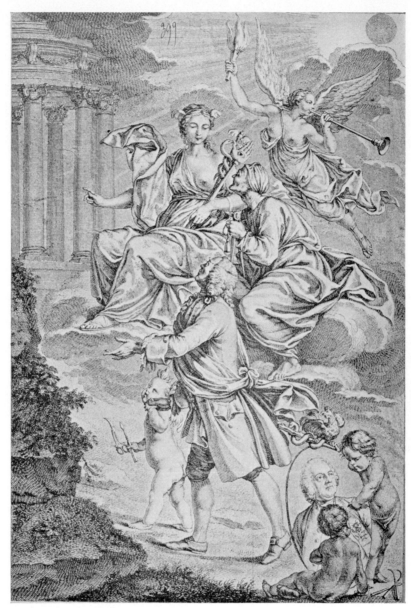

FIG. 1.—DAVIEL'S MARCH TO IMMORTALITY.

For explanation of the allegory, see text.

CHAPTER I

GENERAL CONSIDERATIONS

THE lens is discussed in other volumes of this *System* in some detail. The variations in its morphology in the animal kingdom have been described in Vol. I; its anatomy in man in Vol. II, p. 309; its embryology in Vol. III, p. 127, and its post-natal development on p. 307; the many congenital anomalies which may occur, in Vol. III, p. 688, and the occurrence of colobomata on pp. 472 and 706; its normal metabolism in Vol. IV, Chapter 6; and the techniques of clinical examination in Vol. VII, p. 260.

From the *historical* point of view, a rational understanding of the nature of diseases of the lens is of comparatively recent date. We have already seen in a previous Volume[1] that by Aristotle in classical Greece this structure

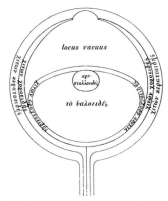

FIG. 2.—THE EYE AFTER CELSUS (*c.* 25 B.C.–A.D. 50).

The outer coat is the cornea and sclera (*keratoides*); within this, the uvea is pierced by the pupil (*vascular choroides*), within which is a web-like *arachnoides* (retina) of unknown function containing the *hyaloides* (vitreous); in front of this is the *crystalloides* (lens), a drop of humour resembling the white of an egg, the seat of the faculty of vision. In front of it is an empty space (the *locus vacuus*) (reconstructed by Magnus, *Die Augenheilkunde der Altern*, Breslau, 1901).

was considered to be an accumulation of phlegm appearing as a post-mortem artefact. In the late Greek learning of the Alexandrian School, although its presence in the eye was recognized, its function and even its location were matters of fancies and prejudices firmly perpetuated by the teaching of Celsus and Galen; it was thought to be the essential organ of vision situated in the centre of the globe and the opacification of cataract was regarded not as lenticular but due to the accumulation and solidification of evil humors in the empty space (*locus vacuus*) between it and the pupil (Fig. 2). Despite

[1] Vol. II, p. 309; Vol. IV, p. 1.

the ancient Hindu teaching of Suśruta[1] that cataract was a disease of the lens itself, the Greek view was accepted as dogma in Europe for 16 centuries. It was not until the late 16th century that Felix Platter (1583)[2] demonstrated that the lens was merely an optical medium, not until the beginning of the next century that it was correctly positioned by Fabricius ab Aquapendente of Padua (1600),[3] and not until a further half century had passed that suggestions were made that cataract was an affection of the lens itself.[4] It was not until a century later when the great and original French surgeon, Jacques Daviel (1748–53),[5] published and demonstrated his technique for the extraction of cataract, that modern concepts of diseases of the lens and their treatment emerged; and for this reason we have chosen for the frontispiece of this Volume the delightful tribute paid to him by the French artist, François de Vogue, blind from the age of 20, whose vision was restored by Daviel in 1756 after his other eye had been rendered useless by unsuccessful surgery.

The allegory of Daviel's March to Immortality depicts in the centre the great surgeon whose right hand leads his genius who has a flame of fire on his forehead and holds Daviel's lancet and scissors. Above, the young female figure of Invention sits upon a cloud holding in her left hand a caduceus, the symbol of medical science, attached to which is a hand in the palm of which is an eye. With her right hand Invention points to the Temple of Memory standing on steep rocks to denote its inaccessibility. Also on the cloud at Invention's left side and a little below her is the aged figure of Experience and behind is Fame with a torch in one hand and blowing her trumpet. On top the sun disperses the clouds of darkness with its beams. At the lower right-hand corner one little genius shows to the other the picture of Daviel above which is a caduceus on which perches a cock to signify Health. It is only fitting that this charming and typically French tribute should introduce this Section on Diseases of the Lens.

Since the lens is devoid of blood vessels and lies suspended in the intraocular fluid as an isolated colony of cells within a capsule, its pathology is more simple than that of most other tissues. Its avascularity makes the typical reaction to pathological injury impossible; primary inflammatory processes do not therefore occur, and the result of trauma is merely passive and degenerative. The only cells in the lens, indeed, capable of regenerative activity or of an active response to irritation are those of the epithelial layer beneath the anterior and equatorial capsule. Since, however, the maintenance of optical transparency—the primary function of the lens —depends upon the smooth working of a complicated metabolism which is precluded from an active response to any insults offered to it, a whole host of conditions—traumatic, toxic or metabolic, local or systemic—is liable to occur wherein its cytochemistry is upset, and degeneration and consequent

[1] *Suśruta Samhita*, Vol. III, Chap. 17, Verses 53–73. See Vol. II, p. 17.
[2] *De corporis humani structura*, Basel (1583).
[3] *De oculo* (1600).
[4] p. 66.
[5] *Mercure de France*, 198 (1748); *Mém. Acad. roy. Chir.*, Paris, **2**, 337 (1753).

opacification result. Thus although limited in their variety, diseases of the lens are not rare; and apart from changes which may occur in the capsule, they are essentially limited to the optical disability of a failure to maintain its transparency, to which must be added a failure to maintain its position; both of these, of course, have serious functional results.

SECONDARY INFLAMMATORY CHANGES

It is to be remembered that although primary inflammation of the lens does not occur, this tissue is affected in many types of intra-ocular infection. Only occasionally does an abscess form in cases of panophthalmitis due either to direct infection from a perforating ulcer or to the development of a

FIGS. 3 to 6. ABSCESS OF THE LENS.

In a 29-year-old patient with an acute bilateral iridocyclitis who developed a vitreous abscess in the left eye; at a later date abscesses appeared in both lenses (G. Goder).

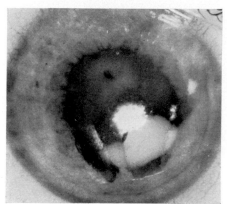 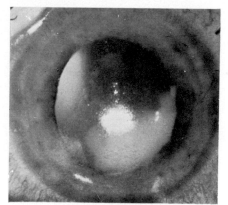

FIG. 3.   FIG. 4.

FIGS. 3 and 4.—The lens in the right eye and in the left eye in the early stage of abscess formation.

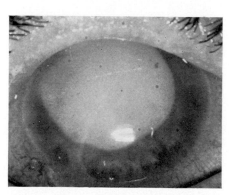 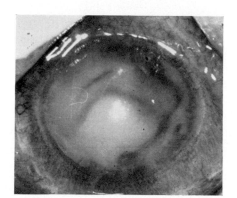

FIG. 5.   FIG. 6.

FIGS. 5 and 6.—The lenses 7 weeks later.

metastatic abscess within the eye (Deutschmann, 1880; Wagenmann, 1896; Higuchi, 1934; Schulte, 1947; Goder, 1967) (Figs. 3–6). In these rare cases the purulent infiltration may seep between the lamellæ of an unbroken capsule, but more usually this protective barrier is eroded and perforated. In less acute cases if the capsule is intact the inward diffusion of toxins causes death and autolysis of the fibres and a complicated cataract results, a subject which will be discussed at a later stage. The pathology of such a development has already been described[1]; in acute inflammations the cytolytic products of the purulent cells dissolve the lens fibres while, if the eye survives, giant cells, granulation tissue and fibroblasts follow in their wake converting the lens into an organized vascularized mass of connective tissue (Fig. 7), and eventually a firm and distorted cicatrix is formed which

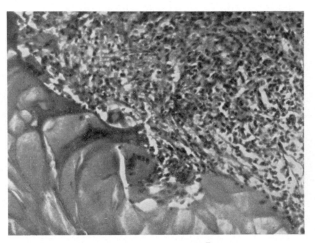

Fig. 7.—Abscess of the Lens.
The abscess of the lens seen in Fig. 6, showing resorptive activity of the granulation tissue (G. Goder).

may finally become calcified; so long as the capsule remains intact it forms an impassable barrier to osteoblasts and true bone formation does not occur. It is important, however, that in these inflammatory reactions the tissues of the lens retain their passive role.

An interesting case was described by Wolter and Bryson (1966) wherein a rupture of the posterior capsule occurred some days after an encircling operation for retinal detachment; a violent phaco-anaphylactic endophthalmitis necessitated enucleation (Figs. 8–10). The anterior capsule was wrinkled, the posterior capsule coiled up, and within the cataractous lens was a massive inflammatory granulomatous reaction with a dense infiltration of pus and giant cells.

We have also seen[2] that a *total cataract* may result as a congenital anomaly particularly when the capsule is ruptured and the lens is invaded by fibro-vascular tissue in

[1] Vol. IX, pp. 96, 107.   [2] Vol. III, p. 752.

FIGS. 8 to 10.—RUPTURE OF THE POSTERIOR LENS CAPSULE IN RETINAL DETACHMENT SURGERY (J. R. Wolter and J. M. Bryson).

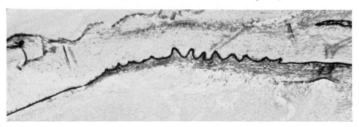

FIG. 8.—The wrinkled anterior lens capsule.

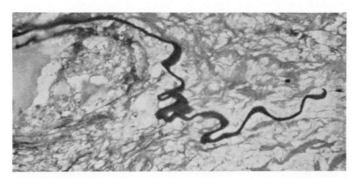

FIG. 9.—Rupture of the posterior lens capsule showing its coiled-up free end.

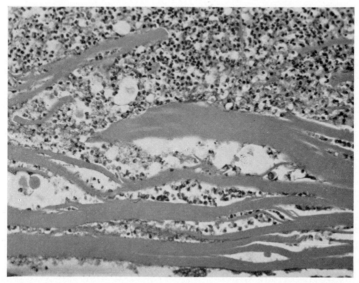

FIG. 10.—Pus cells among the degenerating lens fibres within the cataractous lens in the phaco-anaphylactic endophthalmitis which developed 11 days after surgery.

cases of persistence of the vascular sheath of the lens and the hyaloid vessels; such a lens tends to become shrunken and undergo fibrous, fatty or calcareous degeneration.

A curious case of a HÆMORRHAGE IN THE LENS was reported by Stein (1955). The hæmorrhage remained unchanged beneath the posterior capsule of a child (aged 4) associated with a localized posterior cortical cataract; Stein attributed its origin to the rupture of a posterior hyaloid artery.

NEOPLASMS

It may seem curious that although the cells of the subcapsular epithelium undergo mitosis and division throughout life, neoplasic growths in the lens are unknown. This would appear not to be due to an inherent immunity of

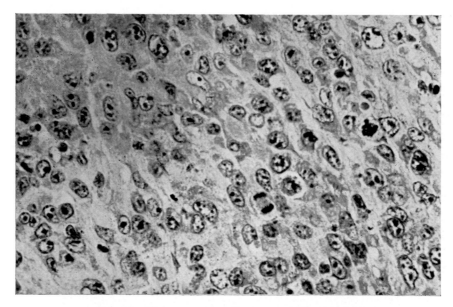

FIG. 11.—TUMOUR OF THE SUBCAPSULAR EPITHELIUM.
Experimental carcinomatous tumour induced subcutaneously in the mouse. Many mitotic figures are seen (Ida Mann).

these cells to cancerous changes, for Ida Mann (1947) showed that if the lens of the mouse were embedded in subcutaneous tissue and the capsule ruptured, the addition of a carcinogenic agent (methylcholanthrene) led to vascularization of the lens and after 2 to 3 months to the formation of a cancerous tumour which gave rise to metastases in the neighbouring lymph nodes and retained its characters through at least eight passages (Fig. 11). The cells showed much mitotic activity and were characteristic of the sub-capsular epithelium and grew readily in tissue-culture. No result, however, was obtained unless the capsule were ruptured and the lens became vas-cularized. The fact that these cells which potentially can become malignant do not do so in life is not understood; it may be due to the avascularity of this tissue and its low metabolic activity (Walther, 1937–39).

A METASTATIC INVASION of the lens by a malignant tumour, however, can occur. Hallermann and Meisner (1954) described a unique case wherein metastases from a malignant melanoma of the ciliary body invaded the

FIGS. 12 and 13.—NEOPLASIC INVASION OF THE LENS.

In a case of malignant melanoma of the ciliary body and choroid (W. Hallermann and G. Meisner).

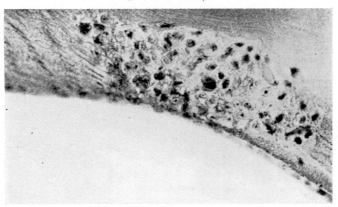

FIG. 12.—A pocket of neoplasic cells showing pigmentation and mitosis within the intact capsule near the equator of the lens.

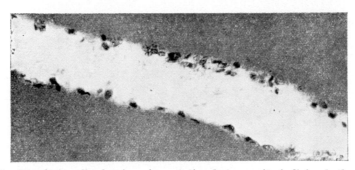

FIG. 13.—Neoplasic cells showing pigmentation but no mitosis lining both sides of a cleft between the nucleus and posterior cortex of the lens.

lens although the capsule remained intact; there was a mass of neoplasic cells underneath the capsule and also groups of pigmented cells in a cleft between the nucleus and cortex (Figs. 12–13).

The DEFORMATION OF THE LENS by a tumour of the anterior uveal tract is a rare phenomenon but is nevertheless more common than an invasion of this tissue. It may cause a localized or complete cataract, but it may also indent the lens without inducing an opacity. This was first described with the slit-lamp by Nordmann (1930) who showed that the cortex and the zones of discontinuity may be deformed while optical clarity is preserved (Figs. 14 and 15). Fuchs (1882) assumed that this deformation was due to an absorption or autolysis of the tissues of the lens. An alternative assumption is that the lens is moulded by pressure without a loss of its substance, a view supported by Nordmann (1965–66) who found that the deformation caused by a ciliary tumour disappeared after the neoplasm had been treated by a cyclectomy so that the lens practically resumed its normal shape. As a rarity the pressure of a tumour may be sufficient to rupture the capsule and produce a traumatic cataract.[1]

FIGS. 14 and 15.—DEFORMATION OF THE LENS (J. Nordmann).

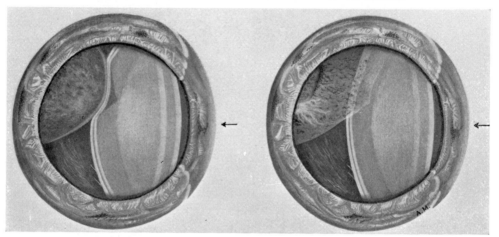

FIG. 14.   FIG. 15.

FIG. 14.—Deformation of the posterior surface of the lens by a ciliary tumour
seen in the beam of the slit-lamp, in a man aged 71.

FIG. 15.—Restoration of the shape of the lens on the relief of pressure after a
cyclectomy; the condition has remained unchanged for $2\frac{1}{2}$ years.

NORMAL AGE CHANGES

A note on the normal changes in the lens with growth and ageing as distinct from the development of senile cataract is apposite here. Its progressive increase in size, weight and density is determined essentially by the continued addition of new tissue which, instead of being cast off from the surface as occurs in other ectodermal tissues which are constantly renewed, accumulates within the lens as the old fibres are enveloped by the new. These additions can be seen with the slit-lamp in the adult lens as successive strata of discontinuity in the optical section so that by the time adult life is reached the successive nuclei—embryonic, foetal, infantile and adult—and the cortex are apparent, while near the capsule lies a strongly

[1] p. 59.

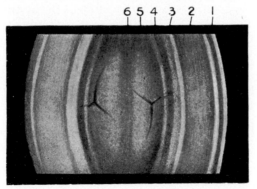

FIG. 16.—THE STRUCTURE OF THE LENS OF AN ADULT OF 40 YEARS AS SEEN IN THE
OPTICAL BEAM OF THE SLIT-LAMP.

1. Anterior capsule.	4. Infantile nucleus.
2. Cortex.	5. Fœtal nucleus.
3. Adult nucleus.	6. Embryonic nucleus.

reflecting zone of disjunction (Vogt, 1931) (Fig. 16); the latter probably
represents a changed state in the lens fibres as they mature when they become
characterized optically by a higher refractive index. The thickness of this
zone thus represents the speed of growth which progressively diminishes
with age; this layer is therefore thinner in the old than in the young and may

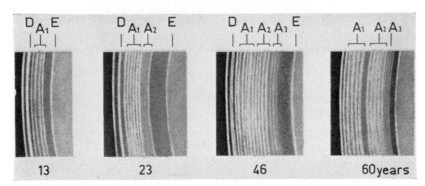

FIG. 17.—ELEMENTARY ZONES IN THE NUCLEUS OF THE LENS.

The elementary zones in the adult nucleus in people of the ages given below
the figures. A_1, formed in childhood; A_2, added after puberty; A_3, added after the
40th year of life; D, zone of disjunction; E, infantile nucleus (H. Goldmann).

even disappear when the growth of the lens has been retarded through
injury (Goldmann, 1964). On the other hand, the thickness of the cortex
and particularly the nucleus increases with age, the progress of which is
seen most dramatically in the adult nucleus wherein many *elementary zones
of discontinuity* up to 20 in number may be visible in a thin optical section;
these are arranged in three groups, the first appearing before puberty, the

second lying anterior to these becoming evident in the third decade, and the third group forming after the fortieth year (Goldmann, 1937–64; Goldmann and Niesel, 1964) (Fig. 17). These iso-indicial reflecting zones probably represent layers of increasing refractivity indicating the state of ageing of the lens fibres as they slowly move inwards towards the centre of the lens; at the same time they are characterized histologically by a change in the cross-section of the lens fibres (Vogt, 1931) and in their staining properties (Cibis, 1956).

It is probable that the shrinkage and optical irregularity of these strips give rise to the appearance known as the *senile nuclear relief*. This peculiar modelling of the surfaces of optical discontinuity of the nuclei of the

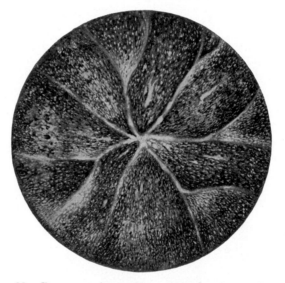

FIG. 18.—RELIEF OF ADULT NUCLEUS IN THE SENILE LENS.

lens is clearly visible only with the slit-lamp. Sometimes it may become distinguishable soon after 20 years of age, but is very common after 50 (Vogt, 1918; Vogt and Lüssi, 1919). The anterior surface of the adult nucleus shows the phenomenon most clearly, particularly in the axial region where the sutures form prominent branching projections throwing shadows on oblique illumination and marking out the design of the lens fibres, while rounded protuberances, presumably vacuoles, are sometimes present (Fig. 18). It is to be noted that this optical effect is not derived from a single internal optical surface but originates somewhat diffusely from zones of varying thickness (Goldmann, 1937).

Occasionally a similar phenomenon is seen on the posterior face of the adult nucleus but here, of course, the relief is reversed; and as a rarity a more simple and less embossed pattern is seen on the anterior surface of the fœtal nucleus. It is to be noted that neither of these senile phenomena impairs the function of vision; they are physiological in nature and are not necessarily a prelude to the development of cataract.

We have already discussed[1] the changes in shape which constantly occur from the almost globular lens of fœtal and infantile life to the lenticular shape of the adult, as well as its progressive increase in size throughout life up to and beyond the age of 80 years until the increment may be three-fold,[2] a phenomenon which results in a shallowing of the anterior chamber and is peculiar to the higher primates and not seen in lower vertebrates. The young lens remains optically clear until maturity; in the ageing lens, apart from the immediately subcapsular layer, there is a slight but progressive increase in its refractive index, especially in the nucleus,[3] and a decrease in the transmissivity particularly of the short waves of the spectrum, largely owing to an increase in the scattering of light and to the presence of a yellow pigment which absorbs short-waved light. This yellow-brown pigment is of common occurrence in the newborn (Vogt, 1931; Cowan, 1959); it increases slowly with age but normally gets no more dense than a light straw-colour even in the aged but clear lens, being always darker in the nucleus than in the cortex (Said and Weale, 1959). The nature of the pigment is unknown but electrospectrographic studies have indicated that it is probably related to melanin (Cowan, 1959; J. and E. Meyer-Arendt, 1960). In senile sclerosis of the lens it may become much more dense and obvious in which connection it will be more fully discussed.[4] The result is that the retina of the aged eye receives less light in general and less blue-violet radiation in particular than the youthful retina. Functionally, although the visual acuity may be little impaired by these changes, the increased consistency diminishes accommodative adaptability and contributes to the development of presbyopia; while the greater density of the central region results in lenticular myopia, a change, however, usually compensated in the absence of marked nuclear sclerosis by the increased flattening of the lens as a whole with age.

A fuller discussion on the normal[5] and abnormal[6] metabolism of the lens will be found elsewhere, but a short summary of the main chemical changes with age may be useful at this stage.[7] It is generally accepted that there is a decrease in its content of water with age, an increase of calcium and sodium, and a decrease in potassium and phosphates. The total content of proteins increases with age, the most important change being the increase of the insoluble (albuminoid) proteins; in the young rat the albuminoid comprises 6 to 7% of the total protein while in the senile animal it amounts to 67% (Dische et al., 1956–59; Lerman et al., 1962). At the same time, the synthesis of soluble proteins decreases as well as the activity of the amino acids, RNA and the

---

[1] Vol. III, p. 307.
[2] Priestley Smith (1883), Raeder (1922), Scammon and Hesdorffer (1937), Johansen (1947), Snydacker (1956), Weale (1962–63).
[3] Woinow (1874), Freytag (1908), Huggert (1948), Nordmann (1954).
[4] p. 127.   [5] Vol. IV, p. 385.   [6] p. 72.
[7] For general summaries, see Bellows (1944), Weekers (1950), Nordmann (1954–65), H. K. Müller et al. (1957), Weale (1963), Thomann (1963), Sippel (1965), Hockwin (1965), Lerman and Zigman (1965).

protein-incorporating systems (Merriam and Kinsey, 1950; Devi *et al.*, 1961; Lerman *et al.*, 1961–62); while the albuminoid RNA increases and the turnover of lenticular RNA shows a progressive decline (Ely, 1949; Virmaux *et al.*, 1958; Praus and Obenberger, 1961; Lerman *et al.*, 1962). The total amount of cystine also increases with age, but the cysteine and glutathione drop considerably, as also does ascorbic acid (Rosner *et al.*, 1938; Pirie *et al.*, 1955). The total lipids decrease in concentration while both the free and total cholesterol increase (Bellows, 1944).

The metabolic activity of the lens shows a progressive decrease during ageing. Most of its energy is derived from anaerobic glycolysis,[1] and the consumption of glucose and oxygen as well as the production of lactate and carbon dioxide all diminish (Sippel, 1962). The whole of the enzymic glycolytic activity also lessens; the hexose-monophosphate pathway is profoundly diminished, a mechanism active in youth but little used in age, while most of the enzymes necessary for metabolism show a lowered activity (carbonic anhydrase, hexokinase, aldolase and the various dehydrogenases). The high-energy labile phosphates (ATP, ADP and creatinine phosphate) which serve as intermediaries of glycolysis decrease in amount indicating a lessened turnover of phosphate (Kleifeld *et al.*, 1956). There is similar evidence of a diminution of the autoxidative capacity and, indeed, a lowering of anaerobic in favour of aerobic activity.

AXIAL PIGMENTATION OF THE LENS is a phenomenon which is rarely seen before the age of 35 but occurs in 30% of people over the age of 60 years (Vogt, 1922–31; O. Müller, 1930; Cowan, 1959–61). A variable density of minute granules of brown pigment of unknown origin but presumably related to melanin[2] appears in the cortex of the lens, at first at the confluence of the sutures just within the anterior line of disjunction in the axial region. The granules are minute (0·001 to 0·005 mm.) and are difficult to see unless under high magnification with the slit-lamp; they spread under the anterior capsule along the sutures and extend more deeply into the cortex, maintaining a remarkably symmetrical arrangement in each eye, but do not penetrate into the nucleus, the posterior cortex remaining free (Figs.19–24). The progression of this pigmentation is usually slow and it does not interfere with vision. It is unrelated to the development of cataract, to the presence of systemic disease, or to the pigmentation of the skin or the outer eye.

CYSTOID SPACES have been described by Reese and Wadsworth (1953) lying beneath the anterior and posterior surfaces of the adult nucleus in some 10% of people above the age of 40 years. Ophthalmoscopically they appear as small round grey opacities, sometimes few in number and sometimes multiple and concentrically arranged. With the slit-lamp they appear as optically empty spaces. These authors have observed their presence for 17 and 19 years without any suggestion of the development of cataract. Histologically the oval spaces contain an eosinophilic granular material, and they interfere little with vision.

Structurally the CAPSULE increases in thickness with age (Clapp, 1942), and in the senile lens Callahan and Klien (1958) found that it tended to become dissociated into layers so that the anterior lamella suffered a *senile exfoliation*. At the posterior pole Alvaro (1953) noted with the slit-lamp a multicoloured iridescence associated with the capsule in 7 to 8% of subjects

---

[1] Vol. IV, p. 357.   [2] p. 127.

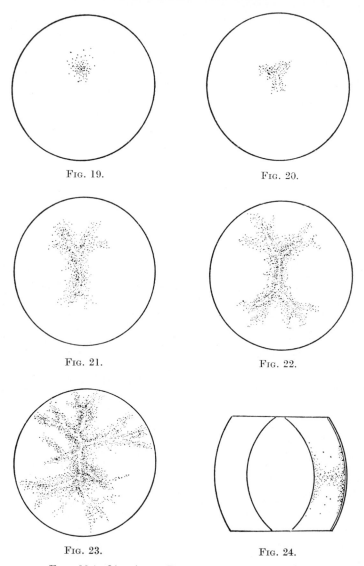

FIG. 19.   FIG. 20.

FIG. 21.   FIG. 22.

FIG. 23.   FIG. 24.

FIGS. 19 to 24.—AXIAL PIGMENTATION OF THE LENS.

The first five figures show the progressive stages of axial pigmentation of the lens. Fig. 24 shows the situation of the granules between the anterior line of disjunction and the adult nucleus (T. H. Cowan).

between the ages of 45 and 65; while its content of glycolytic enzymes is said to be decreased (Dardenne, 1955). The subcapsular epithelium becomes flatter, some cells may show vacuolation, others lipid degeneration, and occasionally lacunæ may be found in this layer. At the same time mitotic activity in the epithelium is decreased and the migration of the equatorial cells into the substance of the lens diminished (Hanna and O'Brien, 1961; Cotlier, 1962; Mikulicich and Young, 1963). The zone of disjunction becomes thinned presumably because the formation of new fibres is retarded or stopped (Goldmann and Niesel, 1964). The cells of the lens themselves, compressed and buried centrally as growth proceeds, become sclerosed, their cytoplasm loses its basophilia, their nuclei become pale and fragmented and suffer pyknosis, the lipid membranes between them disappear so that they have no firm attachment to each other, their edges become serrated and the entire tissue becomes hard and sclerotic, changing into acidophilic fibres without nuclei, a process analogous to keratinization in the skin and when fully developed leading to the formation of a sclerotic nuclear cataract. At the same time there is loss of pliability of the zonular fibres, a change which makes the extracapsular extraction of a cataract more easy in the old than in the young.

THE HEALING OF WOUNDS

As a general rule wounds in the lens of man do not heal, for the only constituent which may show reparative activity is the subcapsular epithelium. If the capsule is perforated, either by accident or design as in the operation of discission, or is torn in a concussive injury, the rent remains open and the lens fibres coming into contact with the aqueous imbibe fluid freely, swell up and become opaque, sometimes within a few hours, a process which we shall consider more fully when dealing with cataract. Occasionally with small punctures, as may occur following the entrance of a small foreign body or may occasionally happen in a discission operation, the wound becomes plugged and a stationary partial cataract results, a sequence more frequently seen in animals such as the rabbit than in man, presumably because with their lower accommodative power the capsule is less taut and elastic and thus tends to gape less when pierced. As a result a scar is left in the capsule. Alternatively, in the anterior polar region the damage is limited by an intense proliferation of the subcapsular epithelium with a regeneration of the capsule, a somewhat unpredictable process which we shall discuss more fully at a later stage.[1] This was first adequately studied by Schlösser (1887) and Schirmer (1889) whose findings have been confirmed by later workers (Sanna, 1931; Brini et al., 1962–63; and others). Somewhat after the same manner as occurs in wounds of the cornea, the surrounding epithelium becomes pushed towards the torn edges of the wound, the cells lose their regular cubical shape, become flattened, undergo mitosis and begin to proliferate. These cells have the appearance and staining reactions of connective-tissue fibroblasts, for which they have sometimes been mistaken. Whatever the response, a localized and often stationary opacity may develop either amorphous, punctate, stellate or

[1] p. 21.

rosette-shaped in design, usually in the vicinity of the wound but sometimes in the region of the posterior pole.

More usually, however, if the laceration has been large, the capsule gapes, the swollen lens material protrudes through the wound and soon becomes disintegrated by proteolytic enzymes; this allows more lens fibres to come into contact with the aqueous until eventually the entire lens becomes tumescent and opaque. In young persons the end-result may be a complete absorption of the lens, apart from the capsule, but in older subjects the sclerosed state of the central fibres forbids this happy termination. When the substance of the lens is exposed to the aqueous humour, no untoward reaction may be excited and a slow solution may occur, while on the surface of the broken capsule the epithelial cells may show an aberrant activity by swelling into large globular shapes (*Elschnig's pearls*, 1911). Sometimes, however, a macrophagic reaction may be excited in which the lens is invaded by epithelioid cells forming a wall in the cortex with aggregations of giant cells around the nucleus. Occasionally the violent immunological reaction of phaco-anaphylactic uveitis is excited wherein mononuclear phagocytes predominate, which frequently leads to disastrous results (Figs. 8 to 10). This has been studied in a previous volume.[1]

All these changes following injury, either from concussion or perforating trauma, and the different types of cataract to which they may give rise will be discussed fully in a subsequent Volume on Injuries.[2] In this context the interesting feature is that in its opacification the lens plays only a passive role; the only constituent which may show evidences of active healing is the subcapsular epithelium.

Alvaro. *Amer. J. Ophthal.*, **86**, 1241 (1953).
Bellows. *Cataract and Anomalies of the Lens*, St. Louis (1944).
Brini, Porte and Stoeckel. *C.R. Acad. Sci.* (Paris), **255**, 3485 (1962).
Bull. Soc. franç. Ophtal., **76**, 193 (1963).
Callahan and Klien. *Arch. Ophthal.*, **59**, 73 (1958).
Cibis. *Amer. J. Ophthal.*, **42**, 278 (1956).
Clapp. *Amer. J. Ophthal.*, **25**, 437 (1942).
Cotlier. *Arch. Ophthal.*, **68**, 801 (1962).
Cowan. *Trans. Amer. ophthal. Soc.*, **57**, 539 (1959).
Surv. Ophthal., **6**, 630 (1961).
Dardenne. *Ber. dtsch. ophthal. Ges.*, **59**, 183 (1955).
Deutschmann. *v. Graefes Arch. Ophthal.*, **26**, 135 (1880).
Devi, Friel and Lerman. *Arch. Ophthal.*, **65**, 855 (1961).
Dische, Borenfreund and Zelmenis. *Arch. Ophthal.*, **55**, 471, 633 (1956).
Dische and Zelmenis. *Amer. J. Ophthal.*, **48** (2), 500 (1959).
Elschnig. *Klin. Mbl. Augenheilk.*, **49**, 444 (1911).

Ely. *Amer. J. Ophthal.*, **32** (2), 215 (1949).
Freytag. *Die Brechungsindices d. Linse*, Wiesbaden (1908).
Fuchs. *Das Sarcom des Uvealtractus*, Wien (1882).
Goder. *Klin. Mbl. Augenheilk.*, **151**, 8 (1967).
Goldmann. *Arch. Augenheilk.*, **110**, 405 (1937).
Amer. J. Ophthal., **57**, 1 (1964).
Goldmann and Niesel. *Ophthalmologica*, **147**, 134 (1964).
Hallermann and Meisner. *Klin. Mbl. Augenheilk.*, **124**, 159 (1954).
Hanna and O'Brien. *Arch. Ophthal.*, **66**, 103 (1961).
Higuchi. *Acta Soc. ophthal. jap.*, **38**, 154 (1934).
Hockwin. *Invest. Ophthal.*, **4**, 496 (1965).
Huggert. *Acta ophthal.* (Kbh.), Suppl. 30 (1948).
Johansen. *Studies in the Inter-relation in Size between the Cornea and Crystalline Lens in Man* (Thesis), Copenhagen (1947).

[1] Vol. IX, p. 500.   [2] Vol. XIV.

Kleifeld, Ayberk and Hockwin. *v. Graefes Arch. Ophthal.*, **158**, 34 (1956).

Lerman, Devi and Banerjee. *Invest. Ophthal.*, **1**, 95 (1962).

Lerman, Devi and Hawes. *Amer. J. Ophthal.*, **51**, 1012 (1961).

Lerman, Donk and Pitel. *Growth*, **26**, 103 (1962).

Lerman and Zigman. *Invest. Ophthal.*, **4**, 643 (1965).

Mann. *Trans. ophthal. Soc. U.K.*, **67**, 141 (1947).

Merriam and Kinsey. *Arch. Ophthal.*, **44**, 651 (1950).

Meyer-Arendt, J. and E. *J. Histochem. Cytochem.*, **8**, 75 (1960).

Mikulicich and Young. *Invest. Ophthal.*, **2**, 344 (1963).

Müller, H. K., Kleifeld, Dardenne *et al.* *Mod. Probl. Ophthal.*, **1**, 85 (1957).

Müller, O. *v. Graefes Arch. Ophthal.*, **124**, 444 (1930).

Nordmann. *Bull. Soc. Ophtal. Paris*, 157 (1930).
Biologie du cristallin, Paris (1954).
Adv. Ophthal., **12**, 1 (1962).
Invest. Ophthal., **4**, 384 (1965).
Bull. Soc. Ophtal. Fr., 655 (1965).
Travaux d'ophtalmologie moderne (dedicated to J. Mawas), Paris, 295 (1966).

Pirie, van Heyningen and Flanders. *Biochem. J.*, **61**, 341 (1955).

Praus and Obenberger. *Folia biol.* (Prague), **7**, 360 (1961).

Raeder. *v. Graefes Arch. Ophthal.*, **110**, 73 (1922).

Reese and Wadsworth. *Trans. Amer. ophthal. Soc.*, **51**, 307 (1953).

Rosner, Farmer and Bellows. *Arch. Ophthal.* **20**, 417 (1938).

Said and Weale. *J. Physiol.*, **145**, 45P (1959).
Gerontologia, **3**, 213 (1959).

Sanna. *Ann. Ottal.*, **59**, 543 (1931).

Scammon and Hesdorffer. *Arch. Ophthal.*, **17**, 104 (1937).

Schirmer. *v. Graefes Arch. Ophthal.*, **34** (3), 147 (1889).

Schlösser. *Experimentelle Studien ü. traumatische Katarakt*, Munich (1887).

Schulte. *Klin. Mbl. Augenheilk.*, **112**, 193 (1947).

Sippel. *Invest. Ophthal.*, **1**, 629 (1962); **4**, 502 (1965).

Smith, Priestley. *Trans. ophthal. Soc. U.K.*, **3**, 79 (1883).

Snydacker. *Trans. Amer. ophthal. Soc.*, **54**, 675 (1956).

Stein. *Acta med. orient.*, **14**, 209 (1955).

Thomann. *Klin. Mbl. Augenheilk.*, **143**, 338 (1963).

Virmaux, Klethi and Mandel. *C.R. Soc. Biol.* (Paris), **152**, 1570 (1958).

Vogt. *Klin. Mbl. Augenheilk.*, **61**, 89 (1918).
v. Graefes Arch. Ophthal., **108**, 192 (1922).
Lhb. u. Atlas d. Spaltlampenmikroskopie d. lebenden Auges, 2nd ed., Berlin, **2** (1931).

Vogt and Lüssi. *v. Graefes Arch. Ophthal.*, **100**, 157 (1919).

Wagenmann. *v. Graefes Arch. Ophthal.*, **42** (2), 1 (1896).

Walther. *Z. Krebsforsch.*, **46**, 313 (1937); **48**, 468 (1939).

Weale. *Brit. J. Ophthal.*, **46**, 660 (1962).
The Aging Eye, London (1963).

Weekers. *Rev. méd. Liège*, **5**, 20, 674 (1950).

Woinow. *Klin. Mbl. Augenheilk.*, **12**, 407 (1874).

Wolter and Bryson. *Amer. J. Ophthal.*, **61**, 1428 (1966).

CHAPTER II

THE CAPSULE AND SUBCAPSULAR EPITHELIUM

No treatise on the lens would be complete without a tribute to ANTON ELSCHNIG [1886–1939] (Fig. 25) on whose work much of our understanding both of the pathology of the lens and of the practical treatment of cataract has depended; in the present connection his studies in 1922–23 on the exfoliation of the lens capsule in glass-blowers were among the first of the major contributions which placed our knowledge of the structure and pathology of the capsule on a sure foundation. To this must be added the great part he played in establishing the value of the intracapsular technique in the extraction of cataract, as well as the popularization of keratoplasty. Born at Leibnitz, he went to Graz and then to Vienna under Schnabel, and in 1907, on the death of Czermak, he became professor of ophthalmology at Prague where he spent the remainder of his working life, eventually becoming Rector of the University. In his youth an able histologist, he excited considerable attention through his explanation of sympathetic ophthalmitis as an anaphylactic phenomenon; but his greatest claim to fame was his exceptional skill and ingenuity as an operating surgeon. Among a multitude of papers, his greatest contributions to our literature were the writing of the third edition of the *Graefe-Saemisch Handbuch* on operative surgery in two volumes, published in 1922, much of which was devoted to the surgery of the lens, and the description of the pathology of glaucoma in the Henke-Lubarsch *Handbuch der speziellen pathologischen Anatomie und Histologie* (1928). He retired in 1933 to live in the former home of Richard Wagner in Marienbad where he spent an idyllic life free from academic and surgical cares, in which his delight in music and art was fully realized until his death in Vienna following an automobile accident.

Changes in the Subcapsular Epithelium

PROLIFERATION OF THE EPITHELIUM

The proliferation of cells in the monolayer of the subcapsular epithelium is interesting and plays an important part in the pathology of the lens. Since the epithelial cells adhere to the capsule when this structure is peeled off, the process can be readily studied microscopically in flat mounts (Howard, 1952; von Sallmann, 1952); a detailed analysis can also be made with the application of high-resolution tritium autoradiography whereby the appearance of the specific tritium-labelled precursors of DNA synthesis (thymidine) can be followed, the process being stopped at the metaphase by the administration of colchicine or at various stages of the mitotic cycle by x-rays or such alkylating agents as busulphan or triethylene melamine (TEM). Such studies have been made on human lenses and on those of several animals (rabbit, rat, frog, fish)[1] and it has been established that while in

---

[1] Harding *et al.* (1960–62), Hanna and O'Brien (1961–63), Cotlier (1962–64), von Sallmann *et al.* (1962), Srinivasan and Harding (1965), Bito and Harding (1965), Bito *et al.* (1965), von Sallmann (1965), and others.

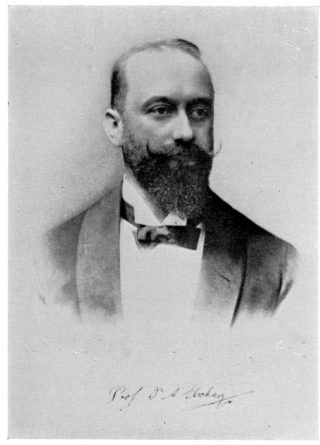

FIG. 25.—ANTON ELSCHNIG [1886–1939].
(Courtesy of Prof. F. Vrabec, Prague.)

the young lens mitosis is diffuse throughout the epithelial sheet, in the adult there is an active germinative zone only around the equator, diminishing in activity towards the axial region. Thus in rabbits von Sallmann and his collaborators (1962) found that the mitotic index in the equatorial zone was 0·26%, in the pre-equatorial zone 0·16%, and in the central area 0·02%; in the rat the turnover (intermitotic) time was 19 days in the first region, 31 days in the second, and as long as 250 days in the axial area. This activity ordinarily precedes the migration of cells from the equatorial zone and their differentiation into fibres which are incorporated into the body of the lens.

There would appear to be periodic fluctuations in animals in this mitotic activity which is increased in the evening in comparison with the morning (von Sallmann, 1952) and in summer compared with winter and spring (Miki, 1961). Moreover, it decreases with age as also does the rate of migration of the cells (Hanna and O'Brien, 1961; Cotlier, 1962; Mikulicich and Young, 1963). It is of interest that in lenses maintained in perfusion experiments the zonular distribution of mitotic activity changes so that instead of its accentuation in the germinative equatorial zone, it becomes more uniformly distributed to include the central area (Kinsey et al., 1955; Schwartz, 1960; Harding et al., 1962; Harding and Thayer, 1964).

This topographical differentiation of the mitotic activity of the epithelium so that it is normally restricted to the equatorial zone is at present unexplained. It is not inconceivable that modifications develop in the DNA of the central cells so that cellular division does not occur or, alternatively, that these are under some form of inhibition. It may be apposite that an unknown water-soluble inhibitor has been discovered in the epithelium and cortex of the lens of rabbits associated with the γ-crystallin fraction; it becomes increasingly concentrated with age (Froomberg and Voaden, 1966), and may have an activity analogous with the chalone which Bullough and Laurence (1964) found to act similarly as a mitotic inhibitor in the mammalian epidermis and the corneal epithelium. However that may be, in addition to its increase in tissue-culture, mitosis and cellular proliferation are stimulated by several factors, the most important of which are mechanical and radiational trauma, a release of tissue-tension or an exposure to toxic conditions and in cataract.

MECHANICAL INJURY

We have already seen[1] that an intense proliferation of the anterior epithelium results from a perforating injury (Schlösser, 1887; Schirmer, 1889; Sanna, 1931; and others) or after massage (Schirmer, 1889) or may occur in the intact lens after a concussion (Vogt, 1931), but an adequate study of the process was not possible until the introduction of the technique of autoradiography to the study of the synthesis of DNA and the observation of mitosis in flat mounts. When a small puncture is made in vivo in the

[1] p. 16.

FIGS. 26 and 27.—PROLIFERATION OF THE SUBCAPSULAR EPITHELIUM AFTER AN
EXPERIMENTAL WOUND IN THE RABBIT (C. V. Harding *et al.*).

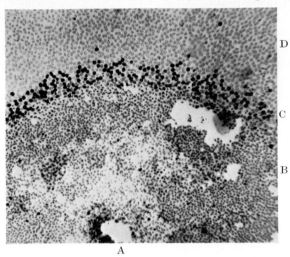

D

C

B

A

FIG. 26.—Thirty-six hours after a needle wound was made at A. The appearance as seen by ³H-thymidine autoradiography indicates the distribution of the cells synthesizing DNA in the subcapsular epithelium. In the region B there is an area of densely-packed cells bordered by a band of radio-active nuclei, C, at the outer edge of which, further from the wound, the cells appear normal, D.

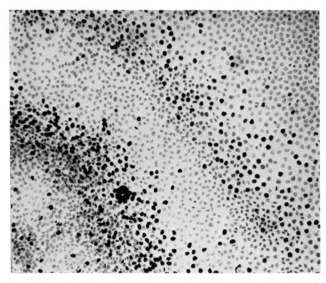

FIG. 27.—An autoradiograph 48 hours after injury, the site of which is out of the field towards the lower left. Two bands of radio-active nuclei are seen encircling the wound.

central area of the lens of the rabbit with a needle, there is a rapid proliferative response in the epithelium at first in the region immediately
surrounding the wound and later becoming propagated throughout a wider
area. Harding and his collaborators (1961) found that after a small wound,
radio-activity of the nuclei owing to the incorporation of radio-active
thymidine becomes evident in 14 hours in the neighbouring cells and extends
over a wide surrounding band within 24 hours when mitotic figures become
evident; nuclear synthetic activity ceases in 48 hours (Fig. 26). When more
extensive wounds are inflicted, this activity persists for a period of upward

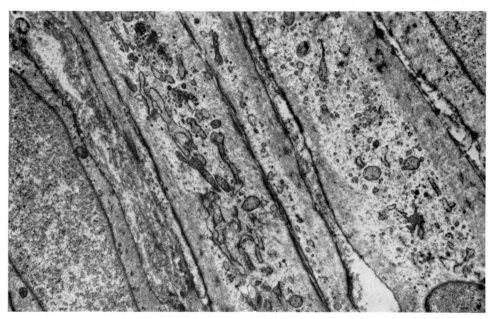

Fig. 28.—The Transformation of Epithelial Cells into Fibres.

In a traumatic cataract in the rabbit. There is a coarse endoplasmic reticulum,
numerous Golgi vesicles and fibrillar material in the hyaloplasm, the cells being
separated by bundles of collagen fibrils (× 9,750) (A. Brini).

of 3 days, occurring in bands suggesting that some cells divide twice, while
the area of the wound itself becomes lined with epithelial cells (Fig. 27);
a somewhat similar reaction is seen in the lenticular epithelium of the frog
but in this animal the division of the cells may be so prolific as to lead to the
formation of a tumour-like mass (Rafferty, 1963; Rothstein et al., 1965).
When the wound is large in the rabbit the cellular proliferation may be
sufficient to form a subcapsular cataract lined anteriorly and posteriorly with
a newly secreted capsule having the characteristic staining properties of the
original capsule, a phenomenon which we shall see presently occurs also in
man.

When the posterior capsule is ruptured a growth of the equatorial

and Waugh, 1954). This activity may assume aberrant forms when the normal whorl-like arrangement of the equatorial cells is lost and cells of irregular shapes and sizes spread underneath the posterior capsule to reach the posterior pole. These vesicular cells (the *bladder-cells* of Wedl, 1861) were considered by Becker (1883) to be due to " hydropic degeneration ", but more probably they represent abortive attempts to realize the inherent capacity of such cells to form lens fibres (Parsons, 1905) (Figs. 30–31). They frequently tend to lose their nuclei and eventually may merge with one another to form large cystic spaces.

FIGS. 30 and 31.—WEDL CELLS (M. J. Hogan and L. E. Zimmerman, *Atlas of Ophthalmic Pathology*, Saunders, Phila.).

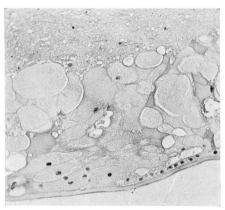 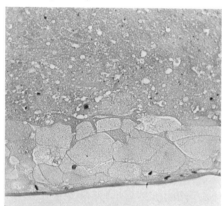

FIG. 30.—The equatorial epithelial cells have proliferated posteriorly to the point where they normally terminate in the nuclear bow.

FIG. 31.—The epithelium has extended back to the posterior pole where the bladder cells are evident.

The occurrence of an aberrant growth of the subcapsular epithelium in posterior lenticonus will be noted subsequently.

The REGENERATION OF LENS FIBRES from the subcapsular epithelium when the lens substance is removed from the capsule is a phenomenon recognized for more than a century and a half (Buchner, 1801), and has been more recently studied in adult animals such as mice and rabbits wherein a relatively complete organ may be reformed. This phenomenon has been discussed in a previous Volume.[1]

COLLOID BODIES. Rounded homogeneous masses staining in the same way as the capsule may be formed on the inner surface of this structure in conditions of senility or in a proliferative phase of epithelial activity such as in cases of chronic iridocyclitis or a necrotic intra-ocular tumour (Becker, 1883 ; Samuels, 1947). Like the colloid bodies (drusen) of Descemet's or Bruch's membrane, they appear to represent deposits of capsular material secreted by the epithelial cells.

[1] Vol. III, p. 71.

DEGENERATION AND ATROPHY OF THE EPITHELIUM

We have already seen that in old age the cells of the subcapsular epithelium tend to atrophy and in some places to disappear (Fig. 32); the process may be seen in the presence of a cataract, often in the immature stage but particularly in maturity when in some areas the cells may be absent while in other regions their nuclei are seen to migrate into the degenerated cortex (Clapp, 1942). The same atrophy and disappearance are sometimes seen in long-standing simple glaucoma. In toxic conditions of sufficient severity, also, the epithelial cells may suffer necrosis, as when a necrotic portion of the iris adheres to the capsule in iridocyclitis, when the capsule is bathed in the pus of a hypopyon or when a necrotic intra-ocular tumour is present (Samuels, 1947). Areas of focal necrosis occurring as a

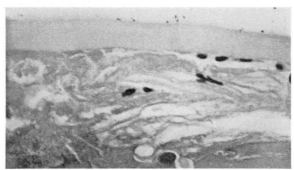

FIG. 32.—ATROPHY OF THE EPITHELIUM.

In a woman aged 57 with cataract complicated by simple glaucoma (C. A. Clapp).

result of pressure may follow an acute attack of glaucoma resulting in the formation of the subcapsular flecks of opacity seen during and after this disease.[1] When the injury is localized and the neighbouring cells survive, these may be stimulated in an endeavour to heal the defect, the proliferating cells sometimes forming irregular tufts dipping into the substance of the lens.

Becker. *Zur Anatomie d. gesunden u. kranken Linse*, Wiesbaden (1883).

Bedell. *J. Amer. med. Ass.*, **88**, 548 (1927).

Bito, Davson and Snider. *Exp. Eye Res.*, **4**, 54 (1965).

Bito and Harding. *Exp. Eye Res.*, **4**, 146 (1965).

Brini, Porte and Stoeckel. *Nature* (Lond.), **200**, 296 (1963).

Bull. Soc. franç. Ophtal., **66**, 193 (1963); **80**, 249 (1967).

Bull. Soc. belge Ophtal., No. 136, 232 (1964).

Buchner. *Waarneming von eene entbinding der crystalvogten*, Amsterdam (1801).

Bücklers. *Klin. Mbl. Augenheilk.*, **89**, 832 (1932); **94**, 289 (1935).

Bullough and Laurence. *Exp. Cell Res.*, **33**, 176 (1964).

Clapp. *Amer. J. Ophthal.*, **25**, 437 (1942).

Collins. *Trans. ophthal. Soc. U.K.*, **10**, 145 (1890).

Cotlier. *Arch. Ophthal.*, **68**, 801 (1962).] *Amer. J. Ophthal.*, **57**, 63 (1964).

Cowan and Fry. *Arch. Ophthal.*, **18**, 12 (1937).

Elschnig. *Klin. Mbl. Augenheilk.*, **49** (1), 444 (1911).

[1] p. 40.

Froomberg and Voaden. *Exp. Eye Res.*, **5**, 1 (1966).

Hanna and O'Brien. *Arch. Ophthal.*, **66**, 103 (1961).
Radiation Res., **19**, 1 (1963).

Harding, Feldherr and Srinivasan. *The Structure of the Eye* (Ed. Smelser), N.Y., 273 (1961).

Harding, Hughes, Bond and Schork. *Arch. Ophthal.*, **63**, 58 (1960).

Harding, Rothstein and Newman. *Exp. Eye Res.*, **1**, 457 (1962).

Harding and Thayer. *Invest. Ophthal.*, **3**, 302 (1964).

Harms. *Klin. Mbl. Augenheilk.*, **78**, 57 (1927).

Hirschberg. *Einführung in d. Augenheilkunde*, Leipzig, 159 (1901).

Howard. *Stain Techn.*, **27**, 313 (1952).

Kinsey, Wachtl, Constant and Camacho. *Amer. J. Ophthal.*, **40** (2), 216 (1955).

Lyda and Waugh. *Amer. J. Ophthal.*, **38** (2), 205 (1954).

Miki. *Acta Soc. ophthal. jap.*, **65**, 2207 (1961).

Mikulicich and Young. *Invest. Ophthal.*, **2**, 344 (1963).

Parsons. *Pathology of the Eye*, London, **2**, 392 (1905).

Rafferty. *Anat. Rec.*, **146**, 299 (1963).

Rothstein, Reddan and Weinsieder. *Exp. Cell Res.*, **37**, 440 (1965).

von Sallmann. *Arch. Ophthal.*, **47**, 305 (1952).
Invest. Ophthal., **4**, 471 (1965).

von Sallmann, Grimes and McElvain. *Exp. Eye Res.*, **1**, 449 (1962).

Samuels. *Amer. J. Ophthal.*, **30**, 1 (1947).

Sanna. *Ann. Ottal.*, **59**, 543 (1931).

Sautter. *Klin. Mbl. Augenheilk.*, **112**, 316 (1947).

Schirmer. *v. Graefes Arch. Ophthal.*, **35** (1), 220; (3), 147 (1889).

Schlösser. *Experimentelle Studien ü. traumatische Katarakt*, Munich (1887).

Schwartz. *Arch. Ophthal.*, **63**, 593 (1960).

Srinivasan and Harding. *Invest. Ophthal.*, **4**, 452 (1965).

Vogt. *v. Graefes Arch. Ophthal.*, **108**, 182 (1922).
Lhb. u. Atlas d. Spaltlampenmikroskopie d. lebenden Auges, 2nd ed., Berlin, **2** (1931).

Wedl. *Atlas d. pathologischen Histologie d. Auges*, Leipzig (1861).

Subcapsular Cataract

When proliferation of the subcapsular epithelium occurs to a marked degree, a clinically evident opacity develops as a plaque lying immediately under the capsule; in its evolution it is not usually progressive. The clinical appearance of such an ANTERIOR SUBCAPSULAR CATARACT was accurately described by Josef Beer (1817) and the histological changes in its develop-

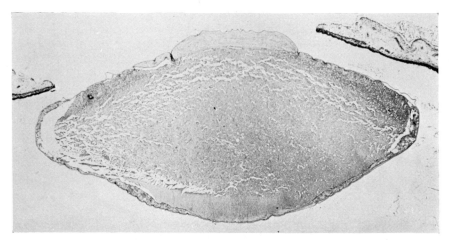

FIG. 33.—ANTERIOR POLAR CATARACT.

In a 12-year-old schizophrenic girl. The lens, showing an anterior subcapsular cataract as well as equatorial fibrous masses (H. & E.; × 20) (P. Henkind and P. Prose).

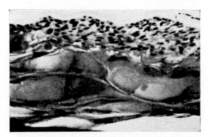

FIG. 34.—ANTERIOR POLAR CATARACT.

Showing the epithelial proliferation and degeneration (J. Friedenwald).

FIGS. 35 and 36.—ANTERIOR POLAR CATARACT (P. Henkind and P. Prose).

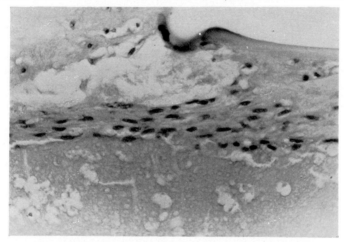

FIG. 35.—The lateral border of the anterior subcapsular cataract seen in Fig. 33. The elongated spindle-shaped cells overlying the degenerate cortex have an appearance resembling fibroblasts (H. & E.; × 330).

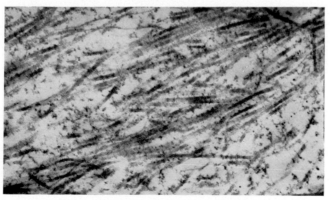

FIG. 36.—Electron-micrograph of the subcapsular material showing typical bundles of collagen (× 35,000).

Figs. 37 and 38.—Regeneration of the Lens Capsule (A. Brini).

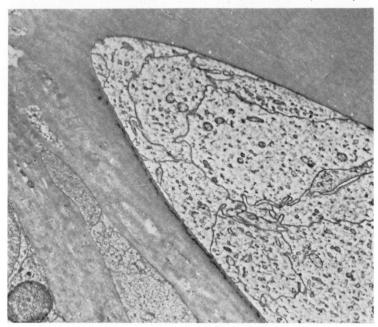

Fig. 37.—In an experimental traumatic cataract in the rabbit. Electron-micrograph showing the formation of a basal substance in connection with the epithelial cells. Inside the newly formed capsule in continuity with the original capsule (above) there is an elimination of the necrotic material.

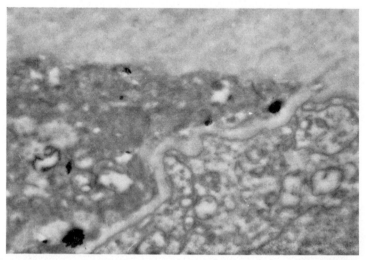

Fig. 38.—In a case of senile cataract. Formation of a new capsule folded from the original capsule (above) separating the healthy epithelium to the right from the necrotic epithelium to the left.

ment have been thoroughly studied[1] (Fig. 33). The essential changes are two-fold: an active proliferation of the subcapsular epithelium and a degeneration of the lens fibres immediately underneath (Fig. 34).

The proliferating subcapsular cells beneath the intact capsule lose their cubical shape and become polygonal, and as they multiply they may form a flat plaque or pile up into a conical projection above the level of the surface of the lens. As they elongate they throw out long processes and assume spindle shapes resembling in every way the cells of fibrous connective tissue, both in their appearance and in their staining properties (Fig. 35);

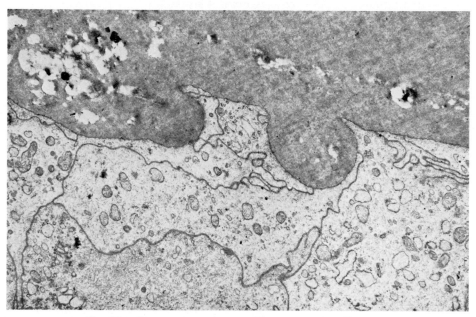

FIG. 39.—REGENERATION OF THE EPITHELIUM AND CAPSULE.

In a traumatic cataract in the rabbit. The regenerated epithelial cells are seen underneath the newly-formed capsule containing necrotic debris within it ($\times$ 10,500) (A. Brini *et al.*).

moreover, they have been shown by electron microscopy to contain fibres of true collagen (Henkind and Prose, 1967; Pau and Caesar, 1967) (Fig. 36). Availing themselves of the known capacity for proliferation in tissue culture, Kirby (1927), Kirby and his colleagues (1929) and Bakker (1936) proved their ectodermal origin by observing their formation from the sub-capsular cells *in vitro*; the phenomenon is therefore a typical example of metaplasia. Eventually, normal cubical cells grow along the posterior surface of the cicatricial mass and slowly secrete a hyaline membrane

[1] H. Müller (1856–57), Knies (1880), Becker (1883), Wagenmann (1889), Schirmer (1889), Gepner (1890), Treacher Collins (1892–1908), Krüger (1903), Peters (1921), Beauvieux and Germain (1922), Maucione (1924), Bücklers (1935), Lamb (1937), Frey (1951), Brini *et al.* (1964), Henkind and Prose (1967), and others.

similar to the normal capsule, so that the appearance suggests that the capsule had split into two layers at the margin of the opacity, one running over it and one underneath. These layers of the capsule eventually enclose the degenerated material, thus isolating the opacity from the lens so that the evidence of epithelial proliferation becomes lost (Brini *et al.*, 1963–64) (Figs. 37–9). In general the cataract may assume three forms: a localized plaque, a raised pyramidal cone or a widespread form extending over a considerable area with undulations or wrinkles on its surface.

After some time degenerative changes tend to occur. The whole tissue may become condensed and converted into a laminated and almost structureless hyaline mass (Figs. 33, 40). Eventually fat or lipid material may be deposited, including a plentiful array of flat or needle-shaped crystals of cholesterol of varying brilliant colours—the DYSTROPHIA EPITHELIALIS

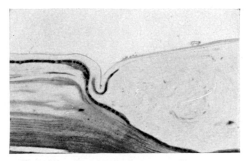

FIG. 40.—ANTERIOR CAPSULAR CATARACT.
Showing ingrowth of cubical epithelium behind the cataract (× 120)
(J. H. Parsons).

LENTIS ADIPOSA of von Szily (1933) (Handmann, 1933; Sagher, 1934). Calcareous degeneration is also relatively common, a process which may give an appearance resembling stalactites (H. Müller, 1856; Krüger, 1903). Sometimes the underlying fibres of the lens are disturbed and degenerate; if this process remains localized normal lens fibres may grow between the subcapsular opacity and the deeper "imprint" so that the picture of a DUPLICATED CATARACT may result. On the other hand, the disturbance which caused the subcapsular opacity may spread to cause a diffuse lenticular cataract.

Such subcapsular cataracts may occur in several conditions.

CONGENITAL SUBCAPSULAR CATARACT has already been described in a previous Volume[1]; it will be remembered that it may be comprised of minute white stationary multiple flecks associated with adhesions of remnants of the primitive vascular system, on the anterior capsule with those of the pupillary membrane, on the pre-equatorial capsule with those of the

[1] Vol. III, p. 716.

capsulo-pupillary membrane, and, more rarely, on the posterior capsule with those of the hyaloid artery or of the posterior fibro-vascular sheath of the lens. Such a FLECK CATARACT is non-progressive and does not affect vision. Alternatively, a more extensive ANTERIOR POLAR CATARACT may form in the axial region which may vary considerably in size and form. It may be a small white plaque or occupy the greater part of the pupillary area, usually it is circumscribed but may show radiating striæ extending outwards, it may be flat or heaped up to form a pyramidal cataract, or it may extend some distance into the substance of the lens or be associated with one and occasionally two imprints within the substance of the lens to form a reduplicated

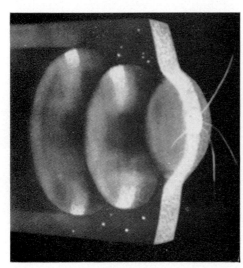
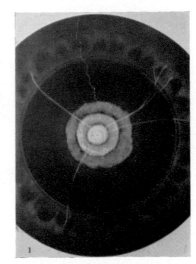

FIG. 41.   FIG. 42.

FIGS. 41 and 42.—ANTERIOR CAPSULAR AND POLAR CATARACT WITH REDUPLICATIONS.
There are remnants of a pupillary membrane (M. Berliner).

cataract (Figs. 41–2). It is interesting that such a condition may be hereditary, the transmission usually being dominant in character. Such a cataract is almost invariably stationary.

Histological examinations of this type of subcapsular cataract were first reported by von Ammon (1852) and more fully by Collins (1892–1908) whose conclusions subsequent observers have merely confirmed; the changes comprise those we have already discussed—a proliferation of the subcapsular epithelium, its transformation into typical fibroblasts and the subsequent degeneration of the mass thus formed (Henkind and Prose, 1967) (Fig. 36).

Several suggestions have been made to explain the development of these opacities—compression of the capsule (Mann, 1937), its rupture by traction (Gifford, 1924; M. van Duyse, 1939), the effects of toxic products carried by the fœtal circulation (Pesme, 1927) or disturbances of the nutrition of the underlying lens fibres through the adherent capsule (Vogt, 1931). None of these, however, is convincing.

A POSTERIOR POLAR CATARACT is rarer.[1] It also may take the form of a localized hyaloid fleck, but adhesions of the posterior fibro-vascular sheath of the lens may lead to more widespread opacities in the lens substance; these may be progressive involving in the worst cases an invasion of the lens by vascular fibrous tissue which may produce a total cataract.[2]

It is to be remembered that adhesions between the hyaloid vessels and the posterior capsule may occur while the lens remains clear; indeed, these adhesions may be so firm that the entire vitreous may be unexpectedly and unfortunately removed with the lens in the extraction of a cataract (Vail, 1954; Reese and Wadsworth, 1958; Wolter, 1961) (Fig. 296).

FIGS. 43 and 44.—PYRAMIDAL CATARACT (J. H. Parsons).

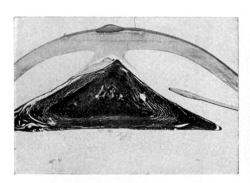 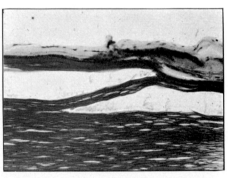

FIG. 43.—From a child, aged 8, after a perforating hypopyon ulcer following measles. A small anterior capsular cataract is to the left of the summit (× 6).

FIG. 44.—The same case as Fig. 43, showing a double hyaline membrane on the surface. The outer membrane is covered by endothelium derived from the cornea and is a cuticular deposit corresponding to Descemet's membrane. The inner membrane is the lens capsule (× 90).

INFECTIVE CONDITIONS. Among these *keratitis* may cause an anterior capsular (polar) cataract which may be present at birth, occur in infancy or appear in later life. That such a cataract could be due to an intra-uterine inflammation of the cornea was suggested by Beck (1838), a theory that has had several subsequent supporters.[3] It is possible in such cases that contact with the inflamed cornea may induce a superficial opacity in the lens, and in this connection it is to be remembered that the spherical lens and the shallow anterior chamber in the fœtus or infant facilitates such contact; but its most frequent cause is a perforating ulcer in cases of ophthalmia neonatorum. These instances are obviously due to a temporary adhesion of the capsule to the inflamed cornea when an ulcer perforates,

[1] Vol. III, p. 723. [2] Vol. III, p. 752.
[3] Mackenzie (1854), Dor (1892), Parsons (1905), Löwenstein (1931), and others.

and when the anterior chamber re-forms the tissue which glues the two together is drawn out into long filaments stretching across the anterior chamber. Usually this is torn and largely disappears, but its traction may distort the lens, drawing its axial area out into a pyramidal cataract (Figs. 43–4).

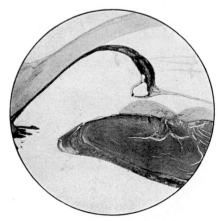

FIG. 45.—IRIS BOMBÉ: SECLUSIO PUPILLÆ.

Extensive peripheral anterior synechiæ. Posterior synechiæ with seclusio pupillæ; inflammatory pupillary membrane with occlusio pupillæ; anterior capsular cataract (J. H. Parsons).

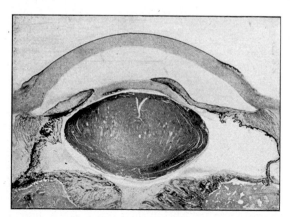

FIG. 46.—OCCLUSIO PUPILLÆ.

Total posterior synechiæ with occlusio pupillæ. There is an anterior capsular cataract and a detachment of the ciliary body and retina (J. H. Parsons).

On the other hand, the connection may remain. In such a case the corneal endothelium may grow over the lens secreting a hyaline layer corresponding to Descemet's membrane, so that the lens eventually becomes clothed by two cuticular membranes, one a new layer covered by endothelium, and the other the true capsule lined by cubical epithelium (Fig. 44) (Haring, 1897; de Vries, 1902; Parsons, 1905). It may be assumed that the toxins from the cornea kill the most severely affected subcapsular cells and excite their neighbours to proliferative activity, although it was suggested by Collins (1898) that the damage might be due to a nutritional upset following an arrest of diffusion through the adherent capsule.

Iridocyclitis is a frequent cause of a subcapsular cataract. In the neighbourhood of pupillary synechiæ the opacity may be localized or extensive depending on the extent of the adhesions (Figs. 45–6), and when the lens is surrounded by a cyclitic membrane it may be widespread and superimposed on a complicated cataract (Fig. 222).

SYSTEMIC CONDITIONS. Among systemic conditions two are associated with a capsular cataract—*syndermatotic (atopic) cataract* as occurs in such

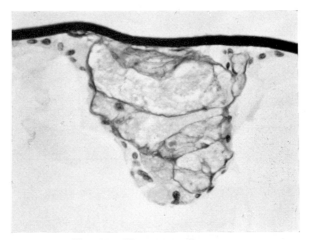

FIG. 47.—MONGOLIAN CATARACT.

To show the wart-like excrescences of the lens capsule associated with aberrations of the epithelium; the mass undergoes progressive displacement into the cortex (D. G. Cogan and T. Kuwabara).

diseases as atopic dermatitis and scleroderma[1] and *mongolian idiocy.* In the latter the peculiar and highly characteristic type of opacity has been fully described in a previous Volume,[2] but one of the most interesting features is the wart-like excrescences of the subcapsular epithelium which are progressively displaced into the cortex, suffering degenerative changes in the meantime (Fig. 47) (Cogan and Kuwabara, 1962). A subcapsular cataract which may appear as a complication of systemic treatment with the *corticosteroids,* commencing at the posterior pole and sometimes affecting the capsule itself, will be discussed at a later stage.[3]

TRAUMA is a further cause of subcapsular cataract. After a *concussion* injury discrete subepithelial opacities may develop, probably as a result of

[1] p. 196.   [2] Vol. III, p. 1135.   [3] p. 230.

FIGS. 48 to 50.—CONCUSSION CATARACT.
Cobweb-like subcapsular opacity (D. M. Rolett).

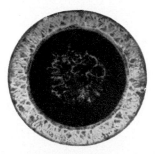

FIG. 48.—The condition as seen by oblique illumination.

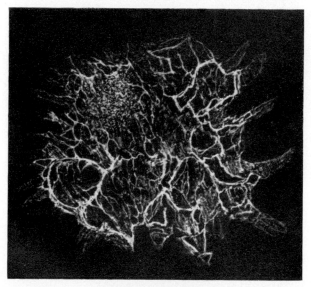

FIG. 49.—Enlargement of the opacity showing that it consists of a delicate framework supporting dust-like spots which, towards the periphery, end in sharply pointed processes.

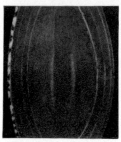

FIG. 50.—The lens in the beam of the slit-lamp showing the opacity lying on the surface immediately under the capsule.

mechanical injury to the epithelial cells or an impairment of the permeability of the capsule. As a result a great variety of forms of opacity may appear differing little in their ætiology and pathology, sometimes transient, sometimes permanent, sometimes few and localized, sometimes widespread and dispersed.[1] Frequently these take the form of minute discrete punctate flecks, axial or peripheral in distribution, or of a diffuse cobweb-like subcapsular opacity (Figs. 48–50), and occasionally small discrete plaques of considerable size may result, the *nodiform cataract* of Vogt (1922), resembling an anterior polar cataract (Fig. 51–2). The appearance of these opacities may occasionally be delayed for a considerable period up to two years after the injury, and eventually they may become separated from the epithelial

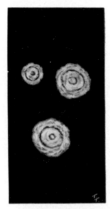   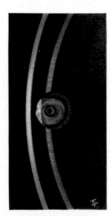

Fig. 51.   Fig. 52.

FIGS. 51 and 52.—CATARACTA NODIFORMIS OF VOGT.
As seen by diffuse illumination (Fig. 51) and in the beam of the slit-lamp (Fig. 52).

zone by the ingrowth of new lens fibres so that they become buried in the clear substance of the lens as an imprint, occasionally united with the subcapsular epithelium by a delicate bridge. In more severe concussion injuries, of course, posterior polar or diffuse opacities may develop in the substance of the lens, changes which will be fully described in a subsequent Volume.[2]

A *massage cataract* has long been known to result from mechanical massage of the anterior lens capsule varying in degree from fine subcapsular opacities to clouding of the entire lens.[3] The same type of change has been noted to follow cases of recurrent dislocation of the lens into the anterior chamber when it repeatedly comes into contact with the posterior surface of the cornea (Schmid, 1946) or may develop after prolonged contact with this tissue as may be seen in a malignant glaucoma (Samuels, 1947).

[1] Whiting (1916), Vogt (1922), Foster (1938), Davidson (1940), Rolett (1940), and others.
[2] Vol. XIV.
[3] Hess (1887), Schirmer (1888), Demaria (1904), Salffner (1904), Bellows and Chinn (1941), and others.

Perforating injuries usually cause widespread opacification of the lens but if the perforation is small and superficial this may be limited to the capsule and the immediately underlying tissue and give rise to the localized non-progressive changes of a *circumscribed traumatic cataract*. We have already seen that the proliferation of the subcapsular epithelium stimulated by the injury may seal up a small perforation and further lenticular damage

FIGS. 53 and 54.—THE END-RESULTS OF CAPSULAR WOUNDS.

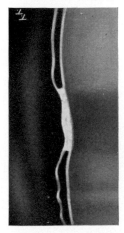 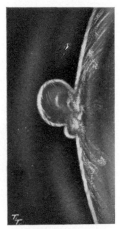

FIG. 53.—Post-traumatic changes, showing a dense capsular scar indenting the lens. There are folds in the capsule around the scar and the anterior line of disjunction disappears at the site of the scar.

FIG. 54.—Blister-like spherule on the anterior lens capsule, seen in optical section with the slit-lamp.

may be averted by the formation of a cicatrix in the capsule; here the anterior zone of disjunction is lost and around the affected area the capsule may show traction folds which radiate outwards (Figs. 53–4) (Davidson, 1940; Rosen, 1945). At a later date degenerative changes may occur in the capsular scar which after some years may rupture with the protrusion of the lens substance into the anterior chamber and the rapid development of a diffuse cataract (Vogt, 1931). Alternatively, the subcapsular opacity may

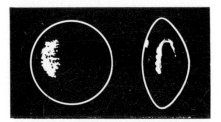

FIG. 55.—PARTIAL STATIONARY TRAUMATIC CATARACT.

A perforating injury of 25 years' standing, seen in diffuse illumination and optical section (M. Davidson).

become buried by the growth of new fibres and migrate into the interior of the lens, still remaining stationary but usually showing no fibrillar design, vacuoles or fluid-clefts (Fig. 55).

Glaucomatous subcapsular flecks, the multiple discrete, stationary sub-capsular opacities appearing after an attack of acute glaucoma, first described by Vogt (1930) as *cataracta disseminata subcapsularis glaucomatosa*, have been extensively studied by many observers.[1] They occur not only in primary acute glaucoma but also in conditions of raised ocular tension after iridocyclitis or a contusion (Vogt, 1931; Pillat, 1957; Schwab, 1957). Their early history has been traced by Jones (1959) (Plate I). He described an initial dirty discoloration in the subcapsular region of the pupillary area which soon shows variations in density so that a reticulated sheet is formed accentuating the shagreen of the lens; thereafter the sheet breaks up into

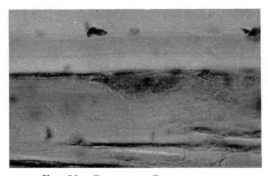

FIG. 56.—CATARACTA GLAUCOMATOSA.
Focal necrosis in the lens epithelium after an attack of closed-angle glaucoma
(J. Winstanley).

multiple discrete subcapsular opacities changing from a fawn to a white colour. After a period varying from one to three weeks these consolidate to form the solid white flecks originally described by Vogt, round, oval, dumb-bell or irregular in shape, discrete and small in size (0·2 to 0·3 mm.), limited to the pupillary area and subcapsular in position. Histologically these are due to areas of focal necrosis of the subcapsular epithelium resembling those occurring in the iris in acute glaucoma[2] and, like them, are due to an acute rise of pressure (Fig. 56). Initially situated immediately under the capsule, they are slowly buried in the lens as new fibres are laid down, but their presence bears permanent testimony to the occurrence of the glaucomatous incident. As they sink into the lens they become bluish in tint but they

---

[1] Weill and Nordmann (1933), Bücklers (1934), van Lint (1936), Kovarskaya and Krolh (1938), Sommer (1940), Seidenari (1940), Sugar (1946–57), Nemetz (1949), Chandler (1952), Krol (1953), Auricchio (1953), Nordmann (1954), Jones (1959), Winstanley (1961), Trantas (1964), and others.
[2] Vol. IX, p. 681.

PLATE I

Glaucomatous Subcapsular Flecks (B. R. Jones)

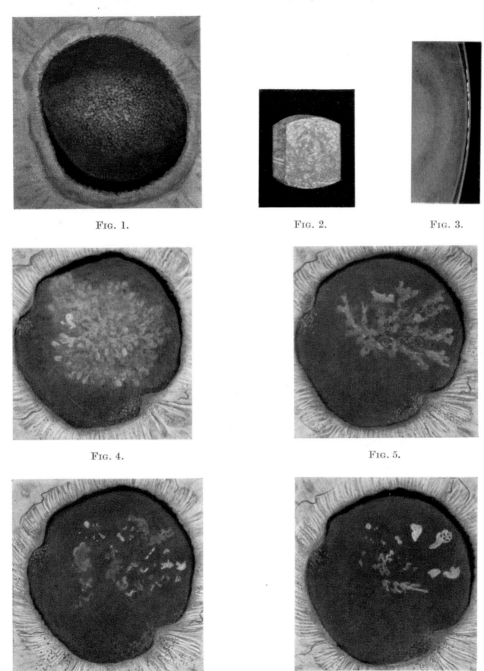

FIG. 1.   FIG. 2.   FIG. 3.

FIG. 4.   FIG. 5.

FIG. 6.   FIG. 7.

FIGS. 1 and 2.—The first stage consists of a diffuse, dirty, subcapsular discoloration.

FIGS. 3 to 5.—In the second stage there is an ill-defined sheet of fawn discoloration showing areas of different density immediately underneath the capsule.

FIG. 6.—In the third stage the sheet breaks up into multiple discrete opacities.

FIG. 7.—In the fourth stage, 1 to 3 weeks later, most of the early opacity has cleared and a few areas have hardened and whitened to give the discrete glaucomatous subcapsular flecks.

remain discrete and do not lead to progressive opacification. Two successive layers were seen by Jones (1959) in a patient who suffered two acute attacks of glaucoma separated by two years of medical treatment.

The *treatment of subcapsular cataract* varies with the extent of the lesion and the condition of the lens itself. If the lens is clear and the opacity is small, vision may not be greatly impeded and specific treatment is not required; if it is necessary, the use of mydriatics or an optical iridectomy limited to the sphincteric portion of the iris may improve the vision. In some cases wherein the opacity is discrete it may be detached from the surface of the lens by a needle or a narrow knife and subsequently removed by forceps through a corneal incision (Selinger, 1932). Alternatively, if it is large, an operation of discission or extraction may be required; but if the lens is cataractous the treatment of the subcapsular lesion takes second place to that of the main lenticular opacity.

von Ammon. *Dtsch. Klin.*, **4**, 97 (1852).
Auricchio. *Rass. ital. Ottal.*, **22**, 50 (1953).
Bakker. *v. Graefes Arch. Ophthal.*, **136**, 166, 333 (1936).
Beauvieux and Germain. *Arch. Ophtal.*, **39**, 285 (1922).
Beck. *Mschr. Med. Augenheilk. Chir.*, **1**, 1 (1838).
Becker. *Zur Anatomie d. gesunden u. kranken Linse*, Wiesbaden (1883).
Beer. *Lehre v. d. Augenkrankheiten*, Vienna (1817).
Bellows and Chinn. *Amer. J. Ophthal.*, **24**, 979 (1941).
Brini, Porte and Stoeckel. *Nature* (Lond.), **200**, 296 (1963).
 Bull. Soc. belge Ophtal., No. 136, 232 (1964).
Bücklers. *Klin. Mbl. Augenheilk.*, **89**, 832 (1932); **94**, 289 (1935).
 Ber. dtsch. ophthal. Ges., **50**, 172 (1934).
Chandler. *Arch. Ophthal.*, **47**, 695 (1952).
Cogan and Kuwabara. *Docum. ophthal.*, **16**, 73 (1962).
Collins. *Trans. ophthal. Soc. U.K.*, **12**, 89 (1892); **18**, 124 (1898).
 Ophthalmoscope, **6**, 577, 663 (1908).
Davidson. *Amer. J. Ophthal.*, **23**, 252, 1358 (1940).
Demaria. *v. Graefes Arch. Ophthal.*, **59**, 568 (1904).
Dor. *Bull. Soc. franç. Ophtal.*, **10**, 1 (1892).
van Duyse. *Traité d'ophtal.*, Paris, **1**, 986 (1939).
Foster. *Trans. ophthal. Soc. U.K.*, **58**, 436 (1938).
Frey. *Kresge Eye Inst. Bull.*, **2**, 62 (1951).
Gepner. *v. Graefes Arch. Ophthal.*, **36** (4), 255 (1890).
Gifford. *Amer. J. Ophthal.*, **7**, 678 (1924).
Handmann. *Klin. Mbl. Augenheilk.*, **91**, 488 (1933).
Haring. *v. Graefes Arch. Ophthal.*, **43**, 25 (1897).

Henkind and Prose. *Amer. J. Ophthal.*, **63**, 768 (1967).
Hess. *Ber. dtsch. ophthal. Ges.*, **19**, 54 (1887).
Jones. *Trans. ophthal. Soc. U.K.*, **79**, 753 (1959).
Kirby. *Arch. Ophthal.*, **56**, 450 (1927).
Kirby, Estey and Tabor. *Arch. Ophthal.*, **1**, 358 (1929).
Knies. *Klin. Mbl. Augenheilk.*, **18**, 181 (1880).
Kovarskaya and Krolh. *Vestn. Oftal.*, **13**, 262 (1938).
Krol. *Vestn. Oftal.*, **32**, 27 (1953).
Krüger. *Z. Augenheilk.*, **9**, 35 (1903).
Lamb. *Arch. Ophthal.*, **17**, 877 (1937).
van Lint. *Bull. Soc. belge Ophtal.*, No. 72, 62 (1936).
Löwenstein. *Klin. Mbl. Augenheilk.*, **87**, 382 (1931).
Mackenzie. *A Practical Treatise on the Diseases of the Eye*, 4th ed., London (1854).
Mann. *Developmental Anomalies of the Eye*, Camb. (1937).
Maucione. *Arch. Ottal.*, **31**, 145 (1924).
Müller, H. *v. Graefes Arch. Ophthal.*, **2** (2), 1 (1856); **3** (1), 55 (1857).
Nemetz. *Klin. Mbl. Augenheilk.*, **115**, 417 (1949).
Nordmann. *Biologie du cristallin*, Paris, 356 (1954).
Parsons. *Pathology of the Eye*, London, **2**, 407; **3**, 808 (1905).
Pau and Caesar. *v. Graefes Arch. Ophthal.*, **171**, 327 (1967).
Pesme. *Arch. Ophtal.*, **44**, 620 (1927).
Peters. *v. Graefes Arch. Ophthal.*, **105**, 154 (1921).
Pillat. *Forsch. u. Praxis*, **10**, 13 (1957).
Reese and Wadsworth. *Amer. J. Ophthal.*, **46**, 495 (1958).
Rolett. *Arch. Ophthal.*, **24**, 1244 (1940).
Rosen. *Brit. J. Ophthal.*, **29**, 370, 373 (1945).

42   DISEASES OF THE LENS

Sagher. *Klin. Mbl. Augenheilk.*, **93,** 355 (1934).
Sallfner. *v. Graefes Arch. Ophthal.*, **59,** 520 (1904).
Samuels. *Amer. J. Ophthal.*, **30,** 1 (1947).
Schirmer. *v. Graefes Arch. Ophthal.*, **34** (1), 131 (1888); **35** (1), 220 (1889).
Schmid. *Ophthalmologica*, **111,** 365 (1946).
Schwab. *Forsch. u. Praxis*, **10,** 20 (1957).
Seidenari. *Rass. ital. Ottal.*, **9,** 216 (1940).
Selinger. *Arch. Ophthal.*, **7,** 109 (1932).
Sommer. *Schw. med. Wschr.*, **21,** 813 (1940).
Sugar. *Amer. J. Ophthal.*, **29,** 1396 (1946).
The Glaucomas, 2nd ed., St. Louis, 315 (1957).
von Szily. *Klin. Mbl. Augenheilk.*, **90,** 607 (1933).
Trantas. *Bull. Soc. franç Ophtal.*, **77,** 659 (1964).

Vail. *Trans. Amer. Acad. Ophthal.*, **58,** 367 (1954).
Vogt. *v. Graefes Arch. Ophthal.*, **109,** 154 (1922).
Klin. Mbl. Augenheilk., **85,** 586 (1930).
Lhb. u. Atlas d. Spaltlampenmikroskopie d. lebenden Auges, 2nd ed., Berlin, **2,** 565 (1931).
de Vries. *v. Graefes Arch. Ophthal.*, **54,** 500 (1902).
Wagenmann. *v. Graefes Arch. Ophthal.*, **35,** 172 (1889).
Weill and Nordmann. *Bull. Soc. Ophtal. Paris*, 295 (1933).
Whiting. *Trans. ophthal. Soc. U.K.*, **36,** 167 (1916).
Winstanley. *Trans. ophthal. Soc. U.K.*, **81,** 23 (1961).
Wolter. *Amer. J. Ophthal.*, **51,** 511 (1961).

Exfoliation of the Capsule

Although it usually appears as a homogeneous structureless membrane on microscopy, it has long been known that the lens capsule is composite. An outer layer was first demonstrated by Berger (1882) after maceration with potassium permanganate; this he called the ZONULAR LAMELLA, a structure which Retzius (1895) termed the PERICAPSULAR MEMBRANE. This

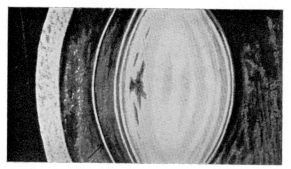

FIG. 57.—THE LENS IN IRIDOCYCLITIS.

To the left the corneal section. There is a marked aqueous flare. The arrow points to a completely detached zonular lamella (drawn thicker than natural). Fluid clefts are seen in the anterior parts of the lens which is subluxated backwards (Harrison Butler).

layering may be demonstrated histologically in the normal capsule by staining with aniline blue (Beauvieux, 1922) or by the use of the silver impregnation method of Bielschowsky (Busacca, 1929), while electron microscopy demonstrates that the entire capsule is made up of a number of faintly fibrillar laminated sheets lying parallel to the surface (Bahr, 1954; Cohen, 1958–65).

In the phenomenon of exfoliation the superficial layers split off from the deep strata to float as a fine membrane in the aqueous humour (Fig. 61), an occurrence which histochemical tests have shown to depend on damage to

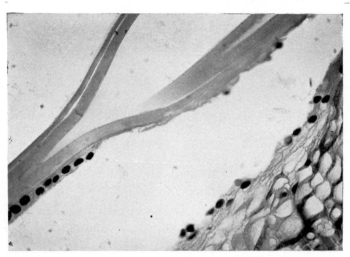

FIG. 58.—THE LENS CAPSULE.

After discission. The separation of the zonular lamella from the capsule proper is well seen, each of the two parts being divided into separate layers. Some of the cuboidal epithelial cells are attached to the cortical remnants (F. Tooke).

the interfibrillary cement substance (Callahan and Klien, 1958). It occurs in four conditions:

1. *Senile exfoliation* occurs occasionally in aged eyes (Callahan and Klien, 1958).

2. *Toxic exfoliation* is seen in atrophic eyes (Elschnig, 1923–29; Butler, 1938), after prolonged iridocyclitis (Rohrschneider, 1936; Butler, 1938) (Fig. 57), or after the lodgment of a metallic foreign body of iron or copper for which the capsule shows an affinity (Vogt, 1932).[1]

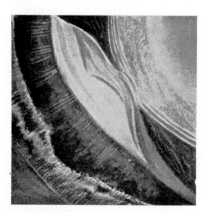

FIG. 59.—DETACHMENT OF THE ZONULAR LAMELLA.

After a blow; the zonular lamella is torn from the subluxated lens and folded back; into it are inserted the zonular fibres (Harrison Butler).

[1] Vol. XIV.

Figs. 60 and 61.—Exfoliation of the Zonular Lamella in Glass-workers.

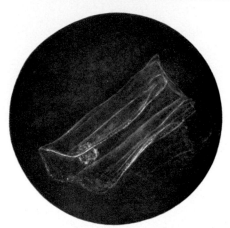 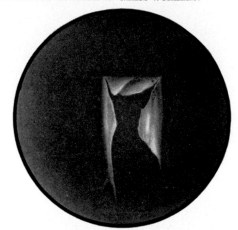

Fig. 60.—W. F. Schnyder.　　　　　　　Fig. 61.—A. Löwenstein.

3. *Traumatic* detachments of the laminæ of the capsule may follow a per-forating injury (Tooke, 1933) (Fig. 58) or may result from a concussion when the zonular lamella attached to the fibres of the suspensory ligament may become separated from a dislocated lens (Meesmann, 1922; Butler, 1938) (Fig. 59).

4. *Heat* acting over a long time may cause the zonular lamella to become shredded in appearance and it may peel off the anterior surface of

Figs. 62 and 63.—Cyst Formation in the Anterior Capsule.
In a man aged 43 (A. Hagedoorn).

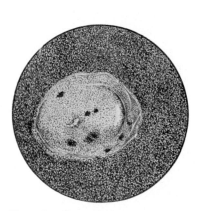 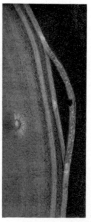

Fig. 62.—General view of the cyst.

Fig. 63.—Slit-lamp section showing the formation of a cyst by splitting of the anterior capsule involving a circumscribed detachment of the zonular lamella.

the lens as a single lamella which may wave about in the anterior chamber or curl up upon itself like a roll of parchment (Figs. 60–1).[1] This will be considered in the Volume devoted to Injuries.[2]

A PARTIAL EXFOLIATION forming a cyst-like structure separating the lamellæ of the capsule is a rarity. Such a transient cyst-like formation between the capsule and the zonular lamella was reported by Hagedoorn (1957) in a man aged 43 (Figs. 62–3). The delicate cyst gave rise to the subjective appearance of glaucomatous haloes around lights, but it disappeared after 4 years leaving a few small glistening dots and irregular lines visible only with the slit-lamp; at this stage the vision had again become normal.

Bahr. *v. Graefes Arch. Ophthal.*, **155**, 635 (1954).

Beauvieux. *Arch. Ophtal.*, **39**, 484 (1922).

Berger. *v. Graefes Arch. Ophthal.*, **28** (2), 28 (1882).

Busacca. *Klin. Mbl. Augenheilk.*, **83**, 737 (1929).

Butler. *Trans. ophthal. Soc. U.K.*, **58**, 575 (1938).

Callahan and Klien. *Arch. Ophthal.*, **59**, 73 (1958).

Cohen. *Amer. J. Anat.*, **103**, 219 (1958). *Invest. Ophthal.*, **4**, 433 (1965).

Cords. *Z. Augenheilk.*, **60**, 251 (1926).

Elschnig. *Klin. Mbl. Augenheilk.*, **69**, 732 (1922); **70**, 325 (1923). *Arch. Augenheilk.*, **100–1**, 760 (1929).

Goldschmidt. *Z. Augenheilk.*, **78**, 341 (1932).

Goulden. *Trans. ophthal. Soc. U.K.*, **45**, 718 (1925).

Hagedoorn. *Brit. J. Ophthal.*, **41**, 442 (1957).

Holloway and Cowan. *Amer. J. Ophthal.*, **14**, 189 (1931).

Kubik. *Klin. Mbl. Augenheilk.*, **70**, 327 (1923).

Meesmann. *Arch. Augenheilk.*, **91**, 261 (1922).

Retzius. *Biol. Untersuch.*, **6**, 67 (1895).

Rohrschneider. *Klin. Mbl. Augenheilk.*, **96**, 31 (1936).

Rotter. *Klin. Mbl. Augenheilk.*, **76**, 71 (1926).

Stein. *Klin. Mbl. Augenheilk.*, **76**, 75 (1926).

Tooke. *Brit. J. Ophthal.*, **17**, 466 (1933).

Vogt. *Schw. med. Wschr.*, **59**, 475 (1929). *Klin. Mbl. Augenheilk.*, **89**, 581, 587 (1932).

Weill and Lévy. *Ann. Oculist.* (Paris), **163**, 748 (1926).

Pseudo-exfoliation

PSEUDO-EXFOLIATION OF THE LENS CAPSULE is *a widespread degenerative condition* usually occurring in old people wherein a substance the nature of which is still unknown accumulates not only upon and within the lens capsule, particularly in its anterior region, but also in association with the internal limiting membranes of the iris and ciliary body, upon their epithelial surfaces and around the vessels of the anterior uvea. It is evident that *the disease is by no means confined to the lens*, but is a generalized exudative phenomenon. Clinically the most important feature is the eventual occurrence of simple glaucoma.

History. The first description of this condition appeared in Scandinavian literature when Lindberg (1917) in Finland reported the appearance of flaky material at the pupillary border of the iris which he interpreted as an old inflammatory exudate in almost half of 60 patients with simple glaucoma, an observation followed by the finding by Malling (1923) in Norway of similar flakes on the anterior surface of the lens; the latter called attention to the possibility of the subsequent development of glaucoma. In the meantime, Vogt (1923–32) published the first accurate description

---

[1] Elschnig (1922–23), Kubik (1923), Goulden (1925), Weill and Lévy (1926), Rotter (1926), Cords (1926), Stein (1926), Vogt (1929), Holloway and Cowan (1931), Goldschmidt (1932), and many others.

[2] Vol. XIV.

of the disease under the name of *superficial exfoliation of the anterior capsule of the lens*, interpreting it as an exfoliation of the superficial layers of the lens capsule and calling the consequential rise in tension *glaucoma capsulare*. This interpretation was accepted by subsequent writers who considered that the exfoliation was essentially senile in type.[1] Some doubts, however, had been expressed regarding the origin of the material deposited; Busacca (1927) who published the first histological study, suggested that this substance, frequently termed " Busacca's deposits ", was derived from the aqueous humour and not from the lens capsule, while Trantas (1929) interpreted the condition as a syndrome affecting all the hyaline membranes of the eye. The matter was considerably clarified in an important paper by Georgiana Dvorak-Theobald (1954) who showed that the depositions were accretions unconnected with exfoliation of the capsule and therefore suggested the term *pseudo-exfoliation*, a name still unsatisfactory and perhaps improved by the suggestion of Weekers and his collaborators (1959) of *senile uveal exudation*, but probably conveniently retained until the nature and origin of the exudative material have been clarified. The view that the condition is not an exfoliation of the capsule but an exudative phenomenon is now generally agreed.[2]

Incidence. Despite its late clinical recognition, pseudo-exfoliation of the lens capsule is not uncommon. In its slighter degrees, however, it is difficult to see and since the changes may be confined to the periphery of the lens, a mydriatic may be necessary for its diagnosis, facts which account for the varied estimates of its incidence; indeed, these depend essentially on the interest and care expended on specifically looking for the condition. It occurs late in life, usually between the ages of 60 and 80, an average being about 70 years (69·4 among 418 patients, Tarkkanen, 1962, in Finland); it is rarely found under the age of 60 and cases occurring in the fifth decade are exceptional (45 years, Trantas, 1929; 46, Gifford, 1957). Among people of the age-group of the 7th and 8th decades, however, it is relatively common; Baumgart (1933) in Italy found it in 7·5% and I. Hørven (1966) in Norway in 8% of people over 50 years of age, and Trantas (1929) in Greece believed that it was present in 25% of those over 55 years. As would be expected it frequently occurs with other senile changes in the eyes but there seems to be no direct correlation with any of these; senile cataract, of course, is common, but in unilateral cases of pseudo-exfoliation the type and degree of cataract is usually similar in both eyes. Some authors have found cataract present in much the same proportion as would be expected in this age-group (E. Hørven, 1937, 18%; Busacca, 1929, 24%; Gradle and Sugar, 1940, 38%) but others record higher figures (Gifford, 1957, 51%; Trantas, 1929, 71%). There is no appreciable sex-preference but it has generally been found to occur some years earlier in males than females. One or both eyes

---

[1] Handmann (1926), Alling (1927), Busacca (1929), Trantas (1929), Rehsteiner (1929), Kirby (1930), Holloway and Cowan (1931), Sobhy Bey (1932), Baumgart (1933), E. Hørven (1937–48), Garrow (1938), Gradle and Sugar (1940–47), Holst (1947), Moffat (1948), Örgen (1949), Thomassen (1949), Bhaduri (1949), Wilson (1953).
[2] Weekers *et al.* (1951), Perlman (1955), Sunde (1956), Gifford (1957–58), Cambiaggi and Pirodda (1957), Cambiaggi (1958–59), Petersen (1958), Paufique and Audibert (1958), Sampaolesi (1959), Bitrán and Villalobos (1959), Blackstad *et al.* (1960), Tarkkanen (1962), Arnesen *et al.* (1963), Ashton *et al.* (1965), Backhaus and Lorentzen (1966), and others.

may be affected but in slightly less than half the cases the condition is unilateral (45%, Gifford, 1957; 48%, Tarkkanen, 1962).

There would appear to be some racial predilection; although the disease has been seen almost all over the world, in Britain and Europe, North and South America, Asia, the Far East and Australia and New Zealand, it has a peculiar racial distribution, the cause of which is at present unknown. Different investigators have found a very variable incidence depending to a considerable extent on whether they have examined all ophthalmological patients or those attending glaucoma clinics where the condition is common, or have made general population studies or, again, on whether the pupil has been dilated.

It is obvious, however, that the disease is particularly common in Norway (E. Hørven, 1935–36), Finland (Lindberg, 1917; Tarkkanen, 1962), the Äland Islands (Forsius and Eriksson, 1961) and in the Isle of Man where the ancestry is Scandinavian (Clements, 1968), but rare in Sweden (Strömberg, 1962) and Denmark (Holm-Pedersen, 1954). It is relatively common in Russia (Pletneva, 1928), Italy (Busacca, 1927; Baumgart, 1933; Travi *et al.*, 1947; Grignolo and Cambiaggi, 1957), Greece (Trantas, 1929–34; Joannides *et al.*, 1961) and Turkey (Örgen, 1949), but rare in Central European countries such as France and Germany (Handmann, 1926; Paufique and Audibert, 1958; Leydhecker, 1960). In India it is common (Irvine, 1940–41) and in the Argentine (Maggi Zavalia and Ferrero, 1950) and Chile (Bitrán and Villalobos, 1959), but in Britain (Thomassen, 1949; Roche, 1968), the U.S.A. (Irvine, 1940), Australia (Gillies, 1962; Lowe, 1964) and New Zealand (Wilson, 1953) it is less frequent. It is interesting that Roche (1968) concluded that it was more common in northern than in southern England and suggested that this was genetically related to the invasion of the northern regions of the country by the Scandinavians. It is rare in Egypt (Maghraby, 1937) and has not been reported in Negroes in any country apart from some cases in the U.S.A. (Gradle and Sugar, 1947). The cause of this peculiar distribution is at present unknown.

A *hereditary* transmission of pseudo-exfoliation is not yet clarified. Tarkkanen (1962) suggested the presence of a gene bearing three characteristics: an abnormality of the drainage channels of the aqueous similar to that determining simple glaucoma, pseudo-exfoliation and degeneration of the pigmentary epithelium of the iris. Variations in the expressivity of this gene would explain why the three events are sometimes found together and why sometimes only two or one is present. With his colleagues (1965) he described a large family wherein certain members had simple glaucoma, myopia and/or pseudo-exfoliation, a finding which suggests that these three manifestations are transmitted by an autosomal dominant gene with incomplete penetrance and variable expressivity.

Clinical Picture. The disease is exceedingly slow and chronic, its course being measured in periods of 10 or 20 years; moreover, it is not static but progresses continuously from an insidious start, a phase very difficult to recognize clinically, to an advanced stage when most of the anterior segment of the eye is obviously affected and glaucoma is far advanced.

The deposits on the anterior lens capsule occur in two areas, a central disc in the pupillary region and a girdle round the periphery; the latter is always present but the former may be missing (18% of cases, Tarkkanen, 1962). It would appear that initially the two are continuous (Gifford, 1957)

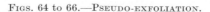

FIGS. 64 to 66.—PSEUDO-EXFOLIATION.

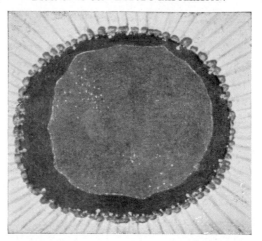

FIG. 64.—Showing the central disc (E. Hørven).

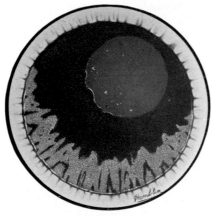

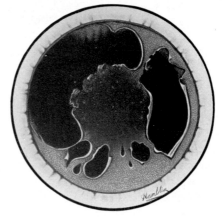

FIG. 65.—With pupillary dilatation, show-ing the central disc completely separated from the peripheral band.

FIG. 66.—Showing a few connections surviving between the two areas of pseudo-exfoliation.

and that the movements of the iris rub off the encrustations immediately under its border so that lacunæ appear in the intermediate area between the two zones; these spaces gradually and slowly enlarge until the two areas are joined merely by bridges or are eventually completely separated from each other by an apparently unaffected zone. This explains the limitation of the central disc to the rim of the pupillary margin; it can be decreased in size if the pupil is kept contracted with miotics and, when the pupil is dilated, part of the granular film attached to the iris has been observed clinically to peel off the capsule forming a segment of the clear intermediate zone (Sunde, 1956).

The *central disc* on the anterior surface of the lens corresponds in extent to the minimum dilatation of the pupil (Fig. 64). It is usually a thin and uniform homogeneous deposit hardly differentiated from the capsule itself and may be difficult to see until the pupil is dilated when a few dandruff-like deposits with sharp rims are found at its boundary. On the other hand, it may be conspicuous, with a clearly defined edge which is often curled inwards so that a ring of tags marks the position of the maximal pupillary

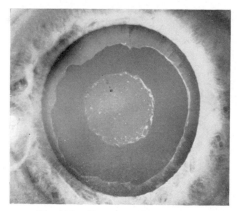

FIG. 67.—PSEUDO-EXFOLIATION.
With a fully dilated pupil the central disc and peripheral band of exudative material are seen with a clear interval between (A. Tarkkanen).

contraction (Fig. 67). Outside this, lying behind the iris usually in the outer third of the distance from the anterior pole to the equator, is a much more conspicuous *peripheral band* of a coarse granular appearance like hoar-frost, looking as if the lens had been sprinkled over with a white powder (Fig. 65). This peripheral band varies in breadth, and although it is separated from the central disc by an area wherein the capsule appears clinically normal, the axial border may be denticulate and bridges may extend across the clear girdle to reach the central disc (Figs. 66–7). At the peripheral border the granular encrustation may gradually fade away merging with normal capsule, or the boundary may be distinct and sharp, in which case it is always festooned with radial projections striking out towards the zonular fibres.

That the zonular fibres become powdered with white crust-like particles was noted incidentally by Trantas (1929) and Vogt (1931), but E. Hørven (1936) first pointed out that this forms an integral part of the clinical picture

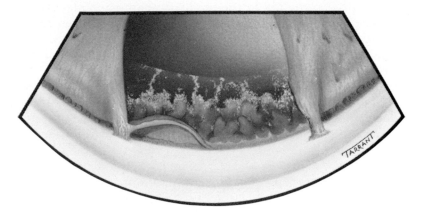

FIG. 68.—PSEUDO-EXFOLIATION.

Gonioscopic view of the precipitation of exudative material over the ciliary body
in an aphakic right eye with glaucoma (Inst. Ophthal.).

on his finding that this appearance was invariably seen when the zonule was
exposed to view by an iridectomy for glaucoma or in enucleated eyes
(Fig. 68).

Such a deposit is a very constant feature, however, on the pupillary
margin of the iris where a powdery accumulation of white flakes is frequently
obvious (Fig. 69). These occur only in the presence of lenticular changes
and seem to be derived from the capsule as if they had been desquamated
spontaneously or rubbed off by the pupillary movements. It is interesting
that Wollenberg (1926) found exfoliation in one eye in which the pupil was
active but none in its fellow wherein the pupil was fixed. The flakes are
constantly changing in quantity, appearing here and disappearing there,
and the fact that they are seen immediately after an iridectomy in dense
masses along the edge of the coloboma suggests
that they may cover most of the posterior surface
of the iris. The flakes are usually not obvious on
the anterior surface of the iris but may be seen in
the crypts; they have also been seen on remnants
of a pupillary membrane, appearing like rime on a
telegraph wire; they float in the anterior chamber;
they become attached to the posterior surface of
the cornea; they accumulate in the angle of the
anterior chamber where they may be seen gonioscopically often with pigmentary deposits (Barkan,
1938); and after the intracapsular extraction of a
cataract the granular material has been found on the
hyaloid surface of the vitreous where it has come
into contact with the posterior surface of the iris.

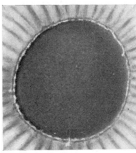

FIG. 69.—PSEUDO-
EXFOLIATION OF THE
CAPSULE.

Powdery deposit on the
margin of the iris (after A.
Garrow).

Pigmentary changes are often prominent (Gradle and Sugar, 1940). When the pupil is dilated some pigment adheres to the capsule and a transient cloud may appear in the anterior chamber, dusting the anterior surface of the iris and becoming deposited over the trabeculæ where an unusually dense accumulation is frequently seen gonioscopically in the angle (Amalric *et al.*, 1960; and others). Sampaolesi (1959) and Tosi (1964) considered that a pigmented line lying on the corneal side of Schwalbe's line was an early sign of the pseudo-exfoliation syndrome; it is not present in eyes with simple glaucoma, but the former author found it in 83% of glaucomatous eyes with pseudo-exfoliation and I. Hørven (1966) in 77%.

Pathology. Histological examinations have been reported by a number of writers[1] and electron-microscopic studies have been fully described.[2] The pseudo-exfoliative material is found in considerable quantity on the capsule of the lens, the zonular fibres, within the iris and ciliary body and in gross accumulations in the posterior chamber, and in many cases in the trabeculæ and drainage channels.

FIGS. 70 and 71.—PSEUDO-EXFOLIATION OF THE LENS CAPSULE
(after A. Garrow and I. C. Michaelson).

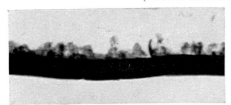 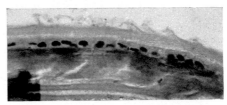

FIG. 70.—Exudative material on the super-   FIG. 71.—Fine strands of exudative material
ficial layers of the capsule.   on the surface of the capsule.

In the lens capsule in the central axial area there are no microscopically visible changes but small amounts of the material may be found on its surface and in its substance (I. Hørven, 1966); the intermediate clear zone is normal. In the peripheral ring the exudative material accumulates in large bush-like aggregations (Figs. 70–1). By electron microscopy a fibrillar substance is clearly seen within the capsule itself, while Bertelsen and his colleagues (1964) found electron-microscopic evidence that these fibrils originated in the subcapsular epithelium. Anterior to the equator the most marked changes are seen; accumulations of exfoliative material become very marked at the insertion of the zonular fibres and changes in the capsule itself are accentuated. Here the deeper layer of the capsule becomes degenerated into a coarsely fibro-granular spongy band, resembling the exfoliated material which accumulates on the surface of the lens and the

[1] Busacca (1927–29), Rehsteiner (1929), Vogt (1930), Blaickner (1932), Sobhy Bey (1932), Garrow and Michaelson (1940), Landolt (1957), Gifford (1957), Calmettes *et al.* (1958), Arnesen *et al.* (1963), I. Hørven (1966), Mikawa (1968).
[2] Blackstad *et al.* (1960), Bertelsen *et al.* (1964), Ashton *et al.* (1965), Shakib *et al.* (1965).

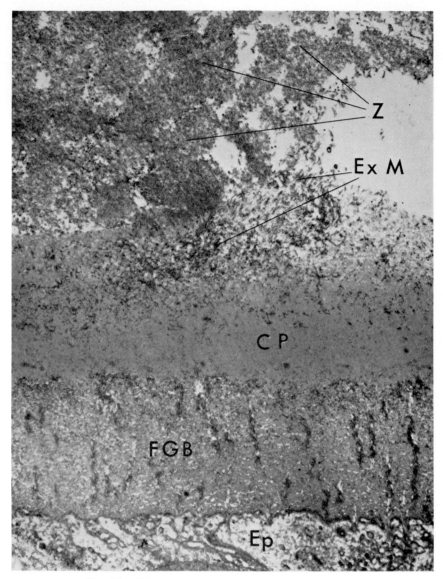

FIG. 72.—PSEUDO-EXFOLIATION OF THE LENS CAPSULE.

CP, the capsule proper; Ep, subcapsular epithelium; Ex M, the exfoliated material; FGB, fibro-granular band between the epithelium and the capsule; Z, the zonule, showing exfoliated material (electron-micrograph; × approx. 5,000) (N. Ashton *et al.*).

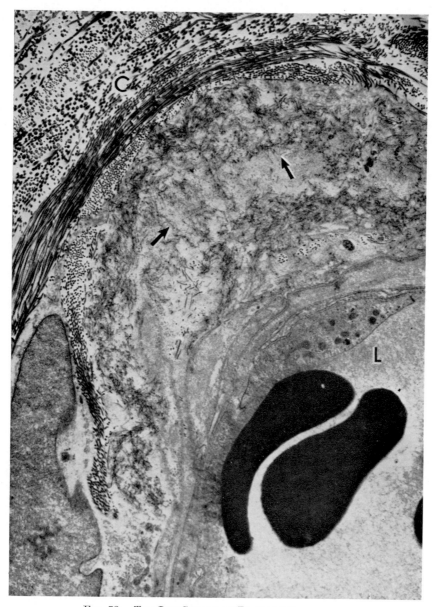

Fig. 73.—The Iris Stroma in Pseudo-exfoliation.

C, collagen fibres; L, lumen of a blood vessel; the arrows indicate the accumulation of exfoliated material around the blood vessel (electron-micrograph; × 12,000) (N. Ashton et al.).

zonule (Fig. 72). Behind the equator the capsule is normal with exudative material lying on its surface and in association with the zonular fibres, while in the posterior central region no abnormality is found.

On the posterior surface of the iris exfoliative material is plentiful, entering deeply into the spaces between the epithelial cells and lying within the internal limiting membrane; the same material is abundant in the stroma, particularly around the vessels and between the basement membrane of the endothelium and the collagen fibres (Fig. 73). It does not, however, appear within intact cells. In the ciliary body the epithelium and stroma are normal but the basement membrane is heavily involved and the greatest accumulations within the eye lie upon the epithelium in the posterior chamber.

The nature of the exudative material is unknown. Morphologically, as seen by the electron microscope, it consists of characteristic interlacing filaments (200 A.U. × 1μ) with a fluffy outline owing to the presence of granules, and is remarkably constant in appearance whether lying in felty masses on a surface or within the capsule or the uveal tissues. Histochemically it contains tyrosine, is resistant to collagenase and hyaluronidase, but can be digested slowly by strong concentrations of trypsin and pepsin and gives negative reactions for hyalin, amyloid, colloid and fat (Busacca, 1927). Most authors agree that it shows the staining reactions of an acid muco-polysaccharide (Gifford, 1957; Arnesen et al., 1963; Bertelsen, 1966; I. Hørven, 1966).

Its origin is equally disputed. That it is not merely an exfoliation of the lens capsule is now clear; its wide distribution throughout the anterior segment cannot be without significance and the prominent involvement of the basement membranes in the iris and ciliary body is suggestive of the original theory of Trantas (1929), as also is the involvement of the substance of the lens capsule. It is possible that an abnormal substance is elaborated in the ciliary body or escapes through the blood-aqueous barrier to be deposited from the aqueous as originally suggested by Busacca (1927); but no abnormal constituent has yet been detected in this fluid (Cambiaggi and Pirodda, 1957; Ashton, 1960). An origin from the uvea has been suggested with considerable reason by several writers (Malling, 1938; Weekers et al., 1951; Goldmann, 1957; Amsler, 1957; Cambiaggi, 1959; Joannides et al., 1961), from the pigmentary epithelium of the iris by others (Caramazza, 1933; Audibert, 1957) or the ciliary epithelium (Ashton, 1957; Étienne, 1960); and the underlying process has been said to be a degenerative uveitis (Joannides et al., 1961), a degeneration of vascular origin (Weekers et al., 1951) or an abiotrophy (Cambiaggi, 1959). These, however, are largely suppositions based on guesswork, and the subject still remains a challenge.

Symptoms of the disease do not exist for throughout its long and insidious course the condition is clinically silent; the only complication which may arise—and it is a serious one—is the development of glaucoma[1].

The relation between capsular pseudo-exfoliation and glaucoma was recognized by the discoverers of the condition. Lindberg (1917) found these changes in 30 out of 60 cases of chronic primary glaucoma, and Malling (1938) in 33 out of 81 glaucomatous eyes. In his first paper on the subject, Vogt (1925) found that of the 12 people affected 9 suffered from advanced

[1] See further, p. 691.

simple glaucoma and, concluding that the glaucoma was in reality secondary, due to the blockage of the angle of the anterior chamber by exfoliated material, he termed it GLAUCOMA CAPSULARE. Although the occurrence of closed-angle glaucoma is a rarity (Ross, 1949), that simple glaucoma is a common occurrence in patients with exfoliation is well established; it may, indeed, be said to occur in some 70% of cases.

The following statistics appear in the literature: 76% Busacca (1927), 75% Pletneva (1928), 35% Trantas (1929), 75% Rehsteiner (1929), 75·5%, and 64% out of 78 published cases, Vogt (1931), 58% out of 156 cases in the literature, Grzedzielski (1931), 54% Sobhy Bey (1932), 16% Garrow (1938), 75% Irvine (1940), 82% Gradle and Sugar (1940), 82% Holst (1947), 79% Thomassen (1949), 77% Maggi Zavalia and Ferrero (1950), 42% Gifford (1957), 48% Audibert (1957), 89% Arentsen and Bitrán (1959), 72% Sampaolesi (1959), 40% Joannides *et al.* (1961), 73% Schwab and Papapanos (1961), 61% Tarkkanen (1962), 50% Zlater (1965), 24% Klouman (1967), 52% Sood and Ratnaraj (1968), and many others.

Similarly, in a considerable proportion of cases, elderly people with simple glaucoma are found to have exfoliation, estimates of which vary from 2 to 93%.

Sixty cases of simple glaucoma included 30 with exfoliation (Lindberg, 1917), 81 eyes included 33 (Malling, 1923), 38 included 16 (Busacca, 1929), 59 included 29 (Baumgart, 1933), 150 operated cases included 128, and 43 cases of glaucoma under treatment included 40 with exfoliation (E. Hørven, 1937), 51 included 8 (Garrow, 1938), 1,112 eyes included 47 affected (Lemoine, 1950), 54 included 24 (Maggi Zavalia and Ferrero, 1950). Again, there seems to be a territorial difference: thus Irvine (1940) found 24% of glaucomatous eyes with pseudo-exfoliation in India and 4% in California, Thomassen (1949) 2% in England and 79% in Norway, the latter figure being confirmed by Sunde (1956), and Clements (1968) 74% in males in the Isle of Man. I. Hørven (1966) found 28% of patients diagnosed as primary glaucoma with exfoliation in Massachusetts, and Roche (1968) 9·2% in England.

Although some authorities deny any close relationship,[1] it must be admitted that the difference between the incidence of exfoliation in glaucomatous patients and in normal subjects seems too great to be incidental and points to a relationship of cause and effect, a subject which will be discussed again in dealing with this disease. The fact that in unilateral cases the glaucoma is often limited to the eye with pseudo-exfoliation also seems significant (43 cases, Tarkkanen, 1962). There is, however, some doubt that the simple explanation originally advanced by Vogt (1925) is correct: that the raised tension was due to obstruction of the drainage channels by flakes of exudative material as well as pigment. Thus in 32 eyes with pseudo-exfoliation and glaucoma, Sunde (1956) found flakes in the angle on gonioscopic examination in only 6, while Tarkkanen (1962) found flakes to be present in this situation almost as frequently (46%) as in non-glaucomatous eyes (50%). It is obvious that the two conditions can occur separately or simultaneously, but the relation between them is not clear. The

[1] Alling (1927), Grzedzielski (1931), Malling (1938), Butler (1938), Thomassen (1949), and others.

variation in the occurrence of the exudative material in the angle as well as the fact that glaucoma may be well advanced before exfoliation, appear to suggest that it is more probable that the same degenerative changes, possibly vascular in origin, which cause the pseudo-exfoliation are themselves responsible for the development of glaucoma, but the question must still remain open. In this event the glaucoma should be regarded as primary in type.

It may be noted here that most surgeons have found that treatment by miotics is rarely satisfactory for the resulting glaucoma, but that a drainage operation is necessary and frequently gives good results. One of the post-operative complications found by Roche (1968) was the profuse showering of the anterior chamber with pigment, sometimes in sufficient quantity to impair vision by its adhering to the anterior surface of the lens. If the lens is cataractous it should be extracted, but it is necessary to continue therapy for the glaucoma which is not affected by removal of the lens.

Alling. *Arch. Ophthal.*, **56**, 1 (1927).

Amalric, Sampaolesi and Bessou. *Bull. Soc. Ophtal. Fr.*, 341 (1960).

Amsler. *Ophthalmologica*, **133**, 318 (1957).

Arentsen and Bitrán. *Arch. chil. Oftal.*, **16**, 74 (1959).

Arnesen, Sunde and Schultz-Haudt. *Acta ophthal.* (Kbh.), **41**, 80 (1963).

Ashton. *Trans. Amer. ophthal. Soc.*, **55**, 189 (1957).
Glaucoma, Macy Fdn. Symp. (Ed. F. W. Newell), N.Y., 197 (1960).

Ashton, Shakib, Collyer and Blach. *Invest. Ophthal.*, **4**, 141 (1965).

Audibert. *La pseudo-exfoliation capsulaire sénile* (Thèse), Lyon (1957).

Backhaus and Lorentzen. *Acta ophthal.* (Kbh.), **44**, 1 (1966).

Barkan. *Trans. ophthal. Soc. U.K.*, **58**, 588 (1938).

Baumgart. *Boll. Oculist.*, **12**, 560 (1933).

Bertelsen. *Acta ophthal.* (Kbh.), **44**, 737 (1966).

Bertelsen, Drablös and Flood. *Acta ophthal.* (Kbh.), **42**, 1096 (1964).

Bhaduri. *Proc. Ind. ophthal. Soc.*, **10**, 55 (1949).

Bitrán and Villalobos. *Arch. chil. Oftal.*, **16**, 79 (1959).

Blackstad, Sunde and Traetteberg. *Acta ophthal.* (Kbh.), **38**, 587 (1960).

Blaickner. *Ber. dtsch. ophthal. Ges.*, **49**, 325, 353 (1932).

Busacca. *v. Graefes Arch. Ophthal.*, **119**, 135 (1927).
Klin. Mbl. Augenheilk., **83**, 737 (1929).

Butler. *Trans. ophthal. Soc. U.K.*, **58**, 575 (1938).

Calmettes, Amalric and Bessou. *Bull. Soc. Ophtal. Fr.*, 447 (1958).

Cambiaggi. *Boll. Oculist.*, **37**, 822 (1958).
G. ital. Oftal., **12**, 520 (1959).

Cambiaggi and Pirodda. *Boll. Oculist.*, **36**, 315 (1957).

Caramazza. *Rass. ital. Ottal.*, **2**, 1299 (1933).

Clements. *Brit. J. Ophthal.*, **52**, 546 (1968).

Dvorak-Theobald. *Trans. Amer. ophthal. Soc.*, **51**, 385 (1953).
Amer. J. Ophthal., **37**, 1 (1954).

Étienne. *Ann. Oculist.* (Paris), **193**, 97, 224 (1960).

Forsius and Eriksson. *Acta ophthal.* (Kbh.) **39**, 318 (1961).

Garrow. *Brit. J. Ophthal.*, **22**, 214 (1938).

Garrow and Michaelson. *Brit. J. Ophthal.*, **24**, 400 (1940).

Gifford. *Trans. Amer. ophthal. Soc.*, **55**, 189 (1957).
Amer. J. Ophthal., **46**, 508 (1958).

Gillies. *Trans. ophthal. Soc. Aust.*, **22**, 120 (1962).

Goldmann. *Ophthalmologica*, **133**, 319 (1957).

Gradle and Sugar. *Amer. J. Ophthal.*, **23**, 982 (1940); **30**, 12 (1947).

Grignolo and Cambiaggi. *L'Année thér. Ophtal.*, **8**, 99 (1957).

Grzedzielski. *v. Graefes Arch. Ophthal.*, **126**, 409 (1931).

Handmann. *Klin. Mbl. Augenheilk.*, **76**, 482 (1926).

Hørven, E. *Om den senile eksfoliasjon av linsekapselen*, Oslo, 166 (1935).
Acta ophthal. (Kbh.), **14**, 231 (1936); **26**, 231 (1948).
Brit. J. Ophthal., **21**, 625 (1937).

Hørven, I. *Arch. Ophthal.*, **76**, 505 (1966).
Acta ophthal. (Kbh.), **44**, 790 (1966); **45**, 294 (1967).

Holloway and Cowan. *Amer. J. Ophthal.*, **14**, 189 (1931).

Holm-Pedersen. *Ugeskr. f. Laeg.*, **116**, 655 (1954).

Holst. *Amer. J. Ophthal.*, **30**, 1267 (1947).

Irvine. *Arch. Ophthal.*, **23**, 138 (1940); **25**, 992 (1941).

Joannides, Katsourakis and Velissaropoulos. *Ophthalmologica*, **142**, 160 (1961).

Kirby. *Arch. Ophthal.*, **4**, 93 (1930).

Klouman. *Acta ophthal.* (Kbh.), **45**, 822 (1967).

Landolt. *Ophthalmologica*, **133**, 309 (1957).

Lemoine. *Amer. J. Ophthal.*, **33**, 1353 (1950).

Leydhecker. *Glaukom*, Berlin, 163 (1960).

Lindberg. *Klin. undersökningar över depigmenteringen av pupillarranden och genomlysbarheten av iris*, Helsingfors (1917).

Lowe. *Brit. J. Ophthal.*, **48**, 492 (1964).

Maggi Zavalia and Ferrero. *Arch. Oftal. B. Aires*, **25**, 547 (1950).

Maghraby. *Bull. ophthal. Soc. Egypt*, **30**, 42 (1937).

Malling. *Acta ophthal.* (Kbh.), **1**, 97 (1923); **16**, 43 (1938).

Mikawa. *Rinsho Ganka*, **22**, 317 (1968).

Moffat. *Proc. roy. Soc. Med.*, **41**, 750 (1948).

Örgen. *Oto nörö oftal.*, **4**, 1 (1949).

Paufique and Audibert. *Act. Latinee Ophtal.*, Paris, 213 (1958).

Perlman. *Acta med. orient.*, **14**, 211 (1955).

Petersen. *Acta ophthal.* (Kbh.), **36**, 375 (1958).

Pletneva. *Russ. Arch. Oftal.*, **4**, 68 (1928).

Rehsteiner. *Klin. Mbl. Augenheilk.*, **82**, 21 (1929).

Roche. *Brit. J. Ophthal.*, **52**, 265 (1968).

Ross. *Acta ophthal.* (Kbh.), **27**, 475 (1949).

Sampaolesi. *Ber. dtsch. ophthal. Ges.*, **62**, 177 (1959).

Ann. Oculist. (Paris), **192**, 839 (1959).

Schwab and Papapanos. *Wien. klin. Wschr.*, **73**, 878 (1961).

Shakib, Ashton and Blach. *Invest. Ophthal.*, **4**, 154 (1965).

Sobhy Bey. *Brit. J. Ophthal.*, **16**, 64 (1932).

Sood and Ratnaraj. *Orient. Arch. Ophthal.*, **6**, 62 (1968).

Strömberg. *Acta ophthal.* (Kbh.), Suppl. 69 (1962).

Sunde. *Acta ophthal.* (Kbh.), Suppl. 45 (1956).

Tarkkanen. *Acta ophthal.* (Kbh.), Suppl. 71 (1962); **43**, 514 (1965).

Thomassen. *Acta ophthal.* (Kbh.), **27**, 423 (1949).

Tosi. *Arch. Oftal. B. Aires*, **39**, 114 (1964).

Trantas. *Arch. Ophtal.*, **46**, 482 (1929).

Ann. Oculist. (Paris), **171**, 610 (1934).

Travi, Bellouard and Rebay. *Arch. Soc. oftal. Litoral*, **1**, 128 (1947).

Vogt. *v. Graefes Arch. Ophthal.*, **111**, 91, 110 (1923).

Klin. Mbl. Augenheilk., **75**, 1 (1925); **84**, 1 (1930); **86**, 736 (1931); **88**, 248; **89**, 581, 587 (1932); **90**, 842 (1933); **95**, 92 (1935); **101**, 703, 705 (1938).

Z. Augenheilk., **58**, 379 (1926); **66**, 105 (1928).

Lhb. u. Atlas d. Spaltlampenmikroskopie d. lebenden Auges, 2nd ed., Berlin, **2**, 572 (1931).

Weekers, L. and R., and Dedoyard. *Docum. ophthal.*, **5–6**, 555 (1951).

Weekers, R., Prijot, Delmarcelle, Lavergne et al. *Bull. Soc. belge Ophtal.*, No. 121, 1 (1959).

Wilson. *Trans. ophthal. Soc. N.Z.*, **7**, 8 (1953).

Wollenberg. *Klin. Mbl. Augenheilk.*, **77**, 128 (1926).

Zlater. *Ophthalmologica*, **150**, 175 (1965).

Folding and Rupture of the Capsule

FOLDING OF THE CAPSULE

This is a rare condition which has been noticed sporadically in several circumstances. Folds in the anterior or posterior capsule sometimes associated with localized subcapsular opacities were described by Bignell (1951) due to a traumatic partial rupture of the zonule; in these cases there were also a subluxation of the lens and astigmatic changes in refraction (Figs. 74–5). Kittel (1960) recorded the occurrence of capsular folds appearing after operations such as iridectomy and iridencleisis. Pau (1950) also noted similar folds in the posterior capsule in a case of heterochromic cataract which had been operated on for glaucoma; there were many corneal precipitates and he interpreted the phenomenon as due to a shrinkage of the lens owing to a decrease in osmotic pressure following a leakage of proteins from the lens.

FLOATING FOLDS of the anterior lens capsule are an exceptional occurrence. A unique case was reported by Pünder (1956) associated with a complicated cataract. On histological examination fan-shaped folded extensions of the capsule were found floating freely in the anterior chamber (Fig. 76).

Bignell. *Brit. J. Ophthal.*, **35**, 234 (1951).

Kittel. *Ber. dtsch. ophthal. Ges.*, **63**, 372 (1960).

Pau. *Ber. dtsch. ophthal. Ges.*, **56**, 361 (1950).

Pünder. *Klin. Mbl. Augenheilk.*, **129**, 98 (1956).

Figs. 74 and 75.—Folds in the Lens Capsule after Trauma (J. L. Bignell).

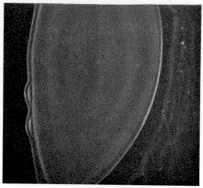 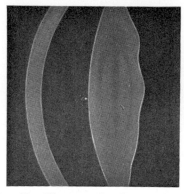

Fig. 74.—The lens of a man aged 42 who was struck by a squash ball with a resulting hyphæma and iridodonesis with partial subluxation of the lens and posterior sub-capsular opacities. The undulations of the anterior capsule are seen, beneath each of which is a slight opacity.

Fig. 75.—The eye of a boy aged 9 was struck by an arrow resulting in a prolapse of the iris. The lens showed a slight subcortical opacity and was dislocated medially. The folds in the posterior capsule are well seen.

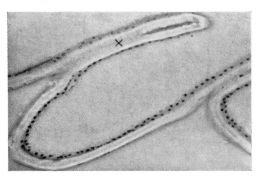

Fig. 76.—Folding of the Lens Capsule.

In a case of complicated cataract. Histological specimen after extraction of the lens showed folds of the lens capsule, X, protruding into the anterior chamber with the deposition of pigment (H. Pünder).

RUPTURE OF THE LENS CAPSULE

Rupture of the lens capsule may occur in the course of a suppurative in-flammation,[1] as a result of trauma or spontaneously. TRAUMATIC RUPTURE of the capsule will be discussed in a subsequent Volume,[2] but it may be noted here that it may follow a concussion or result from a perforating injury. In the first case the rupture is due either to the sudden to-and-fro movements of the lens following a blow on the eye, or to the strain put upon the zonule by the enforced antero-posterior contraction and the associated circumferential expansion of the equatorial region of the globe; the subsequent tear may

[1] p. 6.   [2] Vol. XIV.

occur in the anterior capsule, in the attenuated region near the posterior pole or, less frequently, in the equatorial region near the attachment of the zonule. A perforating injury to the capsule is frequently associated with the entrance of a foreign body into the globe or may be an intentional or inadvertent result of ocular surgery. In either case the result is a localized or diffuse cataract.

SPONTANEOUS RUPTURES occur mainly in two circumstances: in association with a hypermature cataract or a lenticonus; an exceptional cause is pressure from an intra-ocular tumour. In the two former cases the capsular tear results from a rapid swelling of the lens. The capsule has sufficient elasticity to contain a considerable increase in intralenticular swelling, but that this can be exceeded and spontaneous bursting result was dramatically demonstrated by Bellows and Chinn (1941) who altered the physical conditions by subjecting lenses to various chemical solutions. In pathological states it is, of course, possible that the elasticity of the capsule is impaired so that a tear will more readily result. Exceptional instances of spontaneous rupture have been reported in hydrocephalic epilepsy (Orlansky, 1952) and in dislocation of the lens,[1] while the accident has occurred with the development of phaco-anaphylactic uveitis after an encircling operation for retinal detachment (Wolter and Bryson, 1966).

SPONTANEOUS RUPTURE IN HYPERMATURE CATARACT

This is an uncommon event, but since its first description by Arlt (1881) it has been described by a number of observers.[2] The lens is typically hypermature or morgagnian when the capsule always becomes thin and fragile; the accident of rupture is marked by the sudden appearance of a milky fluid in the anterior chamber and the development of glaucoma and is associated with sudden and severe pain, usually with considerable circumcorneal injection; and occasionally it is followed by a shrinkage or dislocation of the lens itself. The subsequent dissolution of the lens substance may explain some cases of the apparently spontaneous disappearance of a cataract.

An INTRA-OCULAR NEOPLASM in the ciliary region may occasionally rupture the capsule by direct pressure on the lens and produce a traumatic cataract.[3]

LENTICONUS

In marked cases of *anterior lenticonus*[4] (Figs. 77–80) which show rapid progression, a spontaneous rupture of the capsule may occur; it will be

---

[1] p. 305.
[2] Ulrich (1882), von Szily (1884), Rollet and Genet (1913), Gonzales (1919), Kaufman (1933), Knapp (1937), Box (1941), Sugar (1949), Bonavolontà (1950), Scott (1953), Raptis and Sapountzis (1953), Ming (1963), and others.
[3] Becker (1883), Lange (1890), Mitvalsky (1894), Treacher Collins (1896), Groenouw (1899), Symens (1901), Nordmann (1930), Merrill (1933), and others.
[4] Vol. III, p. 696.

FIGS. 77 to 80.—ANTERIOR LENTICONUS.

In a male aged 27 with familial hæmorrhagic nephritis (R. D. Brownell and J. R. Wolter).

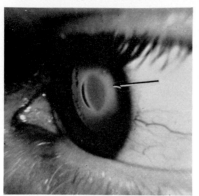

FIG. 77.—The lenticonus (arrowed) seen clinically.

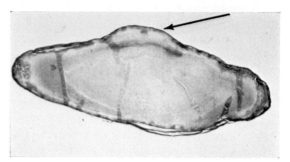

FIG. 78.—Section of the lens showing abnormal thinning of the capsule, a decrease of the epithelial cells and a slight punctate subcapsular cataract at the anterior pole.

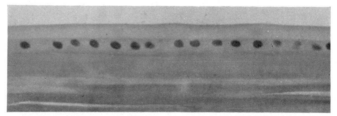

FIG. 79.—The epithelium of a normal lens.

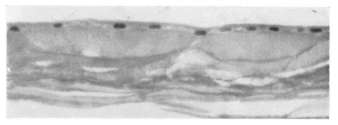

FIG. 80.—The irregular lens epithelium in the present case with small areas of subcapsular cataract.

remembered that the most generally accepted theory to account for the development of this deformity in otherwise normal eyes is a thinning and consequent stretching of the capsule with a diminution of the epithelial cells (Fig. 80) (Elschnig, 1895; Hess, 1911; Knobloch, 1937; Petronio, 1941; Brownell and Wolter, 1964; and others). The rupture occurs near the apex of the cone and a localized anterior polar cataract results. This sequence was observed by Ehrlich (1946) and may result in a cessation of the progress

of the lenticonus (Figs. 81–2); it may be that those cases of anterior lenticonus which have developed an opacity at the anterior pole and have
stabilized are of this nature (Jaworski, 1910; Tsukahara, 1930; Feigenbaum,
1932; Urrets Zavalia and Obregon Oliva, 1939; and others). The lesion
may be congenital and also occurs in familial hæmorrhagic nephritis (Alport's
syndrome, 1927) (Mettier, 1961; Gregg and Becker, 1963; Brownell and
Wolter, 1964).

In *posterior lenticonus*,[1] a condition which may also be accompanied by
cataractous changes, the earlier pathological investigators found a tear in
the posterior capsule (Collins, 1908); that this may have been an artefact
in histological preparation is suggested by the finding by later observers
that a capsule has been seen to be intact although so thin as to be almost

FIGS. 81 and 82.—ANTERIOR LENTICONUS (after L. H. Ehrlich and M. Berliner).

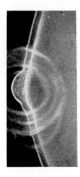   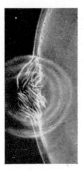

FIG. 81.—Optical section of the conus.   FIG. 82.—Optical section after rupture of
the conus.

invisible over the cone (Makley, 1955). It is interesting that in this condition
an aberrant growth of the subcapsular epithelium has been found to overlie
the lenticonus (Franceschetti and Rickli, 1954; Makley, 1955).

A HEREDITARY SPONTANEOUS RUPTURE OF THE LENS CAPSULE has been described
in mice by Smelser and von Sallmann (1949) and Fraser and Herer (1950). The
"lens rupture" gene is transmitted as a simple recessive factor with no sex-linkage.
In its homozygous state the mutant gene is associated with changes which become
evident about the second or third week of life; these include a distortion of the
nucleus of the lens, the formation of a posterior lenticonus, a rupture of the lens capsule
in this situation, the development of cataract and the expulsion of the nucleus with
varying amounts of the cortex into the vitreous chamber. Thereafter the lens shrinks
and the suspensory ligament gives way so that the remains of the lens may pass through
the pupil into the anterior chamber, a series of events which occurs within the first
three months of life. It would seem probable that the lesion is due to a mutation of a
gene involved in the morphogenesis of the capsule and not of the proteins of the fibres
of the lens (Moser and Gluecksohn-Waelsch, 1967).

[1] Vol. III, p. 700.

A *thickening and friability of the capsule* have been found in diabetic patients, as occur in most basement membranes in this disease. Such a capsule contains a considerably higher proportion of collagenous glyco-protein as indicated by its content of hydroxyproline (Paterson and Heath, 1967). An unusual friability is indicated by the higher proportion of capsular ruptures during an attempted intracapsular extraction (20% compared with 12% in non-diabetic cases, Townes and Casey, 1955; 28% compared with 16%, Ramsell, 1969).

Alport. *Brit. med. J.*, **1**, 504 (1927).
Arlt. *Ber. dtsch. ophthal. Ges.*, **13**, 130 (1881).
Becker. *Zur Anatomie d. gesunden u. kranken Linse*, Wiesbaden (1883).
Bellows and Chinn. *Amer. J. Ophthal.*, **24**, 979 (1941).
Bonavolontà. *Rass. ital. Ottal.*, **19**, 326 (1950).
Box. *Med. J. Aust.*, **1**, 451 (1941).
Brownell and Wolter. *Arch. Ophthal.*, **71**, 481 (1964).
Collins. *Researches*, London (1896).
  Ophthalmoscope, **6**, 577, 663 (1908).
  J. Amer. med. Ass., **51**, 1051 (1908).
Ehrlich. *Amer. J. Ophthal.*, **29**, 1274 (1946).
Elschnig. *Klin. Mbl. Augenheilk.*, **33**, 239 (1895).
Feigenbaum. *Folia ophthal. orient.*, **1**, 103 (1932).
Franceschetti and Rickli. *Arch. Ophthal.*, **51**, 499 (1954).
Fraser and Herer. *J. Hered.*, **41**, 3 (1950).
Gonzales. *Amer. J. Ophthal.*, **2**, 742 (1919).
Gregg and Becker. *Arch. Ophthal.*, **69**, 293 (1963).
Groenouw. *v. Graefes Arch. Ophthal.*, **47**, 282, 398 (1899).
Hess. *Graefe-Saemisch Hb. d. ges. Augenheilk.*, 3rd ed., Leipzig, **9** (2) (1911).
Jaworski. *Arch. Augenheilk.*, **65**, 313 (1910).
Kaufman. *Arch. Ophthal.*, **9**, 56 (1933).
Knapp. *Amer. J. Ophthal.*, **20**, 820 (1937).
Knobloch. *Csl. Ofthal.*, **3**, 67 (1937).
Lange. *v. Graefes Arch. Ophthal.*, **36** (3), 247 (1890).
Makley. *Amer. J. Ophthal.*, **39**, 308 (1955).

Merrill. *Klin. Mbl. Augenheilk.*, **91**, 598 (1933).
Mettier. *Arch. Ophthal.*, **65**, 386 (1961).
Ming. *Singapore med. J.*, **4**, 127 (1963).
Mitvalsky. *Arch. Augenheilk.*, **28**, 152 (1894).
Moser and Glueksohn-Waelsch. *Exp. Eye Res.*, **6**, 297 (1967).
Nordmann. *Bull. Soc. Ophtal. Paris*, 157 (1930).
Orlansky. *Arch. Pediat.*, **69**, 247 (1952).
Paterson and Heath. *Exp. Eye Res.*, **6**, 233 (1967).
Petronio. *Arch. Ottal.*, **48**, 153 (1941).
Ramsell. *Brit. J. Ophthal.*, **53**, 98 (1969).
Raptis and Sapountzis. *Arch. ophthal. Soc. N. Greece*, **2**, 123 (1953).
Rollet and Genet. *Rev. gén. Ophtal.*, **32**, 1 (1913).
Scott. *Brit. J. Ophthal.*, **37**, 58 (1953).
Smelser and von Sallmann. *Amer. J. Ophthal.*, **32**, 1703 (1949).
Sugar. *Amer. J. Ophthal.*, **32**, 1509 (1949).
Symens. *Klin. Mbl. Augenheilk.*, **39** (2), 863 (1901).
von Szily. *Zbl. prakt. Augenheilk.*, **8**, 17 (1884).
Townes and Casey. *Sth. med. J.* (Bham, Ala.), **48**, 844 (1955).
Tsukahara. *Acta Soc. ophthal. jap.*, **34**, 370 (1930).
Ulrich. *Klin. Mbl. Augenheilk.*, **20**, 230 (1882).
Urrets Zavalia and Obregon Oliva. *Arch. Oftal. B. Aires*, **14**, 848 (1939).
Wolter and Bryson. *Amer. J. Ophthal.*, **61**, 1428 (1966).

THE PRESENCE OF NON-LENTICULAR STRUCTURES ON THE LENS CAPSULE is well known; all have been dealt with elsewhere. The most common are congenital remnants of the pupillary membrane sometimes in relatively gross forms, sometimes as minute pigmentary dots or stars and often associated with localized subcapsular opacities,[1] pupillary adhesions and inflammatory exudates which may become organized in iridocyclitis,[2] blood after a hyphæma,[3] pigment after a concussion to form a Vossius's ring,[4] and new blood vessels (rubeosis) from such conditions as thrombosis of the central retinal vein, retinal vasculitis and Eales's disease[5] and particularly diabetes.[6] In this last disease a unique case was reported by Alfano and Sidrys (1957) wherein vessels apparently containing aqueous travelled along the anterior lens capsule in association with a heavily vascularized iris in diabetic rubeosis.

Alfano and Sidrys. *Amer. J. Ophthal.*, **43**, 972 (1957).

[1] Vol. III, p. 778. [2] Vol. IX, p. 99. [3] Vol. IX, p. 88.
[4] Vol. XIV. [5] Vol. IX, p. 34. [6] Vol. IX, p. 651.

CHAPTER III

CATARACT

CATARACT may be simply defined as denoting any opacity in the lens. It is the most common—and fortunately one of the most easily remedied— cause of visual incapacity and blindness; indeed, apart from its occurrence as a developmental anomaly and in various diseases, senile cataract may be looked upon as a normal evidence of senescence, occurring to some degree in 65% of people in the sixth decade and in over 95% above 65 years of age.

From among the multitude of people who have made classical contributions to our knowledge of cataract, we have chosen the photograph of OTTO BECKER [1828–1890] (Fig. 83) to introduce this chapter since he was the first to consolidate scientific knowledge of the subject on a firm basis. He will always be regarded as one of the great masters of ophthalmology and many of his investigations were centred on the lens and cataract. Born in Domhof, he studied much at home, learning Latin from an old lady who was his neighbour; thereafter he studied theology at Erlangen but fortunately for us he turned to medicine. At Vienna he was converted to ophthalmology by von Arlt who influenced him greatly, and after serving as his assistant, when Herman Knapp migrated from Heidelberg to America, Becker was appointed to the Chair of Ophthalmology at that University where he worked until his death, when he was succeeded by Theodor Leber. His energy and enthusiasm for life and work were enormous, and the results of his painstaking and accurate investigations have survived all subsequent criticism. Interested in all aspects of ophthalmology, his writings are voluminous but of these his most important concerned the lens, summarized in the *Pathologie und Therapie des Linsensystems* in the *Graefe-Saemisch Handbuch* (1875) and *Zur Anatomie der gesunden und kranken Linse* (Wiesbaden, 1883). In addition to this he was one of the most popular teachers of his age, attracting many students from all over the world, and he maintained a home filled with art treasures. His original work on the lens is a sufficient memorial but, in addition, his memory is perpetuated by a tablet on the house in Domhof where " the master of the vision " was born and by a bust in the ophthalmic hospital at Heidelberg.

History

It is natural that a condition so common and obvious associated with effects so dramatic upon vision should have been known as early as historical records survive; indeed, the history of cataract goes back some 4,000 years and probably further. Thus the disease and its treatment are frequently said to have been known to the Sumerians of Mesopotamia and also to have figured in the medicine of Ancient Egypt, but these suggestions are possibly erroneous.[1] In ancient Hindu medicine, however, it occupied a prominent place, being interpreted as a type of corrupt humor, and the teaching of Suśruta[2] on its relief by couching was remarkably precise and detailed.

[1] See Feigenbaum, *Amer. J. Ophthal.*, **49**, 305 (1960).
[2] Vol. II, p. 18.

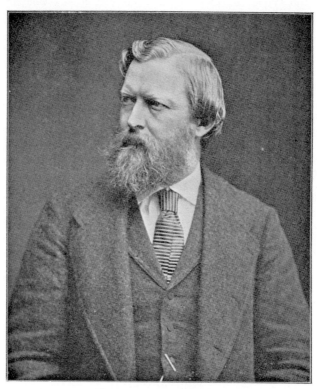

FIG. 83.—OTTO BECKER
[1828–1890]

It is interesting that while in Hindu medicine cataract was defined by Suśruta as an opacity due to a derangement of the intra-ocular fluid, subsequent history is full of fantasies and prejudices concerning its nature. The Hippocratic writings, for example, made no clear distinction between cataract and glaucoma and the acceptance of the humoral theory of disease caused much confusion, but it would seem likely that the knowledge of the Hindus filtered westward to Alexandria. To the Romans, who derived their medical learning from the Alexandrian School as exemplified in the writings of Celsus [25 B.C. to A.D. 50] and Galen [A.D. 131–210], the essential source of the disease lay in the brain and the visual nerves, from which there was derived a corrupt inspissated humour which collected in the empty space between the pupil and the lens, a structure which was regarded as the essential organ of sight and was said to be situated in the centre of the globe (Fig. 2); this ill-humour obstructed the visual spirits, but sight could be restored by removing it either by displacing it with a needle to another part of the eye or by breaking it up. The later classical writers maintained and developed this view—glaucoma was a drying up of the lens itself and was incurable, but cataract was a humour in front of the lens which could be removed. Thus Paulus of Ægina [c. 625–690][1] in his *Hypomnema* wrote that with the latter the patient perceived light while with glaucoma and amaurosis he did not. The same opinion was adopted in Arabian writings and, largely through the immense authority of Galen, was maintained throughout Europe for centuries. Guy de Chauliac [1300–1368] of Avignon, for example, the most eminent surgical authority in the Middle Ages, wrote in his *Chirurgia Magna* (1363) that cataract was " a skin-like spot in front of the pupil which interferes with vision due to an extensive moisture which gradually penetrates into the eye and, in consequence of cold, coagulates. Whether this humour collects between the cornea and the iris (as Jesus proves) or between the aqueous humour and the crystalline lens (as Galen pretends) does not interest me."

In this connection the terminology is interesting. The Greek term first used in the Hippocratic writings, as we have seen, was γλαύκωμα (glaucoma), probably meaning a glazed appearance without lustre[2]; in Alexandrian medicine the humoral concept was expressed in the term ὑπόχυσις (hypochysis), which was translated into Latin as *suffusio*. This was in turn translated by the Arabic scholars as *nuzul-el-ma*, a flowing down of water, and even today the popular term in Arabian countries for cataract is " the blue water ".[3] It is commonly believed that the Carthaginian monk, Constantinus Africanus [1018–85],[4] one of the most famous scholars of the School of Salerno, translating Arabian manuscripts at Monte Cassino into mediæval Latin for the benefit of European learning, converted the Arabian expression in his *Liber de Oculis* into the word *cataracta* (to rush down, as a waterfall or portcullis), a term derived from Greek that had never been used in this medical sense by the classical writers.

[1] Vol. II, p. 17.   [2] p. 380.
[3] In Sindhi cataract is termed *moti pāni* (pearl water) and glaucoma *karo pāni* (black water).
[4] Vol. II, p. 28.

The German word, *Star* (Anglo-Saxon, *staar*) belongs to the root of the verb *starren*, to be stiff or motionless. The German word, *Starblind* corresponds to the English term " stone-blind ".

The position of the lens in the centre of the globe was maintained even by such anatomists as Andrea Vesalius [1514–64] in his *De humani corporis fabrica* (1543), and although Fabricius ab Aquapendente [1537–1619] placed it correctly immediately behind the iris in his book *De Oculo* (1600), clinicians retained the old humoral theory. Dissenting opinions, however, began to appear in the 17th century, particularly in France. About the middle of that century François Quarré taught that cataract was an opacity of the lens itself and not a corrupt humour inspissated in front of it ; so also did Pierre Borclo Rémi Lasnier whose views were discounted " as dreams " by the Parisian College of Surgeons, for the lens was still regarded as the essential organ of vision. These surgeons did not publish their revolutionary opinions, but hearing of them, Werner Rolfinck, the anatomist who dissected executed criminals at Jena, demonstrated in 1656 that cataract was due to a clouding of the lens itself. For half a century, however, these heretical teachings excited little attention. It is true that about 1685 the French surgeon Antoine Maître-Jan, on couching two patients, noted that the rounded lens and not an inspissated membrane appeared in the anterior chamber, an observation which he confirmed in 1692 in the dissection of dead patients whose eyes he had previously couched ; this, however, he did not publish at the time. In the beginning of the next century a French physician, Michel Pierre Brisseau, repeated the observation on April 6th, 1705, on a dead soldier who had cataract, and on November 17th of the same year he communicated to the *Académie Royale des Sciences* in Paris the fact that cataract was indeed an opaque lens and that this and not an opaque humour in front of it was depressed in the operation of couching. It is interesting that on Brisseau's discovery, his teacher, Duverney, strongly advised him against publication lest he jeopardize his professional future by arousing prejudice ; but nevertheless, holding with excellent spirit that " those who opposed his view had more at stake ", he maintained his point[1] with the support of Antoine Maître-Jan and later of Jean Méry, but not without a bitter fight which cost him his position in the French Academy.

Owing to the strong advocacy of Maître-Jan and Méry, however, the battle in the Academy was eventually won, but for a considerable time this controversy ranged throughout Europe, sometimes with much acrimony. On the one side, many surgeons, such as John Thomas Woolhouse, the celebrated English quack-oculist who followed his monarch, James II, in his exile to Paris, stormed against " the new doctrine concerning cataract "[2] ; less fashionably prominent opponents of the new idea were Jacob Hovius

---

[1] Michel Brisseau, médecin major des Hôpitaux du Roy et pensionnaire de la ville de Tournay : *Traité de la cataracte et du glaucoma*. À Paris chez Laurent d'Houry 1709 avec Approbation et Privilège du Roy.

[2] *Diss. savantes et critiques sur la cataracte et le glaucome*, Paris (1717).

and Johann Heinrich Freytag. On the other hand, Hermann Boerhaave, the first teacher since Arabic times to give systematic courses of lectures on diseases of the eye, taught the hundreds of students who flocked to his school in Holland his views that cataract was not an inspissated humour but a hardened and clouded lens and so disseminated the doctrine all over Europe; similarly, Lorenz Heister, the master-surgeon of Germany, propounded the same scientific fact, as also did Giovanni Battista Morgagni in Italy. Nevertheless, scepticism prevailed until Jacques Daviel (Fig. 266) published his classical paper on the deliberate extraction of cataract in 1753 and this operation eventually began to be accepted. This aspect of the story will be continued at a later stage when we consider the history of the operative treatment of the condition.

The remainder of the history of cataract, apart from the evolution of the methods of its treatment, devolved on a rapid increase in our knowledge of the various systemic conditions and the many forms in which it may appear, a study consolidated by Otto Becker of Heidelberg (Fig. 83) and greatly facilitated on the advent of the slit-lamp wherewith the greatest early observer was Alfred Vogt[1] of Zürich, whose accurate and painstaking observations laid the foundations for modern knowledge. Finally, progress has taken the form of research on the normal and abnormal metabolism of the lens in an endeavour to elucidate the cause of the condition with the hope of eventually preventing its occurrence—immensely complex biochemical problems still largely unknown but rapidly becoming clarified as the years pass. Each of these will be discussed in the following pages.

THE ÆTIOLOGY OF CATARACT

At the present time no complete and satisfying description can be given of the ætiology of cataract, for our knowledge of the metabolism of the lens is still so incomplete that an analysis of the still more complex problem of its derangement is impossible. Fundamentally the loss of transparency is due to a disturbance of the intimate structure of the lens, the fibres of which form a colloid system into which a large amount of water is bound. The disturbance may be of two types: a *swelling opacity*, a potentially reversible change producing a diffractive effect by the accumulation of water between the fibres or its intracellular absorption into the protein micellæ usually determined by osmotic forces, or a *coagulative opacity*, an irreversible chemical change whereby the proteins become coagulated and insoluble. In the present state of our knowledge all we can do is to describe what is known of the chemical pathology of the cataractous lens and to discuss the various ways in which lenticular opacities can be experimentally produced.

[1] Vol. II, p. 310.

The Chemical Pathology of the Lens

A description of the chemical composition and metabolism of the normal lens can be found in a previous Volume[1] to which the reader is referred. In this discussion we shall confine ourselves to the changes known to occur in the constituents and the metabolism of the ageing and cataractous lens; some of these may be important, others are probably inconsequential.

CHANGES IN THE CONSTITUENTS OF THE LENS

PROTEINS. The changes in the PROTEINS of the cataractous lens have excited considerable interest and certain general tendencies applicable to many types of cataract have emerged, many of which are common to the process of ageing.[2] We have seen that as the lens grows its protein constituents are constantly being synthesized by the incorporation of amino acids derived from the serum through the aqueous, a process carried out essentially by high-energy phosphates (ATP) and activating enzymes probably located in the microsomes. While in age the protein content of the normal lens thus increases,[3] in all types of cataract which have been investigated, as was first pointed out by Cahn (1881), sooner or later there is a decrease in the total proteins compared with a normal lens of the same age. In this change the insoluble protein (albuminoid) remains comparatively stable so that its concentration is relatively increased, while the soluble proteins are markedly decreased and their synthesis diminished or arrested.[4] No common or consistent pattern has yet been observed with respect to the various constituent proteins but the loss of the β-crystallin fraction is always conspicuous and this involves a diminution of protein sulphydryl groups. In consequence, the active soluble proteins give place to inactive substances, thus tending to metabolic inertia. This change may be caused to some extent by a transference of soluble to insoluble protein owing to denaturation and an alteration in the molecular configuration rather than by a radical alteration in chemical structure (Bühler and Witmer, 1959; Thomann, 1963; Waley, 1965). The evidence suggests, however, that all these changes occur not in the early but in the later phases of the development of cataract when opacification has developed; it would seem likely, therefore, that they are not causal in nature.

In the later stages of the development of cataract, *proteolysis* occurs whereby the soluble proteins are broken down by proteolytic enzymes. Such enzymes are present in the normal lens since sterile lens-homogenates

---

[1] Vol. IV, Chapter VI.

[2] Jess (1913), Tsuji (1932), Salit (1939), Smelser and von Sallmann (1949), Dische and Zil (1951), Pirie *et al.* (1953), François *et al.* (1954), Pirie and van Heyningen (1956), Dische *et al.* (1956), Dische and Zelmenis (1959), Lessinger and Mandel (1960), Lerman and Zigman (1965), Charlton and van Heyningen (1968), and many others.

[3] p. 13.

[4] Jess (1913), Labbé and Lavagna (1925), Krause (1933), Salit (1939), Dische *et al.* (1956–59), Mach (1963), Charlton and van Heyningen (1968).

undergo proteolysis on incubation,[1] first into peptides by the action of proteinases and then to amino acids by peptidases. It has been found that the activity of the peptidases increases markedly in the cataractous lens (de Berardinis, 1950). At this stage, therefore, there is an increase of amino acids in the lens and the aqueous humour (Burdon-Cooper, 1914; Goldschmidt, 1914; Labbé and Lavagna, 1925). The proteinases become much more active in an acidic reaction which tends to develop in cataract[2] so that in these circumstances all the proteins may be thrown out of action, the soluble proteins being hydrolysed to amino acids and the others being coagulated. Since the amount of albuminoid is small in young lens fibres, in these practically all the proteins are thus broken up. Since complete hydrolysis increases the osmotic pressure some 400 times, the initial effect is an enormous imbibition of water with a consequent swelling, which may be followed as diffusion proceeds by an almost complete disappearance of the lenticular substance. In older fibres the presence of the insoluble protein makes disappearance impossible, although the lens as a whole shrinks owing to the loss of β-crystallin and albumin, the shrinkage being necessarily most apparent in the superficial layers. If, as occurs in hypermature cataract, the capsule becomes impermeable, the soluble moiety cannot escape and the lens assumes the form of a sac holding a protein-rich fluid in which a solid albuminoid nucleus floats. If, on the other hand, the capsule is ruptured, the proteases in the aqueous as well as phagocytic cells reach the fibres, and these extra-lenticular enzymes, although they play no part in the primary cataractous changes, help to complete the breakdown of the proteins (Rodigina, 1932).

PEPTIDES. The most important of these substances in the metabolism of the lens is *glutathione*, which by virtue of its sulphydryl group ($SH \rightleftharpoons SS$) is involved in the oxidation-reduction system of the lens, perhaps in association with ascorbic acid.[3] It is enzymically synthesized by the lens and is found, particularly in the cortex, in a higher concentration here than in any other tissue, remaining fairly constant in concentration after the first few months of life. It tends to decrease, however, with age and diminishes markedly in all the forms of cataract investigated, senile or experimental.[4] This reduction is possibly due to a failure in synthesis since the adenosine triphosphate and enzymes necessary for this process have been found to be

[1] Clapp (1911–24), Jess (1920), Krause (1933), Waley and van Heyningen (1962), van Heyningen and Waley (1962–63), Spector (1962–63), Hanson (1962), Glässer and Hanson (1963), Wolff and Resnik (1963), Shoch and Zeller (1964), Hanson *et al.* (1965), Kretschmer and Hanson (1965).

[2] Buglia (1925), Sauermann (1933), Krause (1933), Reiss and Nordmann (1938), Malatesta (1952), Reddy and Kinsey (1962), Dardenne and Kirsten (1962), Calam (1962), Bürger (1964), Calam and Waley (1964), Graeber (1964), Ciusa *et al.* (1965), Reddy (1965).

[3] Vol. IV, p. 389.

[4] Reis (1912), Goldschmidt (1917), Jess (1921), Shoji (1927), Cohen *et al.* (1928), Tassman and Karr (1929), Weinstein (1931), Gifford (1932), Cordero (1933), Rosner *et al.* (1938), Thomann and Tilling (1962), Zygulska-Machowa (1966), Mach (1966), and others.

lacking in certain types of experimental cataract (Daisley, 1955; Cliffe and Waley, 1958). A close association of the lack of glutathione with the development of cataract is that in age and the types of experimental cataract that have been investigated the diminution in concentration precedes the development of opacities, while at a late stage the fall becomes more marked and can be correlated with the degree of opacification; moreover, in those types of experimental cataract which may resolve, its concentration increases again as the opacities disappear (Dische and Zil, 1951; Pirie *et al.*, 1953). Nothing is known of the relation of the tripeptides, *ophthalmic acid* and *norophthalmic acid*, to the cataractous process. *Ascorbic acid*, which may participate with glutathione in the oxidation-reduction reactions and is also found in very high concentration in the cortex, shows a comparable diminution in age or with the development of cataract but this is slight and does not occur at an early stage.[1]

The NUCLEOTIDES, which are particularly important in the phosphorylation of glucose, particularly adenosine triphosphate (ATP) and the diphosphopyridine (DPN, DPNH) and triphosphopyridine nucleotides (TPN, TPNH), also become deficient in age and decrease in cataract.[2]

The total LIPIDS increase in age and in cataract; this principally affects the free lipids, especially cholesterol, for the glycerides and protein-bound lipids decrease.[3] In the later stages of opacification the free lipids may appear in visible crystalline deposits.[4]

The INORGANIC MATERIALS also suffer changes. All observers agree that the cataractous lens is rich in *calcium*[5]; moreover, the deposition of calcium in non-diffusible form increases progressively as the cataract matures so that crystalline deposits may form and the tissue may eventually suffer almost complete calcification.[6] It is probable, however, that this accumulation is secondary and not primary, a passive and inert process in a damaged tissue corresponding to that occurring in an atheromatous artery, a degenerated cornea, or a tuberculous focus in the lung.

The content of *potassium* simultaneously decreases (Burge, 1909; Burdon-Cooper, 1928; Mackay *et al.*, 1932). In the normal lens only a small proportion of this ion is diffusible, the remainder being combined with protein and other complexes; on the death of the cells, however, it becomes liberated and diffuses away concurrently with other vital constituents of

---

[1] Müller (1933–37), Gurewitsch (1934), Nordmann and van Wien (1934), B. and O. Nakamura (1935), Bietti (1935), Bellows (1936), and others.

[2] Müller (1937), Nordmann and Mandel (1952), Klethi and Mandel (1957–65), Praus and Obenberger (1961).

[3] Salit (1935–37), Kirsten and Muradow (1963), Tronche and Mandel (1963), Bürger (1963), G. and L. Feldman (1965).

[4] von Graefe (1854), Tweedy (1873), Lang (1895), Wessely (1922), Kranz (1927), Bunge (1936), and others.

[5] Burge (1909), Burdon-Cooper (1928–33), Adams (1929), Salit (1930–33), Kirby (1931), Evans and Kern (1931), Mackay *et al.* (1932), Updegraff (1932), Campbell (1933), Grabar and Nordmann (1933), Lo Cascio (1937), Rinaldi (1937), and many others.

[6] Wessely (1922), Kranz (1927), Boente (1930), Mackay *et al.* (1932).

the lens. Contemporaneously, the *sodium* increases in the cataractous lens.[1] This increase is probably a diffusion phenomenon, the lens assuming a constitution similar to the aqueous and plasma. The potassium/sodium ratio may be taken as an index of tissue vitality and, while in the normal cortex and nucleus it is 1·65 and 1·34 respectively, in cataract it falls to 0·41 and 0·32 (Lebensohn, 1936). Correspondingly the *chlorides* become increased (Mackay *et al.*, 1932), as also do the *inorganic phosphates* (Müller, 1936). It has been suggested that this shift in the content of cations due to free permeability of the cellular membranes, in place of their control by the mechanism of active transport and cellular activity, may lead to an increase in osmotic pressure as necessitated by the Donnan equilibrium and this participates in the intumescence of the lens (Harris and Gehrsitz, 1951; Pau, 1954).

The *enzymes* and co-enzymes associated with metabolic activity show a considerable diminution in the cataractous lens (Zeller *et al.*, 1951; Pütter and Dardenne, 1958; Zinkham, 1961; Maraini *et al.*, 1966; Friedburg, 1967; and others).

TRANSPORT IN THE CATARACTOUS LENS

Since the entire metabolic activity of the lens depends on biological interchange through the capsule, abnormalities in the permeability of this membrane have from time to time been considered as being ætiologically concerned with the formation of cataract. On the one hand, Löwenstein (1925–34), and Löwenstein and Haurowitz (1929), basing their conclusions on the fact that a rupture of the capsule led to the development of traumatic cataract, postulated that lenticular opacities were due to an increased permeability of the capsule in old age, a view supported by observations that soluble substances diffused out of the cataractous lens. It was shown by Friedenwald (1930), however, and has since been amply confirmed that the permeability of the capsule decreases in age and in early cataract, presumably by the structural constriction of its pores, although it probably increases sufficiently to allow the passage of proteins when the cataract becomes mature (Orzalesi *et al.*, 1961). There is now ample experimental evidence[2] that the capsule acts as an inert membrane, permeable to small and impermeable to large molecules. It may be that a slight decrease in permeability may be a minor factor in the development of senile sclerosis and cataract by decreasing metabolic exchange; but the available evidence seems to indicate that no constant and significant change in capsular permeability such as could exercise any primary and determinant effect can be claimed in cataract, either of the senile type or that produced by toxic

[1] Burge (1909), Evans and Kern (1931), Mackay *et al.* (1932), Lebensohn (1936).
[2] Vol. IV, p. 379.

substances (Gifford *et al.*, 1932; Borley and Tainter, 1937; Bellows and Rosner, 1938; and others).

It is true that substances with small molecules pass through the capsule by simple diffusion depending on the difference in their concentration in the aqueous and the lens (Kaiser and Maurice, 1964; Kinsey and Reddy, 1965), but there is abundant evidence that the entrance of cations, glucose, phosphates and amino acids is controlled by a process of active transport.[1] This occurs at all the boundaries of the lens and probably between its fibres, but the most important mechanism is the subcapsular epithelium, although on the posterior surface the lenticular fibres which are derived from these epithelial cells play a similar although less active part. The process is determined by the activity of enzymes, the energy being ultimately derived from anaerobic glycolysis; experimentally this transport is affected by temperature and can be diminished or abolished by metabolic inhibitors such as ouabain and has been found to be abnormal in certain types of experimental cataract (Becker, 1962; Kinoshita and Merola, 1964; Thoft and Kinoshita, 1965; Cotlier and Becker, 1965). Indeed, it would appear that the failure of this mechanism to maintain a high content of potassium in the lens fibres and a low content of sodium, and the resulting equilibration of these cations with the aqueous humour may contribute to the development of intumescence in a cataractous lens (Harris and Gehrsitz, 1951; Pau, 1954).

THE PATHOLOGICAL METABOLISM OF THE LENS

Despite the intensive research conducted during recent years on the metabolism of the pathological lens, we still know relatively little about the fundamental changes which determine the cataractogenic process. Most experimental work has been concerned with the biochemical changes occurring in the sugar cataracts which will be discussed subsequently; but few anomalies common to all types, senile and experimental, have come to light. We do know, however, that opacification is essentially due to metabolic changes, but although we know something of the general disturbances in the main pathways involved, we are still uncertain of the precise nature of the blocks which inhibit them and presumably depend on failure in the activities of the enzymes which control these complex processes.

The facts that experimental cataract occurs most readily in young animals and the earliest and most acute changes appear in the subcapsular and equatorial regions suggest that the interruption of metabolism affects most acutely the actively dividing epithelial cells. Again, the importance of this factor is suggested by the recovery which may ensue when the cataractogenic agent is removed in several types of opacification induced by metabolic agents, whereas radiational cataract wherein the epithelium is permanently damaged has never been known to be reversed.

[1] Vol. IV, p. 381.

CARBOHYDRATE METABOLISM provides the chief source of energy in the metabolism of the lens and, as would be expected, the most dramatic changes in cataract occur in the various metabolic pathways by which this may take place. In general, both in the aged and cataractous lens it is retarded. It will be remembered[1] that four pathways are involved: anaerobic glycolysis by the Embden-Meyerhof pathway, the aerobic Krebs citric acid cycle, the hexose-monophosphate shunt and the sorbitol (polyol) pathway. Anaerobic glycolysis, which is least active in the fœtal lens, gradually falls with age by a factor of 3 or 4, but in most types of experimental cataract investigated the fall is late (Maraini *et al.*, 1967); with this fall there is a diminution in the production of high-energy phosphates, particularly adenosine triphosphate (ATP) from which energy is normally produced for a variety of purposes. The final stage in this metabolic pathway also tends to fail, for the enzyme, lactic dehydrogenase, which ultimately converts pyruvic into lactic acid, is deficient both in the senile and cataractous lens (Dardenne and Drechsler, 1961; Friedburg, 1966). On the other hand, the part played by the direct oxidative pathway by the hexose-monophosphate shunt which is active in the young lens falls markedly with age by a factor of 10, and is seen to diminish at an early stage in several types of experimental cataract. The aerobic Krebs cycle with its generation of high-energy phosphate bonds probably mainly concerns the epithelium, while we shall see that the sorbitol pathway by which sugars are converted into polyols which are re-oxidized to their corresponding ketoses, is probably of importance in the development of sugar cataracts. Altogether the resulting loss of available energy in diabetic cataract has been estimated by Kuck (1962) at 40%.

The main evidence of a reduction in *oxygenation* is the diminution of glutathione at an early stage in cataractogenesis. Although its precise role in metabolic activity is unknown, its absence probably affects the phosphorylation of glucose and is possibly linked with the decrease in high-energy phosphates that is found in several types of experimental cataract. In this process of gradual asphyxiation the progressive diminution of enzymes associated with oxidation is important (Fischer, 1947).

The principal change in the PROTEIN METABOLISM in age and most types of cataract is a decrease in the synthesis of the metabolically active soluble proteins owing to a diminution of the transport and incorporation of amino acids; Dische and his colleagues (1957) found that this was an early phenomenon which lowered the synthesis of the crystallins by 40%. This process must entail a decrease in the synthesis of enzymes; at some stage it could be speculated that a situation might arise when the concentration of one or more of these substances becomes so low that the normal metabolism could no longer be maintained. Of the relatively unimportant LIPID METABOLISM, little of significance is known.

---

[1] Vol. IV, p. 385.

The only assessment that can be made of the metabolism of the pathological lens is that we know little of it; what we do know is that there is a
progressive loss of the necessary active substances so that it suffers a
gradual diminution, particularly in the important process of glycolysis
and in the activity of its oxidation-reduction systems. In the most
general terms, it could be said that the cataractous lens—certainly in the
later stages of opacification—is on the whole a metabolically sluggish
asphyxiated organ.

SYSTEMIC CHEMICAL CHANGES

Chemical changes in the blood have long been thought to be associated with the
development of cataract. At various times it has been claimed that ætiological factors
may be hyper- or hypo-calcæmia, a hypercholesterolæmia, an alkalosis, an increase in
urea, creatine or creatinine and many other such factors; but these findings have been
inconstant and incidental and most of them slight and to be expected in the type of
patient usually affected with this condition. It is true that certain well-defined
alterations are causative factors in specific types of cataract, such as hyperglycæmia,
galactosæmia or a low calcium/phosphorus ratio. These will be discussed subsequently;
but the general conclusion can safely be reached that a gross disturbance of the
chemistry of the blood is not consistently associated with the development of cataract.

It has recently been suggested that an abnormality in the metabolism of
tryptophan may be associated with the development of senile cataract since opacification follows the ingestion of quinoid substances,[1] and quinonimine was demonstrated
in the urine of patients with senile cataract by Ogino and Yasukura(1957); this has
not been substantiated (Tojo and Uenoyama, 1960–61), and that it is a causal condition
seems unlikely.

Adams. *Biochem. J.*, **23**, 902 (1929).
Becker. *Invest. Ophthal.*, **1**, 502 (1962).
Bellows. *Arch. Ophthal.*, **15**, 78; **16**, 58, 762 (1936).
Bellows and Rosner. *Arch. Ophthal.*, **20**, 80 (1938).
de Berardinis. *Ann. Ottal.*, **76**, 91 (1950).
Bietti. *Boll. Oculist.*, **14**, 3 (1935).
Boente. *Arch. Augenheilk.*, **102**, 261 (1930).
Borley and Tainter. *Arch. Ophthal.*, **18**, 908 (1937).
Bühler and Witmer. *Ophthalmologica*, **137**, 188 (1959).
Bürger. *Vision Res.*, **3**, 227 (1963).
  Klin. Mbl. Augenheilk., **144**, 169 (1964).
Buglia. *Arch. Ottal.*, **32**, 193 (1925).
Bunge. *Arch. Augenheilk.*, **109**, 503 (1936).
Burdon-Cooper. *Ophthal. Rev.*, **33**, 129 (1914).
  Trans. ophthal. Soc. U.K., **48**, 340 (1928); **53**, 401 (1933).
Burge. *Arch. Ophthal.*, **38**, 435 (1909).
Cahn. *Hoppe-Seyl. Z. physiol. Chem.*, **5**, 214 (1881).
Calam. *Exp. Eye Res.*, **1**, 436 (1962).
Calam and Waley. *Biochem. J.*, **93**, 526 (1964).
Campbell. *Trans. ophthal. Soc. U.K.*, **53**, 391 (1933).

Charlton and van Heyningen. *Exp. Eye Res.*, **7**, 47 (1968).
Ciusa, Cristini and Barbiroli. *Minerva oftal.*, **7**, 95 (1965).
Clapp. *J. Amer. med. Ass.*, **56**, 807 (1911).
  Amer. J. Ophthal., **7**, 131 (1924).
Cliffe and Waley. *Biochem. J.*, **69**, 649 (1958).
Cohen, Kamner and Killian. *Proc. Soc. exp. Biol. (N.Y.)*, **25**, 677 (1928).
Cordero. *Rass. ital. Ottal.*, **2**, 69 (1933).
Cotlier and Becker. *Exp. Eye Res.*, **4**, 340 (1965).
Daisley. *Biochem. J.*, **60**, xl (1955).
Dardenne and Drechsler. *v. Graefes Arch. Ophthal.*, **164**, 156 (1961).
Dardenne and Kirsten. *Exp. Eye Res.*, **1**, 415 (1962).
Dische, Borenfreund and Zelmenis. *Arch. Ophthal.*, **55**, 471, 633 (1956).
Dische, Elliott, Pearson and Merriam. *Amer. J. Ophthal.*, **47** (2), 368 (1959).
Dische and Zelmenis. *Amer. J. Ophthal.*, **48** (2), 500 (1959).
Dische, Zelmenis and Youlus. *Amer. J. Ophthal.*, **44** (2), 332 (1957).
Dische and Zil. *Amer. J. Ophthal.*, **34** (2), 104 (1951).
Evans and Kern. *Amer. J. Ophthal.*, **14**, 1029 (1931).

[1] p. 106.

Feldman, G. and L. *Invest. Ophthal.*, **4**, 162 (1965).
Fischer. *Ophthalmologica*, **114**, 1 (1947).
François, Rabaey, Wieme and Neetens. *Ann. Oculist.* (Paris), **187**, 593 (1954).
Friedburg. *v. Graefes Arch. Ophthal.*, **170**, 365 (1966); **173**, 309 (1967).
Friedenwald. *Arch. Ophthal.*, **3**, 182; **4**, 350 (1930).
Gifford, H. *Arch. Ophthal.*, **7**, 763 (1932).
Gifford, S. R., Lebensohn and Puntenny. *Arch. Ophthal.*, **8**, 414 (1932).
Glässer and Hanson. *Naturwissenschaften*, **50**, 595 (1963).
Goldschmidt. *Münch. med. Wschr.*, **61**, 657 (1914).
v. Graefes Arch. Ophthal., **93**, 447 (1917).
Grabar and Nordmann. *C.R. Soc. Biol.* (Paris), **112**, 1534 (1933).
Graeber. *Ber. dtsch. ophthal. Ges.*, **66**, 397 (1964).
von Graefe. *v. Graefes Arch. Ophthal.*, **1** (1), 323 (1854).
Gurewitsch. *Arch. Augenheilk.*, **108**, 572 (1934).
Hanson. *Exp. Eye Res.*, **1**, 468 (1962).
Hanson, Glässer and Kirschke. *Hoppe-Seyl. Z. physiol. Chem.*, **340**, 107 (1965).
Harris and Gehrsitz. *Amer. J. Ophthal.*, **34** (2), 131 (1951).
van Heyningen and Waley. *Exp. Eye Res.*, **1**, 336 (1962).
Biochem. J., **86**, 92 (1963).
Jess. *Z. Biol.*, **61**, 93 (1913).
Hoppe-Seyl. Z. physiol. Chem., **110**, 266 (1920); **112**, 160 (1922).
v. Graefes Arch. Ophthal., **105**, 428 (1921); **109**, 463 (1922).
Kaiser and Maurice. *Exp. Eye Res.*, **3**, 156 (1964).
Kinoshita and Merola. *Invest. Ophthal.*, **3**, 577 (1964).
Kinsey and Reddy. *Invest. Ophthal.*, **4**, 104 (1965).
Kirby. *Arch. Ophthal.*, **5**, 754, 856, 868 (1931).
Kirsten and Muradow. *Ber. dtsch. ophthal. Ges.*, **65**, 311 (1963).
Klethi and Mandel. *Biochim. biophys. Acta*, **24**, 642 (1957); **37**, 549 (1960).
Nature (Lond.), **205**, 1114 (1965).
Kranz. *v. Graefes Arch. Ophthal.*, **118**, 571 (1927).
Krause. *Arch. Ophthal.*, **10**, 631, 788 (1933).
Kretschmer and Hanson. *Hoppe-Zeyl. Z. physiol. Chem.*, **340**, 126 (1965).
Kuck. *Invest. Ophthal.*, **1**, 390 (1962).
Labbé and Lavagna. *C.R. Acad. Sci.* (Paris), **180**, 1186 (1925).
Lang. *Trans. ophthal. Soc. U.K.*, **15**, 117 (1895).
Lebensohn. *Arch. Ophthal.*, **15**, 217 1936).
Lerman and Zigman. *Invest. Ophthal.*, **4**, 643 (1965).
Lessinger and Mandel. *J. Physiol.* (Paris), **52**, 150 (1960).

Lo Cascio. *Ann. Ottal.*, **65**, 801 (1937).
Löwenstein. *Klin. Mbl. Augenheilk.*, **74**, 786 (1925).
v. Graefes Arch. Ophthal., **116**, 438 (1926); **132**, 224 (1934).
Löwenstein and Haurowitz. *v. Graefes Arch. Ophthal.*, **122**, 654 (1929).
Mackay, Stewart and Robertson. *Brit. J. Ophthal.*, **16**, 193 (1932).
Mach. *Klin. Mbl. Augenheilk.*, **143**, 689 (1963); **149**, 897 (1966).
Malatesta. *Boll. Oculist.*, **31**, 685, 691, 762, 765 (1952).
Maraini, Carta and Santori. *Ann. Ottal.*, **92**, 482 (1966).
Maraini, Santori and Carta. *Exp. Eye Res.*, **6**, 126 (1967).
Müller, H. K. *Arch. Augenheilk.*, **108**, 41 (1934); **109**, 304, 434, 497 (1936); **110**, 321 (1937).
Nature (Lond.), **132**, 280 (1933).
Nakamura, B. and O. *v. Graefes Arch. Ophthal.*, **134**, 197 (1935).
Nordmann and Mandel. *Ann. Oculist.* (Paris), **185**, 929 (1952).
Nordmann and van Wien. *Bull. Soc. Ophtal. Paris*, 136 (1934).
Ogino and Ichihara. *Amer. J. Ophthal.*, **43**, 754 (1957).
Ogino and Yasukura. *Amer. J. Ophthal.*, **43**, 936 (1957).
Orzalesi, Miglior and DeRosa. *G. ital. Oftal.*, **14**, 108 (1961).
Pau. *Klin. Mbl. Augenheilk.*, **124**, 1, 129 (1954).
Pirie and van Heyningen. *Biochemistry of the Eye*, Oxon. (1956).
Pirie, van Heyningen and Boag. *Biochem. J.*, **54**, 682 (1953).
Praus and Obenberger. *Csl. Ofthal.*, **17**, 431 (1961).
Pütter and Dardenne. *Hoppe-Seyl. Z. physiol. Chem.*, **310**, 59 (1958).
Reddy. *Invest. Ophthal.*, **4**, 700 (1965).
Reddy and Kinsey. *Invest. Ophthal.*, **1**, 635 (1962).
Reis. *Arch. Augenheilk.*, **72**, 156 (1912).
v. Graefes Arch. Ophthal., **80**, 588 (1912).
Reiss and Nordmann. *C.R. Soc. Biol.* (Paris), **128**, 111 (1938).
Rinaldi. *Ann. Ottal.*, **65**, 667 (1937).
Rodigina. *Vestn. oftal.*, **1**, 121 (1932).
Rosner, Farmer and Bellows. *Arch. Ophthal.*, **20**, 417 (1938).
Salit. *Amer. J. Ophthal.*, **13**, 1072 (1930); **14**, 523 (1931); **20**, 157 (1937); **22**, 413 (1939).
Arch. Ophthal., **5**, 354, 623 (1931); **16**, 271 (1936); **18**, 403 (1937).
Brit. J. Ophthal., **19**, 663 (1935).
Acta ophthal. (Kbh.), **17**, 81 (1939).
Sauermann. *Amer. J. Ophthal.*, **16**, 985 (1933).
Shoch and Zeller. *Amer. J. Ophthal.*, **57**, 737 (1964).
Shoji. *Ann. Oculist.* (Paris), **164**, 344 (1927).

Smelser and von Sallmann. *Amer. J. Ophthal.*, **32**, 1703 (1949).

Spector. *Exp. Eye Res.*, **1**, 330 (1962).
J. biol. Chem., **238**, 1353 (1963).

Tassman and Karr. *Arch. Ophthal.*, **2**, 431 (1929).

Thoft and Kinoshita. *Invest. Ophthal.*, **4**, 122, 800 (1965).

Thomann. *Klin. Mbl. Augenheilk.*, **143**, 338 (1963).

Thomann and Tilling. *Klin. Wschr.*, **40**, 109 (1962).

Tojo and Uenoyama. *Acta Soc. ophthal. jap.*, **64**, 1375 (1960).
Jap. J. Ophthal., **5**, 67 (1961).

Tronche and Mandel. *C.R. Soc. Biol.* (Paris), **157**, 380 (1963).

Tsuji. *J. Biochem.* (Tokyo), **15**, 33 (1932).

Tweedy. *Lancet*, **2**, 519 (1873).

Updegraff. *Proc. Soc. exp. Biol.* (N.Y.), **29**, 964 (1932).

Waley. *Biochem. J.*, **96**, 722 (1965).
Exp. Eye Res., **4**, 293 (1965).

Waley and van Heyningen. *Exp. Eye Res.*, **1**, 343 (1962).
Biochem. J., **83**, 274 (1963).

Weinstein. *Klin. Mbl. Augenheilk.*, **87**, 393 (1931).

Wessely. *Arch. Augenheilk.*, **91**, 158 (1922).

Wolff and Resnik. *Biochim. biophys. Acta*, **73**, 588, 613 (1963).

Zeller, Daily, Wakim and Herrick. *Proc. Mayo Clin.*, **26**, 194 (1951).

Zinkham. *Bull. Johns Hopk. Hosp.*, **109**, 206 (1961).

Zygulska-Machowa. *Klin. oczna*, **36**, 189 (1966).

Experimental Cataract

Much work has been done on the subject of experimental cataract for more than a century, dating from the experiments of Kunde in 1857 on osmotic cataract. The long list of contributors to our knowledge, which includes physicists, biochemists and immunologists as well as ophthalmologists, will be noted in the subsequent pages, and from their number we have chosen the photograph of LUDWIG K. J. VON SALLMANN [1892———] (Fig. 84) whose work on this subject has not been surpassed by anyone in this generation. Born in Vienna, his early ophthalmological studies were undertaken in that city with a short interlude at the Medical School at Pekin (1930–31) until he went to New York. Here he first directed the laboratory at the Herman Knapp Eye Hospital (1939) and then continued research at Columbia University and the Presbyterian Hospital (1940) until he was called to direct ophthalmological research at the Branch of Ophthalmology of the National Institutes of Health at Bethesda (1956). Apart from his work on experimental cataract, he made many outstanding contributions to ophthalmology on such subjects as the physico-chemical properties of the vitreous, antibiotics, the central control of the intra-ocular pressure and other applications of the basic sciences to our specialty.

The highly speculative status of the ætiology of cataract lends special interest to its experimental production. This may be accomplished in many ways, but unfortunately none of these has yet offered a definite clue to the intimate mechanism involved in the occurrence of the usual lenticular opacities in man. It is known that some types of experimental cataract are due to a frank coagulation of the lenticular proteins, others to an abnormal ionic interchange, others to injury to the subcapsular epithelium with consequent damage to the lenticular fibres, others to osmotic hydration following abnormal metabolic changes, a process which may ultimately result in proteolysis, others to an upset of the metabolism of the lens as by enzyme inhibitors or the loss of a substance essential in the biochemical chain of events usually affecting the glycolytic but occasionally the lipid or the protein metabolism, and still others to purely cytotoxic causes. Since, however, this ætiological problem will eventually be solved, and almost certainly through the experimental approach, these studies are of more

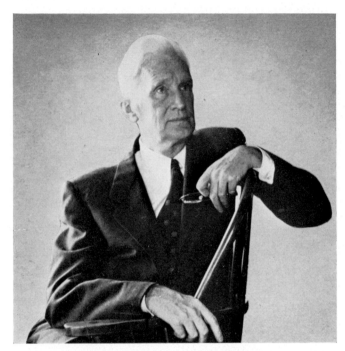

Fig. 84.—Ludwig von Sallmann
[1892———]

than academic interest. The various experimental methods of producing cataract may be summarized thus:

1. Mechanical injury.
      Concussion, contusion, massage, rupture of the capsule.
2. Physical causes.
      Osmotic influences, cold and heat, acidity, electric precipitation.
3. Radiational cataract.
      Micro-wave, thermal, ultra-violet and ionizing radiation.
4. Decrease of the semi-permeability of the capsule.
5. Interference with nutrient supplies.
6. Anoxia and asphyxia.
7. Sugar cataract.
      Galactose, xylose, glucose.
8. Deficiency cataract.
      Lack of proteins, specific amino acids, and vitamins.
9. A low calcium/phosphate ratio in the blood.
      Parathyroidectomy and tetany.
10. Endocrine cataract.
11. Toxic cataract.
      Naphthalene, dinitrophenol, paradichlorobenzene, thallium, cobalt,
          anti-mitotic agents, enzyme inhibitors, cataractogenic drugs.
12. Cataract due to systemic infections.

CATARACT DUE TO MECHANICAL INJURY, whether involving concussion, contusion or induced by massage or rupture of the lens capsule, will be dealt with in the Volume devoted to injuries.[1] Various ætiological factors are operative. In concussion injuries the proteins are coagulated by the energy imparted through mechanical shock and agitation which disrupts the integrity of the epithelial cells and the fibres; these aggregates may be dispersed again with the return of translucency, or necrosis of the cells may follow with the production of cataract. With a rupture of the capsule different conditions arise owing to the entrance of the aqueous, the loss of essential diffusible substances, and rapid proteolysis with the development of a localized or a complete opacity.

CATARACT DUE TO PHYSICAL CAUSES

OSMOTIC CATARACT

It has long been known that an osmotic hydration or dehydration of the lens could bring about an opacity which in its less degrees, so long as only the amount of water in the lens is involved, is reversible; if, however, coagulation of the proteins occurs, the opacity is irreversible. Thus if the isolated lens is kept in physiological saline at body temperature, its transparency is maintained for a considerable time, but in anisotonic solutions opacification appears initially in the superficial regions of the cortex; while the lens gains or loses in weight according to whether it is immersed in hypo-

[1] Vol. XIV.

or hypertonic solutions, an occurrence first demonstrated by Kunde (1857) and confirmed by numerous other experimenters.[1] In the extreme case of immersion in distilled water the swelling may be so great that the nucleus may take up 84% of its own weight of water (von Jäger, 1861). Similarly *in vivo*, temporary lens opacities can be induced in animals by the injection of concentrated solutions of various crystalloids and sugars such as dextrose and lactose by rectum, intraperitoneally, subconjunctivally or into the eye itself.[2] A similar effect has been produced by concentrating the aqueous humour by allowing its evaporation through the cornea after opening the palpebral fissure for long periods in rats (Ewald, 1898; Goldmann and Rabinowitz, 1928; Fraunfelder and Burns, 1962). As would be expected, an injection of concentrated saline into the lens itself has the same effect (in rabbits, Selenkowsky, 1925). The profound dehydration of cholera as well as the prolonged deprivation of drinking water (Kudo, 1921) may also be followed by the development of a cataract.

For these experiments the frog acts as the best osmometer. Thus if 0·2 G. NaCl is injected subcutaneously the lens becomes opaque, and if the animal is then immersed in water the lens regains its transparency (Kunde, 1857). Again, frogs dehydrated in an atmosphere of calcium chloride develop cataract in one day (Köhnhorn, 1858). It is interesting that the opacity produced by the abstraction of water may immediately clear up on mechanical trauma as by massage of the cornea or by a sharp blow on the head (Ewald, 1898). In mammals the production of an osmotic cataract is more difficult, but it has been accomplished in cats and rabbits by hypertonic injections (Richardson, 1860; Heubel, 1879).

That these processes are purely physical and not chemical in nature is shown by the fact that practically any crystalloid in comparably effective concentration produces the same effect. The changes, moreover, depend not directly on the molecular concentration of the blood but of the aqueous immediately in contact with the lens (Heubel, 1879). Ultramicroscopic examinations have shown that the initial reversible opacity is due essentially to the state of the water bound to the proteins (Cattaneo, 1927; Fischer, 1934); when these are merely salted out or their state of turgescence altered, recovery can take place, but this cannot occur if their structure has been destroyed and they have become coagulated.

The clinical importance of the osmotic opacities lies in their relation to changes in the refraction and the development of cataract in diabetes, wherein the osmolarity of the blood is subject to gross variations.

COLD CATARACT

If the isolated lens of a young animal is frozen, it turns completely opaque and on thawing clears up from the periphery (von Michel, 1882)

---

[1] Deutschmann (1877), Heubel (1879), Magnus (1890), Burge (1918), Bergami (1927), Löwenstein and Haurowitz (1929), Fischer (1934), Tron (1939), Pau (1952).

[2] Kunde (1857), Köhnhorn (1858), Mitchell (1860), Richardson (1860), Manca and Ovio (1897), Panico (1929), Collevati (1930), Nordmann (1934–53), von Szily (1937), Weekers (1941), Bellows and Chinn (1941), Sbordone (1953).

(Fig. 85).[1] Similarly, if a young animal is cooled, a cataract develops
which clears up on thawing, although the lens may become hazy again
when the animal begins to move (Kunde, 1857; Grünhagen, 1875; Ritter,
1876; von Michel, 1882). Here again the reaction occurs most easily in the
frog, but can be produced in young mammals (rats, rabbits, calves), particularly if they are rendered prone to lenticular changes as by the deprivation
of vitamins.[2] The reaction is due to the precipitation of gamma-crystallin
when cooling reaches a temperature below 10°C, a reaction reversed on
warming above this temperature. The cold-precipitation possibly occurs

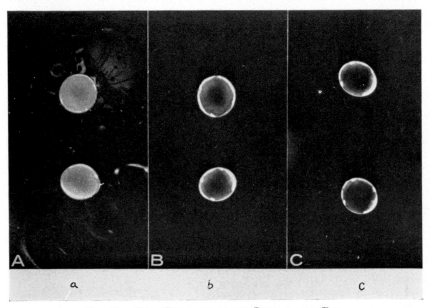

FIG. 85.—COLD CATARACT IN THE LENS OF THE RAT.
A, precipitation of the γ-crystallin at −10° C. B and C, the gradual reversibility
on warming (S. Lerman).

because this protein possesses a large number of exposed hydrophobic groups;
it can occur in aqueous extracts of lens proteins in a test-tube only if the
fraction of gamma-crystallin is greater than 0·3%, perhaps because the other
proteins increase the solubility of the total protein by hydrophobic bonding
with the gamma-crystallin. In the lens, precipitation can occur only if the
relative concentration of the gamma variety is greater than that of either
alpha- or beta-crystallin or of both combined; it is for this reason that the
cataract can be produced only in young animals or in their isolated lenses since

[1] Buglia (1926), Bergami (1927), Löwenstein and Haurowitz (1929), Fischer (1934),
Nordmann (1935), Pau (1952), Lerman (1966), and others.
[2] Henle (1856–78), Ritter (1876–77), Hess (1911), von Szily and Eckstein (1923), Goldschmidt (1927), Yoshimoto (1928), Nordmann (1935), Bon (1959), Stanković and Andjus
(1959).

at an early age the gamma-crystallin constitutes the major part of the proteins of the lens (van Heyningen, 1962; Lerman, 1966). Conversely, a high concentration of urea prevents precipitation of the gamma-crystallin and it may be that the dogfish, in the lens of which cold-precipitation cannot be induced, protects itself from cataract in its naturally cold environment by the unusually high content of urea in its aqueous and lens.[1] The protein-fraction precipitated by cold has been found to be comprised of the three major crystallins, but particularly the γ-fraction, combined with a small but significant amount of RNA (Lerman and Zigman, 1965–67; Lerman et al., 1966).

HEAT CATARACT. The lens becomes opaque on warming above 65° C (von Michel, 1882; Daddi, 1898), an effect due to an irreversible coagulation of the proteins.

CATARACT OF ACIDIFICATION. If the pH of the lens is reduced to between 4·5 and 5 it turns opaque owing to the precipitation of the proteins (Botazzi and Scalinci, 1908–10; Kuwabara, 1909; de Haan, 1922; Burky and Woods, 1928; Gonçalvès, 1930; and others). Löwenstein and Haurowitz (1929) found that the lenticular opacities began to appear at pH 6 and were marked at pH 5, while Bergami (1927) noted the maximum precipitation at pH 4·2. It is interesting that Nordmann (1953) found a second opacification in the alkaline region at pH 8·5.

ELECTRIC CATARACT has been known since it was produced experimentally by Hess (1888) by the electric oscillations in the discharge of a Leyden jar, and by Brixa (1900) from an electric shock. Clinical cases of lenticular opacities arising from a high-tension conductor, from lightning stroke or even from electric-shock therapy have not been very uncommon; these will be fully discussed in the Volume on Injuries.[2] The cause is unknown and is probably composite but may depend largely on the direct coagulation of the proteins and on osmotic changes following damage to the sub-capsular epithelium.

The precipitation of proteins in the lens has resulted in the production of cataract of the complicated type in rabbits after the experimental injection of electro-positive proteins into the vitreous (Orzalesi, 1956; Orzalesi and Miglior, 1956).

A RADIATIONAL CATARACT may be caused by many wavelengths in the electromagnetic spectrum—high-frequency, micro-waves (largely a thermal effect), infra-red, visible (if in sufficient concentration and particularly after the administration of photosensitizing drugs), ultra-violet and ionizing radiations. These will be discussed in the Volume on Injuries where full details with the appropriate bibliographies will be found.[3] In our present study of the general ætiology of cataract the most interesting type is that caused by ionizing radiation (x-rays, β-rays, γ-rays and neutrons). Histo-logically the capsular epithelium is primarily involved, particularly in the germinative equatorial zone, an effect produced more rapidly and extensively in young compared with adult animals. Initially mitosis is inhibited and subsequently is increased with at the same time considerable nuclear fragmentation. These are the cells which constantly form new lens fibres;

[1] Vol. IV, p. 153.   [2] Vol. XIV.   [3] Vol. XIV.

the damaged cells form abnormal opaque fibres which first become clinically evident after a period varying from some months to some years depending on the dose of radiation, the opacity appearing first at the posterior pole of the lens whither these cells migrate. Cysteine or glutathione administered systemically provides some protection against the injury caused by ionizing radiation, an action perhaps due to these SH-compounds preferentially accepting the radiation and thus shielding the tissues from a proportion of the total dose.

The *biochemical effects* of ionizing radiation on the lens are largely unknown but include in the early stages a reduction of DNA, an increased turnover of albuminoid RNA, while the soluble RNA remains unchanged, followed by a slow but progressive decline in the concentration of soluble proteins and an increase in insoluble albuminoid.[1] Other early changes include a decrease in the concentration of lactic acid and then a decline in glycolytic enzymes, particularly glucose-6-phosphate dehydrogenase, accompanied by a loss of adenosine triphosphate (ATP) and a fall in the concentration of glutathione, together with the enzymes associated with its synthesis and metabolism which are almost completely absent when the cataract becomes fully developed.[2] It is thus probable that the early changes following radiation are due to a disturbance of the protein metabolism and the later to a disorientation of the carbohydrate metabolism.

Bellows and Chinn. *Arch. Ophthal.*, **25**, 796 (1941).
Bergami. *Atti reale Accad. naz. Lincei*, Roma, **6**, 117 (1927).
Bon. *Ophthalmologica*, **138**, 35 (1959).
Botazzi and Scalinci. *R.C. reale Accad. Lincei*, **17** (2), 305, 445, 566 (1908); **18** (1), 225, 326, 379; (2), 327, 423 (1909); **19** (2), 162 (1910).
Brixa. *Klin. Mbl. Augenheilk.*, **38**, 759 (1900).
Buglia. *Arch. Fisiol.*, **24**, 454 (1926). *Arch. ital. Biol.*, **77**, 23 (1926).
Burge. *Arch. Ophthal.*, **47**, 12 (1918).
Burky and Woods. *Arch. Ophthal.*, **57**, 464 (1928).
Cattaneo. *Atti reale Accad. naz. Lincei*, Roma, **5**, 711 (1927).
Collevati. *Saggi Oftal.*, **5**, 85 (1930).
Daddi. *Ann. Ottal.*, **27**, 375 (1898).
Daisley. *Biochem. J.*, **60**, xl (1955).
Deutschmann. *v. Graefes Arch. Ophthal.*, **23** (3), 112 (1877).
Dische, Elliott, Pearson and Merriam. *Amer. J. Ophthal.*, **47** (2), 368 (1959).
Ewald. *Pflügers Arch. ges. Physiol.*, **72**, 1 (1898).
Fischer. *Arch. Augenheilk.*, **108**, 80, 517 (1934).
Fraunfelder and Burns. *Proc. Soc. exp. Biol.* (N.Y.), **110**, 72 (1962).

Goldmann and Rabinowitz. *Klin. Mbl. Augenheilk.*, **81**, 771 (1928).
Goldschmidt. *Klin. Wschr.*, **6**, 635 (1927).
Gonçalvès. *Arch. Phys. biol.*, **8**, 5 (1930).
Grünhagen. *Berl. klin. Wschr.*, **12**, 21 (1875).
de Haan. *Arch. néerl. Physiol.*, **7**, 245 (1922).
Henle. *Hb. d. systematischen Anatomie*, Braunschweig, **1** (1856).
Zur Anatomie d. Crystallinse, Göttingen (1878).
Hess. *VII int. Cong. Ophthal.*, Heidelberg, 308 (1888).
Graefe-Saemisch Hb. d. ges. Augenheilk., 3rd ed., Leipzig, Kap. IX (2), 249 (1911).
Heubel. *Pflügers Arch. ges. Physiol.*, **20**, 114 (1879).
van Heyningen. Davson's *The Eye*, London, **1**, 254 (1962).
van Heyningen, Pirie and Boag. *Biochem. J.*, **56**, 372 (1954).
von Jäger. *Ueber d. Einstellungen d. dioptrischen Apparates*, Wien (1861).
Köhnhorn. *De cataracta aquæ inopia effecta* (Diss.), Gryphiæ (1858).
Kudo. *Amer. J. Anat.*, **28**, 399 (1921).
Kunde. *Z. Zool.*, **8**, 466 (1857).
Kuwabara. *Arch. Augenheilk.*, **63**, 121 (1909).
Lerman. *N.Y. St. J. Med.*, **62**, 3075 (1962). *Basic Ophthalmology*, N.Y., 218 (1966).
Lerman, Devi and Banerjee. *Invest. Ophthal.*, **1**, 95 (1962).

[1] Pirie (1956), Dische *et al.* (1959), Lerman (1962), Lerman *et al.* (1962–63), Orekhovich *et al.* (1962).
[2] Pirie *et al.* (1953), van Heyningen *et al.* (1954), Daisley (1955), Pirie (1956), Lerman (1962).

Lerman and Zigman. *Invest. Ophthal.*, **2**, 626 (1963); **4**, 643 (1965).

Acta ophthal. (Kbh.), **45**, 193 (1967).

Lerman, Zigman and Forbes. *Biochem. biophys. Res. Commun.*, **22**, 57 (1966).

Löwenstein and Haurowitz. *v. Graefes Arch. Ophthal.*, **122**, 654 (1929).

Magnus. *v. Graefes Arch. Ophthal.*, **36** (4), 150 (1890).

Manca and Ovio. *Arch. Ottal.*, **5**, 112, 141 (1897).

von Michel. *Ueber natürliche u. künstliche Linsentrübung (Festchr. z. 3 Sœcularfeier d. med. Fac. Würzb.)*, Leipzig, **1**, 53 (1882).

Mitchell. *Amer. J. med. Sci.*, **39**, 106 (1860).

Nordmann. *Arch. Ophtal.*, **51**, 76, 203, 297 (1934); **52**, 78, 170 (1935).

Biologie du cristallin, Paris, 368 (1953).

Orekhovich, Firfarova, Kedrova and Levdikova. *Exp. Eye Res.*, **1**, 324 (1962).

Orzalesi. *G. Geront.*, **4**, 195 (1956).

Orzalesi and Miglior. *Boll. Oculist.*, **35**, 5 (1956).

Panico. *Ann. Ottal.*, **57**, 613 (1929).

Pau. *v. Graefes Arch. Ophthal.*, **152**, 532 (1952).

Pirie. *Trans. ophthal. Soc. U.K.*, **76**, 461 (1956).

Pirie, van Heyningen and Boag. *Biochem. J.*, **54**, 682 (1953).

Richardson. *Med. Times Gaz.*, **1**, 319, 412 (1860).

Ritter. *v. Graefes Arch. Ophthal.*, **22** (2), 255 (1876); **23** (2), 44 (1877).

Sbordone. *Ann. Ottal.*, **79**, 55 (1953).

Selenkowsky. *Klin. Mbl. Augenheilk.*, **75**, 67 (1925).

Stanković and Andjus. *Acta med. jugoslav.*, **13**, 19 (1959).

von Szily. *Hb. d. spez. path. Anat.*, Berlin, **11** (3), 1 (1937).

von Szily and Eckstein. *Klin. Mbl. Augenheilk.*, **71**, 545 (1923).

Tron. *Vestn. Oftal.*, **14**, 59 (1939).

Weekers. *Recherches expér. et clin. concernant la pathogénie des cataractes* (Thèse), Liège (1941).

Yoshimoto. *Arch. Augenheilk.*, **99**, 160 (1928).

A DECREASE IN THE PERMEABILITY OF THE CAPSULE by the precipitation upon it of non-toxic dyes has been shown by Friedenwald (1930) and Monahan (1953) to result in the rapid formation of lenticular opacities.[1] Such a procedure stops the normal traffic of nutrient and metabolic material, and probably produces a condition of acidosis; it is comparable to the effects of the deposition of inflammatory exudates in causing the complicated cataract of cyclitis when the lens becomes plastered with exudates.

AN INTERFERENCE WITH NUTRIENT SUPPLIES, as by the ligation of the posterior ciliary arteries, has been shown to produce posterior cataract (Wagenmann, 1890); a similar reaction follows extirpation of the iris and ciliary body in rabbits (Deutschmann, 1880) and more slowly and less dramatically after ligation of the vortex veins (Koster, 1895; van Geuns, 1899). It has also been found that an ipsilateral posterior cataract develops in many animals after ligation of the common carotid artery (Craviotto, 1965). The effects of these circulatory disturbances probably resemble those determined by a decreased permeability of the capsule and have their clinical counterparts in pulseless disease and in conditions of uveal vascular stasis or congestive glaucoma—decreased anabolism, increased catabolism, increased acidity, and necrosis.

CATARACT IN ANOXIA AND ASPHYXIA

Cataract due to anoxia and asphyxia is unknown in man but can occur in experimental animals. The first workers to produce such a cataract due to ANOXIA were Bellows and Nelson (1943–44) who subjected rats to an atmospheric pressure equivalent to an altitude of 30,000 ft. and above so that 50% of the animals died, controlled experiments being performed to ensure that anoxia and not asphyxia or a lowered pressure was the causal factor; 75% of the dead animals and 10% of those surviving had lenticular opacities accompanied by a three-fold increase in the concentration of lactic acid in the aqueous although the reaction of this fluid remained

[1] p. 71.

unchanged. A decrease in the ascorbic acid and chloride of the lenses of such rats was demonstrated by Morone and Citroni (1951). The cataract thus produced was transient in survivors, resembling that caused by other physical influences such as osmotic changes and cold. Histologically vacuoles appeared under the epithelium and diffuse feathery opacities associated with the sutures in the anterior cortex but less marked in the posterior region. The reversibility of the cataract is interesting; Duguet (1948) produced an anoxic cataract three times in the same rats, with complete regression each time. In anoxia the mitosis of the capsular epithelium is inhibited but this does not run parallel with the cataractous changes (Hoshina and Konishi, 1958; Takagi et al., 1959).

ASPHYXIA, that is a decrease in the available oxygen and an increase of the carbon dioxide in the tissues, also induces a reversible cataract. In the course of extensive studies on asphyxia in rats produced by keeping them in a confined space, Amantea (1934) and Biozzi (1935) noted the development of bilateral cataract affecting the anterior cortex. The latter observer studied particularly the phenomenon in an animal which had been incompletely asphyxiated every day for a month, the most interesting features being the rapid development and the high degree of reversibility of the changes in the lenses. The other notable ocular change was a vaso-dilatation so marked that it led to a massive increase in the protein content of the aqueous such that it assumed exudative properties. He concluded that the cataract was the result of the uncompensated acidosis which accompanies asphyxia. In rabbits and guinea-pigs Bonavolontà (1953) also found that the cataract regressed in 2 to 3 hours after the animals had been restored to a normal atmosphere and noted that while at this stage there was an increase in oxygen and a deficiency of carbon dioxide in the aqueous, the lens had a notably lowered oxygen-quotient. The presumption is that the lenticular opacities are directly due to the deprivation of available oxygen to the lens.

Amantea. *Atti reale Accad. Lincei*, Roma, **6** (A), 20 (1934).

Bellows and Nelson. *Proc. Soc. exp. Biol.* (N.Y.), **54**, 126 (1943).

Arch. Ophthal., **31**, 250 (1944).

Biozzi. *v. Graefes Arch. Ophthal.*, **133**, 423 (1935).

Bonavolontà. *Arch. Ottal.*, **57**, 369 (1953).

Craviotto. *Riv. Anat. pat.*, **27**, 740 (1965).

Deutschmann. *v. Graefes Arch. Ophthal.*, **26** (1), 135 (1880).

Duguet. *Méd. Aéro.*, **13**, 323 (1948).

Friedenwald. *Arch. Ophthal.*, **3**, 182 (1930).

von Geuns. *v. Graefes Arch. Ophthal.*, **47**, 249 (1899).

Hoshina and Konishi. *Acta Soc. ophthal. jap.*, **62**, 1413 (1958).

Koster. *v. Graefes Arch. Ophthal.*, **41** (2), 30 (1895).

Monahan. *Amer. J. Ophthal.*, **36** (2), 24 (1953).

Morone and Citroni. *Riv. Med. aeronaut.*, **14**, 464 (1951).

Takagi, Hoshina, Konishi and Miki. *Tokushima J. exp. Med.*, **6**, 31 (1959).

Wagenmann. *v. Graefes Arch. Ophthal.*, **36** (4), 1 (1890).

SUGAR CATARACT

After the production of cataract was first observed by Mitchell and Dodge (1935) and Yudkin and Arnold (1935) on feeding rats with a diet rich in lactose, its occurrence was rapidly and amply confirmed both with D-galactose and D-xylose (Fig. 86). When the disaccharide, lactose, is ingested it is hydrolysed by enzymes into glucose and galactose before being absorbed by the blood so that the cataractogenic action of lactose is effective only in producing a galactose cataract. When glucose is fed to normal animals it fails to raise the level of the blood-sugar and is therefore not cataractogenic, but it produces a cataract in animals rendered diabetic by such toxic agents such as alloxan or after pancreatectomy. A high blood-sugar level cannot be obtained by feeding with L-arabinose, so that this sugar is not cataractogenic, but when given with galactose it acts synergically and hastens the development of lenticular opacities (Bellows and Chinn, 1941; Patterson, 1955). Mannose, fructose and sorbitol also fail to raise the level

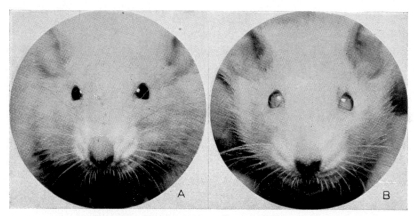

FIG. 86.—EXPERIMENTAL LACTOSE CATARACT.
A, normal rat, B, on a lactose diet (H. S. Mitchell and W. M. Dodge).

of blood-sugar and are not cataractogenic, nor have they been shown to potentiate the action of other sugars (Darby and Day, 1939; Patterson, 1955). The three sugars known to produce this effect are therefore D-galactose, D-xylose and (in diabetic animals) D-glucose.

It is interesting that in man galactose cataract occurs only in galacto-saemic infants with a congenital absence of the enzyme, galactose-1-P uridyl transferase, necessary for the metabolism of this sugar[1] (Kalckar, 1957); a specific type of cataract occurs in young diabetics; but xylose cataracts have not been demonstrated in man even in congenital pentosuria, a condition characterized by an inability to metabolize this sugar which is formed as a constituent of the uronic acid pathway.

All these three conditions—galactosaemia, xylosaemia and diabetes—produce much the same type of experimental cataract (Figs. 87–91); in this the three sugars all act synergically (Patterson, 1955), the speed and develop-

[1] p. 90.

Figs. 87 to 91.—Sugar Cataracts.

Experimental sugar cataracts in the rat (W. Buschke).

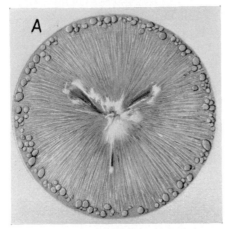

Fig. 87.

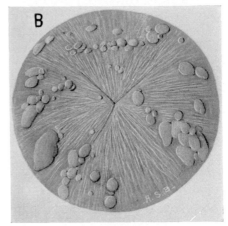

Fig. 88.

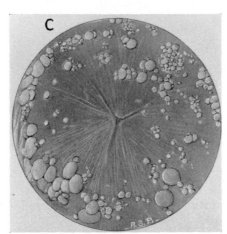

Fig. 89.

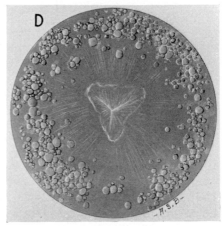

Fig. 90.

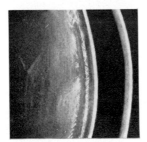

Fig. 91.

Figs. 87 and 88.—Cataract in diabetic rats after pancreatectomy. The optical section is seen in Fig. 91.

Figs. 89 and 90.—Cataract in rats fed a 50% galactose diet. Fig. 89.—Eight days after 4 days' feeding. Fig. 90.—Five days after 6 days' feeding.

ment of the opacification of the lens vary directly with the degree of hyperglycæmia and therefore with the concentration of the sugar in the aqueous
humour (Mitchell and Dodge, 1935; Patterson, 1951–54), the formation of
the opacities and their extent are ameliorated by lowering the blood-sugar

FIGS. 92 and 93.—EXPERIMENTAL GALACTOSE CATARACT.

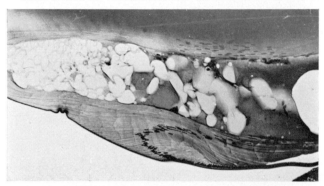

FIG. 92.—Extensive degeneration of the lens fibres at the equator 10 days after a
galactose diet was started in the rat (L. von Sallmann).

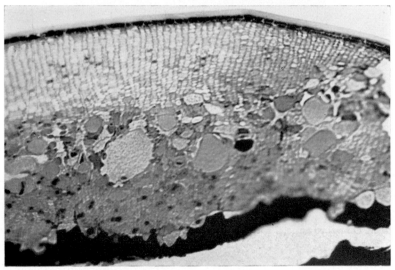

FIG. 93.—In a rat which had received 25% galactose in its diet for 18 days after
weaning. The massive degeneration of the cortical zone is seen (A. Patz).

(Patterson, 1953–54), and in all cases the appearance of the cataract is
similar. Galactose cataract has been produced mainly in rats, among which
there is a considerable variation in susceptibility in different strains (Mitchell,
1936), but Schrader (1961) produced anomalous lenticular changes in albino
rabbits and in cats, while experimental diabetic cataract has also been induced
in other animals such as mice, rabbits and dogs. In all cases the opacification

develops more rapidly and completely in young animals, and with xylose only in weaning rats, other animals being resistant (Booth *et al.*, 1953); it is interesting that in man galactosæmic and diabetic cataracts occur only in the young.

The *clinical appearance* of the changes in the lens induced by these sugars is essentially similar and in all cases young animals are more susceptible than adults (Buschke, 1943; Babel, 1953) (Figs. 87–91). The earliest change is the appearance of vacuoles in the periphery of the lens and in the anterior cortex, which is followed by a posterior polar opacity and a nuclear

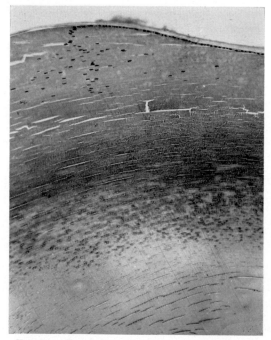

FIG. 94.—EXPERIMENTAL GALACTOSE CATARACT.

In a litter-mate of the white rat of Fig. 93. The animal received 25% galactose in its diet for 18 days after weaning and then a stock diet for 22 months. Note the normal superficial cortex with the old damaged fibres compressed centrally (A. Patz).

opacity before complete maturation. As a general rule the growing fibres are first affected, the cortex in adult animals, and the whole lens in the young.

Histologically the most careful observations have been made on galactose cataract in rats. In these the earliest changes are seen in the subcapsular epithelium of the germinative zone wherein an increase in mitosis occurs 24 hours after feeding commences, to attain a rate 12 times the normal on the 3rd day and reach a maximum in 4 to 6 days when this activity is not confined to the germinal area but involves the entire layer; at the same time a similar mitosis is observed in the ciliary epithelium (Hanna and O'Brien,

1960).   This early change in mitotic activity may explain to some extent the greater susceptibility of young animals to the development of cataract.   In the meantime, about the 3rd day vacuoles appear in the cortex in the equatorial area; at this stage the cataract is reversible.   Thereafter, underneath the proliferating and regenerating epithelium cataractous changes begin to develop when the cell-membranes of the fibres rupture and the fibres themselves break up into granules held in suspension in the vacuoles; the cataract is now irreversible and rapidly becomes complete (von Sallmann, 1957; Patterson and Bunting, 1964; Schrader and Beneke, 1965) (Fig. 92). With the electron microscope Brini and Porte (1961) found that in the affected fibres the fibrillar structure disappeared as they became granular, while they lost their cellular membranes and became confluent.   Eventually the degenerative changes in the cortex become massive and the epithelium sometimes proliferates to an unusual extent (14 layers, Gifford and Bellows, 1939; Patz, 1953) (Fig. 93).   If the artificial diet of galactose is stopped, the DNA synthetic rate again becomes normal and is confined to the equatorial region and the damaged fibres become buried beneath normal superficial cortex (Fig. 94).   It is interesting that the addition of galactose or other foreign sugars to the medium used for culturing lenses reduces the rate of metabolism and does not stimulate mitotic activity (Wachtl and Kinsey, 1957).

GALACTOSE CATARACT

The production of cataract by feeding animals on galactose has been studied by many investigators[1] (Figs. 89–90). The development of lenticular opacities becomes apparent with considerable regularity if the animals are fed on an adequate diet in which galactose is the sole carbohydrate constituent, provided this substance comprises from 25 to 70% of the whole; the younger the animal and the higher the dose, the more rapidly the cataract appears.   It is delayed by the administration of insulin (Quaranta, 1962). A proper supplement of normal diet prevents or delays its occurrence (Patterson, 1953; Dische et al., 1957), as also does a diet rich in protein and fat (Mitchell and Cook, 1940; Patterson, 1955; Patterson et al., 1962–65), although injections of protein are without effect (Rouher and Tronche, 1954); the development of opacities is also delayed by exercise (Mitchell and Cook, 1940) and is hastened by the topical or systemic administration of steroids (Cotlier and Becker, 1965; Bettman et al., 1968).   In the young rat peripheral opacities usually appear about the 3rd day, a complete superficial

[1] Dodge (1935), Jansen (1935), Mitchell and Dodge (1935), Mitchell (1935–36), Day (1936), Bellows (1936), Bellows and Rosner (1937–38), Yudkin (1938), Borley and Tainter (1938), Jess (1938), Mitchell and Cook (1938), Sasaki (1938), Rosner et al. (1938), Gifford and Bellows (1939), Cashell and Kon (1939), Yudkin and Geer (1940), Buschke (1943), Bannon et al. (1945), Patterson (1952–55), Nordmann and Mandel (1953), Craig and Maddock (1953), Hörmann (1954), Tojo (1954–55), Friedenwald and Rytel (1955), von Sallmann (1957), Dische et al. (1957), van Heyningen (1959), Testa and Botti (1961), Quaranta (1961), Korc (1961), Nordmann (1962), Korc and Calcagno (1963), Patterson and Bunting (1964), Patterson et al. (1965), Wilson (1967), and others.

opacity is apparent by the 9th to the 11th day, and the cataract has become mature by the 30th day. If the diet is stopped within a week, the changes in the lens are reversible, but after 10 to 14 days of galactose feeding they are permanent (Patterson *et al.*, 1965). Cataract has developed in the offspring of mothers fed on galactose during pregnancy (Bannon *et al.*, 1945; de Meyer, 1959); but the intraperitoneal (Yudkin, 1938) or hypodermic injection of galactose has no effect (Selle, 1940).

The *biochemistry* of galactose cataract is not by any means yet understood. In the normal animal this sugar can be metabolized to some extent by specific enzymes to glucose and glycogen, but fed in large quantities it is undoubtedly toxic for such animals survive little longer than starved controls probably owing to a fall in the glucose-content of the blood and a depletion of glycogen in the liver (Richter, 1941; Handler, 1947). When fed with galactose, rats show an increase of this substance in the aqueous and a smaller increase in the lens suggesting that it penetrates into the extracellular spaces but not into the fibres (van Heyningen *et al.*, 1955). The sugar appears to be metabolized to some extent (Pirie and van Heyningen, 1956; Wachtl and Kinsey, 1957), but since galactose-1-phosphate accumulates, it is possible that the same metabolic block to the breakdown of galactose exists as in galactosæmia owing to a lack of the enzyme, galactose-1-P uridyl transferase[1] (Schwarz and Goldberg, 1955; Lerman, 1959). Instead, the excess of sugar is reduced by aldose reductase to produce large quantities of sugar alcohols, particularly dulcitol (van Heyningen, 1962; Kinoshita, 1963–65; Kinoshita *et al.*, 1965); this change results in a high osmolarity in the lens which presumably accounts for the early appearance of vacuolation (Kinoshita *et al.*, 1962). This simple explanation, however, is complicated by the fact that the lenses of older rats similarly accumulate dulcitol but do not swell or develop cataract so readily. At the same time there is a diminution of amino acids in the lens which occurs independently of the osmotic dilution (Patterson *et al.*, 1965), an arrest of the synthesis of soluble protein (Dische *et al.*, 1956–57), the fibre-membranes lose their semipermeability (Patterson and Bunting, 1964), and the proteins are precipitated. In mature cataract the osmotic equilibration of the lens is thus entirely dependent upon the permeability of the capsule through which all small molecules find free passage and not on the relatively impermeable membranes of the lenticular fibres; there is therefore a diminution in dry weight owing to a loss of the more permeable proteins and a rapid diffusion outwards of sugar and RNA, an upset of the ionic equilibrium and a great increase in hydrolysis (Mitchell, 1935–36; Nordmann and Mandel, 1953; Klein *et al.*, 1961; van Heyningen, 1962; Kinoshita *et al.*, 1968).

In the meantime, there is a major disturbance of the carbohydrate metabolism in the form of an inhibition of the important hexose-mono-phosphate shunt, possibly by a degradation product of galactose (galactose-

---

[1] p. 172.

1-phosphate), while anaerobic glycolysis remains unimpaired until the cataract is far advanced. The former oxidative pathway is particularly important in the young lens whereas as age increases anaerobic glycolysis becomes more important (and the development of sugar cataract more difficult). This block probably depends on an inhibition of the enzyme glucose-6-phosphate dehydrogenase and results in a marked fall in the high-energy adenosine triphosphate (ATP) normally derived from the oxidation of glucose until little remains[1] (Lerman, 1960–62; Lerman and Ishida, 1960; Korc, 1961).

Apart from these two gross disturbances in the carbohydrate metabolism, other changes occur which are probably of less significance. There is a loss of glutathione and ascorbic acid, first in the cortex and then in the nucleus (Bellows, 1936; Bellows

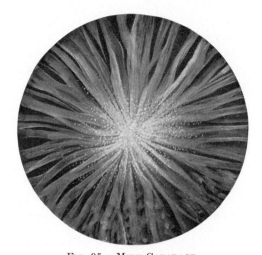

FIG. 95.—MILK CATARACT.

In a rat fed on human milk. The opacities affected the subcapsular layers of the cortex before the nucleus was involved (R. Vozza).

and Rosner, 1937; Rosner et al., 1938), an accumulation of uridine diphosphogalactose (Klethi and Mandel, 1962), a deficiency of amino acids and an apparent cessation in the synthesis of soluble proteins (Dische et al., 1956–57; Lerman, 1960).

It has been shown that young albino rats fed on *human milk* develop cataract within 20 to 30 days, the onset of which can be delayed by adding cow's milk to the diet (Burgio, 1948) (Fig. 95). It is probable that the cataractogenic action of human milk is due to the high lactose and low protein content (Vozza, 1957).

XYLOSE CATARACT

XYLOSE CATARACT as an experimental entity has been equally firmly established.[2] The condition can be produced in rats only during the weaning stage when it develops in 8 to 12 days (Booth et al., 1953) but has also been

[1] Vol. IV, p. 357.
[2] Darby and Day (1939), Sterling and Day (1951), Patz (1953), Booth et al. (1953), Babel (1953).

induced in albino rabbits and cats (Schrader, 1961). A diet of 25 to 50% xylose is required. The changes in the lens are comparable to those occurring in galactose cataract but differ in the fact that the cataract tends to regress even if the diet is continued for the animal apparently adapts itself to it (Booth *et al.*, 1953).

Biochemically the same two changes occur in the carbohydrate mechanism as in galactose cataract, although to a less degree. Xylose, like galactose, readily penetrates the blood-aqueous barrier and enters the lens. In the early stages there is no derangement of anaerobic carbohydrate metabolism (Lerman and Heggeness, 1961). There is, however, an accumulation of sugar-alcohols, initially xylitol and then sorbitol, which presumably give rise to the same osmotic effects as does dulcitol in galactose cataracts, the same rapid inhibition of the hexose-monophosphate pathway in the oxidation of glucose and a considerable fall in the high-energy ATP (van Heyningen, 1959; Lerman and Heggeness, 1961). It is significant, however, that after a period of about 3 weeks when the lenticular opacity begins to disappear, this pathway resumes its normal activity as if the lens becomes able to deal effectively with the xylose.

GLUCOSE (DIABETOGENIC) CATARACT

DIABETOGENIC CATARACT was first produced in experimental animals by pancreatectomy (Figs. 87–8)[1] but is more easily brought about by administering substances which induce coagulative necrosis of the beta-cells of the islets of Langerhans and thus cause diabetes. The first substance to be thus used was ALLOXAN (2,4,5,6-tetra-oxypyrimidine) which may be given in single or repeated doses by subcutaneous, intraperitoneal or intravenous injection,[2] while other effective compounds are DEHYDROASCORBIC ACID, DEHYDRO-GLUCOASCORBIC ACID (Patterson, 1949–51) and DIPHENYL-THIOCARBAZONE (Dithizone) (Inoue, 1952; Butturini *et al.*, 1953). A similar effect by alloxan on the beta-cells of man has not been demonstrated (Brunschwig *et al.*, 1943–44) and its mode of action in animals is unknown, as is the relation of alloxan diabetes to human diabetes; it has been suggested that this substance inactivates an essential enzyme by an irreversible combination with a sulphydryl group (Lazarow, 1947–49; Lazarow *et al.*, 1948), and an inhibition of the citric acid cycle in carbohydrate metabolism has been demonstrated (Younathan, 1962).

The cataract never develops without the onset of diabetes and its extent depends on the severity of the general disease. It appears earlier and develops more rapidly if dextrose or galactose is given as a supplement to the diet (Yaso, 1951; Sterling and Day, 1951), its course is aggravated by the administration of cortisone (Alagna,

[1] Wessely (1922), Chaikoff and Lachman (1933), Foglia and Cramer (1944), Cramer and Foglia (1948), Kajikawa (1955), Kurimoto (1959).
[2] Dogs, Goldner and Gomori (1943), Kajikawa (1955), Kurimoto (1959); rabbits, Dunn *et al.* (1943), Bellows and Shoch (1950), Babel (1951–53), Arizawa (1951), Quaranta *et al.* (1959), Kanzaki (1959); rats, monkeys, Charalampous and Hegsted (1950), Beach *et al.* (1951).

1954) and its incidence can be determined by the injection of anterior pituitary extract (Dohan *et al.*, 1941). Its development is moderated or prevented by lowering the blood-sugar by insulin (Alphen and Cohen, 1950; Rodriguez and Krehl, 1951; Alphen, 1952; Patterson, 1953; Rodriguez, 1954), hypoglycæmic sulphonamides (Quaranta *et al.*, 1959), a reduction in the carbohydrates in the diet (Charalampous and Hegsted, 1950; Rodriguez and Krehl, 1951) or partial starvation (Patterson, 1954), by a diet rich in fat, casein and fructose (Patterson, 1955) or in fat and protein (Patterson *et al.*, 1965), and by the administration of riboflavine (Zivkov and Andreeva, 1960). The animal acquires complete protection against diabetes if the alloxan is prevented from reaching the pancreas by the occlusion of the blood supply to this organ for a very short period (6 minutes only) after the injection (Gomori and Goldner, 1943–45).

The development of alloxan diabetes has been observed to be followed by the formation of cataract within 9 to 17 days (Arizawa, 1951; Sterling and Day, 1951), becoming complete before the 200th day. The lenticular opacities usually begin equatorially and subcapsularly in the posterior cortex, taking the same morphological form as other sugar cataracts.[1] There is an increase in the fluorescence of the lens, an atrophy of the Golgi apparatus and a decrease in the mitochondria in the ciliary epithelium in the rabbit (Karaki, 1954–56; Brolin, 1954–55).

The *biochemical changes* occurring in diabetogenic cataract resemble those in other sugar cataracts (Nordmann and Mandel, 1953; Patterson, 1956; Katsumori, 1956; Mandel and Quaranta, 1958; Lerman, 1962; Sippel, 1962); and again our knowledge is very inadequate. In order to produce lenticular opacities the level of glucose in the blood must be high (above 250 mg. per 100 ml.) with a corresponding level in the aqueous, a concentration approximately the same as that required to bring about an opacity in the incubated isolated lens. In the lens the concentrations of glucose, fructose and sorbitol rapidly become correspondingly high (van Heyningen, 1959; Kuck, 1961; Kinoshita *et al.*, 1962; Lerman, 1962; Patterson and Bunting, 1965), as does sorbitol in the lens of the human diabetic (Pirie and van Heyningen, 1964; Pirie, 1965). The accumulation of sorbitol probably accounts for the osmotic hydration of the lens, while in the oxidation of glucose the hexose-monophosphate shunt is impaired (Fitch *et al.*, 1959; Levari *et al.*, 1961; Lerman, 1962). As in other sugar cataracts there is a decrease of free amino acids and protein synthesis (Lerman, 1962; Reddy and Kinsey, 1963; Reddy, 1965), but the fall in glutathione is late (Bellows and Shoch, 1950).

Alagna. *Arch. Ottal.*, **58**, 203 (1954).

Alphen. *Ophthalmologica*, **123**, 186 (1952).

Alphen and Cohen. *Acta physiol. pharm. néerl.*, **1**, 400 (1950).

Arizawa. *Acta Soc. ophthal. jap.*, **55**, 1239 (1951).

Babel. *Bull Soc. franç. Ophtal.*, **64**, 112 (1951).
  v. Graefes Arch. Ophthal., **153**, 520 (1953).

Bailey, C. and O., and Leech. *New Engl. J. Med.*, **230**, 533 (1944).

Bailey, O and C., and Hagan. *Amer. J. med. Sci.*, **208**, 450 (1944).

Bannon, Higginbottom, McConnell and Kaan. *Arch. Ophthal.*, **33**, 224 (1945).

Beach, Bradshaw and Blatherwick. *Amer. J. Physiol.*, **166**, 364 (1951).

Bellows. *Arch. Ophthal.*, **16**, 762 (1936).

Bellows and Chinn. *Arch. Ophthal.*, **25**, 796 (1941).

Bellows and Rosner. *Amer. J. Ophthal.*, **20**, 1109 (1937).
  Arch. Ophthal., **20**, 80 (1938).

Bellows and Shoch. *Amer. J. Ophthal.*, **33**, 1555 (1950).

[1] Bailey *et al.* (1944), Duffy (1945), Chesler and Tislowitz (1945), Lewis *et al.* (1947), Shipley and Meyer (1947), Simonelli and Andreani (1948), Simonelli and Esente (1948), Fleming (1950), Charalampous and Hegsted (1950), Babel (1951), Janes and Bounds (1952), Gerritzen *et al.* (1957), von Sallmann *et al.* (1958), and others.

Bettman, Fung, Webster *et al. Amer. J. Ophthal.*, **65**, 581 (1968).

Booth, Wilson and De Eds. *J. Nutrit.*, **49**, 347 (1953).

Borley and Tainter. *Amer. J. Ophthal.*, **21**, 1091 (1938).

Brini and Porte. *Bull. Soc. Ophtal. Fr.*, 340 (1961).

Brolin. *Acta ophthal.* (Kbh.), **32**, 83 (1954). *Acta physiol. scand.*, **33**, 359 (1955); **34**, 303 (1955).

Brunschwig, Allen, Owens and Thornton. *J. Amer. med. Ass.*, **124**, 212 (1944).

Brunschwig, Goldner, Allen and Gomori. *J. Amer. med. Ass.*, **122**, 966 (1943).

Burgio. *Boll. Soc. ital. Biol. sper.*, **24**, 650 (1948).

Buschke. *Arch. Ophthal.*, **30**, 735 (1943).

Butturini, Grignolo and Baronchelli. *G. clin. Med.*, **34**, 1253 (1953).

Cashell and Kon. *Trans. ophthal. Soc. U.K.*, **59**, 199 (1939).

Chaikoff and Lachman. *Proc. Soc. exp. Biol.* (N.Y.), **31**, 237 (1933).

Charalampous and Hegsted. *Amer. J. Physiol.*, **161**, 540 (1950).

Chesler and Tislowitz. *Science*, **101**, 468 (1945).

Cotlier and Becker. *Invest. Ophthal.*, **4**, 806 (1965).

Craig and Maddock. *Arch. Path.*, **55**, 118 (1953).

Cramer and Foglia. *Arch. Oftal. B. Aires*, **23**, 101 (1948).

Darby and Day. *Proc. Soc. exp. Biol.* (N.Y.), **41**, 507 (1939).

Day. *J. Nutrit.*, **12**, 395 (1936).

Dische, Borenfreund and Zelmenis. *Arch. Ophthal.*, **55**, 633 (1956).

Dische, Zelmenis and Youlus. *Amer. J. Ophthal.*, **44** (2), 332 (1957).

Dodge. *Arch. Ophthal.*, **14**, 922 (1935).

Dohan, Fish and Lukens. *Endocrinology*, **28**, 341 (1941).

Duffy. *J. Path. Bact.*, **57**, 199 (1945).

Dunn, Sheehan and McLetchie. *Lancet*, **1**, 484 (1943).

Fitch, Hill and Chaikoff. *J. biol. Chem.*, **234**, 2811 (1959).

Fleming. *Trans. Canad. ophthal. Soc.*, **13**, 123 (1950).

Foglia and Cramer. *Proc. Soc. exp. Biol.* (N.Y.), **55**, 218 (1944).

Friedenwald and Rytel. *Arch. Ophthal.*, **53**, 825 (1955).

Gerritzen, Noach, von Wijke and Valk. *Acta endocrin.* (Stockh.), **35**, 91 (1957).

Gifford and Bellows. *Arch. Ophthal.*, **21**, 346 (1939).

Goldner and Gomori. *Endocrinology*, **33**, 297 (1943).

Gomori and Goldner. *Proc. Soc. exp. Biol.* (N.Y.), **54**, 287 (1943); **58**, 232 (1945).

Handler. *J. Nutrit.*, **33**, 221 (1947).

Hanna and O'Brien. *Arch. Ophthal.*, **64**, 708 (1960).

van Heyningen. *Biochem. J.*, **73**, 197 (1959). *Nature* (Lond.), **184**, Suppl. 4, 194 (1959). *Exp. Eye Res.*, **1**, 396 (1962).

van Heyningen, Pirie and Blackwell. *Brit. J. Ophthal.*, **39**, 37 (1955).

Hörmann. *v. Graefes Arch. Ophthal.*, **154**, 561 (1954).

Inoue. *Acta Soc. ophthal. jap.*, **56**, 588 (1952).

Janes and Bounds. *Anat. Rec.*, **112**, 347 (1952).

Jansen. *Acta brev. néerl. Physiol.*, **5**, 165 (1935).

Jess. *Klin. Mbl. Augenheilk.*, **101**, 761 (1938).

Kajikawa. *Acta Soc. ophthal. jap.*, **59**, 907 (1955).

Kalckar. *Science*, **125**, 105 (1957).

Kanzaki. *Acta Soc. ophthal. jap.*, **63**, 3712 (1959).

Karaki. *Acta Soc. ophthal. jap.*, **58**, 1073 (1954); **60**, 251 (1956).

Katsumori. *Acta Soc. ophthal. jap.*, **60**, 407 (1956).

Kinoshita. *Arch. Ophthal.*, **70**, 558 (1963). *Invest. Ophthal.*, **4**, 786 (1965).

Kinoshita, Merola and Dikmak. *Exp. Eye Res.*, **1**, 405 (1962).

Kinoshita, Merola and Hayman. *Fed. Proc.*, **23**, 536 (1964). *J. biol. Chem.*, **240**, 310 (1965).

Kinoshita, Merola and Tung. *Exp. Eye Res.*, **7**, 80 (1968).

Klein, Mandel and Nordmann. *C.R. Soc. Biol.* (Paris), **155**, 617 (1961).

Klethi and Mandel. *Biochim. biophys. Acta*, **57**, 379 (1962).

Korc. *Arch. Biochem.* (N.Y.), **94**, 196 (1961).

Korc and Calcagno. *Nature* (Lond.), **197**, 690 (1963).

Kuck. *Arch. Ophthal.*, **65**, 840 (1961).

Kurimoto. *Yonogo Acta med.*, **4**, 23 (1959).

Lazarow. *Proc. Soc. exp. Biol.* (N.Y.), **61**, 441 (1946); **66**, 4 (1947). *Physiol. Rev.*, **29**, 48 (1949).

Lazarow, Patterson and Levey. *Science*, **108**, 308 (1948).

Lerman. *Arch. Ophthal.*, **61**, 88 (1959); **63**, 128, 132 (1960); **65**, 334 (1961). *Invest. Ophthal.*, **1**, 507 (1962). *N.Y. St. J. Med.*, **62**, 785 (1962). *Basic Ophthalmology*, N.Y. (1966).

Lerman and Heggeness. *Biochem. J.*, **79**, 224 (1961).

Lerman and Ishida. *Arch. Ophthal.*, **63**, 136 (1960).

Levari, Wertheimer, Berman and Kornblueth. *Nature* (Lond.), **192**, 1075 (1961).

Lewis, Moses and Schneider. *Amer. J. med. Sci.*, **213**, 214 (1947).

Mandel and Quaranta. *J. Physiol.* (Paris), **50**, 394 (1958).

de Meyer. *Ann. Endocrin.* (Paris), **20**, 203 (1959).

Mitchell. *Proc. Soc. exp. Biol.* (N.Y.), **32**, 971 (1935). *J. Nutrit.*, **12**, 447 (1936).

Mitchell and Cook. *Arch. Ophthal.*, **19,** 22 (1938).

Proc. Soc. exp. Biol. (N.Y.), **43,** 85 (1940).

Mitchell and Dodge. *J. Nutrit.*, **9,** 37 (1935).

Nordmann. *Bull. Acad. roy. Méd. Belg.*, **2,** 511 (1962).

Nordmann and Mandel. *C.R. Acad. Sci.* (Paris), **236,** 426 (1953).

Patterson, J. *Endocrinology*, **45,** 344 (1949).

J. biol. Chem., **183,** 81 (1950).

Science, **111,** 724 (1950).

Amer. J. Physiol., **165,** 61 (1951); **172,** 77 (1953); **177,** 541 (1954); **180,** 495 (1955).

Amer. J. Ophthal., **35** (2), 68 (1952).

Arch. Biochem. (N.Y.), **58,** 23 (1955).

Proc. Soc. exp. Biol. (N.Y.), **90,** 706 (1955).

Diabetes, **5,** 93 (1956).

Invest. Ophthal., **4,** 667 (1965).

Patterson, J., and Bunting. *Proc. Soc. exp. Biol.* (N.Y.), **115,** 1156 (1964).

Invest. Ophthal., **4,** 167 (1965).

Docum. ophthal., **20,** 64 (1966).

Patterson, J. and M., and Bunting. *Exp. Eye Res.*, **1,** 411 (1962).

Patterson, J. and M., Kinsey and Reddy. *Invest. Ophthal.*, **4,** 98 (1965).

Patz. *Amer. J. Ophthal.*, **36,** 453 (1953).

Pirie. *Invest. Ophthal.*, **4,** 629 (1965).

Pirie and van Heyningen. *Biochemistry of the Eye*, Oxon., 103 (1956).

Exp. Eye Res., **3,** 124 (1964).

Quaranta. *Atti Cong. Soc. oftal. ital.*, **19,** 258 (1961).

Boll. Oculist., **41,** 89, 595, 687 (1962).

Quaranta, Tedeschi, Tittarelli and Vozza. *Boll. Oculist.*, **38,** 41 (1959).

Reddy. *Invest. Ophthal.*, **4,** 700 (1965).

Reddy and Kinsey. *Invest. Ophthal.*, **2,** 237 (1963).

Richter. *Amer. J. Physiol.*, **133,** 29 (1941).

Rodriguez. *Arch. Oftal. B. Aires*, **29,** 207 (1954).

Rodriguez and Krehl. *Yale J. Biol. Med.*, **24,** 103 (1951).

Rosner, Farmer and Bellows. *Arch. Ophthal.*, **20,** 417 (1938).

Rouher and Tronche. *Bull. Soc. franç. Ophtal.*, **67,** 37 (1954).

von Sallmann. *Amer. J. Ophthal.*, **44,** 159 (1957).

von Sallmann, Caravaggio, Grimes and Collins. *Arch. Ophthal.*, **59,** 55 (1958).

Sasaki. *v. Graefes Arch. Ophthal.*, **138,** 351, 365 (1938).

Sasaki and Kodama. *Acta Soc. ophthal. jap.*, **56,** 581 (1952).

Schrader. *v. Graefes Arch. Ophthal.*, **163,** 422 (1961).

Ber. dtsch. ophthal. Ges., **64,** 282 (1961).

Schrader and Beneke. *v. Graefes Arch. Ophthal.*, **168,** 341 (1965).

Schwarz and Goldberg. *Biochim. biophys. Acta*, **18,** 310 (1955).

Selle. *Arch. Ophthal.*, **23,** 369 (1940).

Shipley and Meyer. *Amer. J. Physiol.*, **148,** 185 (1947).

Simonelli and Andreani. *G. ital. Oftal.*, **1,** 132 (1948).

Simonelli and Esente. *G. ital. Oftal.*, **1,** 520 (1948).

Sippel. *Exp. Eye Res.*, **1,** 368 (1962).

Invest. Ophthal., **5,** 568, 576 (1966).

Sterling and Day. *Proc. Soc. exp. Biol.* (N.Y.), **78,** 431 (1951).

Testa and Botti. *Arch. Ottal.*, **65,** 181 (1961).

Tojo. *Acta Soc. ophthal. jap.*, **58,** 556 (1954); **59,** 933 (1955).

Vozza. *Amer. J. Ophthal.*, **44,** 387 (1957).

Wachtl and Kinsey. *Amer. J. Ophthal.*, **44** (2), 318 (1957).

Wessely. *Arch. Augenheilk.*, **91,** 158 (1922).

Wilson. *Trans. Amer. ophthal. Soc.*, **65,** 661 (1967).

Yaso. *Acta Soc. ophthal. jap.*, **55,** 383 (1951).

Younathan. *J. biol. Chem.*, **237,** 608 (1962).

Yudkin. *Amer. J. Ophthal.*, **21,** 871 (1938).

Yudkin and Arnold. *Arch. Ophthal.*, **14,** 960 (1935).

Yudkin and Geer. *Arch. Ophthal.*, **23,** 28 (1940).

Zivkov and Andreeva. *Nauc. trudove, VMI* (Sofia), **39,** 301 (1960).

DEFICIENCY CATARACT

Cataract due to deficiency in the diet has been brought about experimentally by depriving animals either of certain essential amino acids or of vitamins, the former being necessary for the elaboration of lenticular proteins and the latter for the continuance of the metabolism.

A DEFICIENCY IN PROTEINS is responsible for several ocular disabilities[1] but its cataractogenic effect is less clear. We have already seen that a lack of proteins hastens the development of a galactose cataract; and it has been claimed that a diet deficient in protein produces cataract in young rats (Rezende and de Moura Campos, 1942; Hall *et al.*, 1948; Bertolani, 1948), but equivocal results were obtained by Morone (1950). Bagchi (1958) and McLaren (1959) produced opacification of the lenses of

[1] Vol. III, p. 372.

pigs with a protein-deficient diet (Figs. 96–7). The former found a reduction of glutathione and protein-bound sulphydryl groups and made the suggestion that the frequency of cataract in India might be due to this type of dietary deficiency.

The occurrence of deficiency cataract due to lack of essential AMINO ACIDS is more firmly established. Most of the experimental work has been

FIGS. 96 and 97.—CATARACT DUE TO PROTEIN DEFICIENCY IN THE PIG
(D. S. McLaren).

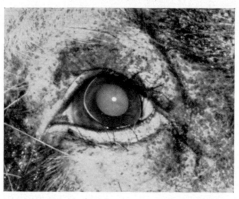

FIG. 96.—The eye of a pig after more than one year on a diet deficient in protein.

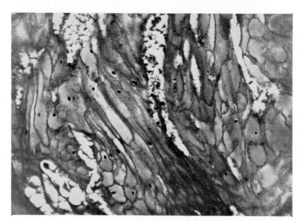

FIG. 97.—The histology of the lens of the pig showing the involvement of all the fibres and the amorphous debris in the interfibrillar clefts.

done on rats and, as would be expected, young and rapidly growing animals are much more susceptible than adults. In this connection the most important amino acid is *tryptophan*[1] (Figs. 98–103). Less dramatic results have been reported following the lack of other indispensable amino acids, with the

[1] Curtis *et al.* (1932), Totter and Day (1942), Albanese and Buschke (1942), Buschke (1943), Ferraro and Roizin (1947), Schaeffer and Geiger (1947), Hall *et al.* (1948), de Berardinis (1949), Schaeffer and Murray (1950), Ogino and Ichihara (1957), von Sallmann *et al.* (1959), Dische *et al.* (1959).

FIGS. 98 to 101.—EXPERIMENTAL CATARACT DUE TO TRYPTOPHAN DEFICIENCY IN THE RAT (W. Buschke).

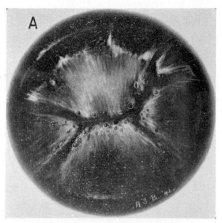

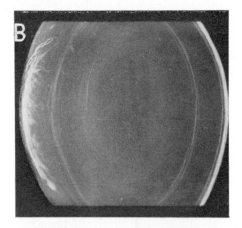

FIG. 98.—Composite drawing of the posterior cortex in the early stage.

FIG. 99.—Optical section in the early stage.

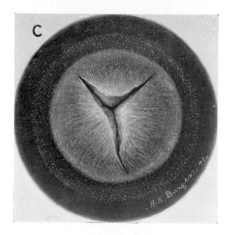

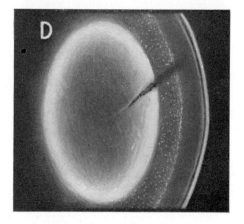

FIG. 100.—The posterior cortex at a later stage.

FIG. 101.—Optical section at a later stage.

exception of arginine: *phenylalanine* (Bowles *et al.*, 1947; Hall *et al.*, 1948), *histidine* (Sydenstricker *et al.*, 1947), and also *methionine* (Cristini, 1950), particularly when the deficiency is produced by administering an antimetabolite of this substance (Bagchi, 1959). It would seem that the occurrence of cataract is due to the arrest of the synthesis of soluble proteins (Dische *et al.*, 1959), and is associated with a general arrest of growth, cutaneous lesions and vascularization of the cornea; restoration of tryptophan to the diet may or may not restrain the development of the lenticular opacities in rats or even clarify the lens (Buschke, 1943; Ferraro and Roizin, 1947), but since the administration of tryptophan separately from the rest of the diet has no beneficial effect (Schaeffer and Geiger, 1947) and a diet containing tryptophan as the sole amino acid still produces cataract (Schaeffer and Murray, 1950), it would seem that protein synthesis can occur only if all the essential amino acids are simultaneously available.

Lack of cystine, a constituent of glutathione, is not generally cataractogenic or only very slightly so (Bietti, 1935), but Patch (1934–43) found that the larvæ of the tiger salamander fed on a diet deficient in this amino acid developed cataract and that this could be prevented by adding it to the food. A diet deficient in methyl groups was found by Cristini (1950) to cause cataract as well as necrotic and hæmorrhagic lesions in several organs in rats.

FIGS. 102 and 103.—EXPERIMENTAL CATARACT DUE TO TRYPTOPHAN DEFICIENCY IN THE RAT (W. Buschke).

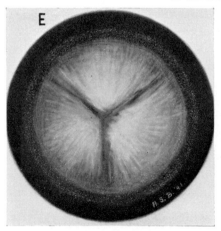

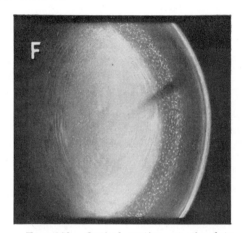

FIG. 102.—Composite drawing of the posterior cortex at the late stage.

FIG. 103.—Optical section at the late stage.

A DEFICIENCY OF VITAMINS, particularly those of the B₂ group, has been claimed to result in the development of cataract.

It was found by Day and his colleagues (1931) that rats fed on a diet deficient in the *vitamin B₂ complex* developed cataract in 94% of cases in from 60 to 87 days, a complication which was prevented by adding the vitamin to the diet; this observation has been confirmed by several other investigators.[1] Apparently the deficiency must be complete since to be effective the diet must start on the weaning of the animals (O'Brien, 1932; Yudkin, 1933), presumably to avoid the accumulation of reserves in the body. Other workers, however, have not obtained by any means the same consistency of results. Sen and his colleagues (1935) obtained cataract in only 5 out of 41 rats, Bourne and Pyke (1935) in 15 out of 98 rats, Eckardt

[1] Langston *et al.* (1933), Langston and Day (1933), Yudkin (1933–38), Day and Langston (1934), Day *et al.* (1937), de Moura Campos and Rezende (1942), Baum *et al.* (1942), Krukowska (1951), El-Sadr (1955).

and Johnson (1939) in 10% of rats, while Jansen (1935), György (1935), Scardaccione (1937), Tainter and Borley (1938) and Suda (1939) saw no lens changes in their animals, and Yudkin (1933) obtained negative results in dogs, but a diet deficient in riboflavine has been found to be cataractogenic in the pig (Wintrobe and his colleagues, 1944) (Fig. 104) and also, when supplemented by a high fatty diet, in the cat (Gershoff *et al.*, 1959). It is obvious that the occurrence of experimental cataract with ariboflavinosis is doubtful. The rarity of the occurrence of cataract in patients with pellagra suggests that a deficiency of nicotinic acid is similarly ineffective. Moreover, in all

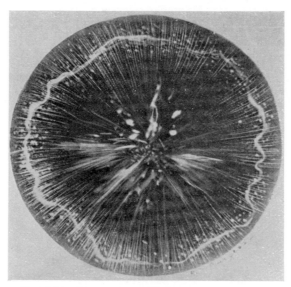

FIG. 104.—RIBOFLAVINE DEFICIENCY IN THE PIG.

A composite slit-lamp drawing of the lens. There is a dense white wave-like opacity near the equator, separation of the fibres in the anterior and posterior cortex and a multitude of dot-like opacities with minute vacuoles near the anterior and posterior poles. The deep cortex and the nucleus are clear (M. M. Wintrobe *et al.*).

these conditions it is difficult to exclude other cataractogenic factors such as a lack of tryptophan or some other essential amino acid. It seems necessary to conclude, therefore, that while cataract may form on a diet deficient in riboflavine, it does not do so regularly, a circumstance which suggests that the essential factor involved may be related to other anomalies in the diet or to as yet unidentified influences. It is noteworthy that deficiency of maternal folic acid in the rat may result in the complete disorganization of the fœtal lens.[1]

A lack of *vitamin A* was claimed by von Szily and Eckstein (1923), Schreiber (1925) and Levina (1926) to lead to the formation of cataract, and Lahiri (1938)

[1] Vol. III, p. 379.

reported its occurrence accompanied by night-blindness in bullocks fed on a diet deficient in carotene; but the observations of Jess (1925) indicated that this was a secondary effect of concomitant severe changes in the cornea and anterior segment. Stepp and Friedenwald (1924) obtained negative results in rats, while McLaren (1963) could trace no evidence that cataract was associated with the deprivation of this vitamin. A condition of maternal hypervitaminosis-A in rats, however, frequently leads to the formation of cataract in the young.[1]

A deficiency in maternal *vitamin E* was found by Ferguson and his colleagues (1956–60) to result in liquefaction and opacification of the lenses in chicks. The cataract obtained by Demole and Knapp (1941) and Corrado (1953) in rats subjected to avitaminosis-E may have been caused by the iridocyclitis and retinal degeneration which developed. There is also some evidence that deprivation of certain vitamins may facilitate the development of cataract by disturbing the metabolism of proteins. Thus a lack of vitamin E has been found to lead to a disordered metabolism of the proteins and nucleic acids in the lenses of rabbits with the formation of opacities (Devi *et al.*, 1965).

Although there is no evidence that lack of *vitamin C* gives rise to cataract, its absence certainly predisposes to the development of lenticular opacities from other causes which may be as slight as a paracentesis of the anterior chamber (Monjukowa and Fradkin, 1935; Mouriquand and Rollet, 1936; Ferrara, 1940); thus a cataract following the administration of sodium butyrate and tyrosine occurs only in scorbutic guinea-pigs, possibly due to the abnormal metabolism of tyrosine, and is preventable by the administration of ascorbic acid and anthranilic acid (Yamada, 1953; Uyama *et al.*, 1955).

Albanese and Buschke. *Science*, **95**, 584 (1942).
Bagchi. *J. Ind. med. Ass.*, **31**, 271 (1958). *Ind. J. med. Res.*, **47**, 437 (1959).
Baum, Michaelree and Brown. *Science*, **95**, 24 (1942).
de Berardinis. *G. ital. Oftal.*, **2**, 260 (1949).
Bertolani. *Boll. Soc. ital. Biol. sper.*, **24**, 1152 (1948).
Bietti. *Boll. Oculist.*, **14**, 938 (1935).
Bourne and Pyke. *Biochem. J.*, **29**, 1865 (1935).
Bowles, Sydenstricker, Hall and Schmidt. *Proc. Soc. exp. Biol.* (N.Y.), **66**, 585 (1947).
Buschke. *Arch. Ophthal.*, **30**, 735 (1943).
Corrado. *Ann. Ottal.*, **79**, 211 (1953).
Cristini. *G. ital. Oftal.*, **3**, 405 (1950).
Curtis, Hauge and Kraybill. *J. Nutrit.*, **5**, 503 (1932).
Day, Darby and Langston. *J. Nutrit.*, **13**, 389 (1937).
Day and Langston. *J. Nutrit.*, **7**, 97 (1934).
Day, Langston and O'Brien. *Amer. J. Ophthal.*, **14**, 1005 (1931).
Demole and Knapp. *Ophthalmologica*, **101**, 65 (1941).
Devi, Raina and Singh. *Brit. J. Ophthal.*, **49**, 271 (1965).
Dische, Elliott, Pearson and Merriam. *Amer. J. Ophthal.*, **47** (2), 368 (1959).
Eckardt and Johnson. *Arch. Ophthal.*, **21**, 315 (1939).
El-Sadr. *J. Egypt. med. Ass.*, **38**, 601 (1955).

Ferguson, Rigdon and Couch. *Arch. Ophthal.*, **55**, 346 (1956).
Ferguson, Swanson, Couch *et al.* *Amer. J. Ophthal.*, **49**, 1165 (1960).
Ferrara. *Ann. Ottal.*, **68**, 529 (1940).
Ferraro and Roizin. *Arch. Ophthal.*, **38**, 331 (1947).
Gershoff, Andrus and Hegsted. *J. Nutrit.*, **68**, 75 (1959).
György. *Biochem. J.*, **29**, 741, 760, 767 (1935).
Hall, Bowles, Sydenstricker and Schmidt. *J. Nutrit.*, **36**, 277 (1948).
Jansen. *Acta brev. néerl. Physiol.*, **5**, 165 (1935).
Jess. *Klin. Mbl. Augenheilk.*, **74**, 49 (1925).
Krukowska. *Klin. oczna*, **21**, 113 (1951).
Lahiri. *Ind. vet. J.*, **15**, 55 (1938).
Langston and Day. *Sth. med. J.*, **26**, 128 (1933).
Langston, Day and Cosgrove. *Arch. Ophthal.*, **10**, 508 (1933).
Levina. *Festschr. f. Prof. Awerbach*, 157 (1926). See *Zbl. ges. Ophthal.*, **17**, 539 (1927).
McLaren. *Brit. J. Ophthal.*, **43**, 78 (1959). *Malnutrition and the Eye*, London (1963).
Monjukowa and Fradkin. *v. Graefes Arch. Ophthal.*, **133**, 328, 378 (1935).
Morone. *Rass. ital. Ottal.*, **29**, 209 (1950).
de Moura Campos and Rezende. *An. IV Cong. bras. Oftal.*, **3** (1942). See *Ophthal. ib.-amer.*, **4**, 192 (1942).
Mouriquand and Rollet. *C.R. Soc. Biol.* (Paris), **122**, 1118 (1936).

[1] Vol. III, p. 377.

O'Brien. *Arch. Ophthal.*, **8**, 880 (1932).

Ogino and Ichihara. *Amer. J. Ophthal.*, **43**, 754 (1957).

Patch. *Science*, **79**, 57 (1934). *Arch. Ophthal.*, **29**, 69 (1943).

Rezende and de Moura Campos. *Arch. Ophthal.*, **28**, 1038 (1942).

von Sallmann, Reid, Grimes and Collins. *Arch. Ophthal.*, **62**, 662 (1959).

Scardaccione. *Atti Cong. Soc. oftal. ital.*, **34**, 655 (1937).

Schaeffer and Geiger. *Proc. Soc. exp. Biol.* (N.Y.), **66**, 309 (1947).

Schaeffer and Murray. *Arch. Ophthal.*, **43**, 202 (1950).

Schreiber. *Ber. dtsch. ophthal. Ges.*, **45**, 272 (1925).

Sen, Das and Guha. *Science and Culture* (Calcutta), **1**, 59 (1935).

Stepp and Friedenwald. *Klin. Wschr.*, **3** (2), 2325 (1924).

Suda. *Acta Soc. ophthal. jap.*, **43**, 743 (1939).

Sydenstricker, Schmidt and Hall. *Proc. Soc. exp. Biol.* (N.Y.), **64**, 59 (1947).

von Szily and Eckstein. *Klin. Mbl. Augenheilk.*, **71**, 545 (1923).

Tainter and Borley. *Arch. Ophthal.*, **20**, 30 (1938).

Totter and Day. *J. Nutrit.*, **24**, 159 (1942).

Uyama, Ogino and Yamada. *Med. J. Osaka Univ.*, **6**, 519 (1955).

Wintrobe, Buschke, Follis and Humphreys. *Johns Hopk. Hosp. Bull.*, **75**, 102 (1944).

Yamada. *Acta Soc. ophthal. jap.*, **57**, 1004 (1953).

Yudkin. *J. Amer. med. Ass.*, **101**, 921 (1933). *Arch. Ophthal.*, **19**, 366 (1938). *Amer. J. Ophthal.*, **21**, 871 (1938).

CATARACT DUE TO A LOW CALCIUM/PHOSPHATE RATIO

It has been known since the observations of Logetschnikow (1872) that cataract may develop in children who suffer from muscular cramps, or of Landsberg (1888) that the same sequence occurred in patients after a thyroidectomy which included an accidental parathyroidectomy. The clinical occurrence of cataract of this type will be noted subsequently,[1] but in the meantime, it is sufficient to state that the lenticular opacities have been traced not to a hormonal influence but to a low calcium/phosphate ratio in the serum and are always accompanied by tetany, obvious or latent (Buschke, 1943; Bellows, 1944).

When cultured *in vitro* in a medium poor in calcium the lens develops opacities more rapidly than controls (von Bahr, 1940; Harris and Gehrsitz, 1951). In young experimental animals (dogs, rats, rabbits) cataract can also be induced by parathyroidectomy or by the deprivation of calcium from the diet to an extent sufficient to produce tetany, a change which can be stopped by the administration of calcium.[2] It will be remembered that the administration of the parathyroid hormone increases the calcium in the serum and the secretion of inorganic phosphates in the urine, while parathyroidectomy lowers the Ca/P ratio by decreasing the calcium in the serum and increasing its content of inorganic phosphates. von Bahr (1936) found on feeding animals on a rachitogenic diet, that if the Ca/P ratio were 4 : 1 in the diet no cataract developed, but if it were 1 : 1, a sudden fall of serum-calcium resulted and cataract immediately appeared. In his parathyroidectomized dogs, Rauh (1937) found that if the blood-calcium were kept at a normal level by the administration of irradiated ergosterol, no cataract resulted.

[1] p. 175.

[2] Erdheim (1906), Pfeiffer and Mayer (1908), Adler and Thaler (1908), Edmunds (1916), Luckhardt and Blumenstock (1923), Hiroishi (1924), Dragstedt *et al.* (1924), Siegrist (1927–28), Goldmann (1929), von Pellathy (1929), Rauh (1931–41), Borsellino (1934), von Bahr (1936), Campos (1937), Lo Cascio (1937), Bietti (1940–53), Rauh and Wagner (1941–50), Swan and Salit (1941), Fedrizzi (1948–55), Brolin (1953), and others.

FIGS. 105 to 108.—EXPERIMENTAL TETANIC CATARACT AFTER PARATHYROIDECTOMY
(H. Goldmann).

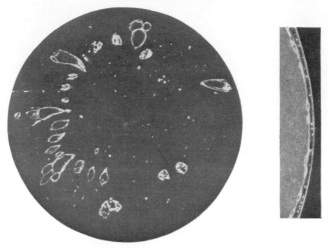

FIG. 105.   FIG. 106.

FIGS. 105 and 106.—Early changes of vacuoles and punctate opacities in the rat, 5 weeks
after the commencement of the experiment.

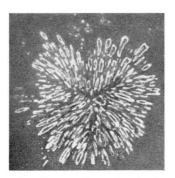

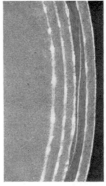

FIG. 107.—Rosette formation in the rat at   FIG. 108.—In the dog, after 21 months
a later stage.   during which time the animal was periodically
                                                 relieved by the administration of calcium.
                                                 Note the clear subcapsular interval.

The experimental cataract is characterized by the appearance of a
multitude of small discrete opacities in the subcapsular region and at a
later stage it spreads centrally along the sutures (Figs. 105–8). Goldmann
(1929), who was able to keep his parathyroidectomized dogs alive for some
months during which time he allowed periods of tetany to come and go by
withholding and administering calcium, found that during the periods of
deprivation subcapsular opacities developed, but when tetany was kept
away, clear fibres were laid down so that he was able to establish alternate

layers (in one case, six) of affected and clear zones in the cortex (Fig. 108). Histological examination showed signs of degeneration of the subcapsular epithelium and necrosis of the fibres in the underlying region, with the formation of vacuoles and the aggregation of cellular detritus, while the remainder of the eye was normal.

The ætiology of this type of cataract is unknown. The early explanation that the cataract was caused mechanically by a tetanic spasm of the ciliary muscle (Schmidt-Rimpler, 1883; Wettendorfer, 1897; Peters, 1900) is unlikely (Fedrizzi, 1954); equally implausible is the suggestion that some toxin such as tyramine, histamine and guanidine liberated from the muscles at the time of spasms affected the subcapsular epithelium and the fibres thereunder (Pineles, 1906; Goldmann, 1929; Weinstein, 1933). In the lens itself the content of calcium may not differ from that in control animals on a normal diet (Swan and Salit, 1941). A lack of glutathione has been reported (Lo Cascio, 1937), a decrease in anaerobic glycolysis and a reduction in the ability of the lens to produce lactic acid (Firschein, 1962), while the oxygen-uptake remains relatively normal (Campos, 1937). Possibly the action lies in the cellular ionic balance in the lens which is disturbed when calcium is withdrawn from the incubating fluid (Harris and Gehrsitz, 1951).

Adler and Thaler. *Z. Geburtsh. Gynäk.*, **62**, 194 (1908).
von Bahr. *Hygiea*, **98**, 797 (1936).
　Ber. dtsch. ophthal. Ges., **51**, 369 (1936).
　Acta ophthal. (Kbh.), **18**, 170 (1940).
Bellows. *Cataract and Anomalies of the Lens*, St. Louis (1944).
Bietti. *Klin. Mbl. Augenheilk.*, **105**, 299 (1940).
　Studi sassaresi, **19**, 134 (1941).
　Année thér. en ophtal., **4**, 261 (1953).
Borsellino. *Arch. Ottal.*, **41**, 57 (1934).
Brolin. *Acta ophthal.* (Kbh.), **31**, 485 (1953).
Buschke. *Arch. Ophthal.*, **30**, 735 (1943).
Campos. *Ann. Ottal.*, **65**, 481 (1937).
Dragstedt, Sudan and Phillips. *Amer. J. Physiol.*, **69**, 477 (1924).
Edmunds. *Proc. roy. Soc. Med.*, **9**, Sect. Ophthal., 53 (1916).
Erdheim. *Mitt. Grenzgeb. Med. Chir.*, Jena, **16**, 632 (1906).
Fedrizzi. *Atti Cong. Soc. oftal. ital.*, **10**, 439 (1948).
　Atti Soc. oftal. Lomb., **9**, 256 (1954); **10**, 128 (1955).
Firschein. *Invest. Ophthal.*, **1**, 788 (1962).
Goldmann. *v. Graefes Arch. Ophthal.*, **122**, 146 (1929).
Harris and Gehrsitz. *Amer. J. Ophthal.*, **34** (2), 131 (1951).
Hiroishi. *v. Graefes Arch. Ophthal.*, **113**, 381 (1924).

Landsberg. *Zbl. prakt. Augenheilk.*, **12**, 39 (1888).
Lo Cascio. *XV int. Cong. Ophthal.*, Cairo, **3**, 401 (1937).
Logetschnikow. *Klin. Mbl. Augenheilk.*, **10**, 351 (1872).
Luckhardt and Blumenstock. *Amer. J. Physiol.*, **63**, 409 (1923).
von Pellathy. *Klin. Mbl. Augenheilk.*, **83**, 438 (1929).
Peters. *Z. Augenheilk.*, **4**, 337 (1900).
Pfeiffer and Mayer. *Mitt. Grenzgeb. Med. Chir.*, Jena, **18**, 377 (1908).
Pineles. *Zbl. prakt. Augenheilk.*, **30**, 235 (1906).
Rauh. *Ber. dtsch. ophthal. Ges.*, **51**, 357 (1936).
　XV int. Cong. Ophthal., Cairo, **4** (Comm. libres), 36 (1937).
　v. Graefes Arch. Ophthal., **126**, 256 (1931).
　Klin. Mbl. Augenheilk., **107**, 59 (1941).
Rauh and Wagner. *v. Graefes Arch. Ophthal.*, **143**, 85 (1941).
　Ber. dtsch. ophthal. Ges., **56**, 233 (1950).
Schmidt-Rimpler. *Klin. Mbl. Augenheilk.*, **21**, 181 (1883).
Siegrist. *Ber. dtsch. ophthal. Ges.*, **46**, 217 (1927).
　Der graue Altersstar, Berlin (1928).
Swan and Salit. *Amer. J. Ophthal.*, **24**, 611 (1941).
Weinstein. *Brit. J. Ophthal.*, **17**, 236 (1933).
Wettendorfer. *Wien. med. Wschr.*, **47**, 469, 528, 1656 (1897).

ENDOCRINE CATARACT

Apart from the conditions of hypoparathyroidism and diabetes, which are recognized as causing endocrine cataracts, several other ductless glands are associated with disturbances in the lens, particularly the adrenals and the thyroid.

THE CORTICOSTEROIDS

Although it has been established that the systemic administration of the corticosteroids may lead to the development of a cataract commencing subcapsularly near the posterior pole of the lens, attempts to reproduce this condition in animals have not been successful. It is true that Bonavolontà and de Berardinis (1951) claimed that after large doses of cortisone administered subcutaneously in rats there was some increase in the optical density of the nucleus of the lens, and that Haour and Rougier (1950) and Thorn and his colleagues (1959) obtained some cataractous changes, but this slight effect was not reproduced in these animals by von Sallmann and his colleagues (1960) nor by Bettman and his co-workers (1964) in chicks. That these substances may have some effect on the metabolism of the lens, however, is suggested by the finding of Yuge (1962) that bovine lenses cultured

FIGS. 109 and 110.—EXPERIMENTAL STEROID CATARACT (E. Cotlier and B. Becker).

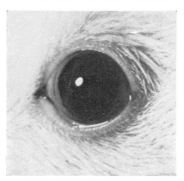 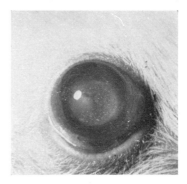

FIG. 109.—The normal eye of the rat receiving 40% galactose in the diet for 30 days.

FIG. 110.—The eye of the same rat treated with betamethasone.

in a solution containing prednisone showed some inhibition of glycolysis affecting the hexose-monophosphate shunt, as well as a disturbance of the transport mechanisms for sodium (Harris and Gruber, 1962) and rubidium (Becker and Cotlier, 1965). Moreover, it has been found that the action of other cataractogenic agents could be intensified if steroids were also administered ; this has been observed after subcataractous doses of dinitrophenol in chicks (Bettman et al., 1964) and in rats fed galactose whether the steroid were given systemically (Bettman et al., 1964–68) or topically (Cotlier and Becker, 1965) (Figs. 109–10). It would thus seem that the steroids have a minimal cataractogenic action of an unknown nature ; the only pointer so far suggested is some small upset of glycolytic metabolism or fluid transport.

ADRENALINE has been found to produce lenticular opacities in the mouse (tum Suden, 1940) and the rat (tum Suden and Wyman, 1940), while Redslob (1927) produced a cataract by its intravitreal or retrobulbar injection. It has also been induced in the fœtus of the rat by the intra-uterine injection of adrenaline, an action unlikely to be due to a vasoconstrictor action on the hyaloid vessels since drugs with a similar action have no cataractogenic effect (Pitel and Lerman, 1962; Lerman *et al.*, 1962).

THYROXINE administered to pregnant rats results in the formation of congenital cataract in the young,[1] and given to 5-week-old rats causes an increase in the synthesis of albuminoid (Dische and Zelmenis, 1959). It may be noted that partial destruction of the thyroid by radiation in pregnant rats soon after conception leads to fœtal absorption and the production of multiple deformities including cataract in the young (Coulaud and Rochon-Duvigneaud, 1926); partial thyroidectomy has the same effect (Chu, 1945; Langman and van Faassen, 1955).

INSULIN is capable of producing lenticular opacities both in man and experimental animals (Cristini, 1946; Bietti and Siliprandi, 1951; de Conciliis, 1956); the opacities can be reversed on the administration of glucose and are probably determined by an osmotic effect more marked than that causing the refractive changes which accompany a chronic state of hypoglycæmia.

Becker and Cotlier. *Invest. Ophthal.*, **4**, 117 (1965).

Bettman, Fung and Noyes. *Invest. Ophthal.*, **3**, 678 (1964).

Bettman, Fung, Webster *et al.* *Amer. J. Ophthal.*, **65**, 581 (1968).

Bettman, Noyes and DeBoskey. *Invest. Ophthal.*, **3**, 459 (1964).

Bietti and Siliprandi. *Ann. Oculist* (Paris), **184**, 346 (1951).
Ophthalmologica, **121**, 67 (1951).

Bonavolontà and de Berardinis. *Boll. Soc. ital. Biol. sper.*, **27**, 1339 (1951).

Chu. *J. Endocr.*, **4**, 109 (1945).

de Conciliis. *Ann. Ottal.*, **82**, 465 (1956).

Cotlier and Becker. *Invest. Ophthal.*, **4**, 806 (1965).

Coulaud and Rochon-Duvigneaud. *Clin. Ophthal.*, **15**, 706 (1926).

Cristini. *Riv. Oftal.*, **1**, 156 (1946).

Dische and Zelmenis. *Amer. J. Ophthal.*, **48** (2), 500 (1959).

Giroud and Martinet. *C.R. Soc. Biol.* (Paris), **147**, 997 (1953); **148**, 1742 (1954).
Arch. Ophtal., **14**, 247 (1954).

Giroud and de Rothschild. *C.R. Soc. Biol.* (Paris), **145**, 525 (1951).
Bull. Soc. Ophtal. Fr., 543 (1951).

Giroud, de Rothschild and Lefebvres-Boisselot. *Ann. Endocr.* (Paris), **12**, 610 (1951).

Haour and Rougier. *Bull. Soc. Ophtal. Fr.*, 518 (1950).

Harris and Gruber. *Exp. Eye Res.*, **1**, 372 (1962).

Langman and van Faassen. *Ned. T. Geneesk.*, **99**, 2119 (1955).
Amer. J. Ophthal., **40**, 65 (1955).

Lerman, Donk and Pitel. *Growth*, **26**, 103 (1962).

Martinet, Baron and Guillon. *C.R. Soc. Biol.* (Paris), **147**, 1911 (1953).

Pitel and Lerman. *Invest. Ophthal.*, **1**, 406 (1962).

Redslob. *Bull. Soc. franç. Ophtal.*, **40**, 373 (1927).

von Sallmann, Caravaggio, Collins and Weaver. *Amer. J. Ophthal.*, **50**, 1147 (1960).

tum Suden. *Amer. J. Physiol.*, **130**, 543 (1940).

tum Suden and Wyman. *Endocrinology*, **27**, 628 (1940).

Thorn, Renold and Camill. *Diabetes*, **8**, 337 (1959).

Tusques. *C.R. Soc. Biol.* (Paris), **149**, 1170 (1955).

Yugc. *Folia ophthal. jap.*, **13**, 64 (1962).

TOXIC CATARACT

Several toxic substances of a variety of types are cataractogenic when administered systemically; these may be classified as hydrocarbons or substituted hydrocarbons (particularly naphthalene and dinitrophenol), the salts of certain metals (thallium, cobalt, selenium), anti-mitotic agents, enzyme-inhibitors (such as iodoacetic acid), and a number of drugs.

[1] Giroud and de Rothschild (1951), Giroud *et al.* (1951), Giroud and Martinet (1953–54), Martinet *et al.* (1953), Tusques (1955).

Hydrocarbons and Substituted Hydrocarbons

NAPHTHALENE CATARACT

NAPHTHALENE administered systemically is a potent cataractogenic
agent, an effect initially communicated to the French Academy of Medicine
as a chance occurrence by Bouchard and Charrin in 1886, and subsequently
experimentally produced usually in rabbits but also in cats, rats, guinea-
pigs and chicken by many workers[1]; such a lesion, however, occurs only
exceptionally in man.

The rare occurrence of naphthalene cataract in man is interesting. Lezenius
(1902) reported a case in a man following the ingestion of 5 G. of naphthalene. It has
developed in a worker in an explosives factory (Caspar, 1917) and in a dye-plant
(Ghetti and Mariani, 1956); in van der Hoeve's (1902) patient lenticular opacities
appeared after the prolonged use of an ointment containing naphthalene.

To induce the formation of an experimental cataract and yet maintain
the health of the animal the optimum dose should not exceed 1 G. of naphthalene per kg. body-weight, but animals vary greatly in the dosage and
time required to develop lenticular changes. These usually appear within
2 or 3 weeks after the commencement of the feeding; but cataract may be
obvious in a day or two after a single large dose, or may not develop even
if large doses are given over prolonged periods (Panas, 1887). During the
diet in the majority of cases the animals remain relatively healthy, but
hæmorrhagic and exudative changes may appear in the eye, and signs of a
general toxæmia, particularly of a gastro-intestinal nature, are common; in
some cases these have been so severe as to cause death before the development of the lens opacities.[2] Jess (1921–30) claimed to have produced a
similar type of cataract after the subcutaneous injection of a 20% naph-
thalene-paraffin emulsion. It is also interesting that when pregnant rabbits
are fed with naphthalene, the offspring may develop cataract, and if the
diet is commenced before the separation of the lens vesicle has occurred
(11th day of gestation) the changes in the lens are associated with other
gross ocular anomalies (Pagenstecher, 1911; Vasilev *et al.*, 1960). The
production of naphthalene cataract has been found to be inhibited by a diet
rich in cabbage (Bourne and Campbell, 1933); this is coincident with a high
blood-calcium, ascribed by Bellows (1936) to the richness of ascorbic acid
in these vegetables, a finding corroborated by Yoritaka and his colleagues
(1958).

[1] Hess (1887), Dor (1887), Panas (1887), Kolinsky (1889), Magnus (1890), Faravelli
(1893), Manca and Ovio (1896–98), Ovio (1898), Salffner (1904), van der Hoeve (1907), Takamura (1912), Lindberg (1922), Cade and Barral (1928), Adams (1930), Bourne (1933), von Euler
and Malmberg (1934), Müller *et al.* (1934), Bourne and Young (1934), Stekol (1935–37), Basile
(1939), Weekers (1941), Simonelli (1948), Fitzhugh and Buschke (1949), Brolin (1950), Ogino and
Sobagaki (1951), Nordmann and Mandel (1952), Uyama *et al.* (1955), Uyama and Ogino (1956),
Nakamura (1956), Pirie (1968), and others.
[2] Kolinsky (1889), Klingmann (1897), Igersheimer and Ruben (1910), Michaïl and Vancea
(1926–40), Panico (1928), and others.

The lenticular changes in the rabbit after the administration of naphthalene are bilateral and remarkably consistent; an initial increase in
weight and volume of the lens due to the imbibition of fluid is followed
within 24 hours by the appearance of fluid vacuoles, which are rapidly
succeeded by the development of a true opacity of the lenticular fibres
beginning at the periphery, spreading through the cortex, and finally
involving the nucleus. Before the opacities appear the fluorescence of the
lens is increased (Brolin, 1950). Within 5 days from its onset the cataract
is usually complete (Fig. 111); both lenses are milky-white but they eventually tend to develop a grey or brown pigmentation. Lindberg (1922) noted

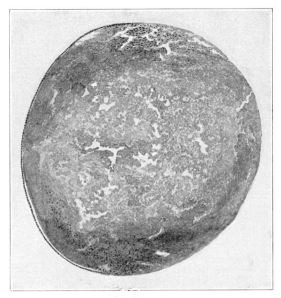

Fig. 111.—Naphthalene Cataract.
In the rabbit, showing complete destruction of the fibres (A. von Szily).

that the opacity first became evident in the portion of the lens covered by
iris, that it was more peripheral when the pupil was kept dilated, and that
a colobomatous area remained free for some time after an iridectomy.

The histological changes resemble very closely those of senile cataract
and include a derangement of mitoses in the subcapsular epithelium (Fukuhara, 1959), a subcapsular accumulation of fluid, the separation of the fibres
by homogeneous material, the appearance of vacuoles in the fibres, and
eventually a proliferation of the epithelium and complete destruction of the
fibres.[1] Unless the naphthalene is stopped before the stage at which actual
opacities first appear, discontinuance of the chemical does not prevent the

[1] Hess (1887), Klingmann (1897), Salffner (1904), Busacca (1927), Panico (1928), Adams
(1930), Ogino et al. (1957), Pirie (1968).

full development of cataract. Coincidental changes, mainly exudative in nature, may be found in the uveal tract and retina.

Several derivatives of naphthalene have been found to be similarly cataractogenic: TETRA-HYDRO NAPHTHALENE (Tetralin) (Badinand *et al.*, 1947), DECA-HYDRO NAPHTHALENE (Basile, 1939; Badinand *et al.*, 1947; Smyth *et al.*, 1951), β-TETRALOL, which is twice as potent (Fitzhugh and Buschke, 1949), β-NAPHTHOQUINONE (in guinea-pigs, Uyama *et al.*, 1955; Ogino *et al.*, 1957; but not in rabbits, Kiuchi, 1959). This last substance causes opacities to develop in incubated lenses, an action which Yuge (1962) ascribed to a prevention of the formation of reduced glutathione.

The cause of the development of lenticular opacities is still unknown, but they would appear to be due to a disturbance of the lenticular metabolism rather than to the production of a specific toxin. Naphthalene has not been demonstrated to penetrate into the aqueous humour, while no significant changes have been observed in the serum with the exception of an increase in its content of conjugated glucuronic acid, a metabolite of naphthalene, coincidentally with the development of lenticular opacities; this substance has also been found in the eye and it is probably a cataractogenic agent in view of the fact that its diminution in the serum after the exhibition of carbon tetrachloride appears to suppress the development of cataract (Takagi and Okamura, 1961; Okamura, 1962).

Certain changes have been observed in the lens which may or may not be apposite: a decrease in its content of protein, especially β-crystallin (Tsuji, 1932), a diminution of glutathione at a very early stage even before the development of opacities (Gifford, 1932; Tsuji, 1932; Müller, 1939; Kinsey and Merriam, 1950), a decrease in the high-energy phosphates and in the concentration of glucose (Müller, 1939; Nordmann *et al.*, 1952; Kusuki, 1958) and an increase in lactic acid (Kinsey and Merriam, 1950; Nordmann *et al.*, 1952) together with a decrease in lactic dehydrogenase and malic enzyme (Salmony, 1960). It has been claimed that the topical injection of glutathione has no inhibitory effect (Dorello, 1952). van Heyningen and Pirie (1966) found that one of the breakdown-products of naphthalene in the blood, 1,2-naphthoquinone, combined with the proteins of the lens. In incubated lenses taken from experimental animals there is an initial rise and subsequent fall in the consumption of glucose and an increase in the output of CO_2 (Nordmann *et al.*, 1952), an effect found to be widespread by Ponte and Pandolfo (1957) in experimental animals, affecting particularly aerobic glycolysis.

It has been suggested that animals fed on naphthalene used up their available cysteine with which this chemical becomes conjugated so that the stock of this amino acid in the lens was depleted and the activity of its oxidative mechanism was thus diminished (Bourne and Young, 1934; White, 1936; Bourne, 1937), but the evidence for this is by no means conclusive. It would appear, however, that whatever its mechanism, before there are any visible changes in the lens there is an unexplained increase in its glycolysis, while the combination of the proteins of the lens with the breakdown-products of naphthalene which reach the eye by way of the blood is probably significant.

Adams. *Brit. J. Ophthal.*, **14**, 49, 545 (1930).
Badinand, Paufique and Rodier. *Arch. Mal. prof.*, **8**, 124 (1947).
Basile. *Boll. Oculist.*, **18**, 951 (1939).
Bellows. *Arch. Ophthal.*, **16**, 762 (1936).
Bouchard and Charrin. *C.R. Soc. Biol.* (Paris), **8**, 614 (1886).
Bourne. *Brit. J. Ophthal.*, **17**, 210 (1933). *Physiol. Rev.*, **17**, 1 (1937).

Bourne and Campbell. *Brit. J. Ophthal.*, **17**, 220 (1933).
Bourne and Young. *Biochem. J.*, **28**, 803 (1934).
Brolin. *Acta ophthal.* (Kbh.), **28**, 163 (1950).
Busacca. *Atti reale Accad. naz. Lincei*, Roma, **6**, 175 (1927).
Cade and Barral. *C.R. Soc. Biol.* (Paris), **99**, 520 (1928).

Caspar. *Klin. Mbl. Augenheilk.*, **59**, 142 (1917).

Dor. *Bull. Soc. franç. Ophtal.*, **5**, 150 (1887).

Dorello. *Boll. Soc. ital. Biol. sper.*, **28**, 2013 (1952).

von Euler and Malmberg. *Hoppe-Seyl. Z. physiol. Chem.*, **230**, 225 (1934).

Faravelli. *Ann. Ottal.*, **22**, 8 (1893).

Fitzhugh and Buschke. *Arch. Ophthal.*, **41**, 572 (1949).

Fukuhara. *Folia ophthal. jap.*, **10**, 37 (1959).

Ghetti and Mariani. *Med. d. Lavoro*, **47**, 533 (1956).

Gifford. *Arch. Ophthal.*, **7**, 763 (1932).

Hess. *Ber. dtsch. ophthal. Ges.*, **19**, 54 (1887).

van Heyningen and Pirie. *Biochem. J.*, **100**, 70P (1966).

van der Hoeve. *v. Graefes Arch. Ophthal.*, **53**, 74 (1902).

Arch. Augenheilk., **56**, 259 (1907).

Igersheimer and Ruben. *v. Graefes Arch. Ophthal.*, **74**, 467 (1910).

Jess. *v. Graefes Arch. Ophthal.*, **104**, 48 (1921).

Kurzes Hb. d. Ophthal., Berlin, **3**, 170 (1930).

Kinsey and Merriam. *Arch. Ophthal.*, **44**, 370 (1950).

Kiuchi. *Shikoku Acta med.*, **14**, 110 (1959).

Klingmann. *Pflügers Arch. ges. Physiol.*, **149**, 12 (1897).

Kolinsky. *v. Graefes Arch. Ophthal.*, **35** (2), 29 (1889).

Kusuki. *Folia ophthal. jap.*, **9**, 85 (1958).

Lezenius. *Klin. Mbl. Augenheilk.*, **40** (1), 129 (1902).

Lindberg. *Klin. Mbl. Augenheilk.*, **68**, 527 (1922).

Magnus. *v. Graefes Arch. Ophthal.*, **36** (4), 150 (1890).

Manca and Ovio. *Arch. Ottal.*, **4**, 167 (1896); **5**, 112, 141 (1897); **6**, 69 (1898).

Michaïl and Vancea. *C.R. Soc. Biol.* (Paris), **94**, 291 (1926); **96**, 63, 65, 1456; **97**, 1097, 1569 (1927); **134**, 309 (1940).

Müller. *v. Graefes Arch. Ophthal.*, **140**, 171 (1939).

Müller, Buschke, Gurewitsch and Brühl. *Klin. Wschr.*, **13**, 20 (1934).

Nakamura. *Acta Soc. ophthal. jap.*, **60**, 291, 924 (1956).

Nordmann and Mandel. *Bull. Soc. belge Ophtal.*, No. 102, 524 (1952).

Nordmann, Zimmer and Mandel. *C.R. Soc. Biol.* (Paris), **146**, 1804 (1952).

Ogino and Sobagaki. *Acta Soc. ophthal. jap.*, **55**, 606 (1951).

Ogino, Tojo, Fujishige and Katumori. *Amer. J. Ophthal.*, **44**, 94 (1957).

Okamura. *Acta Soc. ophthal. jap.*, **66**, 290 (1962).

Ovio. *Arch. Ottal.*, **6**, 69 (1898).

Pagenstecher. *Ber. dtsch. ophthal. Ges.*, **37**, 44 (1911).

Panas. *Ann. Oculist.* (Paris), **97**, 247, 313 (1887).

Panico. *Ann. Ottal.*, **56**, 799 (1928).

Pirie. *Exp. Eye Res.*, **7**, 354 (1968).

Ponte and Pandolfo. *Boll. Soc. ital. Biol. sper.*, **33**, 1792, 1794, 1796 (1957).

Salffner. *v. Graefes Arch. Ophthal.*, **59**, 520 (1904).

Salmony. *Brit. J. Ophthal.*, **44**, 29 (1960).

Simonelli. *G. ital. Oftal.*, **1**, 47 (1948).

Smyth, Carpenter and Weil. *Arch. indust. Hyg. occup. Med.*, **4**, 119 (1951).

Stekol. *J. biol. Chem.*, **110**, 463 (1935); **113**, 475 (1936); **117**, 147 (1937).

Takagi and Okamura. *Acta Soc. ophthal. jap.*, **65**, 1162 (1961).

Takamura. *Arch. Augenheilk.*, **70**, 335 (1912).

Tsuji. *J. Biochem.* (Tokyo), **15**, 33 (1932).

Uyama and Ogino. *Med. J. Osaka Univ.*, **6**, 813 (1956).

Uyama, Ogino and Ichihara. *Med. J. Osaka Univ.*, **6**, 229 (1955).

Uyama, Ogino, Ichihara *et al.* *Med. J. Osaka Univ.*, **6**, 771 (1955).

Vasilev, Dabov and Rankov. *Nauc. trudove*, ISUL, **7**, 143 (1960).

Weekers. *Recherches expér. et clin. concernant la pathogénie des cataractes* (Thèse), Liège (1941).

White. *J. biol. Chem.*, **112**, 503 (1936).

Yoritaka, Tominaga, Semba and Hiwaki. *Folia ophthal. jap.*, **9**, 1 (1958).

Yuge. *Acta Soc. ophthal. jap.*, **66**, 1135 (1962).

DINITROPHENOL CATARACT

Although dinitrophenol has long been recognized as cataractogenic to man, particularly to women when taken as a drug to reduce the body-weight by increasing metabolic activity,[1] the effect is readily produced among animals only in avians. If 0·25% dinitrophenol is added to the feed of ducklings and young chicks, fine vacuoles appear in the anterior lens fibres in 4 to 6 hours and marked degeneration of the fibres near the posterior pole occurs in 3 to 5 days (Robbins, 1944; Dietrich and Beutner, 1946; Buschke, 1947).

[1] Vol. XIV.

Even although dinitrophenol produces the same increase in the oxidative metabolism in mammals as in man, most attempts to produce lenticular opacities in the former have been futile even if animals susceptible to experimental cataract have been dosed with the drug up to fatal concentrations continuously from weaning until death (rats, rabbits, guinea-pigs).[1] This failure persists even when every other encouragement to the formation of cataract is afforded, such as by feeding with a vitamin-deficient diet (Borley and Tainter, 1938) or with lactose (Borley and Tainter, 1938) or after thyroidectomy (Smelser, 1941). Exceptional positive results, however, were obtained in albino rats (Cordero, 1937–38), hypocalcæmic rabbits with tetany (Zilliacus, 1941), obese mice (Bettman, 1946), and vitamin-C-deficient guinea-pigs (Ogino and Yasukura, 1957). It has also been produced by the direct injection of dinitrophenol into the anterior chamber of rabbits as well as chicks (de Conciliis, 1955) and axial posterior subcapsular opacities have been seen in the offspring of pregnant rabbits dosed with dinitrophenol (Vassilev *et al.*, 1959) as well as in chicks after injection into the eggs (Feldman *et al.*, 1958–60).

The rationale of dinitrophenol cataract is presumably a disturbance of the oxidative metabolism (Field *et al.*, 1937). It has been shown that dinitrophenol administered orally finds its way into the lens (Horner, 1936) but it has no precipitating effect *in vitro* upon the lenticular proteins (D. and F. Cogan, 1935), nor does it change the permeability of the capsule either *in vivo* or *in vitro* (Borley and Tainter, 1937). In acute poisoning with the drug, anoxia of all the tissues may occur with an accumulation of lactic acid when the demand for oxygen exceeds consumption (Tainter, 1935; MacBryde and Taussig, 1935). The cataract might therefore be due to anoxia following an increase of cellular metabolism above the level at which it can be adequately met, acting by changing the phosphate metabolism of the lens so as to affect oxidative phosphorylation (D. and F. Cogan, 1935), as well as by reducing the oxygen-uptake [and increasing the lactic acid (Kleifeld and Hockwin, 1956). Yasukura (1955), Ogino and Yasukura (1957) and Ogino and his colleagues (1957) considered that one of the metabolites of dinitrophenol, 2-amino-*p*-quinonimine, was the cataractogenic agent.

PARADICHLOROBENZENE, a moth-repellant and insecticide, is known to produce cataract in man on inhalation after a delay of some months; Berliner (1939) was unable to produce an experimental cataract with it except in one rabbit which was fed orally with this substance. The insecticide, HEPTACHLOR, however, has been found to produce cataracts not only in 22% of rats when added daily to their food for 18 months but also in up to 16% of their sucklings (Mestitzová, 1967).

Basile. *Ann. Ottal.*, **67**, 223 (1939).
Berliner. *Arch. Ophthal.*, **22**, 1023 (1939).
Bettman. *Amer. J. Ophthal.*, **29**, 1388 (1946).
Borley and Tainter. *Arch. Ophthal.*, **18**, 908 (1937); **20**, 30 (1938).
    Amer. J. Ophthal., **21**, 1091 (1938).
Buschke. *Amer. J. Ophthal.*, **30**, 1356 (1947).
Cogan, D. and F. *J. Amer. med. Ass.*, **105**, 793 (1935).

de Conciliis. *Boll. Oculist.*, **34**, 65 (1955).
Cordero. *Arch. Ottal.*, **44**, 152, 213, 294 (1937); **45**, 105, 203, 295, 331 (1938).
Dietrich and Beutner. *Fed. Proc.*, **5**, 174 (1946).
Feldman, Ferguson and Couch. *Amer. J. Ophthal.*, **49**, 1168 (1960).
Feldman, Ferguson, Rigdon *et al.* *Proc. Soc. exp. Biol.* (N.Y.), **98**, 646 (1958).

[1] Helminen (1937), Tainter (1938), Sohr (1938), Basile (1939), Vannas (1939), Meyer (1940).

Field, Tainter, Martin and Belding. *Amer. J. Ophthal.*, **20**, 779 (1937).

Helminen. *Acta ophthal.* (Kbh.), **15**, 490 (1937).

Horner. *Arch. Ophthal.*, **16**, 447 (1936).

Kleifeld and Hockwin. *v. Graefes Arch. Ophthal.*, **158**, 54 (1956).

MacBryde and Taussig. *J. Amer. med. Ass.*, **105**, 13 (1935).

Mestitzová. *Experientia* (Basel), **23**, 42 (1967).

Meyer. *Klin. Mbl. Augenheilk.*, **104**, 339 (1940).

Ogino, Tojo, Fujishige and Katumori. *Amer. J. Ophthal.*, **44**, 94 (1957).

Ogino and Yasukura. *Amer. J. Ophthal.*, **43**, 936 (1957).

Robbins. *J. Pharm. exp. Therap.*, **80**, 264; **82**, 301 (1944).

Smelser. *Amer. J. Ophthal.*, **24**, 680 (1941).

Sohr. *v. Graefes Arch. Ophthal.*, **138**, 332 (1938).

Tainter. *J. Pharm. exp. Therap.*, **51**, 45, 143 (1934); **63**, 51 (1938). *J. Amer. med. Ass.*, **104**, 1071 (1935).

Vannas. *Orvosképzés*, **29**, 416 (1939). See *Zbl. ges. Ophthal.*, **44**, 363 (1939).

Vassilev, Dabov and Rankov. *Arch. Ophtal.*, **19**, 13 (1959).

Yasukura. *Acta Soc. ophthal. jap.*, **59**, 72, 925 (1955).

Zilliacus. *Nord. Med.*, **11**, 2388 (1941).

Metallic Salts

THALLIUM

In experiments on rats fed on thallium acetate, widespread damage has occurred in many epithelial structures throughout the body, involving alopœcia, gastro-intestinal symptoms, polyneuritis and optic neuritis, and several animals have been found to develop cataract, occasionally bilaterally.[1] Thallium appeared to be the responsible agent although other unexplained individual or genetic factors seemed to determine its incidence. The lenticular changes appeared as subcapsular opacities which remained stationary if the diet were stopped but proceeded to complete opacification if it were continued (Figs. 112–15). At the stage of total cataract, but not before, there are sometimes evidences of iridocyclitis and corneal vascularization. Microscopic examination has shown that the subcapsular epithelium of the lens is absent or has proliferated into several layers, and that the most marked changes in the lenticular fibres are in the axial region where accumulations of homogeneous or granular material may be considerable (Donski, 1932 (Fig. 115)).

A cataract of this type may occur occasionally in man; Kubesova (1949) reported a case wherein lenticular opacities developed in the deeper parts of the anterior and posterior cortex.

COBALT. In rabbits and rats intoxication with cobalt chloride has been found to be accompanied by the development of cataract somewhat resembling that induced by alloxan along with hepatic and splenic lesions, all of which could to some extent be reduced by the simultaneous administration of cysteine (Alagna and d'Aquino, 1956). The same investigators (1957) found in rabbits that cataract and degenerative changes in the uveal tract and nervous tissues accompanied SELENIUM intoxication.

Alagna and d'Aquino. *Arch. Ottal.*, **60**, 5 (1956); **61**, 55 (1957).

Alvarez-Castelao. *Med. españ.*, **5**, 395, 501 (1941).

Buschke. *Arch. Ophthal.*, **30**, 735 (1943).

Buschke, Löwenstein and Joel. *Klin. Wschr.*, **7**, 1515 (1928).

Buschke and Peiser. *Dtsch. med. Wschr.*, **48**, 1466 (1922).

[1] Buschke and Peiser (1922), Ginsberg and Buschke (1923), Buschke *et al.* (1928), Donski (1932), Puglisi-Durante (1933), Tanaka (1938), Alvarez-Castelao (1941), Buschke (1943).

FIGS. 112 TO 115.—THALLIUM CATARACT IN RATS.

A white rat, 4 weeks old, 40 G. weight, given thallium acetate 1 in 10,000 1 ml. daily for 46 days; 2 ml. daily for 116 days; nil for 10 days; 3 ml. daily for 5 days (J. Donski).

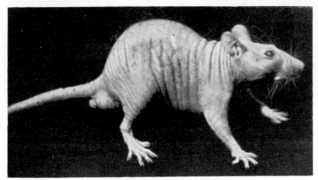

FIG. 112.—The cataract is macroscopically visible; alopœcia is complete.

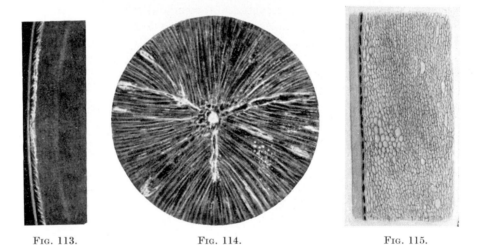

FIG. 113.   FIG. 114.   FIG. 115.

FIGS. 113 TO 115.—The lens of such an animal, showing a dense opacity which is largely subcapsular (Fig. 113). The lens is seen in microscopic section in Fig. 115.

Donski.   *v. Graefes Arch. Ophthal.*, **128**, 294 (1932).

Ginsberg and Buschke.   *Klin. Mbl. Augenheilk.*, **71**, 385 (1923).

Kubesova.   *Csl. Ofthal.*, **5**, 149 (1949).

Puglisi-Durante.   *Rass. ital. Ottal.*, **2**, 1158 (1933).

Tanaka.   *Acta Soc. ophthal. jap.*, **42**, 1615 (1938).

Anti-mitotic Agents

Several RADIOMIMETIC ANTI-MITOTIC AGENTS have been found to be cataractogenic to experimental animals. Of these the most fully explored has been 1,4-dimethanesulphonoxybutane (busulphan; Myleran) (Solomon *et al.*, 1955; Light *et al.*, 1956; von Sallmann, 1957; Kandori and Kurimoto,

1960).   In rats the first changes are degeneration and nuclear fragmentation of the cells of the subcapsular epithelium followed after 5 to 7 weeks by the subcapsular opacities progressing from the equator to the posterior and anterior subcapsular zones, the whole somewhat resembling a radiational cataract (Fig. 116).   Hammar and Brolin (1959) found an increase in the fluorescence of the lens, and del Pianto and his colleagues (1958) a decrease in the sulphydryl groups.

Other radiomimetic chemicals have been found to produce lenticular opacities after systemic administration: nitrogen mustard, triethylene melamine (TEM), 4-(p-dimethylaminostyryl) quinoline (Conklin *et al.*, 1963; Christenberry *et al.*, 1963) and

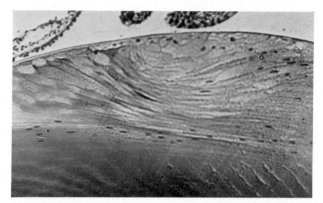

FIG. 116.—EXPERIMENTAL MYLERAN CATARACT.
The lens of a rat, showing moderate displacement of the bow nuclei and hydrops of the equatorial fibres 7 weeks after starting a diet with Myleran (L. von Sallmann).

2,3,5 triethylenamino-1-4-benzoquinone (Trenimon) which causes a unilateral cataract 30 to 40 days after the intracarotid injection of the drug in mice (Apponi *et al.*, 1964).   A clouding of the lens has been seen in rabbits after intravitreal injections of nitrogen mustard, cyclophosphamide (Endoxana), methotrexate and other anti-mitotic agents by Ericson and his colleagues (1964).

MIMOSINE (LEUCENOL) CATARACT.   A cytotoxic agent, β[3-hydroxy-4-pyridone]-α-amino propionic acid, was isolated from the leaves and seeds of *Leucœna glauca* by Mascré (1937), who called it *leucenol*, and from *Mimosa pudica* by Kleipool and Wibaut (1950) who called it *mimosine*.   Administered to rats it causes stunted growth and loss of hair, transient inflammatory signs in the cornea and iris, and a permanent and complete cataract (Yoshida, 1944; von Sallmann *et al.*, 1959; Tittarelli *et al.*, 1961). The changes in the lens are unique.   The first effect is anti-mitotic in the equatorial zone of the subcapsular epithelium, appearing dramatically within 3 days of adding the agent to the feed, and this is rapidly followed by a hydropic swelling of the superficial lenticular fibres, particularly in the equatorial area, and in the later stages by a complete disorganization of the fibres throughout the lens (Fig. 117).   It seems probable that the toxic agent reaches the eye from the blood, attacks first the epithelium and then diffuses throughout the lens causing destruction of the fibres, proteolysis and opacification.

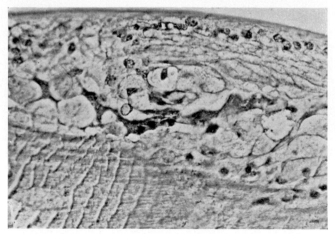

Fig. 117.—Experimental Mimosine Cataract.

The lens of a rat, showing advanced changes in the equatorial area with degenerated cells and hydrops of the superficial fibres on the 7th day of mimosine feeding (L. von Sallmann *et al.*).

Apponi, Rinaldi and de Simone. *Ann. Ottal.*, **90**, 224 (1964).

Christenberry, Conklin, Upton and Cosgrove. *Arch. Ophthal.*, **70**, 250 (1963).

Conklin, Upton, Christenberry and McDonald. *Rad. Res.*, **19**, 156 (1963).

Ericson, Karlberg and Rosengren. *Acta ophthal.* (Kbh.), **42**, 721 (1964).

Hammar and Brolin. *Acta ophthal.* (Kbh.), **37**, 344 (1959).

Kandori and Kurimoto. *Acta path. jap.*, **10**, 35 (1960).

Kleipool and Wibaut. *Rec. trav. chim.*, **69**, 37 (1950).

Light, Solomon and de Beer. *J. Nutrit.*, **60**, 157 (1956).

Mascré. *C.R. Acad. Sci.* (Paris), **204**, 890 (1937).

del Pianto, Bozzoni and Valesini. *Boll. Oculist.*, **37**, 40 (1958).

von Sallmann. *Amer. J. Ophthal.*, **44**, 159 (1957).

von Sallmann, Grimes and Collins. *Amer. J. Ophthal.*, **47** (2), 107 (1959).

Solomon, Light and de Beer. *Arch. Ophthal.*, **54**, 850 (1955).

Tittarelli, Catalino and Bucci. *Boll. Oculist.*, **40**, 619 (1961).

Yoshida. *A Chemical and Physiological Study on the Toxic Principle of* Leucæna glauca (Thesis), Minnesota (1944).

Enzyme Inhibitors

IODOACETIC ACID, the most representative of this group of agents, acts by disturbing the carbohydrate metabolism by inhibiting enzymes containing sulphydryl groups; it has interesting and specific effects on the metabolism of the retina and causes exudative changes in the aqueous humour. Some months after injecting iodoacetic acid intravenously into rabbits, cataracts have been produced initially in the posterior cortex with vacuoles and granular and iridescent opacities. The condition is characterized histologically first by the inhibition of mitosis in the subcapsular epithelium and later by swelling and disorganization of the lenticular fibres particularly near the equator and their migration as swollen Wedl balloon cells to the posterior cortex resulting in the deposition of granular material (Cibis and Noell, 1955; Cibis *et al.*, 1957; Ricci, 1957)

Figs. 118 to 121. Experimental Iodoacetate Cataract (P. Cibis *et al.*).

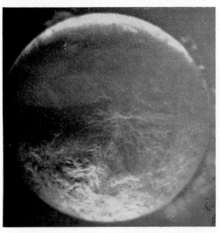

Fig. 118.

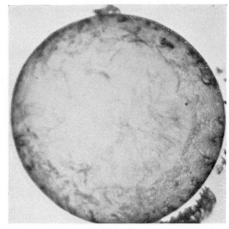

Fig. 119.

Figs. 118 and 119.—Photographs of the posterior region of the lens of the rabbit 7 months after the administration of iodoacetate. Fig. 118.—Seen by transillumination. Fig. 119.—Seen by dark-field illumination.

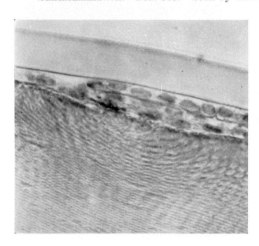

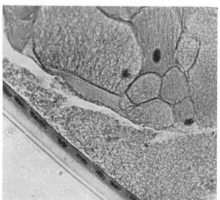

Fig. 120.—The anterior portion of the lens of the rabbit 4 months after the administration of 4 mg./kg. of iodoacetate. There is swelling of the capsule, proliferation and duplication of the subcapsular epithelium and distortion of the structure of the lens.

Fig. 121.—Balloon cells resulting in the deposition of granular debris in the subcapsular zone 4 months after the administration of 40 mg./kg. of iodoacetate.

(Figs. 118–21). These changes occur only in the ipsilateral eye two months after intracarotid injection (Tieri and Vecchione, 1963). Lenses cultured in a solution containing iodoacetic acid rapidly cloud, an effect associated with a reduction in the oxygen-uptake, a diminution of lactic acid, adenosine triphosphate and phosphocreatine, indicating an inhibition of anaerobic

FIGS. 122 to 124.—TRIPARANOL CATARACT (L. von Sallmann *et al.*).

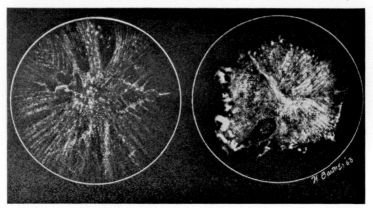

FIG. 122.—Composite drawing of triparanol cataract in man, showing the opacities in the anterior and posterior cortex.

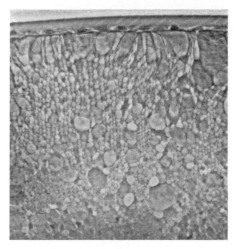

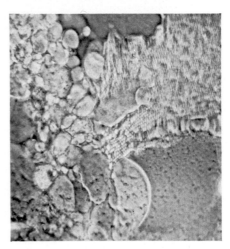

FIG. 123.—The fibres in the anterior cortex of the lens of a rat fed on triparanol. The fibres are swollen and in the deeper layers they are irregularly distributed.

FIG. 124.—The lens fibres in the posterior cortex of a rat fed on triparanol, showing islands of normal fibres and advanced cataractous changes.

glycolysis (Nordmann *et al.*, 1954; Hockwin *et al.*, 1956). Injections into the lens have a similar result (Zeller and Shoch, 1961).

A somewhat similar blocking of glycolysis has been found in cultured lenses after the addition of POTASSIUM CYANIDE to the medium (Hockwin *et al.*, 1956) or of SODIUM FLUORIDE which possibly acts by inhibiting the enzyme emolase (Kleifeld *et al.*, 1956).

TRIPARANOL disturbs the metabolism of lipids by blocking the enzymic reduction of dehydrocholesterol to cholesterol, and consequently has been used as a therapeutic agent to lower the cholesterol in the blood; in such patients cataracts have been noted. von Sallmann and his colleagues (1963) and Kirby (1967) induced somewhat similar lenticular opacities in young rats after 3 or 4 months' feeding; there was a swelling and degeneration of the superficial lenticular fibres with the deposition of sudanophilic material and areas of circumscribed proliferation of the epithelium; these changes are presumably due to the derangement of the lipid metabolism associated with a disturbance of the transport of cations (Figs. 122–4).

Cibis, Constant, Pribyl and Becker. *Arch. Ophthal.*, **57**, 508 (1957).

Cibis and Noell. *Amer. J. Ophthal.*, **40**, 379 (1955).

Hockwin, Kleifeld and Arens. *v. Graefes Arch. Ophthal.*, **158**, 47 (1956).

Kirby. *Trans. Amer. ophthal. Soc.*, **65**, 492 (1967).

Kleifeld, Hockwin and Ayberk. *v. Graefes Arch. Ophthal.*, **158**, 39 (1956).

Nordmann, Mandel and Achard. *Brit. J. Ophthal.*, **38**, 673 (1954).

Ricci. *Boll. Oculist.*, **36**, 368 (1957). *Arch. Ottal.*, **61**, 411 (1957).

von Sallmann, Grimes and Collins. *Arch. Ophthal.*, **70**, 522 (1963).

Tieri and Vecchione. *Acta ophthal.* (Kbh.), **41**, 205 (1963).

Zeller and Shoch. *Amer. J. Ophthal.*, **52**, 65 (1961).

Cataractogenic Drugs

A motley of drugs has been found to have a certain cataractogenic effect: the morphine group, the antihistamines, the cholinesterase inhibitors and the sulphonamides.

THE MORPHINE GROUP. A temporary deposit on the surface of the lens has been found to accumulate in rodents within some minutes after the subcutaneous injection of a variety of morphine-like compounds (Figs. 125–8) (Weinstock *et al.*, 1958; Weinstock and Stewart, 1961; Brown *et al.*, 1966).

FIGS. 125 to 128.—MORPHINE CATARACT IN THE MOUSE.

The cataract was induced by 20 mg./kg. bodyweight methadone hydrochloride administered subcutaneously.

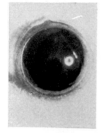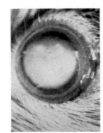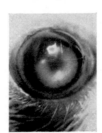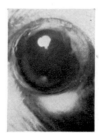

FIG. 125.　　　　FIG. 126.　　　　FIG. 127.　　　　FIG. 128.

FIG. 125.—The eye at the time of injury. FIG. 126.—After 50 minutes. FIG. 127.—After 90 minutes, showing the beginning of clarification. FIG. 128.—After 135 minutes, the lens is clear (M. Weinstock and H. C. Stewart).

The cloudy deposit on the anterior lens capsule is of unknown composition, possibly the narcotic or some catabolite, and in the isolated lens it can be washed away; in the intact animal it rapidly disappears in one or more hours and its development can be prevented or its disappearance hastened by the injection of a morphine-antagonist such as N-allyl-normorphine. It can also be prevented by closure of the lids, suggesting that corneal dehydration and possibly cooling of the aqueous are factors in determining

FIGS. 129 and 130.—EXPERIMENTAL MIOTIC CATARACT.
The lens of a rabbit incubated with a miotic (J. Michon and J. H. Kinoshita).

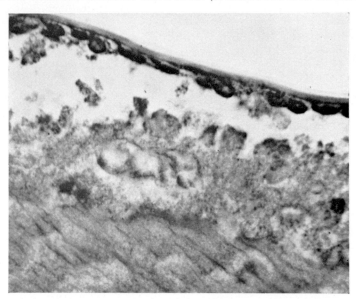

FIG. 129.—The anterior part of the lens after 5 hours' incubation with demecarium bromide, showing swollen epithelial cells detached from the capsule, round vacuole-like bodies and eosinophilic material interposed between the capsule and the cortical fibres.

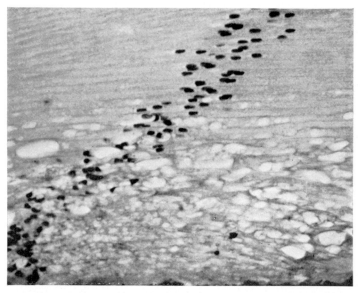

FIG. 130.—The equator of the lens after 18 hours' incubation with echothiophate iodide, showing the formation of numerous vacuoles.

its formation (Fraunfelder and Burns, 1966). It will, indeed, be remembered that a reversible cataract can be induced in young rats merely by keeping the lids open and thus producing dehydration of the lens.[1]

A similar temporary deposit may follow the administration of the related CATE-CHOLAMINES (Smith *et al.*, 1963) or, again in mice, large doses of the phenothiazine derivative, CHLORPROMAZINE (Smith *et al.*, 1966).

MIOTICS, particularly the cholinesterase inhibitors (DFP, TEPP, etc.), on intracarotid injection were found by Diamant (1954) to produce a reversible cataract in guinea-pigs in a significant proportion of animals. Michon and Kinoshita (1968) obtained similar results in the isolated cultured lenses of rabbits with demecarium bromide and echothiophate (Phospholine) iodide; with the former the epithelial cells became disordered and swollen while the cortex remained normal (Fig. 129); with the latter numerous subcapsular vacuoles in the equatorial and posterior cortical regions gave the lens a milky haziness (Fig. 130).

The cause of these changes remains unelucidated. Müller and his associates (1957) reported a decreased consumption of oxygen in the lenses of dogs, pigs and man incubated with such drugs or with pilocarpine, and Harris and his co-workers (1959) demonstrated an abnormal cation balance in the lenses of rabbits incubated with physostigmine, a result confirmed by Michon and Kinoshita in their experiments, who found an increase in hydration and in the content of sodium and a diminution of potassium. Boles-Carenini and Orzalesi (1966) concluded that the effect was due to inhibition of glucose-6-phosphate dehydrogenase in the lens, a finding not verified by Michon and Kinoshita (1968).

Certain SYNTHETIC ANTIHISTAMINE DRUGS injected subconjunctivally or intra-peritoneally were shown by Azzolini and Faldi (1951) to produce bilateral sutural opacities in guinea-pigs but not in rabbits (Azzolini and da Pozzo, 1951).

SULPHANILAMIDE in high concentrations was found by Bakker (1947) to cause opacification in the cultured lenses of rabbits; the action was ascribed to an inhibition of carbonic anhydrase.

STREPTOZOTOCINE, an antibiotic which produces a diabetic state with hyper-glyceridæmia in rats, was said by Verheyden (1967) to produce cataract in these animals after a latent period of 11 to 18 weeks.

IMPURITIES IN DRUGS of an unknown nature have been found to be cataractogenic. Thus Nakagawa and his colleagues (1961) produced lenticular opacities in a significant proportion of laboratory animals on the administration of *quercetrin*, a flavinoid constituent of vitamin P, an effect abolished on removing impurities by filtration through silicone.

Azzolini and Faldi. *Boll. Oculist.*, **30,** 129 (1951).

Azzolini and da Pozzo. *G. ital. Oftal.*, **4,** 353 (1951).

Bakker. *Brit. J. Ophthal.*, **31,** 216 (1947).

Boles-Carenini and Orzalesi. *Boll. Oculist.*, **45,** 847 (1966).

Brown, DeGraw, Ferguson and Skinner. *J. med. Chem.*, **9,** 261 (1966).

Diamant. *Acta ophthal.* (Kbh.), **32,** 357 (1954).

[1] p. 79.

Fraunfelder and Burns. *Arch. Ophthal.*, **76,** 599 (1966).

Harris, Gruber and Hoskinson. *Amer. J. Ophthal.*, **47,** 387 (1959).

Michon and Kinoshita. *Arch. Ophthal.*, **79,** 79, 611 (1968).

Müller, Kleifeld, Hockwin and Dardenne. *Ber. dtsch. ophthal. Ges.*, **60,** 115 (1957).

Nakagawa, Shetlar and Wedner. *Proc. Soc. exp. Biol.* (N.Y.), **108,** 401 (1961).

Smith, Gavitt and Kaplan. *Recent Advances Biol. Psychiat.*, **6,** 208 (1963).

Smith, Gavitt and Karmin. *Arch. Ophthal.*, **75,** 99 (1966).

Verheyden. *Bull. Soc. belge Ophtal.*, No. 147, 479 (1967).

Weinstock and Stewart. *Brit. J. Ophthal.*, **45,** 408 (1961).

Weinstock, Stewart and Butterworth. *Nature* (Lond.), **182,** 1519 (1958).

CATARACT DUE TO SYSTEMIC INFECTIONS

Several infective agents have been found to produce cataract in young animals. Of these the most common are viral infections: in the chick, the rubella virus (van Gilse, 1949), the Newcastle virus (Blattner and Williamson, 1951) and the mumps virus (Williamson *et al.*, 1957; Robertson *et al.*, 1964), in mice the vaccinia virus

FIGS. 131 and 132.—Virus-induced Cataract (C. Hanna *et al.*).

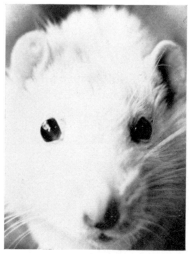 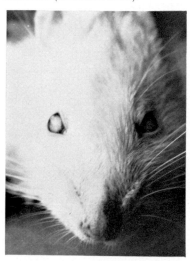

FIG. 131.   FIG. 132.

FIG. 131.—A control rat. FIG. 132.—Bilateral cataracts developing after the intracerebral injection of St. Louis encephalitis virus, when 4 days of age. The rat is now 16 months of age and the cataract developed from the 6th to the 9th month. The virus was present in the eyes. Compared with the control there is marked microphthalmos.

(Thalhammer, 1958) and in rats the St. Louis encephalitis virus (Hanna *et al.*, 1968) (Figs. 131-2). An undescribed virus named "the suckling mouse cataract agent" isolated from ticks on a dead rabbit was found by Clark (1964) and Olmsted and her colleagues (1966) to produce cataract on intracerebral inoculation into suckling mice; the virus could be recovered from the eyes.

Lenticular changes have been found in the offspring of rats infected with toxoplasma (Giroud *et al.*, 1954).

Blattner and Williamson. *Proc. Soc. exp.*
    Biol. (N.Y.), **77**, 619 (1951).
Clark. *J. infect. Dis.*, **114**, 476 (1964).
van Gilse. *Ned. T. Geneesk.*, **93**, 2852 (1949).
Giroud, P. and A., and Martinet. *Bull. Soc.
    Path. exot.*, **47**, 505 (1954).
Hanna, Jarman, Keatts and Duffy. *Arch.
    Ophthal.*, **79**, 59 (1968).

Olmsted, Prasad, Sheffer *et al.* *Invest.
    Ophthal.*, **5**, 413 (1966).
Robertson, Williamson and Blattner. *Amer.
    J. Anat.*, **115**, 473 (1964).
Thalhammer. *Med. Bild*, **1**, 43 (1958).
Williamson, Blattner and Simonsen. *Proc.
    Soc. exp. Biol.* (N.Y.), **96**, 224 (1957).

Ætiological Theories

From a study of the various agents which may cause the development of cataract it has been obvious that a multitude of factors enters into the ætiology of different varieties of opacification of the lens. Several theories, however, have been advanced in an attempt to find a common denominator underlying this process; all have failed in this composite purpose; some of them have been irrelevant, several have fitted peculiar circumstances, and for the sake of completeness they will be shortly discussed under the following headings:

1. Biological (*a*) an expression of senility,
                (*b*) genetic tendencies.
2. Immunological.
3. Functional, due to excessive accommodation.
4. Local disturbances (*a*) of nutrient supply; (*b*) of the chemistry of the lens; (*c*) radiational damage.
5. General metabolic disturbances: (*a*) changes in blood chemistry, (*b*) toxic states, (*c*) conditions of deficiency, or (*d*) endocrine disturbances.

1. Of the *biological theories*, cataract in man has often been primarily associated with *senility*; in conditions of senile sclerosis of the lens it is possibly the sole factor. In this respect the lens merely shows the characteristics of all tissues which grow until maturity is reached and then descend into senescence. This evolution is seen strikingly in epithelial tissues, among which senile cataract may be compared to the whitening of the hair, the brittleness of the nails and the wrinkling of the skin. The changes in the sclerosed lens correspond to those of ageing tissues generally—a diminished metabolism and an accumulation of waste material. These changes, of course, are affected by other conditions particularly the results of the stresses and strains of life acting over a long time, endocrine changes, and the little understood but immensely important effects of constitution and heredity.

That *genetic influences* are responsible for the degenerative phenomena of cataract was stressed by Vogt (1931). In the absence of nuclei in the mature lenticular fibres the primary change must be a genetically induced alteration in the structural configuration of the protein molecules so that their resistance is weakened and they succumb more readily to environmental changes such as may be induced by radiant energy, hormonal, nutritional, or toxic influences. In view of our present ignorance of these problems, such a theory is impossible to prove or disprove, but the undoubted hereditary element in some cases of senile cataract, and the somewhat vague findings in experimental animals that some strains are more susceptible to noxious influences than others, suggest the possible influence of some genetic groundwork. It is arguable, however, whether these hereditary factors act directly upon the lens itself or upon the basic processes which lead to opacification of the lens.

2. *Immunological factors* have been associated with the development of cataract since the discovery of the organ-specificity of the proteins of the lens by Uhlenhuth in 1903.[1] Since the body does not become tolerant during embryonic life to at least 5 organ-specific components of the protein complexes of its own lens (possibly because of the early formation of its capsule) as it does to all other antigenic substances in its constitution, it has been suggested that cataract may sometimes be due to an accidental sensitization to these proteins. Of this theory Römer (1906) was the most ardent advocate; he claimed that the lenticular proteins behaved as an antigen in homologous individuals, producing specific antibodies acting as cytolysins for lenticular tissue, and that these diffused into the clear lens through the capsule, attacked the proteins there and produced a cataract. For this there is no foundation on fact, and it is a concept rendered most improbable by the impermeability of the capsule to cytolysins and other immunological substances. It is true that when the proteins are allowed to escape into the aqueous humour, such an allergic reaction may occur and result in the violent inflammatory response of endophthalmitis phacoanaphylactica[2]; but no such reaction is known when the capsule is intact or its normal semi-permeability is retained. Moreover, despite contrary claims, there is no conclusive evidence that antibodies have ever led to the development of cataract (Halbert *et al.*, 1957–65; Mansky and Halbert, 1965). Although the skin of cataractous patients may occasionally show some degree of sensitivity to lenticular proteins (Verhoeff and Lemoine, 1922), with few exceptions (Vulchanov *et al.*, 1967) most investigators have found that the sera of such patients do not contain detectable antibodies. The evidence is inconclusive that auto-immune factors can induce congenital cataract even although the mother's serum has contained high antibody titres throughout pregnancy; while it would seem that in life antibodies capable of reacting with the lenticular proteins may bathe the lens for long periods without exciting a reaction; either the lens remains impervious to them, or alternatively, they are innocuous to it. Finally, as we shall see at a later stage, all attempts to inhibit the development of cataract by the therapeutic use of such substances have been completely futile.

In any assessment of the influence of the specificity of the protein of the lens in causing cataract, it must be remembered that certain antigenic constituents of the lens are found not only in other ocular tissues such as the

[1] Vol. IV, p. 369.
[2] Vol. IX, p. 501.

cornea, aqueous, vitreous, iris and retina,[1] but also in other organs such as the brain, skin, lung, liver and kidney.[2]   Moreover, Clayton and his associates (1968) decided that this specificity was not a feature peculiar to the lens but was due to a unique selection of genetically available antigens, any one of which may be found in other organs but all of which are present in high concentration in this tissue.   In this event the importance of immunological factors in the ætiology of cataract cannot be admitted.

3. A *functional theory* that the strains of accommodation had a deleterious effect on the lenticular fibres and thus predisposed to opacification was put forward by Meier (1862) on observing the development of cataract in cases of convulsive ergot poisoning, a view supported by others on the basis of the occurrence of opacification in association with tetany and aparathyroidism (Schmidt-Rimpler, 1883; Wettendorfer, 1897; Peters, 1900). Senile cataract in this view is dependent upon the extra accommodative effort required with a sclerosed lens in presbyopia, a suggestion which has received sporadic agreement up to recent times (Schoen, 1889; Römer, 1914; Pau, 1950; and others).   It cannot, however, be supported by any scientific evidence except that lenticular opacities have been reported after prolonged miotic therapy.[3]

4. *Local disturbances* have been claimed as causal factors.   Impairment of the *nutrient supply* to the lens has been blamed, either caused by sclerosis of the supplying blood vessels (von Michel, 1881) or senile changes in the ciliary epithelium (Peters, 1904–5).   The evidence for this is not clear, although Linnér (1954) found an indication of a decrease in the flow of blood through the ciliary body in cataractous in comparison with normal eyes by estimating the content of ascorbic acid in the aqueous humour. Disturbances of the *metabolism of the lens* have a much more solid basis as an ætiological theory and we have already discussed the effect of many such factors.   These, however, are responsible for specific types of opacification and no single metabolic factor can be incriminated as a general ætiological determinant of all types of cataract.

Disturbances of permeability undoubtedly act as a cataractogenic factor.   The diminution of the mechanism of active transport is probably a vital factor and by allowing an ionic equilibrium to exist between the aqueous and the lens it would seem partly to explain the process of intumescence (Harris and Gehrsitz, 1951; Pau, 1954; and others).

The *radiational effect of sunlight* has been quoted as an ætiological factor to explain the prevalence of this lesion in tropical or subtropical countries such as India (Hirschberg, 1898; Smith, 1928; Cowdry, 1942). For this, however, there is little scientific evidence (Duke-Elder, 1926).

5. *General metabolic disturbances* have frequently been arraigned as

---

[1] Rao *et al.* (1955), van Alphen and Robinette (1961), Langman and Maisel (1962), Perkins and Wood (1963), Maisel and Harmison (1963), Little *et al.* (1965).
[2] Perkins and Wood (1963), Maisel (1963), Mehta *et al.* (1964), Davies *et al.* (1965).
[3] p. 232.

causal factors; renal deficiency, hypercholesterolæmia, hypercalcæmia, or focal sepsis and other conditions have been suggested but, as we have seen, such changes are more probably a concomitant expression of senility or disease without any causal relation to the development of cataract with which no gross derangement of the blood chemistry is constantly associated. Owing to the oxidative function of ascorbic acid, a deficiency of *vitamins* has been advanced as an ætiological factor, while several *endocrine glands* have similarly excited attention in the ætiology of senile cataract, particularly the thyroid, the parathyroids, the hypophysis and even the gonads.[1] While some of these are undoubtedly of importance in certain specific types of cataract, their influence as general ætiological factors is completely unproven.

In summary, it must be said that neither the ætiology nor the mechanism of the formation of cataract is known. Probably the causes of opacification are many and various and it may be that they affect the transparency of the lens in different ways. Certainly, at the present time, we have no single clue which could serve as a common denominator to explain the metabolic disturbances which seem to cause the process.

van Alphen and Robinette. *Acta ophthal.* (Kbh.), **39**, 1029 (1961).

Blatt, Brätianu, Jovin and Milcou. *XV int. Cong. Ophthal.*, Cairo, **4**, 109 (1937).

Clayton, Campbell and Truman. *Exp. Eye. Res.*, **7**, 11 (1968).

Cowdry. *Problems of Ageing*, 2nd ed., Baltimore (1942).

Davies, De Sarum, Perkins and Wood. *Exp. Eye Res.*, **4**, 206 (1965).

Duke-Elder. *Lancet*, **1**, 1188, 1250 (1926).

Fischer and Triebenstein. *Klin. Mbl. Augenheilk.*, **52**, 441 (1914).

Fischer-Galati. *Bull. Soc. roum. Neurol.*, **5**, 45 (1928). See *Zbl. ges. Ophthal.*, **23**, 2 (1930).

Greppin. *Schweiz. med. Wschr.*, **52**, 1260 (1922).

Halbert, Locatcher-Khorazo, Swick *et al. J. exp. Med.*, **105**, 439, 453 (1957).

Halbert and Mansky. *Invest. Ophthal.*, **4**, 516 (1965).

Harris and Gehrsitz. *Amer. J. Ophthal.*, **34** (2), 131 (1951).

Hesse and Phleps. *Z. Augenheilk.*, **29**, 238 (1913).

Hirschberg. *Zbl. prakt. Augenheilk.*, **22**, 113 (1898).

Langman and Maisel. *Invest. Ophthal.*, **1**, 86 (1962).

Linnér. *Acta ophthal.* (Kbh.), **32**, 213 (1954).

Little, Ikeda, Zwaan and Langman. *Exp. Eye Res.*, **4**, 187 (1965).

Maisel. *Amer. J. Ophthal.*, **55**, 1208 (1963).

Maisel and Harmison. *Arch. Ophthal.*, **69**, 618 (1963).

Mansky and Halbert. *Invest. Ophthal.*, **4**, 539 (1965).

Mehta, Cooper and Rao. *Exp. Eye Res.*, **3**, 192 (1964).

Meier. *v. Graefes Arch. Ophthal.*, **8** (2), 120 (1862).

von Michel. *Das Verhalten d. Auges bei Störungen im Circulationsgebiete d. Carotis* (Festschr. z. Ehren Prof. Horners), Wiesbaden, 1 (1881).

Pau. *v. Graefes Arch. Ophthal.*, **150**, 340 (1950).
Klin. Mbl. Augenheilk., **124**, 1, 129 (1954).

Perkins and Wood. *Exp. Eye Res.*, **2**, 255 (1963).

Peters. *Z. Augenheilk.*, **4**, 337 (1900).
Klin. Mbl. Augenheilk., **42** (2), 37 (1904); **43** (1), 621 (1905).

Rao, Kulkarni, Cooper and Radhakrishnan. *Brit. J. Ophthal.*, **39**, 163 (1955).

Römer. *Arch. Augenheilk.*, **56**, Erg., 150 (1906); **76**, 120 (1914).

Schmidt-Rimpler. *Klin. Mbl. Augenheilk.*, **21**, 181 (1883).

Schoen. *Arch. Augenheilk.*, **19**, 77 (1889).

Siegrist. *Der graue Altersstar*, Berlin (1928).

Smith. *Trans. ophthal. Soc. U.K.*, **48**, 89 (1928).

Uhlenhuth. *Zur Lehre v. d. Unterscheidung verschiedener Eiweissarten mit Hilfe spezifischer Sera*, Jena, 49 (1903).

[1] Hesse and Phleps (1913), Fischer and Triebenstein (1914), Greppin (1922), Siegrist (1928), Fischer-Galati (1928), Blatt *et al.* (1937).

Verhoeff and Lemoine. *Int. Cong. Ophthal.*,
    Washington, 234 (1922).
Vogt. *Lhb. u. Atlas d. Spaltlampenmikro-
    skopie d. lebenden Auges*, 2nd ed.,
    Berlin, **2**, 528 (1931).

Vulchanov, Nikolov and Kehayov. *Immuno-
    logy*, **12**, 321 (1967).

Wettendorfer. *Wien. med. Wschr.*, **47**, 469,
    1656 (1897).

THE PATHOLOGY OF CATARACT

We are introducing this Section with the portrait of GIOVANNI BATTISTA MORGAGNI [1682–1771] (Fig. 133), a pupil of Valsalva, who became a professor of anatomy in the ancient university of Padua (1715–71). In his 79th year he published the results of his life's work in five books of letters, wherein he may be said to have laid the foundation of modern pathology, for the first time linking it with clinical observations. It is true that he was far ahead of his time in abolishing the classical humoral doctrine for he failed to stimulate a school of followers, but the original observations which he made, in addition to the first description of a hypermature " morgagnian " cataract, were astonishing in their scope and exactness, and included intracranial suppuration, the many systemic manifestations of syphilis, valvular disease of the heart, pneumonia, tuberculosis of the kidney, and a host of others.

Since the lens is composed of a single relatively inactive constituent—epithelial cells and the fibres derived from them—no matter what the ætiology or type of cataract may be, the general pathological changes are essentially the same and relatively simple—degeneration of the lenticular fibres, either of sclerosis or necrosis, associated with some aberrant activity of the epithelium.

THE CHANGES IN THE EPITHELIAL CELLS AND THE CAPSULE have already been discussed at length in the previous Chapter. These include a thickening of the capsule in some cases of senile cataract or, alternatively, a thinning in intumescent or mature cataracts and occasionally its spontaneous rupture with the possible development of an anaphylactic uveitis and a secondary glaucoma. The subcapsular epithelium may proliferate owing to toxic influences or injury and on occasion may suffer metaplasia into fibroblasts, sometimes with the formation of a new hyaline capsule which may encircle the mass of epithelial cells. This proliferative tendency may be accentuated in mature cataracts in which the capsular cells at the equator may make abortive attempts to form new fibres in the posterior cortex resulting in the formation of swollen vesicular cells (the bladder cells of Wedl) or may even line the posterior capsule with a layer of epithelium. Alternatively, degenerative changes may occur involving cloudy swelling, cytoplasmic vacuolation, pyknosis and death of the subcapsular cells.

CHANGES IN THE LENTICULAR FIBRES

The histological changes occurring in the lenticular fibres on the development of cataract were first studied by early investigators such as Becker (1883) and Collins (1896), and to their descriptions few additions

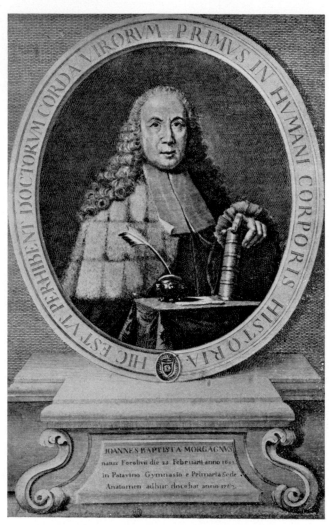

FIG. 133.—GIOVANNI BATTISTA MORGAGNI
[1682–1771].

have been made, although electron-microscopic[1] and histochemical studies (Babel, 1965) have clarified details.   Two types of change occur: a slow process of sclerosis and the more rapid development of coagulation and necrosis, either generally in the cortex or in localized foci.

SCLEROSIS is a characteristic of a common type of senile cataract and occurs normally in the aged nucleus from which it may spread to affect almost the entire tissue (Fig. 134).   This is merely an accentuation of the changes occurring normally in age; these we have already noted.[2]   The change is analogous to the keratinization of the epithelium of the skin, but in the lens the cells cannot be exfoliated and are retained.   The fibres become compressed, their cytoplasm loses its basophilia, their nuclei become pale and suffer pyknosis, and their edges become serrated and lose the lipid

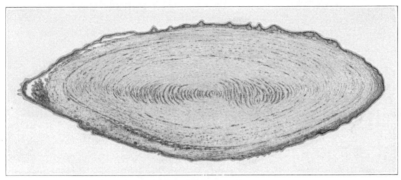

Fig. 134.—HARD CATARACT.
Showing induration of the whole lens (A. von Szily).

membranes separating each from its neighbours.   The process is slow and gradual, leaving no sharp demarcation between the living and dead cells which eventually become fused together into an almost structureless homo-geneous eosinophilic mass of granular or rubber-like consistency.   At the same time, a considerable part of the water-content is lost and, as we have seen, the soluble proteins give place to insoluble albuminoid, a process accompanied by the appearance of a yellow pigment which may develop into a dusky brown (*cataracta brunescens*) (Plate II, Figs. 2 and 3) or even black colour (*cataracta nigra*) (Fig. 135).   Pau (1951) suggested that these changes were not necessarily senile but were often evidences of ocular degeneration since they may be seen in the affected eye in cases of uniocular myopia or other comparable conditions.

The nature of the pigment is unknown[3]; it has been described as an oxidation product of tryptophan (Sauermann, 1933) or protamine or cystine (Bellows, 1935), or as lipofuscin (Puscariu and Nitzulescu, 1936), urochrome formed by the disintegration

[1] Tokunaga (1958), Kitamura (1960), Kimura *et al.* (1961), Okamoto (1961), Tokunaga and Riley (1962), Wanko and von Sallmann (1962), Brini *et al.* (1963).
[2] p. 10.   [3] p. 13.

of proteins (McEwen, 1959) or as products of melanin (F. P. Fischer, 1940; de Berardinis and de Rosa, 1951; Cowan, 1959–61; J. and E. Meyer-Arendt, 1960). The pigment is mainly concentrated in the nucleus and can be extracted with sodium hydroxide but is very inert to chemical tests; spectrophotometric studies, however, have indicated that although it is related to uveal melanin it is not identical with it (Cowan, 1959; J. and E. Meyer-Arendt, 1960). Cowan (1961) suggested that it does not usually appear in quantity since the precursors of melanin are prevented from oxidizing by the abundance of powerful reducing agents in the normal lens such as ascorbic acid and cysteine, but that these are reduced in the sclerosed tissue so that the pigment may appear just as a yellow-brown colour develops in the aged skin. The resulting pigmentation has been said to account for the distortion of colours sometimes seen in the work of artists who have attained a considerable age, as if they viewed the world through amber spectacles (Liebreich, 1872; Angelucci, 1894; Trevor Roper, 1959; and others).

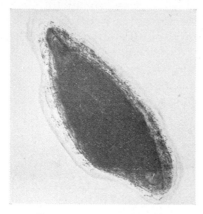

Fig. 135.—Black Cataract.
Unstained section of the lens. The central part of the lens consisted of an amorphous mass of black granules. Stereoscopic examination proved the absence of blood pigment (J. van Heuven).

Although it causes a change in refraction, the process of sclerosis may not seriously impair the transparency of the fibres, but in extreme instances, largely because it occurs irregularly involving the development of multiple irregular refracting surfaces, the transparency of the whole lens may be gravely affected, while the increased refractivity leads to the development of myopia.

The alternative process of coagulation, proteolysis and NECROSIS is more dramatic. It occurs primarily in the cortex but may be associated with the development of nuclear sclerosis. The first change in the cortical fibres is the development of acidification, due to the accumulation of the products of the retarded and altered metabolism,[1] followed by a hydropic swelling of the fibres (Friedenwald and Rytel, 1955). Thereafter there ensues a more rapid death of the cells than occurs in nuclear sclerosis. With the acidic reaction we have already seen that proteolytic enzymes are activated so that the soluble proteins are broken down into smaller fragments, while the insoluble proteins are thrown out of the colloid system. The first process increases the osmotic pressure within the lens so that water in quantity is drawn into it from the aqueous (*intumescent cataract*), a change which may be accentuated by the accumulation of other metabolic products (Fig. 136); the second releases water normally bound in the colloidal system of the fibres and extrudes it into the perifibrillar spaces to add to the accumu-

[1] p. 72.

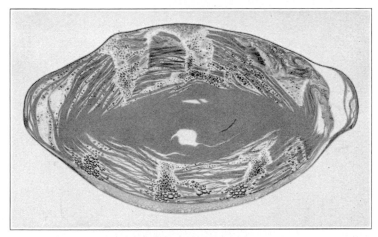

FIG. 136.—SOFT CATARACT.
Intumescent stage (A. von Szily).

lation already there, while at the same time it produces a cloudy swelling of the fibres themselves. The pathological picture thus presented in the lens is therefore one of gaps and fissures of all forms and sizes, filled with fluid between the fibres which themselves are granular, cloudy and swollen, and distorted into grotesque forms (Figs. 137–9). This disarrangement and

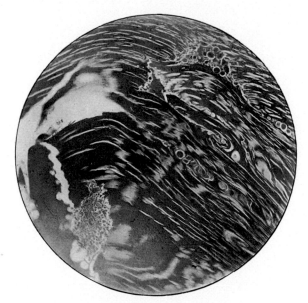

FIG. 137.—CATARACTOUS LENS.
Showing general disintegration and necrosis of the fibres with the formation of morgagnian globules ($\times$ 55) (J. H. Parsons).

FIGS. 138 to 140.—DEGENERATIVE CHANGES IN SENILE CATARACT (A. Brini *et al.*).

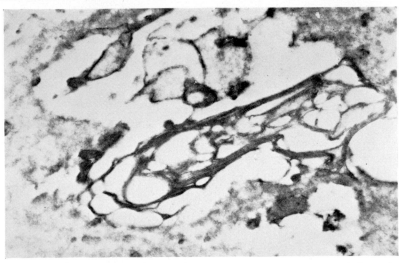

FIG. 138.—Degenerated fibres forming superimposed membranes from their ruptured walls (× 10,000).

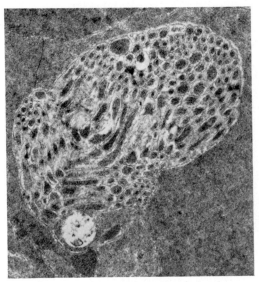

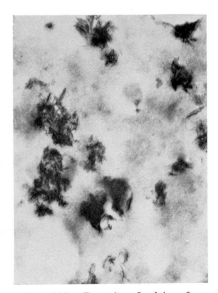

FIG. 139.—Complex 'mosaic' figures formed near the interdigitations of degenerative fibres probably from lateral 'buds' (× 16,000).

FIG. 140.—Deposits of calcium from lenticular fibres (× 44,000).

vacuolization is well seen in electron-micrographs (Kimura *et al.*, 1961; Brini *et al.*, 1963).

In its early stages this state of œdema may be reversible if the metabolic upset can be controlled; the loss of optical transparency thus caused may therefore be restored, as may occur, for example, in early diabetic cataract or after a contusion. If the metabolism is decreased locally to a mild degree, however, clusters of granular material may appear in the fibres while cholesterol esters or calcium in the form of phosphates or carbonates or even proteins may be precipitated by a process similar to that termed infiltration

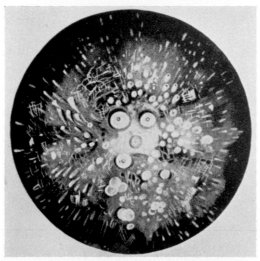

FIG. 141.—CORALLIFORM CATARACT (M. Berliner).

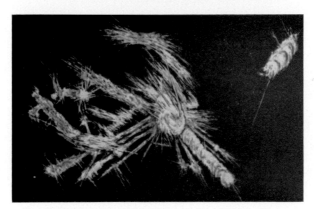

FIG. 142.—NEEDLE-SHAPED CATARACT (after A. Vogt).

in other tissues (Wanko and von Sallmann, 1962; Brini *et al.*, 1963) (Fig. 140). It is interesting that in a clear lens such a precipitation of carbonates (Kranz, 1927; Boente, 1930), cholesterol (Purtscher, 1938) or tyrosine (Braun, 1927) may occasionally occur.

Sometimes the accumulation of crystals forms the greater part or the whole of the opacity as is seen in most dramatic forms in certain types of congenital cataract.[1]

[1] Vol. III, p. 745.

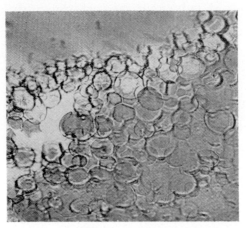

FIG. 143.—MORGAGNIAN GLOBULES.

In an experimental naphthalene cataract in the rabbit, 23 days after the beginning of the experiment when the cataract was mature (S. Ogino *et al.*).

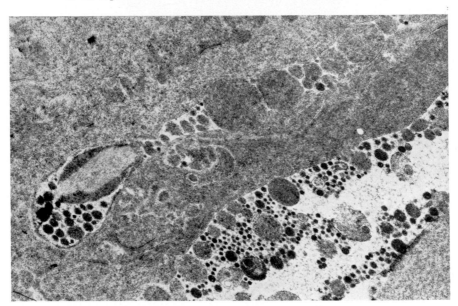

FIG. 144.—LESIONS IN THE SUPERFICIAL FIBRES IN SENILE CATARACT.

Showing the development of morgagnian bodies ($\times$ 13,500) (A. Brini *et al.*).

Such a crystalline congenital cataract in an otherwise transparent lens may present bizarre and beautiful pictures, the accumulations of crystals cutting across the architecture of the lens at random, as in coralliform cataract (Fig. 141) or needle-shaped cataract (Fig. 142); in these the crystals are probably of a protein nature (Verhoeff, 1918; Vogt, 1922; Bücklers, 1938; Rieger *et al.*, 1944) although in the latter type they may be salts of calcium (Gifford and Puntenney, 1937), and in other forms cholesterol deposits (Riad, 1938). In the acquired varieties of cataract crystals may also be present in a relatively clear lens, such as those seen in the localized opacities occurring in thyroid dysfunction, myotonic dystrophy and tetany, while, as in congenital cataracts, crystalline deposits of a protein nature without other opacities may be present (Chatterjee *et al.*, 1962).

More usually, however, the necrotic process proceeds and, although the pathological changes pursue a relatively simple course, the topographical incidence of the changes may result in the appearance of many clinical forms, such as spokes, wedge-shaped or dot-shaped opacities, or lamellar separation of the fibres. Sometimes these changes remain localized in the cortex for a considerable time, occasionally interfering little with vision, but

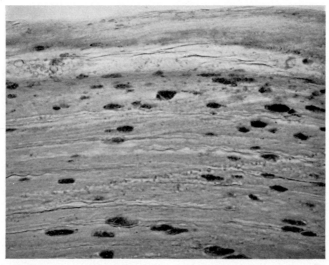

Fig. 145.—Senile Cataract.

There are numerous sudanophilic granular deposits packed in the clefts between the bundles of fibres in the post-cortical region (Sudan black B) (L. von Sallmann *et al.*).

if the metabolic upset has been sufficiently acute to determine a marked imbibition of fluid, complete opacification is usually rapid.

As the necrotic changes proceed, the nuclei, if they are present, disappear from the fibres, vacuoles form which coalesce into large spaces, and eventually the fibres break down into round globules (*morgagnian globules*) frequently lying in rows, staining faintly with eosin and not with hæmatoxylin (Figs. 137, 143–4). As time goes on, homogeneous or granular masses of albuminous coagula are found, staining deeply with hæmatoxylin, and in the later stages the fissures and spaces increase in size becoming filled with an almost infinite variety of the waste products of the original fibres— clear fluid, morgagnian globules, albuminous coagula of insoluble protein, fatty droplets, the detritus of partially disintegrated fragments of fibres, and calcareous and crystalline deposits of various types, some clear and some richly multicoloured (Plate II; Figs. 138–40, 145).

These depositions include cholesterol,[1] calcium phosphate, carbonate and oxalate,[2] and the relatively insoluble amino acids, tryptophan, leucine and tyrosine[3] (Figs. 146–50). Subsequent degenerative changes may take the form of extensive fatty deposits (XANTHOMATOSIS LENTIS, von Szily, 1923; Sala, 1935; CATARACTA ADIPOSA, Franz Fischer, 1955) which have been noted in senile cataract (Toufesco, 1906), in

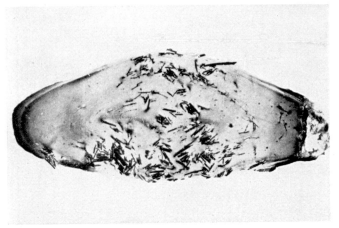

FIG. 146.—CRYSTALS IN A CATARACTOUS LENS (J. Burdon-Cooper).

FIGS. 147 and 148.—CALCIUM OXALATE CRYSTALS (ARROWED) IN THE NUCLEUS OF THE CATARACTOUS LENS.

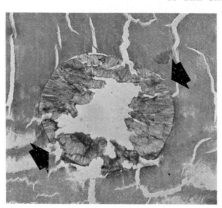 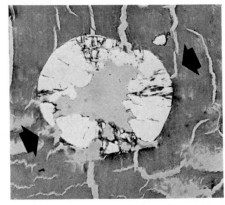

FIG. 147.—Photographed through non-polarized light.

FIG. 148.—Photographed through polarized light (M. F. Goldberg).

[1] von Graefe (1854), Tweedy (1873), Lang (1895), Krautschneider (1897), Leber (1906), Gross (1906), Hoffmann (1913), Vogt (1919), Baratta (1935), Dorello (1953), and others.
[2] Wessely (1922), Busacca (1925), Kranz (1927), Boente (1930), Brini *et al.* (1963), Goldberg (1967).
[3] Becker (1877), Baas (1897), Coats (1912), Burdon-Cooper (1922), Chinaglia and Amidei (1955).

coronary cataract (Metzger, 1931) and in the cataract complicating glaucoma (Jess, 1933); amyloid degeneration is rare (von Szily, 1937). A more usual change, however, is an impregnation with calcium salts. Such a CATARACTA CALCAREA is a common occurrence particularly in cataracts of very long standing (56 years, Cserńak, 1948) and in the later stages of complicated (Becker, 1883; Kahler, 1911; Ribas Valero and Menacho, 1915; and others) or traumatic cataract (Radnót, 1948; Vogler,

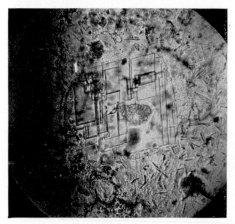

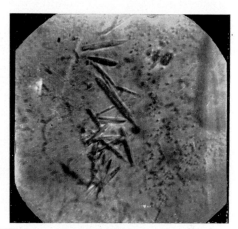

FIG. 149.—CHOLESTEROL AND TYROSINE CRYSTALS IN DIABETIC CATARACT (J. Burdon-Cooper).

FIG. 150.—TYROSINE CRYSTALS IN A CATARACTOUS LENS (J. Burdon-Cooper).

1951; Lombardi, 1956; Schröder, 1957; Hager and Ebel, 1964), and may accompany a widespread calcification or even ossification of the uveal tract[1] (Figs. 151–2). When the lens capsule has been ruptured or disintegrated, changes of a more advanced nature may occur, including the entrance of fully formed vascularized granulation and fibrous tissue with the occasional subsequent formation of true bone showing sometimes haversian systems (CATARACTA OSSEA).[2]

FIGS. 151 and 152.—CALCAREOUS DEGENERATION.

In enucleated eyes which had suffered from chronic relapsing iridocyclitis and had been blind for many years (G. Hager and K. Ebel).

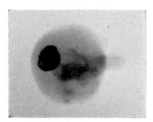

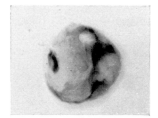

FIG. 151.—Calcification of the lens and diffuse calcification of the uvea.

FIG. 152.—Calcification of the lens and dense calcification of the uvea.

[1] Vol. IX, p. 740.
[2] Gluge (1843), Wagner (1851), Ayres (1882), Dunn and Holden (1898), Aubineau (1904), Roure (1905), Pitsch (1926), Betsch (1927), Kaufmann (1932), Michaïl (1934).

The ultimate fate of the lens substance depends largely upon its age. In the young lens if the injury is severe and general, it frequently happens that owing to the preponderance of soluble and the paucity of insoluble proteins, the process of proteolysis may be so complete that the lens may become entirely absorbed leaving a condition of aphakia with the capsule alone remaining. If the injury is localized, a portion of the lens substance may be destroyed; the debris may be almost entirely absorbed leaving a faceted, flattened lens; or alternatively, a localized area of opacity may be left which is enclosed and buried by the formation of new clear fibres resulting in a lamellar or a punctate cataract (Fig. 153). If, however, the lens is of adult age, there is a considerable residue which resists enzymic proteolysis. In this event, while the nucleus may remain relatively unchanged, showing perhaps large fissures and areas of regional degeneration, the cortex becomes converted into a pultaceous mass. At this stage, owing

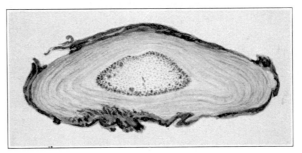

Fig. 153.—Zonular Cataract (after A. von Szily).

to the diffusion away of the products of proteolysis, there is a loss of water and the lens becomes inspissated, wrinkled and shrunken, flat and yellowish, and frequently glistening with scattered cretaceous deposits and bright crystalline accumulations. Such a cataract is termed *hypermature*. If, on the other hand, owing to thickening of the capsule and proliferation of the epithelial cells, permeability is abolished, the water is retained within the capsule, and the cortex, instead of becoming pultaceous, turns fluid. The fluid is of a milky colour and is richly albuminous, holding in suspension globules of lipids and coagulated protein, granular detritus and the remnants of individual fibres with frayed ends and corroded edges. In such a liquefied lens a thermal current has been detected with the slit-lamp as occurs in the aqueous (Siedenbiedel, 1951; Binder, 1954). Meanwhile, the nucleus, which is gradually converted into a homogeneous shrunken mass, sinks to the bottom of the capsular sac (*morgagnian cataract*) (Figs. 154–5). In the most advanced cases the nucleus may also partially or entirely disappear leaving only milky fluid enclosed in a thickened capsule dotted with small white opacities (Herbert, 1915; Gabriélidès, 1924; and others). These spots represent spaces enclosed between layers of the capsule filled with fluid and granular debris which may eventually undergo calcareous degeneration (Fig. 156)

While at one time a morgagnian cataract was a commonplace, so much so, indeed, that Morgagni (1764) looked upon it as the normal form of cataract, since the adoption

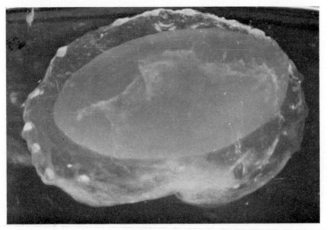

FIG. 154.—MORGAGNIAN CATARACT.
Macroscopic appearance of the lens in a case of phacolytic glaucoma. The nucleus floats within the intact capsule which shows many focal opacities (M. F. Goldberg).

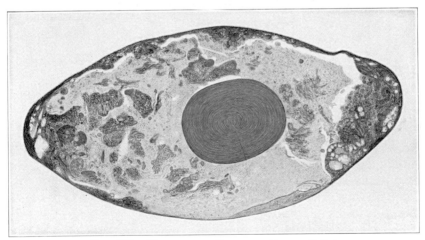

FIG. 155.—MORGAGNIAN CATARACT (A. von Szily).

of widespread operative treatment it has become rare in countries wherein medical care is available. Thus, although it occurs more frequently than the figures indicate, Taylor (1911) recalled that no case had been brought before the Ophthalmological Society of the United Kingdom for 30 years, and Chance (1912) found a similar absence in the American Ophthalmological Society for 22 years.

Although it is the rule in young persons that a cataract is completely absorbed if the capsule is opened, partly through the action of proteolytic enzymes and partly through phagocytosis (Rodigina, 1932), the *spontaneous absorption* of a cataract when the capsule is apparently intact is a rare event; indeed, most instances which have been recorded probably do not legitimately come into this category. Cases reported in the pre-ophthalmoscopic era should doubtless be disregarded (Warnatz, 1835), but early cases were noted by Becker (1877), and von Reuss (1900), and in the present century reports have been more numerous.[1] Dor (1908) gathered 80 known cases

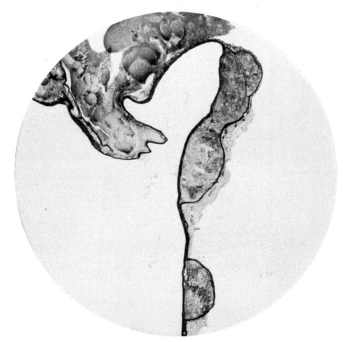

FIG. 156.—CAPSULAR OPACITIES IN MORGAGNIAN CATARACT (× 72) (H. Herbert).

from the literature, Vancea (1932) 30 cases, while Marlow (1952) estimated the number as 129.

Most cases reported as illustrating the spontaneous disappearance of a cataract are probably explained by a spontaneous rupture of the capsule,[2] and it is likely that in some of these the tear may not be recognized; others have been instances of the occurrence of a posterior dislocation of the lens leaving a clear pupillary aperture. Those cases recorded following an iridectomy (Trousseau, 1901; Paterson, 1930; Butler, 1932) probably come

[1] Pyle (1902), Gonzalez (1919), Ballantyne (1926), Ferrer (1928), Butler (1932), Holloway and Cowan (1932), Vancea (1932), Ehrlich (1948), Hallermann (1948), Marlow (1952), Gregersen (1956), Blodi (1957), François (1961).

[2] p. 59.

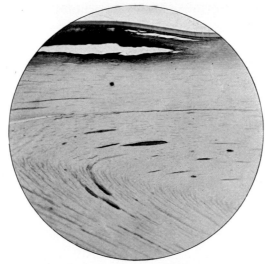

FIG. 157.—PUNCTATE LENTICULAR OPACITIES (J. H. Parsons).

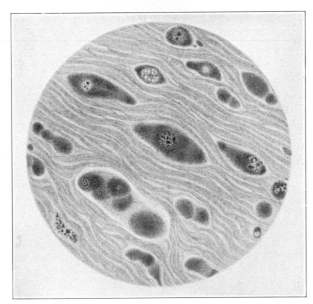

FIG. 158.—FOCAL CATARACT.

Oval homogeneous or flocculated foci with dispersed honeycombed granular
deposits (a drawing by A. von Szily).

into the first category wherein the injury was not noticed.   The sinking of
the nucleus below the visual axis in a morgagnian cataract and the disappearance of the fluid cortex through the abnormally permeable capsule
may also result in an apparently clear pupil (Butler, 1925; Aliquò-Mazzei,

1930). But the complete spontaneous absorption of all the lens substance without injury or advanced degenerative changes is rare except in young patients.[1]

When the hypermature products of lenticular degeneration escape from the lens either through an intact but permeable capsule or because this structure has perforated, a violent phaco-anaphylactic response may be excited in the uvea, producing a macrophagic infiltration and often a phacolytic glaucoma; these inflammatory reactions have been described in a previous Volume[2] and the subject of phacolytic glaucoma is noted elsewhere.[3]

In place of a generalized process of necrosis, the degenerative changes may be localized to discrete areas. Such a FOCAL CATARACT has been traditionally associated with anomalies of the endocrine glands and has frequently been called *endocrine cataract* (Weill and Nordmann, 1926–30), but the evidence for this is somewhat unconvincing. It is true that hypoparathyroidism is a relatively common cause of opacities of this type, but it would appear that in this condition the essential determinant is a low calcium/phosphate ratio in the serum. Similar opacities occur in mongolism, myotonic dystrophy—a genetic disease probably due primarily to metabolic rather than to endocrine disturbances—and in certain dermatoses.

The lenticular opacities in such conditions have a striking morphological similarity. In their pure form—for they are frequently complicated by other changes—the discrete opacities are characterized anatomically by rounded, oval foci with deeply staining contents, sometimes homogeneous, sometimes flocculated and sometimes granular (Bartels, 1906; von Szily, 1938) (Figs. 157–8). Their most striking clinical features are their early onset, their bilateral incidence and their zonular distribution. They are obviously caused by metabolic disturbances, some of which may well be under hormonal control, and around them clear fibres remain which localize the necrotic areas. The general tendency, however, is for opacification of the lens to become complete in the course of time.

Aliquò-Mazzei. *Boll. Oculist.*, **9**, 170 (1930).
Angelucci. *Arch. Ottal.*, **2**, 135 (1894–95).
Aubineau. *Ann. Oculist.* (Paris), **132**, 100 (1904).
Ayres. *Arch. Augenheilk.*, **11**, 323 (1882).
Baas. *v. Graefes Arch. Ophthal.*, **44**, 657 (1897).
Babel. *Bull. Soc. franç. Ophtal.*, **28**, 413 (1965).
Ballantyne. *Brit. J. Ophthal.*, **10**, 202 (1926).
Baratta. *Lett. oftal.*, **12**, 437 (1935).
Bartels. *Klin. Mbl. Augenheilk.*, **44** (1), 374 (1906).
Becker. *Graefe-Saemisch Hb. d. ges. Augenheilk.*, 1st ed., Leipzig, **5**, 186 (1877).

Zur Anatomie d. gesunden u. kranken Linse, Wiesbaden (1883).
Bellows. *Arch. Ophthal.*, **14**, 99 (1935).
de Berardinis and de Rosa. *Arch. Ottal.*, **55**, 145 (1951).
Betsch. *Klin. Mbl. Augenheilk.*, **79**, 48 (1927).
Binder. *v. Graefes Arch. Ophthal.*, **155**, 347 (1954).
Blake. *Amer. J. Ophthal.*, **29**, 464 (1946).
Blodi. *Arch. Ophthal.*, **57**, 593 (1957).
Boente. *Arch. Augenheilk.*, **102**, 261 (1930).
Braun. *v. Graefes Arch. Ophthal.*, **118**, 701 (1927).
Brini, Porte and Stoeckel. *Bull. Soc. franç. Ophtal.*, **76**, 193 (1963).

[1] Jeancon (1945), Long and Danielson (1945), Blake (1946), Ehrlich (1948), Marlow (1952).
[2] Vol. IX, p. 500.   [3] p. 663.

Bücklers. Gutt's *Hb. d. Erbkrankheiten*, Leipzig, **5**, 96 (1938).

Burdon-Cooper. *Brit. J. Ophthal.*, **6**, 385, 433 (1922).

Busacca. *Rev. gén. Ophtal.*, **39**, 439 (1925).

Butler. *Trans. ophthal. Soc. U.K.*, **45**, 657 (1925).
 Brit. J. Ophthal., **16**, 35 (1932).

Chance. *J. Amer. med. Ass.*, **59**, 1013 (1912).

Chatterjee, Mukherji and Sen. *Arch. Ophthal.*, **68**, 468 (1962).

Chinaglia and Amidei. *Rass. ital. Ottal.*, **24**, 3 (1955).

Coats. *Trans. ophthal. Soc. U.K.*, **32**, 153 (1912).

Collins. *Researches*, London (1896).

Cowan. *Trans. Amer. ophthal. Soc.*, **57**, 539 (1959).
 Surv. Ophthal., **6**, 630 (1961).

Cserńak. *Ophthalmologica*, **115**, 187 (1948).

Dor. *Encycl. franç. Ophtal.*, Paris, **7**, 222 (1908).

Dorello. *G. ital. Oftal.*, **6**, 136 (1953).

Dunn and Holden. *Arch. Ophthal.*, **27**, 499 (1898).

Ehrlich. *Arch. Ophthal.*, **39**, 205 (1948).

Ferrer. *Amer. J. Ophthal.*, **11**, 886 (1928).

Fischer, F. P. *Ophthalmologica*, **99**, 425; **100**, 150 (1940).

Fischer, Franz. *Ophthalmologica*, **129**, 160 (1955).

François. *Amer. J. Ophthal.*, **52**, 207 (1961).

Friedenwald and Rytel. *Arch. Ophthal.*, **53**, 825 (1955).

Gabriélidès. *Ann. Oculist.* (Paris), **161**, 561 (1924).

Gifford and Puntenney. *Arch. Ophthal.*, **17**, 885 (1937).

Gluge. *Ann. Oculist.* (Paris), **10**, 226 (1843).

Goldberg. *Brit. J. Ophthal.*, **51**, 847 (1967).

Gonzalez. *Amer. J. Ophthal.*, **2**, 743 (1919).

von Graefe. *v. Graefes Arch. Ophthal.*, **1** (1), 323 (1854).

Gregersen. *Acta ophthal.* (Kbh.), **34**, 347 (1956).

Gross. *Arch. Augenheilk.*, **57**, 107 (1906).

Hager and Ebel. *Klin. Mbl. Augenheilk.*, **144**, 513 (1964).

Hallermann. *Klin. Mbl. Augenheilk.*, **113**, 315 (1948).

Herbert. *Trans. ophthal. Soc. U.K.*, **35**, 349 (1915).

Hoffmann. *Münch. med. Wschr.*, **60**, 741 (1913).

Holloway and Cowan. *Arch. Ophthal.*, **7**, 332 (1932).

Jeancon. *Amer. J. Ophthal.*, **28**, 904 (1945).

Jess. *Klin. Mbl. Augenheilk.*, **91**, 830 (1933).

Kahler. *Beitr. z. pathologischen Anatomie d. Linse* (Diss.), Marburg (1911).

Kaufmann. *Röntgenpraxis*, **4**, 347 (1932).

Kimura, Nishio and Kitamura. *Acta Soc. ophthal. jap.*, **65**, 1165 (1961).

Kitamura. *J. Kurume med. Ass.*, **23**, 7387 (1960).

Kranz. *v. Graefes Arch. Ophthal.*, **118**, 571 (1927).

Krautschneider. *Beitr. Augenheilk.*, **3** (26), 482 (1897).

Lang. *Trans. ophthal. Soc. U.K.*, **15**, 117 (1895).

Leber. *v. Graefes Arch. Ophthal.*, **62**, 85 (1906).

Liebreich. *Brit. med. J.*, **1**, 271, 296, 318 (1872).

Lombardi. *Ann. Radiol. diagn.* (Bologna), **29**, 428 (1956).

Long and Danielson. *Arch. Ophthal.*, **34**, 24 (1945).

McEwen. *Amer. J. Ophthal.*, **47** (2), 144 (1959).

Marlow. *Trans. Amer. ophthal. Soc.*, **50**, 283 (1952).

Metzger. *Klin. Mbl. Augenheilk.*, **87**, 850 (1931).

Meyer-Arendt, J. and E. *J. Histochem. Cytochem.*, **8**, 75 (1960).

Michaïl. *v. Graefes Arch. Ophthal.*, **131**, 390 (1934).

Morgagni. *Epistolæ anatomicæ XVIII, ad scripta pertinentes cel. Valsalvæ*, Padua, Ep. 18, 19, p. 356 (1764).

Okamoto. *Acta Soc. ophthal. jap.*, **63**, 2602 (1959); **65**, 1021 (1961).

Paterson. *Trans. ophthal. Soc. U.K.*, **50**, 617 (1930).

Pau. *Klin. Mbl. Augenheilk.*, **119**, 12 (1951).

Pitsch. *Klin. Mbl. Augenheilk.*, **77**, 636 (1926).

Purtscher. *v. Graefes Arch. Ophthal.*, **139**, 358 (1938).

Puscariu and Nitzulescu. *Brit. J. Ophthal.*, **20**, 531 (1936).

Pyle. *Ophthal. Rec.*, **11**, 398 (1902).

Radnót. *Brit. J. Ophthal.*, **32**, 47 (1948).

von Reuss. *Zbl. prakt. Augenheilk.*, **24**, 33 (1900).

Riad. *Brit. J. Ophthal.*, **22**, 745 (1938).

Ribas Valero and Menacho. *Arch. Oftal. hisp.-amer.*, **15**, 257 (1915).

Rieger, Stark and von Zeynek. *v. Graefes Arch. Ophthal.*, **147**, 426 (1944).

Rodigina. *Vestn. oftal.*, **1**, 121 (1932).

Roure. *Rev. gén. Ophtal.*, **24**, 49 (1905).

Sala. *Boll. Oculist.*, **14**, 266 (1935).

Sauermann. *Amer. J. Ophthal.*, **16**, 985 (1933).

Schröder. *Klin. Mbl. Augenheilk.*, **130**, 385 (1957).

Siedenbiedel. *Klin. Mbl. Augenheilk.*, **119**, 79 (1951).

von Szily. *Klin. Mbl. Augenheilk.*, **71**, 30 (1923).
 Lubarsch-Henke *Hb. d. spez. path. Anat. u. Histol.*, Berlin, **11** (3), 1 (1937).
 Trans. ophthal. Soc. U.K., **58**, 595 (1938).

Taylor. *Trans. ophthal. Soc. U.K.*, **31**, 146 (1911).

Tokunaga. *Acta Soc. ophthal. jap.*, **62**, 1383 (1958).

Tokunaga and Riley. *Nagasaki med. J.*, **37**, 221 (1962).

Toufesco. *Ann. Oculist.* (Paris), **135**, 265; **136**, 1 (1906).

Trevor-Roper. *Proc. roy. Soc. Med.*, **52**, 721 (1959).

Trousseau. *Ann. Oculist.* (Paris), **125**, 184 (1901).

Tweedy. *Lancet*, **2**, 519 (1873).

Vancea. *Arch. Ophtal.*, **49**, 78 (1932).

Verhoeff. *Arch. Ophthal.*, **47**, 558 (1918).

Vogler. *Fortschr. Röntgenstr.*, **74**, 87 (1951).

Vogt. *Klin. Mbl. Augenheilk.*, **63**, 232 (1919).

v. Graefes Arch. Ophthal., **107**, 234 (1922).

Wagner. *Nachr. Ges. Wiss. Göttingen, Math.-phys. Kl.*, No. 8 (1851). Quoted by Panas, *Traité des maladies des yeux*, Paris, **1**, 437 (1894).

Wanko and von Sallmann. *Acta XIX int. Cong. Ophthal.*, Delhi, **1**, 593 (1962).

Warnatz. *v. Ammons Z. Ophthal.*, **5**, 49 (1835).

Weill and Nordmann. *Ann. Oculist.* (Paris), **163**, 401 (1926). *Bull. Soc. franç. Ophtal.*, **43**, 17 (1930).

Wessely. *Arch. Augenheilk.*, **91**, 158 (1922).

THE SYMPTOMATOLOGY OF CATARACT

The SYMPTOMATOLOGY of cataract is essentially concerned with a disturbance, then a diminution, and finally a failure of vision. To a large extent the disability depends on the situation of the opacity. Thus a relatively small opacity at the posterior pole may be incapacitating because it is situated near the nodal point of the dioptric system, while peripheral opacities which leave the axial region free may cause little inconvenience.

FIGS. 159 and 160.—ENTOPTIC APPEARANCES.

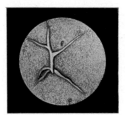 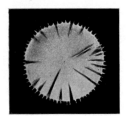

FIG. 159.—Star figures of the lens.   FIG. 160.—Incipient cataract.

Similarly, a nuclear sclerosis interferes with vision much more decisively than an anterior cortical opacity which, indeed, may be compatible with almost normal acuity if clear spaces exist between the opaque areas. Moreover, a patient with an axial opacity sees best in dull light when the pupil is dilated, while in peripheral cataract a bright light improves the vision because of the contraction of the iris.

In general, however, the subjective symptoms are four-fold. First, is *the appearance of black spots* which move only with movements of the eyes and are especially prominent when looking at a bright background. These can be accentuated and rendered more distinct by looking through a stenopæic hole in a black card held at the anterior focus of the eye (15·7 mm. in front of the cornea). In this event lenticular opacities can be clearly seen and their pattern drawn and their progress followed by the patient himself (Figs. 159–60) (Darier, 1895; East, 1922; Priestley Smith, 1924). More accurate optical conditions but relatively little better results are achieved by the use of an entoptoscope[1] (Barrett, 1918; Scheerer, 1924–25).

These lenticular opacities if diffuse can produce an apparent generalized reduction in the *visual fields* which may be diminished by increasing the illumination or the size of the perimetric test-object, and if they are localized they can give rise to scotomata. Being in front of the nodal point, an opacity in the anterior cortex will give rise to a defect in the same side of the visual field but, since it lies behind the nodal point, a posterior cortical opacity produces a defect in the opposite side. These scotomata may decrease in size if the pupil is dilated owing to the admission of more light around the opacity, but it is to be remembered that their growth may cause the apparent progression of a glaucomatous scotoma while localized paraxial opacities may cause asymmetrical defects in the visual fields resembling hemianopic or quadrantic defects.

Secondly, *uniocular polyopia* is frequently an early symptom, whereby the images of objects are distorted or reduplicated; the phenomenon is due to irregular refraction within the lens, a development which also produces stars and beams and coloured diffraction haloes around lights. The differential diagnosis of such haloes from those due to glaucoma has already been considered.[2] Thirdly, the development of *lenticular myopia* is due essentially to nuclear sclerosis; this may be relatively slight, and in so far as the presbyopic person may become able to read without his glasses, it may be interpreted by the patient as an actual strengthening of vision (*second sight*), but when it attains marked dimensions (up to -20 D and more) may be extremely incapacitating; at other times the increased refractive power of the nucleus may give rise to the condition of double focus. At the same time, changes in astigmatism, sometimes marked in degree, tend to occur rapidly, causing much visual disturbance. Finally, a generalized *impairment of vision* eventually appears. Reversible œdematous and refractive changes may cause considerable variations in the visual acuity from time to time, but eventually as the opacification progresses, the vision decreases until finally quantitative perception of light only may be left.

An incidental feature which is not often remarked is the *change in colour values*. The sclerosing lens absorbs the shorter wavelengths of the spectrum, first the violet and blue, and eventually sometimes up to the yellow, so that the resultant effect is as if looking through a colour-filter with the blue and violet excluded.[3] The effect may be accentuated by an increase in the yellow pigmentation of the lens. Conversely, after an extraction of cataract, the sudden influx of short-waved light in the presence of an established adaptation to the yellow and longer wavelengths, frequently results in a fleeting blue vision (cyanopsia).

THE OBJECTIVE sign of cataract is the presence of opacities in the lens. By direct illumination these appear grey or white, but in judging the condition of the lens it must be remembered that, owing to internal reflection

[1] Vol. VII, p. 447.   [2] Vol. VII, p. 451.   [3] Vol. IV, p. 461.

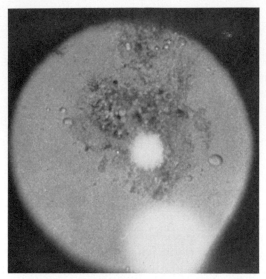

FIG. 161.—SENILE POSTERIOR CATARACT.
Seen by silhouette photography (J. C. Long).

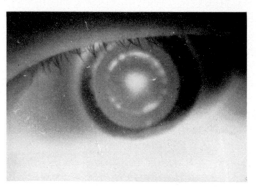

FIG. 162.—PHOTOGRAPHY OF SENILE CORTICAL AND NUCLEAR OPACITIES.
Seen by trans-scleral illumination (A. J. Ogg).

and refraction and the absorption of the shorter wavelengths, the senile lens may appear grey and relatively opaque when in reality it is highly transparent and interferes little with visual acuity. While an advanced cataract is obvious, a more accurate assessment of early opacities is made by transmitted light when actual opacities, obstructing the light reflected from the fundus, appear black in the pupillary reflex.

THE OBJECTIVE CLINICAL EXAMINATION is therefore most satisfactorily started by observing the fundus reflex with the ophthalmoscope or retino-scope, at first at a distance of about $\frac{1}{3}$ metre, and then with a + 20 D lens at close focus. Such an examination should always be done under full mydriasis since the earlier opacities are frequently peripheral. Not only by this method are the opacities recognized as such, but their position in the lens can be assessed by the phenomenon of parallax.[1]

Examination with the slit-lamp, however, provides information of more value, allowing a detailed microscopic view by direct or transmitted light and by indirect lateral illumination by which fine changes and vacuoles can be detected, as well as permitting a study of the specular reflection from the surfaces.[2] By its means not only can an accurate knowledge of the type and form of any opacity be gained but more subtle effects, such as the presence of subcapsular iridescence and the relief of the adult nucleus, can be appreciated; moreover, pathological changes can be accurately localized topographically in the cortex, the adult, infantile or fœtal nucleus.

Photographic records of the extent and progress of a cataract may be of considerable value, but the technique is not easy. An estimation of the changes in the progression of a cataract was made by Dekking (1936–48) whereby the density can be estimated photometrically when the eye is illuminated by a beam of light of constant and known intensity. In the focal beam of the slit-lamp lenticular opacities may be photographed (Goldmann, 1940) but the most satisfactory method is to photograph them against the glow of the fundus caused by an axial illuminating system either by the fundus camera appropriately focused (Douvas and Allen, 1950; Lubkin, 1950) or by the slit-lamp (Fincham, 1955; Long, 1963) (Fig. 161). Ogg (1960), on the other hand, elaborated a technique using trans-scleral illumination (Fig. 162).

In the clinical examination certain objective and subjective tests are of importance in assessing the operability of the case and the prognosis. Of the objective questions the most important are:

1. The state of the nucleus: whether it shows evidence of senile sclerosis and how far the sclerotic process extends towards the periphery, questions which affect the ease of delivery of the lens in extraction.

2. The state of the cortex: whether it is still clear (in which case the cataract is clinically *immature*), whether complete opacification extends to the capsule (*mature cataract*), or whether it is liquefied (*hypermature cataract*). To estimate the depth of clear cortical substance, a useful rough clinical test depends upon the observation of the depth of the shadow cast by the iris on oblique illumination; if clear substance still remains, the iris throws a shadow of itself upon the grey opacity in the pupil, but if the cortex is completely opaque so that the pupillary margin lies almost in contact with the opacity, no shadow appears (Figs. 163–4). A more accurate assessment can, however, be obtained by direct observation of the optical section of the lens with the slit-lamp; if the cortex is liquefied the dense grey nucleus may be seen by direct illumination occupying the lower area of the pupil (Fig. 186).

3. The presence or absence of any signs of inflammation should be carefully determined to eliminate a possible complicated ætiology—corneal bedewing or endothelial deposits, cells and debris in the aqueous, or iridic synechiæ and patches of atrophy. With the relatively immobile pupil of old persons, the freedom of the iris cannot sometimes be adequately established without dilatation with a mydriatic.

4. Every cataract, no matter how dense, transmits light freely, so that a pupillary

[1] Vol. VII, p. 316. [2] Vol. VII, p. 260.

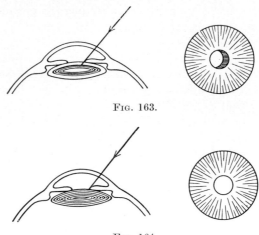

FIG. 163.

FIG. 164.

FIGS. 163 and 164.—THE CLINICAL DETERMINATION OF MATURITY.

In immature cataract a shadow of the iris appears by oblique illumination (Fig. 163), which is absent in mature cataract (Fig. 164).

glow should be obtained on transillumination: its absence indicates a neoplasm or the presence of organized material or blood in the vitreous.

THE FUNCTIONAL TESTS for the demonstration of a healthy retina and optic nerve are of importance; if the lens is opaque the fundus cannot be seen and such knowledge is essential if the extreme disappointment is to be avoided of undertaking an operation which may lead to no useful result owing to the existence of other disease. For this reason the careful and complete examination of the fundus under full mydriasis of every case of incipient cataract should be scrupulously undertaken for the purpose of future reference. If, however, the lens is already opaque, the following tests are of value:

1. The pupil should always react promptly and normally to light.

2. A point of light should be immediately and accurately located in every part of the visual field. Such a test should be undertaken in a dark room when a small point of light should be easily seen and should be accurately localized by pointing with the finger when held in all quadrants of the visual field. It may happen, particularly with older patients when the opacity is dense, that the projection of light may be poorly indicated; indeed, after the careful testing of 64 cases with dense senile cataract, Braendstrup (1948) contended that in this type of case the prognostic value of this test was small.

3. Macular function can be assessed by holding in front of the eye a black disc perforated with two or three pinholes, behind which a light is shining; the ability to count the holes and recognize their pattern indicates a healthy macula (Young, 1917–23). Other entoptic tests may be useful: the red line seen with the Maddox rod, for example, should appear intact without a central distortion or break.

4. With an intelligent patient considerable information may be obtained by the method of auto-ophthalmoscopy described by Eber (1922) and Friedman (1931); it

will be remembered[1] that by rubbing the lower lid with the electric bulb of an ophthalmoscope pressed against the globe, an inverted image of the fundus is seen by the patient wherein macular or peripheral lesions or field defects appear as black patches in an illuminated ground (Goebel, 1922; Paterson, 1948; Ehrich, 1957–58).

The entoptic appearance of Haidinger's brushes[2] has been accepted as indicating a functional macula (Goldschmidt, 1950; Kondziela-Brzykowa, 1966).

5. Electroretinographic records[3] may be of value in assessing the function of the retina, particularly of the macula.[4]

The COMPLICATIONS OF CATARACT are few, the most important being a secondary rise of tension. Such a SECONDARY GLAUCOMA occurs either at the intumescent or the hypermature stage. This complication in the *intumescent* stage was first clearly recognized by von Graefe (1869) and has now been fully established as being due to a blockage of the filtration angle by the swelling of the lens. The progressive narrowing of the angle in such cases has been directly measured by Weekers and his colleagues (1963). The mechanism of the glaucoma and its treatment are discussed in a subsequent Section.[5]

A second complication of a cataract in the advanced stage is due to the anaphylactic irritation of the products of *hypermaturity;* this condition of lens-induced uveitis and phacolytic glaucoma has been described in a previous Volume[6]; it will be remembered that it is caused by an anaphylactic reaction to lenticular proteins escaping through a capsule which has become permeable or occurring occasionally after the spontaneous rupture of this membrane.

A further complication of hypermature cataract is *subluxation or dislocation* of the lens[7] owing to atrophy of the zonular fibres; if the dislocation is backwards no reactive catastrophe may result, at any rate for a considerable time; but if the luxation is forwards and the lens is arrested in the pupil or becomes dislocated into the anterior chamber, a severe secondary glaucoma is a common sequel.[8]

Barrett. *Trans. ophthal. Soc. U.K.*, **38**, 349 (1918).
Braendstrup. *Acta ophthal.* (Kbh.), **26**, 337 (1948).
Darier. *Ann. Oculist.* (Paris), **114**, 198 (1895).
Dekking. *v. Graefes Arch. Ophthal.*, **135**, 90 (1936).
Ophthalmologica, **115**, 219 (1948).
Douvas and Allen. *Amer. J. Ophthal.*, **33**, 291 (1950).
East. *Brit. J. Ophthal.*, **6**, 365 (1922).
Eber. *Amer. J. Ophthal.*, **5**, 973 (1922).
Ehrich. *Ber. dtsch. ophthal. Ges.*, **61**, 286 (1957).

Klin. Mbl. Augenheilk., **133**, 396 (1958).
Fincham. *Brit. J. Ophthal.*, **39**, 85 (1955).
Friedman. *Arch. Ophthal.*, **5**, 636 (1931).
Goebel. *Arch. Augenheilk.*, **90**, 245 (1922).
Goldmann. *Ophthalmologica*, **98**, 257 (1940).
Goldschmidt. *Arch. Ophthal.*, **44**, 129 (1950).
von Graefe. *v. Graefes Arch. Ophthal.*, **15** (3), 153 (1869).
Kondziela-Brzykowa. *Klin. oczna*, **36**, 505 (1966).
Long. *Amer. J. Ophthal.*, **56**, 761 (1963).
Lubkin. *Amer. J. Ophthal.*, **43**, 718 (1950).
Ogg. *Brit. J. Ophthal.*, **44**, 374 (1960).
Paterson. *Trans. ophthal. Soc. U.K.*, **68**, 265 (1948).

[1] Vol. VII, p. 454.
[3] Vol. VII, p. 431.
[5] p. 662.
[7] p. 298.

[2] Vol. VII, p. 457.
[4] Vol. IV, p. 512.
[6] Vol. IX, p. 500.
[8] p. 307.

Scheerer.   *Klin. Mbl. Augenheilk.*, **73**, 67   Weekers, Grieten and Lekeux.   *Ophthal-*
    (1924); **74**, 688 (1925).   *mologica*, **146**, 57 (1963).
Smith, Priestley.   *Brit. J. Ophthal.*, **8**, 145   Young.   *Brit. J. Ophthal.*, **1**, 362 (1917); **7**,
    (1924).   167 (1923).

THE CLINICAL TYPES OF CATARACT

A very large number of clinical types of cataract is encountered differing considerably in their ætiology, pathology, symptomatology and clinical course.   For descriptive purposes we shall divide them into 11 categories:

1. Congenital cataract.
2. Evolutionary cataract.
3. Senile cataract.
4. Metabolic cataract.

   (*a*) Diabetic, (*b*) galactosæmic, (*c*) hypocalcæmic, (*d*) hypothyroidic, (*e*) myotonic, (*f*) deficiency, (*g*) organic aciduria, (*h*) other metabolic anomalies.

5. Syndermatotic cataract.

   Atopic   dermatitis,   Rothmund's   and   Werner's   syndromes, anhidrotic ectodermal dysplasia, other diseases of the skin.

6. Cataract in osseous disease.
7. Osmotic cataract.
8. Multiple syndromes with cataract.
9. Complicated cataract.

   Inflammatory, embryopathic, degenerative, anoxic, with systemic disease, in prematurity.

10. Toxic cataract.

11. Traumatic cataract.

In this Volume we shall confine ourselves to the various manifestations of senile cataract and the lenticular opacities associated with systemic and ocular diseases. **Congenital cataract** in its many forms has been discussed in a previous Volume[1] and **traumatic cataract** will be subsequently described.[2]

Evolutionary Cataract

Several varieties of cataract are essentially developmental in nature; they are composed of minute, limited, discrete opacities which, although visible on oblique illumination, are frequently so small as to disappear in transmitted light, rarely so gross as to cause visual symptoms, and to a large extent are stationary and non-progressive in type and call for no treatment.

[1] Vol. III, p. 715.
[2] Vol. XIV.

Only exceptionally is vision impaired and the opacities seldom multiply as life proceeds. They cannot be called physiological, nor can they be classed with progressive cataracts of a pathological nature of which they do not even form a premonitory sign.

In so far as these opacities are circumscribed, discrete and show little or no tendency to develop, they resemble the congenital types of lenticular opacity. They may appear at all stages of growth, and it will be remembered that the lens continues to develop until adult life. The date of their appearance determines their site: they are represented in pre-natal development by such conditions as PUNCTATE NUCLEAR CATARACT, FLORIFORM CATARACT, and SUTURAL CATARACT.[1] While similar in their clinical appearance and pathology, the developmental opacities appearing in post-natal life differ from those of ante-natal life only in their site; they represent the result of the same type of process, a failure in development or a degeneration of lenticular fibres occurring, however, after birth and therefore, instead of affecting the central area, appearing in the infantile or adult nucleus or in the cortex. Their persistence is due to the fact that the lens is what may be designated as a " permanent organ " (von Szily, 1938) because it consists of imperishable elements, so that any disturbances in the course of development, no matter how trivial, may give rise to permanent changes.

The most dramatic of these are PUNCTATE (BLUE-DOT) CATARACT, composed of a cloud of fine, minute spots invisible with the ophthalmoscope but presenting a beautiful picture with the slit-lamp, which has already been described,[2] as well as other irregular forms of opacity including the DILACERATED CATARACT of Vogt (1922) which appears as a piece of teased-out moss.[3] The former is usually most marked in the deep cortex representing late-formed fibres which have degenerated and turned granular and have been surrounded by healthy fibres; the latter of similar origin usually lies in the superficial zone of the infantile and the deep layers of the adult nucleus. The most common and clinically apparent condition, however, is coronary cataract.

CORONARY CATARACT

This type of developmental punctate cataract appears usually just after puberty. The older writers considered it a rare form, but after the advent of the slit-lamp its common occurrence was noted by Vogt (1917–18) who found such changes present in some degree in 25% of persons; from the crown-like arrangement of the opacities he termed the condition CORONARY CATARACT (Figs. 165–7). His observations have been amply confirmed (Weissenbach, 1917; Krenger, 1918; Horlacher, 1918; Gjessing, 1920; Foster and Benson, 1934; and others). The opacities are arranged as a regular corona in a peripheral zone in the outer layers of the adult

---

[1] Vol. III, p. 732.   [2] Vol. III, p. 744.
[3] Vol. III, p. 743.

nucleus and the inner layers of the cortex, the axial region and the extreme periphery remaining free; frequently, therefore, they are behind the iris and do not become apparent until the pupil is dilated. They are of all shapes, the most common being a club-shape with the head of the club pointing

FIGS. 165 to 167.—CORONARY CATARACT (J. Foster and J. Benson).

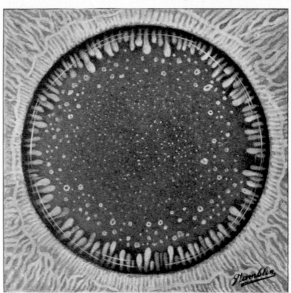

FIG. 165.—Early stage.

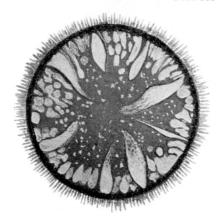

FIG. 166.—Advanced stage.

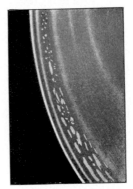

FIG. 167.—Slit-lamp section.

centrally, but punctiform, ring-shaped and disciform types are common, while they vary in colour from white to grey, yellow, brown, red, or blue. They may be associated with punctate or nummular opacities scattered throughout the axial region of the lens, for they differ from other developmental punctate opacities only in the lateness of their appearance in life and not in their nature. Like these they are non-progressive, or so slowly progressive as never to lead to complete opacification of the lens; in elderly people the regular process of senile cortical cataract must be superimposed upon them if a complete opacity is to develop.

The blue colour of these opacities, as in blue-dot cataract (CATARACTA CÆRULEA), is a physical phenomenon depending on the dispersion of light. In any opalescent medium minute particles disperse the light irregularly to an extent varying inversely as the fourth power of the wavelength, so that the major part of the dispersed light is made up of the short blue and violet waves. The cataract is blue, therefore, for the same reason as the sky is blue owing to dispersion by the atmosphere.

The anatomical basis of punctate cataract of the pre-senile type and coronary cataract is the presence of round, elliptical or fusiform lacunæ between the fibres in the deeper layers of the cortex (Hess, 1893–1905) (Fig. 157). These spaces are filled with homogeneous or finely granular coagula which stain deeply with hæmatoxylin, while the fibres themselves and the entire nucleus remain normal.

The *hereditary occurrence* of coronary cataract as a dominant characteristic has been well established (Vogt, 1930; Vogt *et al.*, 1940; O. and R. Wolfe, 1943) (Fig. 168). The topographical distribution of the opacities, however, may not be constant in a family: thus coronary lesions may be interchanged with nuclear and perinuclear opacities (Halbertsma, 1928).

The cause of a developmental cataract of this type is unknown. Some writers[1] have associated it with infantile or juvenile tetany,[2] others with an endocrine origin (Nordmann, 1928) depending particularly on the gonads at puberty (Fischer-Galati, 1930). Noting that in a case of complete uveal coloboma at the site of which the zonular fibres were lacking, coronary opacities were absent while being abundant elsewhere, Pau (1950) considered that the strains of accommodation were a causal factor. Nothing approaching conclusive evidence, however, has been advanced in support of these hypotheses.

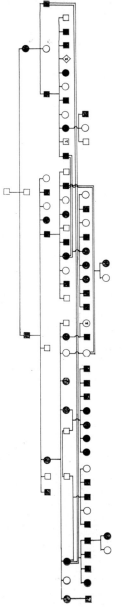

FIG. 168.—CORONARY CATARACT (after K. T. A. Halbertsma, 1928).

[1] Peters (1901–5), Hesse and Phleps (1913), Fischer and Triebenstein (1914), Greppin (1922), Romanowa (1934), and others.

[2] p. 175.

Fischer-Galati. *Clinique*, **25**, 119 (1930).
Fischer and Triebenstein. *Klin. Mbl. Augen-
    heilk.*, **52**, 441 (1914).
Foster and Benson. *Trans. ophthal. Soc.
    U.K.*, **54**, 127 (1934).
Gjessing. *Klin. Mbl. Augenheilk.*, **65**, 233
    (1920).
Greppin. *Schweiz. med. Wschr.*, **52**, 1260
    (1922).
Halbertsma. *Klin. Mbl. Augenheilk.*, **80**, 794
    (1928).
Hess. *v. Graefes Arch. Ophthal.*, **39** (1), 183
    (1893).
    Graefe-Saemisch Hb. d. ges. Augenheilk.,
    2nd ed., Leipzig, **6** (2), Kap. 9 (1905).
Hesse and Phleps. *Z. Augenheilk.*, **29**, 238
    (1913).
Horlacher. *Z. Augenheilk.*, **40**, 33 (1918).
Krenger. *Klin. Mbl. Augenheilk.*, **60**, 229
    (1918).
Nordmann. *Ann. Oculist.* (Paris), **165**, 29
    (1928).

Pau. *Klin. Mbl. Augenheilk.*, **117**, 290
    (1950).
Peters. *Z. Augenheilk.*, **4**, 337 (1900); **5**, 89
    (1901).
    Klin. Mbl. Augenheilk., **43** (1), 621 (1905).
Romanowa. *v. Graefes Arch. Ophthal.*, **133**,
    143 (1934).
von Szily. *Trans. ophthal. Soc. U.K.*, **58**, 595
    (1938).
Vogt. *Klin. Mbl. Augenheilk.*, **58**, 579 (1917).
    Z. Augenheilk., **40**, 123 (1918).
    v. Graefes Arch. Ophthal., **107**, 196 (1922).
    *Lhb. u. Atlas d. Spaltlampenmikroskopie
    d. lebenden Auges*, Berlin (1930).
Vogt, Wagner and Sclapfer. Just's *Hb. d.
    Erbbiologie d. Menschen*, Berlin, **3** (1940).
Weissenbach. *Klin. Mbl. Augenheilk.*, **59**,
    527 (1917).
Wolfe, O. and R. *Amer. J. Ophthal.*, **26**, 404
    (1943).

Senile Changes

PATHOLOGICAL SENILE CHANGES

A group of senile changes must now be considered which cannot be called physiological; they may, however, remain for an indefinite time without progression, but the eventual frequent superimposition of cataract upon them justifies their being looked upon as forerunners of this condition. They are all indicative of hydration of the cortex and are the expression of the accumulation of fluid which is probably largely derived from without, but may partly be abstracted from colloid combination in the fibres.[1] This fluid may collect in globules and vacuoles, or forcing itself between the fibres of the lens, may make great clefts in a radial direction or force the sutures apart or, separating the radial lamellæ, it may cause lines of cleavage between them.

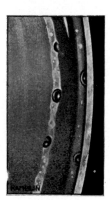

FIG. 169. FLUID VACUOLES IN THE LENS.

Subcapsular and on the surface of the adult nucleus.

VACUOLE FORMATION. Isolated vacuoles filled with fluid occurring either under the capsule or in the interior of the lens, particularly on the surface of the adult nucleus, are not infrequent, and carry no grave prognostic significance (Fig. 169).[2] They occasionally occur in young people and may remain stationary for years; in age they tend to multiply; and in early cortical cataract they may appear in enormous numbers under the capsule forming a veritable carpet.

THE FORMATION OF CLEAR CLEFTS. The formation of clear radial clefts (*Wasserspalten; fissured cataract*) is of graver prognostic significance, a fact which was

[1] p. 67.   [2] p. 14.

noted by the earlier observers (Becker, 1883; Magnus, 1890). Such spaces rarely appear before the age of 50, but become relatively common thereafter (Pfeiffer, 1921; Vogt, 1922). They occur most frequently in the cortex, usually just underneath the capsule, but occasionally they penetrate into the adult nucleus; Pfeiffer (1921) found that they usually occurred in the anterior cortex (53%), quite frequently both in the anterior and posterior cortex (42%), and only rarely in the latter alone (5%). They

FIGS. 170 TO 174.—CLEAR FLUID CLEFTS.

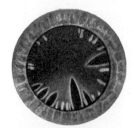
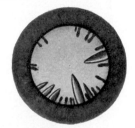

FIG. 170.—In focal   FIG. 171.—By the plane
illumination.   mirror.

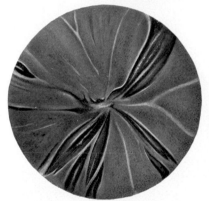
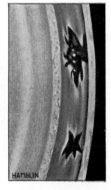
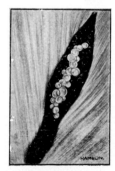

FIG. 172.—In oblique illumina-   FIG. 173.   FIG. 174. With
tion.   Optical section.   granular debris.

may occur anywhere in the lens but, as would be expected, they have a predilection for the sutures which consequently appear to gape (*dehiscence of the sutures*), a phenomenon readily seen in the isolated lens on maceration (Vogt, 1914; von der Heydt, 1930) (Fig. 170). Although they are transparent in transmitted light, being filled with a homogeneous fluid, in focal illumination they appear dark or black because of the lack of optical density (Figs. 170–2), and in the optical beam of the slit-lamp they are seen as irregularly angulated spaces (Fig. 173). As cataractous changes develop, however, they become filled with debris and fatty droplets so that they become opaque (Fig. 174).

FIGS. 175 to 177.—LAMELLAR SEPARATION.

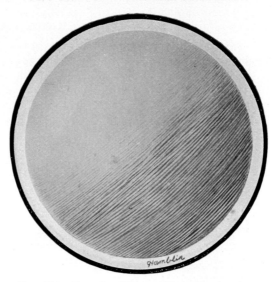

FIG. 175.—Seen by diffuse oblique illumination.

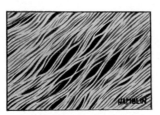

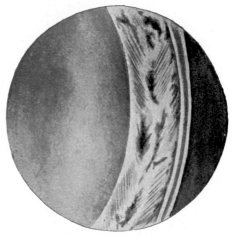

FIG. 176.—Surface view of the anterior   FIG. 177.—Optical section (T. Harrison
cortex with the slit-lamp.   Butler).

LAMELLAR SEPARATION. This is a senile phenomenon which begins to
appear usually in the anterior cortex after the age of 50 (in 7% of lenses)
and is found in 50% of people above 80 years (Schild, 1921); it is intimately
associated with early cortical cataract, evidences of which are usually
present. It represents a separation of the radial lamellæ in a series of fine
parallel lines, usually occupying a whole sector of the lens and running
upwards and outwards from the infero-nasal region, but sometimes forming

two or more systems in separate bands cutting each other at right angles (Vogt, 1914–19) (Figs. 175–7).

SENILE CATARACT

Incidence. Senile cataract is very common and may, indeed, be said to be the rule in advanced age. Thus Horlacher (1918) found that 65% of all persons between 51 and 60, and Barth (1914) that 96% of those above 60 years of age have some lenticular opacities visible with the slit-lamp; but it is to be remembered that in the majority of cases the condition is extremely slowly progressive, and the proportion of people in whom the process becomes so advanced before death as to cause visual disability is comparatively small. Three estimates of the incidence of lenticular changes in the various age-groups, one of them taken from Scandinavia and two from America, are seen in Table I.

TABLE I

Age	41–50 %	51–60 %	61–70 %	70+ %
Andersen (1924)	38·2	65·1	85·0	92·0
Gradle (1926)	34·1	66·2	68·4	90·9
Cinotti and Patti (1968) . .	63·3	58·6	83·2	93·1

It is not therefore surprising that cataract is one of the most common causes of blindness. This is so even in highly developed countries. In Britain it accounted for 22·6% of those registered blind between 1955 and 1960 (Sorsby, 1966), and in the excellently annotated figures for Canada it represented 15·94% of the total causes of blindness (MacDonald, 1965) and in the United States 15·6% (Kinsey, 1967). This may seem surprising for a condition that is eminently rectifiable by surgery, but in many such cases the cataract is complicated in type or occurs in patients considered (perhaps often unnecessarily) medically unsuitable for a surgical ordeal or who are content to suffer the visual disability in the peace or lassitude of old age. In under-developed countries, largely because of the unavailability of surgical treatment, the percentage of the blind from this cause is much higher (45 % in Kenya, Bisley, 1963), and in a country such as India those blind from this reason are numbered in hundreds of thousands, while in Pakistan 60,000 people are said to be blind from this cause, only one-third of whom receive surgical attention (Refatullah, 1953). Nevertheless, in a typical English population, partly urban and partly rural, approximately one per 2,000 individuals over 20 years of age present themselves for cataract surgery per year (Caird *et al.*, 1965). In every country in the world for which statistics are known, operations for cataract are much more numerous than for any other ophthalmological condition (A. Fuchs, 1962).

Heredity. There can be no doubt that the early and rapid development of cataract has a hereditary tendency, a feature common to all the phenomena of senescence, but we are ignorant as yet whether the cataract itself or the influences which determine it are genetically conditioned; moreover, in a change characteristic of age affecting over 65% of the population over 50 years, the establishment of heredity is difficult. In a previous Volume we have seen the extraordinary hereditary influence in many types of congenital lenticular opacities[1]; juvenile and pre-senile opacities have the same tendency (Nettleship, 1909–12; Rowan and Wilson, 1921; Halbertsma, 1928). This influence may not be so potent in senile cataract, but it was sufficiently apparent to attract the attentions of as early an observer as Belivier (1818), who noted its preferential incidence in a family over a period of 100 years. In the subsequent literature there are numerous reports of

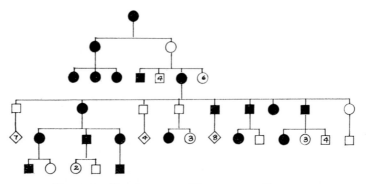

FIG. 178.—THE DOMINANT HEREDITY OF CATARACT
(after J. Green, 1890).

families showing a high incidence over several generations (Fig. 178).[2] Thus Nettleship (1905) collected 122 families of which 375 persons comprising 145 males (38%) and 230 females (62%) had advanced cataract, the tendency not only appearing in a sibship but being transmitted up to 5 generations. Vogt and his colleagues (1931–39) and Nordmann (1954) claimed that not only is the type of cataract hereditary, whether nuclear or cortical, but also its architecture and its rate of clinical progress. Moreover, a concordance in expression has been seen in monozygous twins with a tendency for the lesion to appear at approximately the same age (Waardenburg, 1932; Oguchi, 1936; Vogt *et al.*, 1939). The heredity shows a *direct, continuous and dominant transmission,* either sex transmitting but the female sex showing the highest

[1] Vol. III, p. 715.
[2] Bastard (1850), Green (1890), Groenouw (1904), Nettleship (1905–12), Casey Wood (1906), Zydek (1915), Parker (1916), Vogt (1918), Garfunkel (1926), Terrien and Blum (1928), Rollet (1929), Moretti (1931), Waardenburg (1932), Hornback and de Garis (1933), Vinsonhaler and Cosgrove (1936), Bücklers (1936–38), Biro (1936), Hedinger (1939), Johnstone (1947), Abreu Fialho (1953), Orlowski (1966), and many others.

incidence. Only occasionally is the dominance irregular, one or more generations being skipped (Nettleship, 1909; Andrassy, 1921; Garfunkel, 1926).

Clinical Forms. The clinical forms in which senile cataract may appear are numerous, and although arguments may be put forward against their differentiation into separate categories, and despite the fact that different forms may appear simultaneously in the two eyes and that frequently more than one form is seen together in the same lens, it is convenient for purposes of description to study them separately. Following Elschnig's (1911) classification, they may be divided into two large classes, nuclear and cortical: some 20 to 25% are nuclear and the majority cortical in type. Nuclear cataracts vary only in the degree of sclerosis, being either uniform over the whole central zone, or affecting the fœtal nucleus when a lens with a double focus results, or becoming extreme in degree and extent in which case the rare condition of brown or black cataract develops. Cortical cataract may be divided into three main types which differ in their site and evolution —cuneiform, in the peripheral cortex; punctate perinuclear; and cupuliform occurring usually in the posterior cortex.

The relative incidence of these types has been variously assessed. Knapp (1916) estimated nuclear cataracts at 1·5% of the total, cuneiform at 33%, peripheral equatorial opacities at 50%, and posterior cortical at 6·3%. Kirby (1932) found 29% nuclear cataracts, 52% in the peripheral cortex and 3·5% in the posterior cortex, with a mixture of nuclear and cortical in 9%, nuclear and posterior cortical in 4%, and peripheral and posterior cortical in 2·5%. Foster and Benson (1934) found 22% nuclear, 37% cuneiform, 17% punctate, 6% cupuliform, and 18% mixed in which category the nuclear cataract predominated. They also found that the cupuliform type occurred earliest with a maximum incidence between 50 and 60 years, cuneiform and punctate between 60 and 70, and nuclear between 70 and 75. Over most parts of the world it has been said that the average age for operation is 65 years (Gradle, 1930) or (in Norway) over 70 years (Waaler, 1961).

NUCLEAR CATARACT

(HARD CATARACT)

A nuclear cataract, as we have seen, is merely the intensification of the physiological change of sclerosis which has progressed to such a degree that vision becomes affected (Figs. 179–180), a process which usually begins about the age of 50 and reaches a maximum incidence between 70 and 75. There is a diffuse increase of the optical density of the nuclei beginning in the deeper layers of the fœtal nucleus and spreading gradually in a peripheral direction to include the whole adult nucleus; the Y-suture and the nuclear relief are particularly obvious. The change is diffuse, for any circumscribed sharply defined opacities in this central area must be of congenital origin. With transmitted light the senile yellow or orange coloration of the lens is particularly marked, but frequently the nuclear opacity remains white

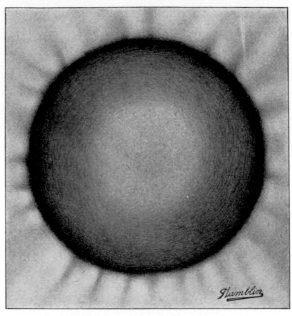

FIG. 179.—NUCLEAR CATARACT.
Seen by oblique illumination (J. Foster and J. Benson).

without trace of pigment (28 cases in 359 of nuclear cataract, Voisin and Piroteau, 1962). Such a sclerotic process is gradual, showing no sudden changes, is usually extremely slow in its progression, and is not associated with the appearance of vacuoles, clefts, lamellar separation or any evidences of hydration of the lens. It is true that cortical changes are often superimposed upon the nuclear sclerosis, in which case the latter process tends to hold the former in check and delays the development of the soft cataract.

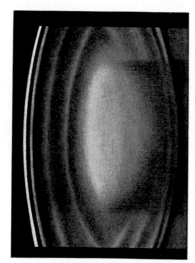

FIG. 180.—NUCLEAR CATARACT.
Slit-lamp section (J. Foster and J. Benson).

Pathologically the lens shows exactly the opposite changes to those which characterize cortical cataract (Fig. 134): there is a dense uniform induration of the affected area which assumes a rubber-like consistency, the whole mass of hardened and compressed fibres showing a regular concentric lamination with only sporadic inter-fibrillar spaces and displaying a resistance to all histological stains (Becker, 1883; v. Szily, 1938; and others). On the whole, therefore, the lens retains its anatomical integrity, suffering a change in certain physiological and physical attributes, particularly its refractive index and density.   The weight of such a lens may increase by one third and the water-content may diminish almost to one half (d'Agostino and Manes, 1960).   We have seen that chemically it differs completely from cortical cataract; clinically the fundus may be seen although it is generally considerably distorted, and the main visual symptoms are a slow and gradual diminution of visual acuity especially in bright light, a distortion of objects, and a progressive myopia.

Two special types deserve separate notice; in the first the sclerosis is limited to the fœtal nucleus, and in the second it progresses to involve practically the entire lens and is associated with marked coloration.

LENS WITH DOUBLE FOCUS

This condition, although noted by L. Müller (1894), was first described by Demicheri (1895) under the name of FALSE LENTICONUS, and it has been variously called FALSE CATARACT (Halben, 1903), CENTRAL HYPER-REFRIN-GENCE (Koby, 1930) or LENS WITH DOUBLE FOCUS (v. Szily, 1903).   Patho-logically the process is a simple sclerosis, but it is limited to the fœtal nucleus; the central interval of the embryonic nucleus is obliterated and the entire fœtal nucleus becomes homogeneous with the Y-sutures alone distinguishable.   Its limits are well marked and are separated from the adult nucleus by a dark space (Vogt, 1923), but eventually this interval disappears and finally the whole adult nucleus becomes homogeneously sclerosed.

The most arresting clinical feature of this type of cataract is the development of a double refraction, the axial area being highly myopic while the peripheral part remains hypermetropic, often with profound visual consequences, sometimes involving diplopia or, if the condition is bilateral, quadrantanopia.   The difference between the two areas may be considerable, variations in refraction of 10 or 12 dioptres being frequently noted, while 27 dioptres have been recorded (Guttmann, 1898; Hess, 1911; Gaiser, 1928; and others).   Demicheri (1895) at first thought that the disparity between the two regions was due to cortical changes involving a peripheral hypermetropia, but the slit-lamp has demonstrated without doubt that the cause is the increased optical density of the nucleus, an effect enhanced by the fact that the curvature of the fœtal nucleus is considerably greater than that of the lens.   Occasionally, also, the refractive effect of the optical surface thus created may be intensified by the development of a true internal lenticonus (Møller, 1927).

It is interesting that a similar condition of " double focus " has been observed to follow the therapeutic administration of dimethylsulphoxide (Kleberger and Gordon, 1967)[1]; a similar change can be produced experimentally in rabbits (Kamiya et al., 1967).

[1] See Vol. XIV.

BLACK CATARACT (CATARACTA BRUNESCENS OR NIGRA)

As the process of senile sclerosis proceeds it gradually spreads towards the periphery of the lens, and although it does not actually reach the capsule, so that some cortical substance always remains, it may eventually occupy practically the entire tissue. In this event the colour of the lens slowly changes from the yellow appearance of nuclear sclerosis, to amber, reddish brown, and finally it may become almost black; strata of these differing colours have been observed in the various layers of the lens (Vogt, 1931) (Plate II, Figs. 1 and 3). This occurrence which was called CATARACTA NIGRA by Wenzel (1786) and CATARACTA BRUNESCENS by Becker (1883), is relatively rare (10 out of 1,500 cataracts, Elschnig and Zeynek, 1913; 23 out of 6,206, Mahieu, 1921–22). The clinical appearance is peculiar, for although the pupil appears black on oblique focal illumination, in marked cases the fundus reflex is absent, a circumstance which makes the condition resemble the effect of a massive hæmorrhage into the vitreous body. The nature of the pigment has already been discussed.[1]

CORTICAL CATARACT
(SOFT CATARACT)

In contrast to the sclerosis of nuclear cataract, the phenomena characteristic of cortical cataract are those of hydration and intumescence. The opacities are typically preceded by the pre-cataractous signs of hydration which we have already studied: the formation of vacuoles, separation of the lamellæ by fluid, and water-splitting of the sutures to form clear clefts. These processes are eventually associated with the development of an ill-defined haze in the cortex, which in its initial stages may be a physical œdema and therefore reversible, but eventually proceeds to denaturation and coagulation of the proteins with the consequent formation of organic opacities. According to the nature and position of these opacities such cataracts may be divided into several types.

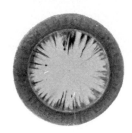

FIG. 181.

CUNEIFORM CATARACT. Seen by direct illumination.

CUNEIFORM CATARACT

This is the most typical form of senile cataract in which the opacities develop in the peripheral parts of the deep cortex, particularly in the lower segment, and run axially both anterior and posterior to the nucleus forming radial " spokes " or " riders " pointing at the centre of the pupil. These, in contrast to water-clefts, appear grey by oblique illumination and black and opaque on transillumination (Figs. 181–3). Sometimes these opaque spokes may be numerous, small and discrete, and at other times

[1] p. 127.

PLATE II

Cataract

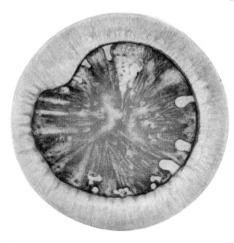

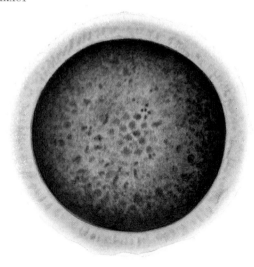

FIG. 1.—SENILE NUCLEAR SCLEROSIS (RED CATARACT) WITH CORONARY AND SENILE PERIPHERAL CHANGES.

FIG. 2.—CUPULIFORM CATARACT.

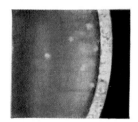

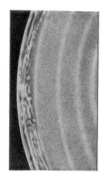

FIG. 3.—SENILE NUCLEAR SCLEROSIS: RED CATARACT.

FIG. 4.—CUPULIFORM CATARACT.

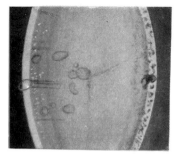

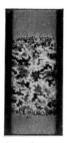

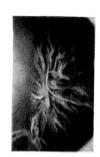

FIG. 5.—EARLY DIABETIC CATARACT.
Punctate opacities and fluid droplets in the cortex.

FIG. 6.—COMPLICATED CATARACT.
Polychromatic lustre at the posterior pole.

FIG. 7.—CRYSTALS IN THE LENS.

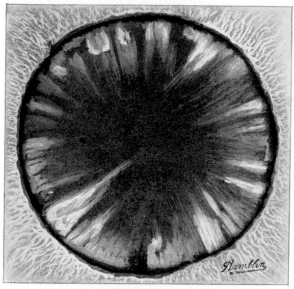

FIG. 182.—CUNEIFORM CATARACT.
Seen by oblique illumination (J. Foster and J. Benson).

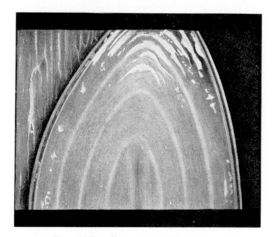

FIG. 183.—CUNEIFORM CATARACT.
Slit-lamp section (J. Foster and J. Benson).

they become fused, losing their individuality to form great plaques occupying a large sector of the periphery. When they occur alone without other changes and are sharply defined, their progress may be exceedingly slow and they may remain stationary for years, or one or two elements may break into the pupillary region or strike right across the lens. At other times, when they are associated with much hydration of the cortex, they may show a stormy progression; in this event the appearance of clear clefts and lamellar separation is followed by a cloudy swelling of the whole cortex which becomes swollen in a state of *intumescence,* often making the anterior chamber shallow. This phase progresses to *maturity* (Fig. 184) and is eventually

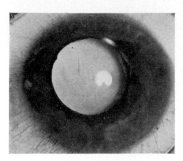

followed by the autolysis of the fibres and loss of fluid resulting in the silvery white, desiccated appearance characteristic of *hypermaturity* (Fig. 185) or, alternatively, the fluid is retained and the *morgagnian* state develops wherein the solid nucleus floats in a white milky fluid cortex. In the erect position the nucleus of such a cataract sinks downwards in the capsular sac and may be seen as a brownish shadow in the milky fluid, changing

FIG. 184.—A MATURE CATARACT

Clinical appearance as seen by diffuse focal illumination (Inst. Ophthal.).

its position with movements of the head, and when the patient is supine it sinks posteriorly and the pupillary area becomes uniformly clouded (Fig. 186).

Pathologically, in the stage of intumescence the most prominent feature is the disintegration and splintering of the swollen lenticular fibres, and the accumulation of their detritus as spherical and granular agglomerations in the gaps and fissures between them (Fig. 136). Beneath the lens

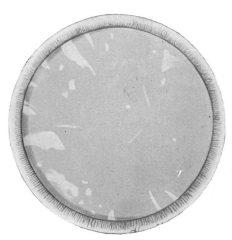

FIG. 185.—HYPERMATURE CATARACT.

capsule there is sometimes a remarkable folding of the fibres, but ultimately the majority becomes fragmented to form globules and granular detritus frequently running in algæ-like formations. The nucleus may be preserved for some time, but eventually it also tends to become fissured, and as the cortex gradually becomes dehydrated and then shrinks to form a pultaceous

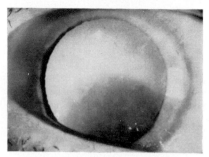

FIG. 186.—MORGAGNIAN CATARACT.

The cortex takes the form of a cloudy fluid like milk and with the patient erect the dark nucleus sinks downwards (P. A. MacFaul).

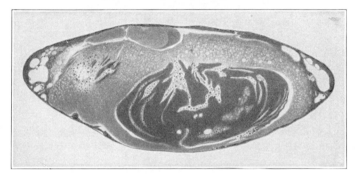

FIG. 187.—HYPERMATURE CATARACT.

Liquefied cortex and displacement of the fissured nucleus (A. von Szily).

mass, the cataract passes into the stage of hypermaturity (Fig. 187) and eventually may reach the morgagnian condition.

PERINUCLEAR PUNCTATE CATARACT

This type of opacity to which several names have been given (DUST-LIKE CATARACT IN CONCENTRIC LAYERS, etc.) appears in elderly people often in association with a coronary cataract. Its onset is recognized by a thickening and intensification of the appearance of the anterior and posterior bands of the adult nucleus, and eventually multiple small opaque dots usually interspersed with larger plaques are seen in the deeper layers, forming aggregations of small foci, concentric lines and cloudy patches (the PERIPHERAL CONCENTRIC OPACITIES of Vogt, 1918). Pathologically these early opacities are seen to represent more or less narrow fissures following generally the course of the lenticular fibres filled with finely granular detritus (von Szily, 1938) (Fig. 188); but although such an appearance may remain relatively unchanged for some considerable time, it usually becomes complicated by the addition of other types of cortical cataract and complete opacification eventually results.

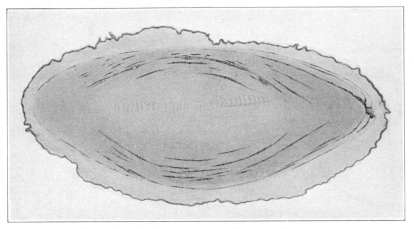

Fig. 188.—Perinuclear and Cortical Cataract.
Interlamellar fissures filled with finely granular detritus (A. von Szily).

CUPULIFORM (SUBCAPSULAR) CATARACT

This type of opacity—the SAUCER-SHAPED CATARACT of Vogt (1919)—is a common form of senile opacification consisting of a thin layer of granules located just beneath the capsule, most commonly confined to the posterior part of the lens with a preference for the lower nasal quadrant but sometimes affecting the anterior region and occasionally both. In the focal illumination of the slit-lamp the affected layer appears distinctly yellow, probably because of the dispersion of the shorter rays of light, and is seen to be made up of a cloud of minute opacities, frequently crystalline in appearance, between which are numerous rounded vacuoles (Plate II, Figs. 2 and 4). The initial change was ascribed by Pau (1956) to alterations in the permeability of the capsule. This form of cataract may be an early change (Sautter, 1963) and progresses very slowly of itself, but it usually becomes complicated by other types; nuclear sclerosis is the most common association, while other cortical opacities accelerate the general opacification of the lens. Such a lesion, being near the nodal point of the dioptric system, obstructs vision at an early stage and may interfere to a surprising degree with the visual acuity when the opacity may be so slight as to be readily overlooked with the ophthalmoscope. Herein lies the clinical importance of its recognition and the value of examining the posterior region of the lens under mydriasis with the slit-lamp in cases of failing vision in elderly persons. A second important clinical matter is the differential diagnosis from a complicated cataract, sometimes a problem of some difficulty which will be discussed when dealing with the latter.[1] Fortunately, however, despite the apparent immaturity, the lens is usually easily extracted even by the extracapsular method, for relatively little cortex is left behind.

[1] p. 217.

Abreu Fialho. *Rev. bras. Med.*, **10**, 251 (1953).

d'Agostino and Manes. *Arch. Ottal.*, **64**, 377 (1960).

Andersen. *Acta ophthal.* (Kbh.), **2**, 250 (1924).

Anderson. *J. Hered.*, **40**, 157 (1949).

Andrassy. *Klin. Mbl. Augenheilk.*, **66**, 568 (1921).

Appenzeller. *Mitt. ophthal. Klin. Tübingen*, **2**, 120 (1884).

Barth. *Z. Augenheilk.*, **32**, 8, 143 (1914).

Bastard. *Considérations pratiques sur la cataracte* (Thèse), Montpellier (1850).

Becker. *Zur Anatomie d. gesunden u. kranken Linse*, Wiesbaden (1883).

Belivier. In Guillé's *Nouvelles recherches sur la cataracte et la goutte sereine*, Paris (1818).

Biro. *Arch. Ophtal.*, **53**, 685 (1936).

Bisley. *E. Afr. med. J.*, **40**, 570 (1963).

Bücklers. *Klin. Mbl. Augenheilk.*, **96**, 119 (1936); **100**, 777 (1938).

Caird, Hutchinson and Pirie. *Brit. J. prev. soc. Med.*, **19**, 80 (1965).

Cinotti and Patti. *Amer. J. Ophthal.*, **65**, 25 (1968).

Demicheri. *Ann. Oculist.* (Paris), **113**, 93 (1895).

Elschnig. *Klin. Mbl. Augenheilk.*, **49** (1), 38 (1911).

Elschnig and Zeynek. *Z. Augenheilk.*, **29**, 401 (1913).

Foster and Benson. *Trans. ophthal. Soc. U.K.*, **54**, 127 (1934).

Fuchs, A. *Geography of Eye Diseases*, Vienna (1962).

Gaiser. *v. Graefes Arch. Ophthal.*, **121**, 145 (1928).

Garfunkel. *Arch. Klaus-Stift. Vererb. Forsch.*, **2**, 71 (1926).

Gradle. *Contribs. to Ophthalmic Science* (Jackson Birthday Vol.; ed. Crisp and Finnoff), Wisconsin, 255 (1926).
Arch. Ophthal., **4**, 588 (1930).

Green. *Trans. Amer. ophthal. Soc.*, **5**, 724 (1890).

Groenouw. *Graefe-Saemisch Hb. d. ges. Augenheilk.*, 2nd ed., Leipzig, **11** (1), 430 (1904).

Guttmann. *Zbl. prakt. Augenheilk.*, **22**, 193 (1898).

Halben. *v. Graefes Arch. Ophthal.*, **57**, 277 (1903).

Halbertsma. *Klin. Mbl. Augenheilk.*, **80**, 108, 794 (1928).

Hedinger. *Beitr. z. Vererbung d. präsenilen Kataract* (Diss.), Zürich (1939).

Hess. *Graefe-Saemisch Hb. d. ges. Augenheilk.*, 2nd ed., Leipzig, **6** (2), Kap. IX (1905); 3rd ed., Kap. IX (1911).

von der Heydt. *Arch. Ophthal.*, **4**, 188 (1930).

Horlacher. *Z. Augenheilk.*, **40**, 33 (1918).

Hornback and de Garis. *J. Morphol.*, **54**, 347 (1933).

Jeaffreson. *Lancet*, **1**, 387, 434, 479 (1886).

Johnstone. *Brit. J. Ophthal.*, **31**, 385 (1947).

Kamiya, Wakao and Nishioka. *Folia ophthal. jap.*, **18**, 387 (1967).

Kirby. *Arch. Ophthal.*, **8**, 97 (1932).

Kinsey. *Vision and its Disorders*, U.S. Public Health Service, Bethesda, 114 (1967).

Kleberger and Gordon. *Fortschr. Med.*, **85**, 171 (1967).

Knapp. *Arch. Ophthal.*, **45**, 600 (1916).

Koby. *Slit-lamp Microscopy of the Living Eye*, London (1930).

MacDonald. *Canad. med. Ass. J.*, **92**, 264 (1965).

Magnus. *v. Graefes Arch. Ophthal.*, **36** (4), 150 (1890).

Mahieu. *Considérations sur la cataracte noire* (Thèse), Lyon (1921).
Arch. Ophtal., **39**, 510 (1922).

Møller. *Acta ophthal.* (Kbh.), **5**, 258 (1927).

Moretti. *Arch. Ottal.*, **38**, 289 (1931).

Müller, L. *Klin. Mbl. Augenheilk.*, **32**, 178 (1894).

Nettleship. *Roy. Lond. ophthal. Hosp. Rep.*, **16**, 179 (1905).
Trans. ophthal. Soc. U.K., **29**, lxxviii, 188 (1909); **32**, 337 (1912).

Nordmann. *Biologie du cristallin*, Paris (1954).

Norrie. *Ugeskr. f. Laeger.*, **3**, 937 (1896).

Oguchi. *Chuo-Ganka-Iho*, **28**, 85 (1936).

Orlowski. *Klin. oczna*, **36**, 195 (1966).

Parker. *J. Michigan med. Soc.*, **15**, 188 (1916).

Pau. *Klin. Mbl. Augenheilk.*, **129**, 371 (1956).

Pfeiffer. *v. Graefes Arch. Ophthal.*, **107**, 71 (1921).

Redl. *Klin. Mbl. Augenheilk.*, **114**, 24 (1949).

Refatullah. *Bull. ophthal. Soc. Egypt*, **46**, 275 (1953).

Rollet. *Ann. Oculist.* (Paris), **166**, 146 (1929).

Rowan and Wilson. *Brit. J. Ophthal.*, **5**, 64 (1921).

Sautter. *Ber. dtsch. ophthal. Ges.*, **65**, 379 (1963).

Schild. *v. Graefes Arch. Ophthal.*, **107**, 49 (1921).

Sorsby. *Blindness in England*, 1951–54, London (1956).
The Incidence and Causes of Blindness in England and Wales, 1948–62, London (1966).

von Szily. *Klin. Mbl. Augenheilk.*, **41** (2), 44 (1903).
Trans. ophthal. Soc. U.K., **58**, 595 (1938).

Terrien and Blum. *Bull. Soc. Ophtal. Paris*, 379 (1928).

Vinsonhaler and Cosgrove. *Arch. Ophthal.*, **15**, 222 (1936).

Vogt. *v. Graefes Arch. Ophthal.*, **88**, 329 (1914); **107**, 196 (1922).
Z. Augenheilk., **40**, 123 (1918); **50**, 145 (1923).

Vogt. *Klin. Mbl. Augenheilk.*, **61**, 89 (1918);
　　62, 396, 582, 593 (1919).
　　Lhb. u. Atlas d. Spaltlampenmikroskopie d.
　　lebenden Auges, 2nd ed., Berlin, **2** (1931).
Vogt, Wagner, Richner and Meyer. *Arch.*
　　Klaus-Stift. Vererb. Forsch., **14**, 475
　　(1939).
Voisin and Piroteau. *Bull. Soc. franç.*
　　Ophtal., **75**, 151 (1962).

Waaler. *Acta ophthal.* (Kbh.), **39**, 182 (1961).
Waardenburg. *Das mensch. Auge u. seine*
　　Erbanlagen, Hague (1932).
Weber. *Schweiz. med. Wschr.*, **1**, 295 (1940).
Wenzel. *Traité de la cataracte*, Paris (1786).
Wood, Casey. *Ophthal. Rec.*, **15**, 142 (1906).
Zydek. *Klin. Mbl. Augenheilk.*, **54**, 482
　　(1915).

Metabolic Cataract

DIABETIC CATARACT

The condition of diabetes mellitus has been fully discussed in its
ætiological, clinical and hereditary aspects in a previous Volume in association with diabetic retinopathy.[1] That sufferers from this disease are
particularly prone to the development of cataract has been recognized for
many years; this was noted, for example, by as early a writer as John
Rollo (1798), while by the time of Berndt (1834), T. Benedict (1842) and
Himly (1843), its recognition was common. In these patients two types
of cataract occur:

1. ORDINARY CHANGES OF THE SENILE TYPE differing in no way from
those usually met with in aged subjects, except that in diabetics they are
generally accepted as occurring more frequently and at an earlier age than
in non-diabetic subjects and tend to progress more rapidly to maturity.

2. A TRUE DIABETIC CATARACT characterized by widespread subcapsular
changes, occurring bilaterally, which tends to run a relatively acute course,
and occurs preferentially in young persons.

The first type of cataract is common; the second rare.

The occurrence of changes resembling senile cataract among diabetics
has given rise to controversy. Some observers have found them no more
frequently than in the non-diabetic adult population,[2] while others have
recorded a higher incidence.[3] Some of the figures recorded have been high:
thus Kirby (1933) found that 64% of all diabetics had lenticular opacities
of some kind, of which 70% were of the senile cortical type, 21% nuclear,
7% posterior cortical, and 2% subcapsular. It has also been said to occur
at a younger age than average (O'Brien *et al.*, 1934; Schulte, 1952), and to
increase with the duration (Kirby, 1933; Janert *et al.*, 1956; Dollfus and
Haye, 1957) and the severity of the diabetes (Pirie, 1965). The percentage
of patients presenting for surgical treatment of cataract has also been found
to be higher among diabetics than non-diabetics (Clegg, 1920; Anthonisen,
1936; Townes and Casey, 1955), while the significant observation has been
made that 3% of all patients presenting at hospital for senile cataract had
an undiagnosed diabetes (Caird *et al.*, 1964; Pirie, 1965); lenticular opacities

---

[1] Vol. X, p. 408.

[2] Andersen (1929), Waite and Beetham (1935), Dollfus (1954), Caird *et al.* (1964).

[3] Kirby (1933), O'Brien *et al.* (1934), Heinsius and Arndt (1950), Kennedy and Kirchbaum
(1951), Kato *et al.* (1960), Tulloch (1962), Burditt and Caird (1968), and others.

may also appear at a relatively early age in people in the pre-diabetic state (Paufique and Michaud, 1965; Brückner, 1965; van Selm, 1966).

   Typical diabetic cataract (the *snow-flake cataract* of O'Brien *et al.*, 1934) tends to occur in patients who, while they have severe diabetes, are yet relatively well and in whom the water-balance is well maintained. It is comparatively rare (3 cases in 7,500 cataracts, Refatullah, 1953). It may appear at an early age in cases of infantile diabetes (11 months, Major and Curran, 1925). In adolescents between 7 and 16 years it becomes more common[1]; it is not met with frequently in adults although cases have been seen between 47 and 52 years of age (Elschnig, 1924; Bücklers, 1939; Franceschetti, 1941; Schlosshardt, 1950), and in the aged the typical subcapsular opacities become

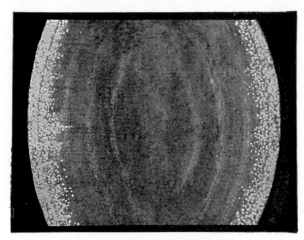

FIG. 189.—DIABETIC CATARACT.
Showing a dense band of subcortical opacities in optical section (C. Goulden).

rare although they may still occur (Komi *et al.*, 1965). Characteristically the cataract matures rapidly, especially in the young, sometimes within a few hours (Litten, 1893; Scheffels, 1898), usually within some days (4 days, Scheffels, 1898; Kirby, 1933; 11 days, Neuburger, 1893) and seldom taking more than a few weeks. In adults, however, its course is less stormy, for progression of the opacities may proceed leisurely presenting periods of arrest and even retrogression with variations in the intensity of the glycosuria.

   As preliminary events, a sudden myopia has been observed to occur prior to the development of an acute cataract (in a youth of 19, Marx, 1940), while an increase in the optical density of the anterior cortex of the lens,

[1] Sherrill (1922), Schnyder (1923), Joslin (1923), Strouse and Gradle (1924), Kirby (1933), Marx (1940), Franceschetti (1941), Lawrence *et al.* (1942), Gordon (1949), Janert *et al.* (1956), Dolének *et al.* (1966), and others.

varying with the level of the blood-sugar, sufficiently great to diminish the brightness of the fundus reflex and perhaps to affect vision was noted by Vere (1952) and Vere and Verel (1955). In juvenile diabetics Huggert (1953) found that a change in the appearance of the zone of disjunction is an early and common change.

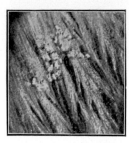

FIG. 190.—CATARACT IN DIABETES.

The superficial fibres of the lens: surface view (C. Goulden).

Clinically the cataract, which invariably occurs bilaterally, has a typical appearance consisting essentially of subcapsular opacities in the superficial layers of the anterior and posterior cortex. This distribution of the early changes was known to the older writers both from clinical (Förster, 1877; Neuburger, 1893; Klein, 1901) and pathological (Deutschmann, 1877–87) observation, while in more recent times the slit-lamp has confirmed its more intimate details (Schnyder, 1923; Goulden, 1928; Weill and Nordmann, 1930; O'Brien et al., 1934; and others). Immediately under the capsule there appears a veritable carpet of vacuoles interspersed with fine punctate and flaky white opacities, and in the cortex underneath extensive hydration of the tissues is usually revealed by the presence of water-clefts and separation of the sutures (Figs. 189–190; Plate II, Fig. 5). Occasionally the vacuoles have been observed deep in the cortex (Marx, 1940). Thereafter more diffuse cloudy opacities appear, usually grey and transparent in front and forming white solid plaques behind, until the stage of general intumescent cataract is reached and the opacification becomes complete and uniform (Fig. 191).

It is to be noted that in the early stages, when the changes are limited

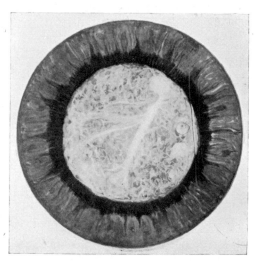

FIG. 191.—MATURE DIABETIC CATARACT (E. O. G. Kirwan).

essentially to œdema without denaturation of the proteins, adequate control of the diabetes may result in a disappearance of the opacities (Nettleship, 1885). This reversal may occur dramatically in the acutely developing cataract,[1] but has also been seen on adequate treatment of the disease when the lenticular opacities have been of some duration (Seegen, 1875; Tannahill, 1885; Fischer, 1925; Osadchey, 1954). Such a happy result, however, is not common although it has been said to occur in 10% in young diabetics (Burditt and Caird, 1968).

Pathological examinations have repeatedly been done on diabetic cataract.[2] The general histological appearances resemble those of other types of lenticular opacity, but the peculiar features are the localization of the opacities to the subcapsular region and the occasional massive œdema of the tissue (*hydrops capsulæ lentis*).

Chemically the most significant change found in diabetic cataracts is an increase of sorbitol, glucose and fructose in the lens (van Heyningen, 1959; Pirie and van Heyningen, 1964; Pirie, 1965). The first sugar is absent from the senile cataractous lens; the last two are present but in smaller quantity than in the diabetic lens. The concentration of potassium has been found to be lower than in senile cataract (Carey and Hunt, 1935). The metabolic and osmotic changes have not been investigated in man but are presumably parallel to those found in experimental glucose cataract in animals.[3]

While it is undoubtedly the case that the operative treatment of cataract in diabetics provides more anxieties than in non-diabetic patients, the presence of diabetes in itself is no contra-indication for dealing with the cataract in the ordinary way. The two complications to be avoided are the occurrence of hæmorrhage and the subsequent development of infection to which uncontrolled diabetics are notoriously prone. In these subjects, therefore, hyperpiesia should receive attention, and the exclusion of obvious focal sepsis should be undertaken; but with these precautions, surgery should lead to good results provided the diabetes has been adequately controlled for some time beforehand. For some weeks prior to operation, therefore, the patient should be under the unremitting care of the physician, and for some days before the operation sugar should be eliminated or as nearly so as may seem advisable, and the dietary conditions and dosage of insulin or other hypoglycæmic agents standardized in the hospital where the operation is to be performed. It is to be remembered, however, that it is inadvisable to push insulin in large doses immediately before the operation since there is evidence that this increases the liability to hæmorrhage (W. L. Benedict, 1925).

It is interesting that the proper use of insulin has completely changed the prognosis of such operations, for surgery in diabetics used to give rise to considerable anxiety.

[1] Neuburger (1893), Alt (1906), Braun (1935), Lawrence (1946), Roberts (1950), Schlosshardt (1950), Jackson (1955), C. and A. Turtz (1958), Neuberg *et al.* (1958).
[2] His (1854), Knapp (1863), Becker (1883), Deutschmann (1887), Kamocki (1887), Görlitz (1894), Kako (1903), Hess (1911), Mitsuhashi and Nambu (1955), and others.
[3] p. 88.

Thus before its introduction, Gifford (1911) found that after extraction 43% of young diabetics lost their eyes from post-operative infection, while Wheeler (1916), over a series of 2,123 extractions, met post-operative hæmorrhages in 5% of ordinary cases and in 28·94% of diabetics. With adequate control of the diabetes, however, with insulin if necessary, hæmorrhages, although still more common among such patients than in others (Kirmani, 1964; Norn, 1967), have become much less frequent.

Ætiology. The reason for the common occurrence of cataract in diabetics has excited much interest and, although several theories have been advanced in explanation, the question cannot be considered by any means as settled. So far as is known, the three most important factors in the production of a true diabetic cataract are osmotic hydration, the development of acidity with consequent proteolysis, and a disturbance of the carbohydrate meta-bolism.[1] From the historical point of view, some of the earlier suggestions, however, are of interest.

1. The oldest suggestion that the lenticular opacities were due to *the presence of sugar* in the aqueous and the lens (Kunde, 1857; Stoeber, 1862; and others) had necessarily to be discarded when it was demonstrated that to be effective a concentra-tion of 5% was required, which is far above that compatible with life; moreover, actual estimations showed that this was never approached in the aqueous, while the cataractous lens itself might be sugar-free (Deutschmann, 1877–87).

2. *The œdematous and degenerated state of the ciliary epithelium* in the diabetic eye[2] was said to interfere with the nutrition of the lens (Peters, 1893).

3. A *photochemical explanation* was advanced by Schanz (1916), who claimed that sugar and acetone sensitized protein to the denaturing action of light.

4. *Endocrine failure*, affecting primarily the internal secretion of the pancreas, was suggested as the primary cause (Schiötz, 1913; Löwenstein, 1926–34; and others).

5. A *decrease in the permeability of the capsule* in the presence of glucose was demon-strated *in vitro* by Bellows and Rosner (1938), who suggested that this might predispose to the development of cataract. It is interesting that Kirby and his colleagues (1933) found that while sugar did not interfere with the growth of the lenticular epithelium *in vitro*, ketone bodies (acetone and oxybutyric acid) were toxic in concentrations such as are met with in moderately severe diabetes.

6. *The hydration of the lens by osmotic influences* may well be an ætiological factor. Systemic changes may exert an influence (Duke-Elder, 1925–26); with a rising blood-sugar, provided the water-balance of the body is reasonably maintained, the effective osmotic pressure of the tissue-fluids tends to fall owing to a loss of salts; these to some extent are replaced by glucose, but the heavy loss of salt in the increased excretion of urine is not adequately replaced since the bulk of fluid is made up by drinking water. The lowered osmotic pressure of the aqueous thus determines an inflow of water into the lens, causing first its deformation with the production of myopia[3] and eventually the œdema and hydration which result in cataract. In addition, local chemical changes, particularly the accumulation of sorbitol, glucose and fructose in the lens, also play a prominent part in inducing an osmotic hydration as they do in experimental sugar cataract.[4]

[1] p. 90.   [2] Vol. IX, p. 649.   [3] Vol. V.   [4] p. 90.

7. *Acidosis* associated with diabetes may have some influence in the rapid development of cataract, for it will be remembered that with a lowering of the pH, proteolytic enzymes become active which may to some extent be directly responsible for opacification; moreover, it may also act indirectly by increasing the osmotic pressure within the lens owing to the breakdown of large osmotically inactive molecules to smaller complexes, thus determining an osmotic inflow of fluid into the lens (Krause, 1934).

Alt. *Amer. J. Ophthal.*, **23**, 294 (1906).
Andersen. *Acta ophthal.* (Kbh.), **7**, 339 (1929).
Anthonisen. *Acta ophthal.* (Kbh.), **14**, 150 (1936).
Becker. *Zur Anatomie d. gesunden u. kranken Linse*, Wiesbaden (1883).
Bellows and Rosner. *Arch. Ophthal.*, **20**, 80 (1938).
Benedict, T. *Abhdl. a. d. Gebiet. d. Augenheilk.*, Breslau, **1**, 38 (1842).
Benedict, W. L. *Ohio St. med. J.*, **21**, 648 (1925).
Berndt. *Klinischen Mitteilungen*, Greifswald (1834).
Braun. *Klin. Wschr.*, **14**, 222 (1935).
Brückner. *Praxis*, **54**, 746 (1965).
Bücklers. *Klin. Mbl. Augenheilk.*, **102**, 465 (1939).
Burditt and Caird. *Brit. J. Ophthal.*, **52**, 433 (1968).
Caird, Hutchinson and Pirie. *Brit. med. J.*, **2**, 665 (1964).
Carey and Hunt. *New Engl. J. Med.*, **212**, 463 (1935).
Clegg. *Trans. ophthal. Soc. U.K.*, **40**, 37 (1920).
Deutschmann. *v. Graefes Arch. Ophthal.*, **23** (3), 112 (1877); **25** (2), 213 (1879); **33** (2), 229 (1887).
Dolének, Takác and Jutzi. *Csl. Ofthal.*, **22**, 155 (1966).
Dollfus. *Bull. Soc. franç. Ophtal.*, **67**, 62 (1954).
Dollfus and Haye. *Bull. Soc. belge Ophtal.*, No. 115, 184 (1957).
Duke-Elder. *Brit. J. Ophthal.*, **9**, 167 (1925). *Lancet*, **1**, 1188, 1250 (1926).
Elschnig. *Med. Klin.*, **20**, 7 (1924).
Fischer. *Z. Augenheilk.*, **55**, 190 (1925).
Förster. *Graefe-Saemisch Hb. d. ges. Augenheilk.*, 1st ed., Leipzig, **7**, 220 (1877).
Franceschetti. *Klin. Mbl. Augenheilk.*, **106**, 236 (1941). *Ophthalmologica*, **101**, 241 (1941).
Gifford. *Ophthal. Rec.*, **20**, 243 (1911).
Görlitz. *Beitr. z. pathologischen Anatomie d. Cataracta diabetica* (Diss.), Freiburg (1894).
Gordon. *Arch. Ophthal.*, **41**, 462 (1949).
Goulden. *Trans. ophthal. Soc. U.K.*, **48**, 97 (1928).
Heinsius and Arndt. *v. Graefes Arch. Ophthal.*, **150**, 555 (1950).

Hess. *Graefe-Saemisch Hb. d. ges. Augenheilk.*, 3rd ed., Leipzig, Kap. IX, 126 (1911).
van Heyningen. *Nature* (Lond.), **184**, 194 (1959).
Himly. *Die Krankheiten u. Missbildungen d. mensch. Auges*, Göttingen (1843).
His. *Virchows Arch. path. Anat.*, **6**, 561 (1854).
Huggert. *Acta ophthal.* (Kbh.), **31**, 227 (1953).
Jackson. *Brit. J. Ophthal.*, **39**, 629 (1955).
Janert, Mohnike and Günther. *Klin. Wschr.*, **34**, 742 (1956).
Joslin. *Treatment of Diabetes Mellitus*, 3rd ed., Phila. (1923).
Kako. *Klin. Mbl. Augenheilk.*, **41** (1), 253 (1903).
Kamocki. *Arch. Augenheilk.*, **17**, 247 (1887).
Kato, Amaha, Hagai and Matusui. *Acta Soc. ophthal. jap.*, **64**, 577 (1960).
Kennedy and Kirchbaum. *Cleveland clin. Quart.*, **18**, 134 (1951).
Kirby. *Arch. Ophthal.*, **9**, 966 (1933).
Kirby, Estey and Wiener. *Arch. Ophthal.*, **10**, 37 (1933).
Kirmani. *Amer. J. Ophthal.*, **57**, 617 (1964).
Klein. *Wien. klin. Wschr.*, **14**, 1097 (1901)
Knapp. *Klin. Mbl. Augenheilk.*, **1**, 168 (1863).
Komi, Taketani, Otsuka and Shimoide. *Rinsho Ganka*, **19**, 159 (1965).
Krause. *Amer. J. Ophthal.*, **17**, 502 (1934).
Kunde. *v. Graefes Arch. Ophthal.*, **3** (2), 275 (1857).
Lawrence. *Brit. J. Ophthal.*, **30**, 78 (1946).
Lawrence, Oakley and Barne. *Lancet*, **2**, 63 (1942).
Litten. *Münch. med. Wschr.*, **40**, 880 (1893).
Löwenstein. *v. Graefes Arch. Ophthal.*, **116**, 438 (1926); **132**, 224 (1934).
Major and Curran. *J. Amer. med. Ass.*, **84**, 674 (1925).
Marx. *Ophthalmologica*, **99**, 286 (1940).
Mitsuhashi and Nambu. *Acta Soc. ophthal. jap.*, **59**, 1686 (1955).
Nettleship. *Trans. ophthal. Soc. U.K.*, **5**, 107 (1885).
Neuberg, Griscom and Burns. *Diabetes*, **7**, 21 (1958).
Neuburger. *Zbl. prakt. Augenheilk.*, **17**, 165 (1893).
Norn. *Acta ophthal.* (Kbh.), **45**, 322 (1967).
O'Brien, Molsberry and Allen. *J. Amer. med. Ass.*, **103**, 892 (1934).

Osadchey. *Vestn. oftal.*, **33**, 40 (1954).
Paufique and Michaud. *Ann. Oculist.* (Paris), **198**, 1 (1965).
Peters. *v. Graefes Arch. Ophthal.*, **39** (1), 221 (1893).
Pirie. *Invest. Ophthal.*, **4**, 629 (1965).
Pirie and van Heyningen. *Exp. Eye Res.*, **3**, 124 (1964).
Refatullah. *Bull. ophthal. Soc. Egypt*, **46**, 275 (1953).
Roberts. *Amer. J. Ophthal.*, **33**, 1283 (1950).
Rollo. *An Account of Two Cases of Diabetes Mellitus*, London (1798).
Schanz. *v. Graefes Arch. Ophthal.*, **91**, 238 (1916).
Scheffels. *Ophthal. Klin.*, **2**, 124 (1898).
Schiötz. *Norsk Mag. Lægevidensk.*, **74**, 1201 (1913).
Schlosshardt. *Klin. Mbl. Augenheilk.*, **116**, 237 (1950).
Schnyder. *Klin. Mbl. Augenheilk.*, **70**, 45 (1923).

Schulte. *Z. ärztl. Fortbild.*, **46**, 338 (1952).
Seegen. *Diabetes Mellitus*, Berlin (1875).
van Selm. *S. Afr. med. J.*, **40**, 801 (1966).
Sherrill. *J. metab. Res.*, **1**, 667 (1922).
Stoeber. *Ann. Oculist.* (Paris), **48**, 192 (1862).
Strouse and Gradle. *J. Amer. med. Ass.*, **82**, 546 (1924).
Tannahill. *Brit. med. J.*, **1**, 226 (1885).
Townes and Casey. *Sth. med. J.*, **48**, 844 (1955).
Tulloch. *Diabetes Mellitus in the Tropics*, London (1962).
Turtz, C. and A. *Amer. J. Ophthal.*, **46**, 219 (1958).
Vere. *Lancet*, **2**, 1017 (1952).
Vere and Verel. *Clin. Sci.*, **14**, 183 (1955).
Waite and Beetham. *New Engl. J. Med.*, **212**, 367, 429 (1935).
Weill and Nordmann. *Bull. Soc. franç. Ophtal.*, **43**, 17 (1930).
Wheeler. *Trans. Amer. ophthal. Soc.*, **14**, 742 (1916).

GALACTOSÆMIC CATARACT

GALACTOSÆMIA is a rare inborn error of metabolism[1] first defined by von Reuss (1908), due to an inability of the infant to metabolize galactose into glycogen owing to an absence of the necessary enzyme, galactose-1-phosphate uridyl transferase (Kalckar, 1957); all other metabolic pathways appear to be intact. In the lens of a 4-week-old boy suffering from the disease, Lerman (1959) found that this enzyme was completely lacking. The condition is said to occur in 1 out of 18,000 births. In the untreated infant the clinical picture is characterized by general malnutrition with an arrest of growth, mental retardation, hepatomegaly appearing during the first week of life due to fatty infiltration and secondary cirrhosis resulting in jaundice with vomiting and diarrhœa, splenomegaly, osteoporosis and the presence of galactose, amino acids and proteins in the urine. Untreated, the condition is incompatible with life.

The *hereditary* nature of galactosæmia is now well established. The number of familial cases reported indicates a recessive inheritance,[2] while consanguinity has been noted in the parents (Flury and Berger, 1955). According to Holzel and Komrower (1955) the disease represents a homozygous condition and the parents of affected siblings, being heterozygotes, show an abnormal galactosæmic curve in the blood. It is interesting, however, that Cristini (1959) and Toselli and Bartalena (1960) noted that a cataract may be the only clinical indication seen in children with " minor " galactosæmia, the diagnosis of which is possible only by a galactosæmic tolerance test.

---

[1] Vol. VII, p. 132.
[2] Göppert (1917), Boer (1932), Goldbloom and Brickman (1946), Bell *et al.* (1950), Townsend *et al.* (1951), Donnell and Lann (1951), Patz (1953), Flury and Berger (1955), and others.

CATARACT develops in about 75% of cases of galactosæmia[1] and progresses dramatically, resembling closely the lesion seen experimentally in young rats fed on a diet in which galactose is the only carbohydrate constituent[2]; it has been observed some days after birth in infants, constituting the first observable symptom of the disease (Bray *et al.*, 1952; Cordes, 1960). Usually about the age of 7 weeks a refractive ring appears in the centre of the lens resembling a drop of oil on ophthalmoscopic examination and due to opacities in the deep cortex; some 2 weeks later this spreads with the appearance of cortical vacuoles and general hydration until complete opacification of the lens results after the child is some 10 weeks old (Figs. 192–4). In cases of minor galactosæmia, however, the lenticular changes

FIGS. 192 and 193.—GALACTOSÆMIC CATARACT (J. Nordmann).

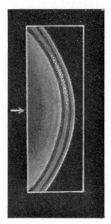

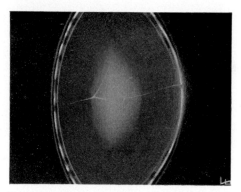

FIG. 192.—At an early stage.   FIG. 193.—Early changes in the nucleus and cortex.

may not appear until the age of about one year (Toselli and Bartalena, 1960). Indeed, it may be that some cases of juvenile cataract may suffer from a latent galactosæmia revealed only by an abnormal galactose-loading test or a raised fasting blood-galactose; Rommel and Cramer (1967) found 9 such cases in a series of 36 young children with juvenile cataract. It is interesting that Hartstein (1958) found that the feeding of large quantities

[1] Fanconi (1933), Mason and Turner (1935), Norman and Fashena (1943), Bruck and Rapoport (1945), Goldbloom and Brickman (1946), Greenman and Rathbun (1948), Goldstein and Ennis (1948), Donnell and Lann (1951), Townsend *et al.* (1951), Falls *et al.* (1951), Enns (1951), DuShane and Hartman (1951), Reiter and Lasky (1952), Holzel *et al.* (1952), Patz (1953), McAuley (1953), Steiner (1953), Paufique and Etienne (1954), Cox and Pugh (1954), Flury and Berger (1955), Ritter and Cannon (1955), Turnbull (1956), Dolcet (1957), Seedorff (1958), Wilson and Donnell (1958), Cordes (1960), Toselli and Bartalena (1960), Boissin (1961), Eurico Ferreira (1961), Appelmans *et al.* (1962), Greaves (1963), Sacrez *et al.* (1964), Mehra and Seth (1965), Nordmann (1965–66), Wilson (1967).
[2] p. 89.

of galactose to normal patients over many months resulted in no damage to the lens.

The *treatment* of the condition rests on the denial of lactose in the form of milk or milk products to the infant and its substitution by a synthetic feed; if this is done sufficiently early the general symptoms may rapidly disappear but most survivors show permanent mental retardation. In general, if treatment is undertaken before the 4th week of life the prognosis is said to be good (Brandt and Tolstrup, 1967). The opacities in the lenses may clear if they are not too advanced (Reiter and Lasky, 1952; McAuley, 1953; Johnson, 1953; Turnbull, 1956), a happy result which, however, does not invariably occur (Wilson and Donnell, 1958). Alternatively, if the process is stopped the opaque zonular opacity is surrounded by new

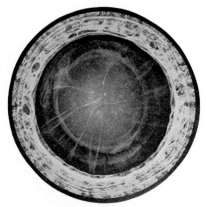

FIG. 194.—GALACTOSÆMIC CATARACT.
In a child aged 4 months, showing a bilateral zonular cataract (F. C. Cordes).

and clear fibres and is thus buried (Steiner, 1953). The ocular prognosis— and indeed the life of the child—thus depends on early diagnosis of the condition, and this may well depend on the recognition and diagnosis of the ocular changes.

The *ætiology* of the cataract has already been indicated in our discussion of the experimental lesion.[1] So far as the lens is concerned, the galactose is reduced by aldose reductase to produce large quantities of sugar alcohols, particularly dulcitol, producing osmotic hydration of the lens, an arrest of the synthesis of soluble protein and a disturbance of permeability. So far as the general condition is concerned, the aminoaciduria may be of significance[2]; it is interesting that in galactosæmia the normal pattern of amino acids in the urine is markedly disturbed with the appearance of threonine, tryptophan, methionine and tyrosine (Bickel and Hickmans, 1952; Holzel *et al.*, 1952), and the urine becomes normal again in this respect quantitatively and qualitatively on a galactose-free diet (Hsia *et al.*, 1954).

[1] p. 89.
[2] p. 192.

The formation of juvenile cataracts has been reported by Gitzelmann (1967) from an aberration of *galactokinase activity*, that is, the inability of the blood cells to oxidize galactose to form phosphorylated intermediates; the anomaly appears to have a recessive mode of inheritance.

Appelmans, Michiels, Cols and Colette. *Bull. Soc. belge Ophtal.*, No. 131, 421 (1962).

Bell, Blair, Lindsay and Watson. *J. Pediat.*, **36,** 427 (1950).

Bickel and Hickmans. *Arch. Dis. Childh.*, **27,** 347 (1952).

Boer. *Maandschr. Kindergeneesk.*, **2,** 15 (1932).

Boissin. *Ann. Oculist.* (Paris), **194,** 422 (1961).

Brandt and Tolstrup. *Acta pœdiat.* (Uppsala), **56,** 85 (1967).

Bray, Isaac and Watkins. *Arch. Dis. Childh.*, **27,** 341 (1952).

Bruck and Rapoport. *Amer. J. Dis. Child.*, **70,** 267 (1945).

Cordes. *Amer. J. Ophthal.*, **50,** 1151 (1960).

Cox and Pugh. *Brit. med. J.*, **2,** 613 (1954).

Cristini. *Rass. ital. Ottal.*, **28,** 3 (1959).

Dolcet. *Arch. Pediat.* (Barcelona), **7,** 681 (1957).

Donnell and Lann. *Pediatrics*, **7,** 503 (1951).

DuShane and Hartman. *Pediatrics*, **7,** 679 (1951).

Enns. *Amer. J. Ophthal.*, **34,** 1268 (1951).

Eurico Ferreira. *Rev. bras. Oftal.*, **20,** 313 (1961).

Falls, Lowrey and Anderson. *Amer. J. Ophthal.*, **34,** 1271 (1951).

Fanconi. *Jb. Kinderheilk.*, **138,** 1 (1933).

Flury and Berger. *J. Génét. hum.*, **4,** 1 (1955).

Gitzelmann. *Pediat. Res.*, **1,** 14 (1967).

Göppert. *Berl. klin. Wschr.*, **54,** 473 (1917).

Goldbloom and Brickman. *J. Pediat.*, **28,** 674 (1946).

Goldstein and Ennis. *J. Pediat.*, **33,** 147 (1948).

Greaves. *Proc. roy. Soc. Med.*, **56,** 24 (1963).

Greenman and Rathbun. *Pediatrics*, **2,** 666 (1948).

Hartstein. *Arch. Ophthal.*, **59,** 406 (1958).

Holzel and Komrower. *Arch. Dis. Childh.*, **30,** 155 (1955).

Holzel, Komrower and Wilson. *Brit. med. J.*, **1,** 194 (1952).

Hsia, D. and H., Green, Kay and Gellis. *Amer. J. Dis. Child.*, **88,** 458 (1954).

Johnson. *Amer. J. Ophthal.*, **36,** 1380 (1953).

Kalckar. *Science*, **125,** 105 (1957).

Lerman. *Arch. Ophthal.*, **61,** 88 (1959).

McAuley. *Brit. J. Ophthal.*, **37,** 655 (1953).

Mason and Turner. *Amer. J. Dis. Child.*, **50,** 359 (1935).

Mehra and Seth. *Orient. Arch. Ophthal.*, **3,** 153 (1965).

Nordmann. *Arch. Ophtal.*, **25,** 43 (1965). *Amer. J. Ophthal.*, **61,** 1257 (1966).

Norman and Fashena. *Amer. J. Dis. Child.*, **66,** 531 (1943).

Patz. *Amer. J. Ophthal.*, **36,** 453 (1953).

Paufique and Etienne. *Bull. Soc. franç. Ophtal.*, **67,** 42 (1954).

Reiter and Lasky. *Amer. J. Ophthal.*, **35,** 69 (1952).

von Reuss. *Wien. med. Wschr.*, **58,** 799 (1908).

Ritter and Cannon. *New Engl. J. Med.*, **252,** 747 (1955).

Rommel and Cramer. *Münch. med. Wschr.*, **109,** 238 (1967).

Sacrez, Juif, Gigonnet *et al.* *Bull. Soc. Ophtal. Fr.*, **64,** 940 (1964).

Seedorff. *Acta ophthal.* (Kbh.), **36,** 658 (1958).

Steiner. *Amer. J. Ophthal.*, **36,** 841 (1953).

Toselli and Bartalena. *Ann. Ottal.*, **86,** 197 (1960).

Townsend, Mason and Strong. *Pediatrics*, **7,** 760 (1951).

Turnbull. *Amer. J. Ophthal.*, **42,** 602 (1956).

Wilson. *Trans. Amer. ophthal. Soc.*, **65,** 661 (1967).

Wilson and Donnell. *Arch. Ophthal.*, **60,** 215 (1958).

HYPOCALCÆMIC CATARACT

TETANY may be of two types, post-operative or idiopathic. *Post-operative tetany* (*tetania strumipriva*) occurs as a rule 2 to 3 days after an operation for removal of the thyroid gland with which the parathyroids have been also removed by mistake. *Idiopathic tetany* usually occurs in young people, particularly in infants (*infantile tetany*) but also in adults, and may result from a low intake of calcium or its excessive excretion either through the bowel or the kidneys, or as a result of an elevation in the serum-phosphate or from a condition of alkalosis. Clinically either type may appear in two forms, latent and manifest. In *latent tetany* (or *spasmophilia*) the only clinical evidences are certain trophic changes in the epithelial structures (falling out of the hair, brittleness of the nails, wrinkling of the skin and dental decay) and a hyperexcitability of the peripheral nervous system (diagnosed by Erb's sign, an increased muscular contraction to the galvanic stimulation of a nerve; Chvostek's sign, facial twitchings produced by tapping the facial nerve in the parotid region; and Trousseau's sign, muscular contractions of the forearm and hand on constriction of the arm). When the condition becomes manifest, cramps and spasms appear in the hands and arms, and later in the feet and legs; these carpo-pedal spasms may be accompanied by laryngospasm, muscular weakness with gastro-intestinal and mental irritability until generalized convulsions may result in death. A constant occurrence is a reduction of the serum-calcium, an increase of phosphates and a relative increase of potassium. In latent tetany the serum-calcium usually varies from 6 to 10 mg. per 100 ml.; if it falls below 5 mg. convulsions occur (see Klotz, 1958).

Spontaneous (non-operative) hypocalcæmia in adults is most commonly due to *idiopathic hypoparathyroidism*, characterized pathologically by the absence of parathyroid tissue or its replacement by fat (Drake *et al.*, 1939). The condition is relatively rare; Steinberg and Waldron (1952) found only 52 cases in the literature. Both sexes are equally affected and the disease usually develops about the age of 17 but may occur much later (60 years, Bronsky *et al.*, 1958). In addition to the symptoms characteristic of tetany, punctate calcifications may occur in the basal ganglia and mental retardation has been noted; lenticular opacities are seen in approximately 50% of patients and papillœdema and increased intracranial pressure may occur.

In addition to idiopathic hypoparathyroidism, two other syndromes have been differentiated: pseudo-hypoparathyroidism (Albright *et al.*, 1942), and a condition designated by the extraordinary name of pseudo-pseudo-hypoparathyroidism (Albright *et al.*, 1952).

Pseudo-hypoparathyroidism (*hypoparathyroid cretinism*, Schüpbach and Courvoisier 1949), a clinical entity probably genetically determined (Elrick *et al.*, 1950), is not at all common: in the literature, Frame and Carter (1955) found 25 cases, Cusmano and his colleagues (1956) 30, in addition to 6 cases of their own, and Cernea and his associates (1965) 67. The feature of this condition is a failure in the response to the normally produced parathyroid hormone probably because of a renal defect, for the parathyroid glands themselves are normal or even hypertrophied. Females are affected twice as frequently as males and the average age of onset is between 8 and 9 years. The hypocalcæmia and hyperphosphatæmia with tetany are associated with extraskeletal calcification, ossification and bony dysplasias, and the combination has been called the *hereditary osteodystrophy* of *Albright* or *Albright's syndrome*. A cataract is relatively common.

Pseudo-pseudo-hypoparathyroidism (*brachymetacarpal dwarfism*, van der Werff ten Bosch, 1959) is the rarest form of this endocrine disturbance: Hanno and Weiss (1961) found 20 cases in the literature. The metabolic abnormalities of hypocalcæmia and hyperphosphatæmia as well as tetany are absent, but the skeletal changes and the ectopic calcification and ossification are present, usually with mental retardation. In the eyes, blue scleræ have been reported but cataract is exceptional.

Over a century and a half ago a relation between the occurrence of zonular cataract and convulsions in infants was noted by Schmidt (1801), a connection corroborated by several subsequent observers (von Arlt, 1853; Eberhardt, 1863). Shortly thereafter a similar incidence of lenticular opacities with clonic muscular spasms in adults was described by Logetschnikow (1872) and Schmidt-Rimpler (1883); and at a later date attention was drawn more vividly to the subject by the recognition by Landsberg (1888) of rapidly developing cataracts in a patient who suffered from epileptiform convulsions after thyroidectomy. Thereafter a large number of observations fully established this post-operative sequence.[1] Lenticular opacities with tetany have also been observed to follow radiational therapy to the thyroid gland for the treatment of exophthalmos (Gilbert-Dreyfus et al., 1958). It must be remembered, however, that the occurrence of lenticular opacities is by no means invariable in cases of hypocalcæmia after surgery; thus Boothby and his colleagues (1931) reported a series of 88 cases of post-operative tetany without a single instance of cataract. The clinical appearance of opacities in the lens sometimes becomes evident a few months after parathyroidectomy (2 months, Goulden, 1928; 3 to 4 months, Jeremy, 1919; 5 months, Matthews, 1920), but may be delayed for some years (7 years, Knüsel, 1924; 11, Eiselsberg, 1921; 20, Heine, 1925); an average interval of 11 years after operation was found by Hamilton (1964); the development of uniocular cataract is rare (Bullerschen, 1951).

Although a zonular cataract in cases of idiopathic tetany in childhood was, as we have seen, an old observation, the development of characteristic lenticular opacities in later life has been amply confirmed.[2] After Albright and his colleagues (1942–52) had differentiated the three types of hypo-parathyroidism, most such cases have been found to occur in the idiopathic condition (Jordan and Kelsall, 1951; Steinberg and Waldron, 1952; Meyer, 1955); in a review of 118 cases, Pohjola (1962) found reports of cataract in 58%. In pseudo-hypoparathyroidism typical lenticular opacities are also common.[3] On the other hand, in pseudo-pseudo-hypoparathyroidism cataract is exceptional (Roche, 1955; Miles and Elrick, 1955; Smuylan and Raisz, 1959) since the typical opacities occur only in the hypocalcæmic forms of tetany (Holtz, 1960).

In the idiopathic cases the appearance of a cataract has been reported as early as in a 2-month-old infant (Zunin, 1952), but it is interesting that although systemic symptoms with tetany may have been intermittently present since childhood, the lenticular opacities may not appear until relatively late in life (50 years, Babel, 1954). They may also be brought on dramatically on the depletion of calcium in the serum which may accompany intestinal diseases such as steatorrhœa (Goulden, 1928; Bennett et al., 1932; Lowe et al., 1950) (Fig. 196) or sprue (Bangerter, 1939), or may occur during pregnancy or lactation (Lo Cascio, 1937; Maxwell and Pi, 1940; Lyle, 1949; Mecca, 1951; Springer, 1951); it is noteworthy that the level of calcium in the

---

[1] Hoffmann (1896), Schiller (1899), Westphal (1901), Possek (1907), Königstein (1907), Purtscher (1909), Jeremy (1919), Matthews (1920), Jaeger (1920), Eiselsberg (1921), Pamperl (1921), van Lint (1922), Sainton and Péron (1922), Sidler-Huguenin (1922), Greppin (1922), Knüsel (1924), Heine (1925), Kast (1926), Aub (1926), Hunter (1928), Jacques (1928), Goulden (1928), Cole (1930), Salvesen (1930), Marcove (1931), Vogt (1931), O'Brien (1932), Ellett (1934), Lo Cascio (1937), Badeaux (1941), Lyle (1947), Lopez et al. (1947), Weiner (1948), Brand (1950), Ramstedt (1957), Hamilton (1964), and others.

[2] Cosmettatos (1927), Hoesch (1937), Meesmann (1938), Martin and Bourdillon (1940), Jaensch (1949), Sautter (1951), and others.

[3] Albright et al. (1942), Barnes (1947), Schüpbach and Courvoisier (1949), Alexander and Tucker (1949), Gsell (1950), Lowe et al. (1950), Elrick et al. (1950), Mackler et al. (1952), Babel (1954), Prentice (1954), Frame and Carter (1955), 7 out of 25 cases, Sorsby (1958), Bergstrand et al. (1958), Hanno and Weiss (1961).

serum is higher in the infant than the adult so that the lens of the baby remains clear even although the mother suffers from tetany (Meesmann, 1955). The occurrence of cataract has also been noted in a child following treatment for nephritis with systemic corticosteroids (Grislain and Bezri, 1959). In contradistinction to the dramatic onset of the post-operative type of cataract, its maturation in idiopathic cases is usually slow.

At first these lenticular changes in young children were associated by some authors with rickets rather than with tetany (von Arx, 1883), but the experimental production of cataract in animals deprived of calcium or after a thyroidectomy and the maintenance of a clear lens with a rachitic diet has amply confirmed the association with hypocalcæmia.[1] On the other hand, on equally slender evidence it has been claimed that latent tetany is a frequent cause of senile cataract (Hesse and Phleps, 1913; Fischer and Triebenstein, 1914; Greppin, 1922; and others).

FIGS. 195 and 196.—HYPOCALCÆMIC CATARACT (C. Goulden).

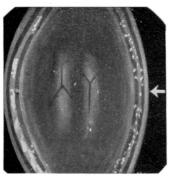
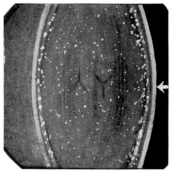

FIG. 195.—In aparathyroidism. In a woman aged 42, 20 years after a thyroidectomy. No signs of myxœdema, but carpo-pedal, laryngeal and oculomotor spasms with positive Chvostek's, Erb's and Trousseau's signs. There are white powdery and red, blue and green crystalline deposits in the cortex.

FIG. 196.—In infantile tetany with steatorrhœa. There are cortical opacities and powdery and crystalline deposits in the nucleus. Vision normal.

The changes in the lens may take on many forms, but the typical appearance is that of numerous small, discrete opacities both in the anterior and posterior cortex lying in a layer separated from the capsule by a clear zone of disjunction (Figs. 195–200); usually these are small, white and punctate, sometimes they are aggregated into larger flakes frequently elongated in shape, and not infrequently they are interspersed with angular iridescent crystals of a blue, green or red colour. A feature stressed by some writers is a lessened antero-posterior diameter of the lens (Kast, 1926; Vogt, 1931; Jaensch, 1949), and sometimes there is a more or less homogeneous opacity of the lamellar type surrounding the nucleus (O'Brien, 1932). The three constituents, punctate spots, flakes and iridescent crystals, may vary in

[1] p. 101.

their relative proportions, one or other may be predominantly present and usually they are most prominent near the posterior pole. In mild cases the condition may remain stationary indefinitely giving rise to little disturbance of vision, and if the hypocalcæmia is intermittent, the lenticular opacities may occur in strata separated by clear lens substance (Jaensch, 1949;

FIGS. 197 to 200.—TETANIC CATARACT.
In a patient aged 51 with idiopathic latent tetany (J. Babel).

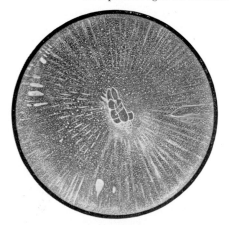

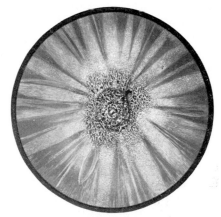

FIG. 197.—Right lens, anterior face.　　　FIG. 198.—Right lens, posterior face.

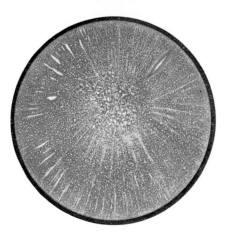

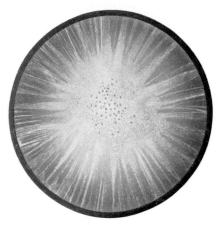

FIG. 199.—Left lens, anterior face.　　　FIG. 200.—Left lens, posterior face.

Kaiser *et al.*, 1960). The nucleus itself is rarely involved (Keerl, 1960); alternatively, the lesions may multiply and opacities of the senile type may supervene. In acute cases or after thyroid surgery the whole lens may become intumescent and uniformly opaque in a comparatively short time. The pathological examination of such a fully developed opacity described by Bartels (1906) showed the outer cortex riddled with fissures, vacuoles and punctate opacities, beneath which was a homogeneous layer of deep cortical opacity, while the nuclear fibres had begun to degenerate and disintegrate.

The *diagnosis* is made upon the history of thyroidectomy and the evidences of tetany or of latent tetany as evinced by hyperexcitability of the nervous system, the low serum-calcium and high serum-phosphate, as well as upon the characteristic morphological appearance of the lenticular opacities occurring bilaterally. It is to be noted that the opacities closely resemble those seen in myotonic cataract.

We have seen that in experimental cataract after removal of the parathyroids in animals the development of opacification is controlled by maintaining a high blood-calcium or by the administration of irradiated ergosterol (Rauh, 1936–37). The *treatment* of tetany is similarly directed to relieving the hypocalcæmia. In acute cases of hypoparathyroidism a rapid response usually follows the administration of parathyroid extract (parathormone); refractoriness to the hormone, however, may readily develop and in chronic cases a good response usually follows the administration of calcium lactate or gluconate with vitamin D or dihydrotachysterol (A.T. 10). A low phosphate diet is important; aluminium hydroxide is useful since it combines with the dietary phosphorus, while ammonium chloride may reduce the alkalinity of the blood. With this treatment it has been claimed that the development of the cataract may be stopped or at least delayed (Meesmann, 1938; Rauh, 1940; Weekers, 1944; Klotz, 1958; Kaiser *et al.*, 1960; Klotz and Fiks, 1962). As would be expected, patients with pseudo-hypoparathyroidism do not respond to parathyroid extract, but react well to vitamin D and dihydrotachysterol. There is no indication that the operative removal of the lens presents any special difficulties, although the occasional reported occurrence of severe post-operative hæmorrhage (Kast, 1926; O'Brien, 1932) is an indication for the administration of calcium and parathyroid hormone before and after surgery.

The cause of the cataract has already been discussed in the section on experimental cataract[1] and the various ætiological views put forward have been detailed—that the opacities are due to excessive muscular action, to a local chemical upset owing to a disturbance of the ionic equilibrium by the calcium deficiency, or to the liberation of a toxin either owing to a deficiency of parathyroid secretion or to a substance such as histamine, guanidine or tyramine liberated during tetanic spasms. It will be remembered that all these views are conjectural. A diminution of anaerobic glycolysis in the lens has been found, but it has been established that the constant factor in such cases is a low calcium/phosphate ratio in the blood and not any specific hormonal defect (von Bahr, 1936–40).

Albright, Burnett, Smith and Parson. *Endocrinology*, **30**, 922 (1942).

Albright, Forbes and Henneman. *Trans. Ass. Amer. Phys.*, **65**, 337 (1952).

Alexander and Tucker. *J. clin. Endocr.*, **9**, 862 (1949).

von Arlt. *Die Krankheiten d. Auges, für praktische Aerzte*, Prague, **2** (1853).

[1] p. 101.

von Arx. *Zur Pathologie d. Schichtstaars* (Diss.), Zürich (1883).

Aub. *Boston med. surg. J.*, **194**, 846 (1926).

Babel. *Bull. Soc. franç. Ophtal.*, **67**, 328 (1954).
  Année thér. en Ophtal., **8**, 9 (1957).

Badeaux. *J. Hôtel-Dieu Montréal*, **10**, 98 (1941).

von Bahr. *Acta ophthal.* (Kbh.), Suppl. 11 (1936); **18**, 170 (1940).

Bangerter. *Ophthalmologica*, **98**, 291 (1939).

Barnes. *Amer. J. Ophthal.*, **30**, 1029 (1947).

Bartels. *Klin. Mbl. Augenheilk.*, **44** (1), 374 (1906).

Bennett, Hunter and Vaughan. *Quart. J. Med.*, **1**, 603 (1932).

Bergstrand, Ekengren, Filipsson and Huggert. *Acta endocr.* (Kbh.), **29**, 201 (1958).

Boothby, Haines and Pemberton. *Amer. J. med. Sci.*, **181**, 81 (1931).

Brand. *Acta ophthal.* (Kbh.), **28**, 372 (1950).

Bronsky, Kushner, Dubin and Snapper. *Medicine* (Balt.), **37**, 317 (1958).

Bullerschen. *Klin. Mbl. Augenheilk.*, **118**, 416 (1951).

Cernea, Floares, Irimiciuc and Zbranca. *Ophthalmologica*, **150**, 409 (1965).

Cole. *Lancet*, **1**, 13 (1930).

Cosmettatos. *Rev. gén. Ophtal.*, **41**, 421 (1927).

Cusmano, Baker and Finby. *Radiology*, **67**, 845 (1956).

Drake, Albright, Bauer and Castleman. *Ann. intern. Med.*, **12**, 1751 (1939).

Eberhardt. *Gaz. Hôp. Paris*, **15**, 254 (1863).

Eiselsberg. *Arch. klin. Chir.*, **118**, 387 (1921).

Ellett. *Arch. Ophthal.*, **11**, 58 (1934).

Elrick, Albright, Bartter *et al. Acta endocr.* (Kbh.), **5**, 199 (1950).

Fischer and Triebenstein. *Klin. Mbl. Augenheilk.*, **52**, 441 (1914).

Frame and Carter. *Neurology* (Minneap.), **5**, 297 (1955).

Gilbert-Dreyfus, Zara and Gali. *Sem. Hôp. Paris*, **34**, 1301 (1958).

Goulden. *Trans. ophthal. Soc. U.K.*, **48**, 97 (1928).

Greppin. *Schweiz. med. Wschr.*, **52**, 1260 (1922).

Grislain and Bezri. *Ophthalmologica*, **137**, 293 (1959).

Gsell. *Dtsch. med. Wschr.*, **75**, 1117 (1950).

Hamilton. *Trans. Asia-Pac. Acad. Ophthal.*, **2**, 363 (1964).

Hanno and Weiss. *Arch. Ophthal.*, **65**, 221, 238 (1961).

Heine. *Z. Augenheilk.*, **55**, 1 (1925).

Hesse and Phleps. *Z. Augenheilk.*, **29**, 238 (1913).

Hoesch. *Dtsch. med. Wschr.*, **63**, 1582 (1937).

Hoffmann. *Dtsch. Z. Nervenheilk.*, **9**, 278 (1896).

Holtz. *Klin. Mbl. Augenheilk.*, Suppl. 34 (1960).

Hunter. *Proc. roy. Soc. Med.*, **21**, 1409 (1928).

Jacques. *Amer. J. med. Sci.*, **175**, 185 (1928).

Jaeger. *Zbl. Chir.*, **47**, 565 (1920).

Jaensch. *Nervenarzt*, **20**, 81 (1949).

Jeremy. *Brit. J. Ophthal.*, **3**, 315 (1919).

Jordan and Kelsall. *Arch. intern. Med.*, **87**, 242 (1951).

Kaiser, Loewe and Ponsold. *Klin. Mbl. Augenheilk.*, **136**, 65 (1960).

Kast. *Z. Augenheilk.*, **59**, 357 (1926).

Keerl. *Ophthalmologica*, **139**, 363 (1960).

Klotz. *Le tétanie chronique du spasmophilie*, Paris (1958).

Klotz and Fiks. *Probl. act. Endocr. Nutrit.*, **6**, 245 (1962).

Knüsel. *v. Graefes Arch. Ophthal.*, **114**, 636 (1924).

Königstein. *Klin. Mbl. Augenheilk.*, **45**, 268 (1907).

Landsberg. *Zbl. prakt. Augenheilk.*, **12**, 39 (1888).

van Lint. *Ann. Soc. Sci. méd. Bruxelles*, **76**, 36 (1922).

Lo Cascio. *XV int. Cong. Ophthal.*, Cairo, **3**, 401 (1937).
  Ann. Ottal., **65**, 801 (1937).

Logetschnikow. *Klin. Mbl. Augenheilk.*, **10**, 351 (1872).

Lopez, Quiñones and Esteva. *Arch. As. Evit. Ceg. Mex.*, **5**, 77 (1947).

Lowe, Ellinger, Wright and Stauffer. *J. Pediat.*, **36**, 1 (1950).

Lyle. *Trans. Amer. ophthal. Soc.*, **45**, 101 (1947).
  Amer. J. Ophthal., **32**, 1183 (1949).

Mackler, Fouts and Birsner. *Calif. Med.*, **77**, 332 (1952).

Marcove. *Amer. J. Ophthal.*, **14**, 887 (1931).

Martin and Bourdillon. *Rev. méd. Suisse rom.*, **60**, 1166 (1940).

Matthews. *Trans. ophthal. Soc. U.K.*, **40**, 440 (1920).

Maxwell and Pi. *Proc. roy. Soc. Med.*, **33**, 777 (1940).

Mecca. *Fracastro* (Verona), **44**, 84 (1951).

Meesmann. *Klin. Mbl. Augenheilk.*, Suppl. 1 (1938).
  Med. Klin., **50**, 29 (1955).

Meyer. *New Engl. J. Med.*, **252**, 622 (1955).

Miles and Elrick. *J. clin. Endocr.*, **15**, 576 (1955).

O'Brien. *Arch. Ophthal.*, **7**, 71 (1932).

Pamperl. *Dtsch. Z. Chir.*, **161**, 258 (1921).

Pohjola. *Acta ophthal.* (Kbh.), **40**, 255 (1962).

Possek. *Klin. Mbl. Augenheilk.*, **45**, Beil., 1 (1907).

Prentice. *J. clin. Endocr.*, **14**, 1069 (1954).

Purtscher. *Zbl. prakt. Augenheilk.*, **33**, 97 (1909).

Ramstedt. *Svenska Läk.-Tidn.*, **54**, 3961 (1957).

Rauh. *Ber. dtsch. ophthal. Ges.*, **51**, 357 (1936).
  XV int. Cong. Ophthal., Cairo, **4**, 36 (1937).
  Med. Klin., **36**, 99 (1940).

Roche. *J. clin. Endocr.*, **15**, 964 (1955).

Sainton and Péron. *Rev. neurol.* (Paris), **29**, 442 (1922).

Salvesen. *Acta med. scand.*, **73**, 511; **74**, 13 (1930).

Sautter. *Die Trübungsformen d. menschlichen Linse*, Stuttgart (1951).

Schiller. *Beitr. klin. Chir.*, **24**, 535 (1899).

Schmidt. *Ueber Nachstaar u. Iritis nach Staaroperationen*, Wien (1801).

Schmidt-Rimpler. *Klin. Mbl. Augenheilk.*, **21**, 181 (1883).

Schüpbach and Courvoisier. *Schweiz. med. Wschr.*, **79**, 887 (1949).

Sidler-Huguenin. *v. Graefes Arch. Ophthal.*, **107**, 1 (1922).

Smuylan and Raisz. *J. clin. Endocr.*, **19**, 478 (1959).

Sorsby. *Systemic Ophthalmology*, London, 346 (1958).

Springer. *Bull. Féd. Soc. Gyn. Obst. Fr.*, **3**, 632 (1951).

Steinberg and Waldron. *Medicine* (Balt.), **31**, 133 (1952).

Vogt. *Lhb. u. Atlas d. Spaltlampenmikroskopie d. lebenden Auges*, 2nd ed., Berlin, **2**, 553 (1931).

Weekers. *Ophthalmologica*, **107**, 257 (1944).

Weiner. *Amer. J. Ophthal.*, **31**, 225 (1948).

van der Werff ten Bosch. *Lancet*, **1**, 69 (1959).

Westphal. *Berl. klin. Wschr.*, **38**, 849 (1901).

Zunin. *Lattante*, **23**, 294 (1952).

HYPOTHYROIDIC CATARACT

Hypothyroidism is a common condition and if it gave rise to cataract it would be expected that such a lesion would be frequent; nevertheless, it has rarely been reported either in cretinism (Jeremy, 1921; Goulden, 1928; Vancea, 1929; Lemoine, 1938; Lowe, 1949; and in a calf, Schiøtz, 1913) or in myxœdema (Callan, 1895; Cantonnet, 1910; Dutoit, 1914; Löwenstein,

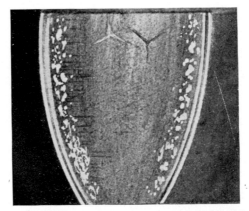

FIG. 201.—CATARACT IN CRETINISM (after C. Goulden).

1926; Vancea, 1929). The lenticular opacities reported have been small and flaky, interspersed with iridescent crystalline deposits in the superficial cortex (Fig. 201); the changes were discernible only with the slit-lamp and did not interfere with vision. It is difficult to say whether the lenticular changes in these cases were due to hypothyroidism; some may have been associated with the very similar opacities seen in hypoparathyroidism.

Callan. *Trans. Amer. ophthal. Soc.*, **7**, 391 (1895).

Cantonnet. *Ann. Oculist.* (Paris), **143**, 475 (1910).

Dutoit. *Z. Augenheilk.*, **32**, 139 (1914).

Goulden. *Trans. ophthal. Soc. U.K.*, **48**, 97 (1928).

Jeremy. *Proc. roy. Soc. Med., Sect. Dis. Child.*, **14**, 11 (1921).

Lemoine. *Arch. Ophthal.*, **19**, 184 (1938).

Löwenstein. *Klin. Mbl. Augenheilk.*, **76**, 539 (1926).

Lowe. *Brit. J. Ophthal.*, **33**, 131 (1949).

Schiøtz. *Norsk Mag. Lægevidensk.*, **11**, 1201 (1913).

Vancea. *Cluj. med.*, **10**, 464 (1929).

MYOTONIC CATARACT

CATARACT IN MYOTONIC DYSTROPHY

MYOTONIA as an isolated symptom was first described in the congenital form as *myotonia congenita* by Ernst Leyden of Berlin in 1874, and the disease, myotonic dystrophy, was fully established as a clinical entity by Batten and Gibb (1909) and Steinert (1909–10). The dystrophy is characterized by myotonia (that is, an excessive contractility and a difficulty in relaxation of the muscles) which at times is widespread and general but is most characteristically present in the hand-grips which show an inability to relax, weakness of the facial and masticatory muscles, atrophy particularly of the sterno-mastoids, the vasti of the thighs, the dorsiflexors of the feet and the flexors of the hands, together with baldness, atrophy of the testes or a premature menopause, and cataract. There is a typical myotonic facies, with an unlined, hollow, expressionless face, a drooping jaw, a slow unrelaxing smile accompanied by a slow thick voice. Mental changes are usually present, the patients being slow, apathetic, unsociable and suspicious; and they show a loss of sexual interest and are sterile. These symptoms may occasionally be seen in young children but usually appear between the ages of 20 and 30 and show a gradual progression, most of the patients dying of some secondary disease at a relatively young age, usually before 45 years. The cause of the disease is unknown, but it is presumably a biochemical aberration; one finding, which may or may not have significance, is a deficiency of the quantitatively predominant immunoglobulin IgG owing to its rapid catabolism (Wochner *et al.*, 1966).

The ocular symptoms are manifold. The most common and dramatic is a characteristic form of bilateral cataract; the less common features are a lowering of the ocular tension,[1] tapeto-retinal degenerations resembling pigmentary dystrophy[2] with a diminution of the retinal electrical responses, and sometimes macular degeneration or optic atrophy. In addition, the myotonia itself affects particularly the levator palpebræ muscles, the orbicularis oculi and the extra-ocular muscles giving rise to ptosis, ectropion, lacrimation and an impairment of mobility, while involvement of the intra-ocular muscles results in abnormal pupillary reflexes. Full accounts of the ocular complications are found in the comprehensive works of Thomasen (1948), Vos (1961) and Junge (1966).

The first to draw attention to the occurrence of cataract in myotonia was Greenfield (1911), who pointed out that presenile cataracts seen in these

[1] p. 732.　　　　[2] Vol X, p. 615.

patients were not a fortuitous but an essential part of the clinical picture, and occurred not only in the victims of the general disease but also in otherwise unaffected members of the same family.

Incidence. Before the slit-lamp was introduced cataract was recognized as a common complication of myotonic dystrophy; its occurrence is now accepted as being almost universal, estimates varying from 90% (Simon, 1962), 93% (Pendefunda *et al.*, 1964), 97% (de Jong, 1955; Klein, 1958) and 100% of patients over 20 years of age (Sautter, 1941; Vos, 1961; Junge, 1966). Exceptional cases occur wherein the lens remains clear (Paulian and Tudor, 1939; Waring *et al.*, 1940; Ladekarl and Stürup, 1940; Maas and Paterson, 1950), but it must be remembered that the opacities may not occur until late in the disease (Franceschetti *et al.*, 1947; Thomasen, 1948; Klein, 1958).

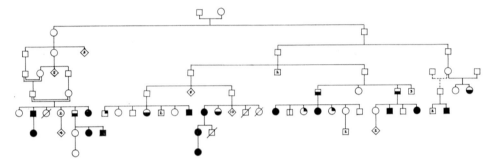

■ ● Myotonic dystrophy and cataract.
◨ ◑ Cataract.
◪ ◔ Abortive or probable myotonic dystrophy.
⊞ Oligophrenia.
⊘ ⊘ Died young.

FIG. 202.—MYOTONIC DYSTROPHY (after D. Klein, 1954).

The youngest age at which it usually occurs is 14 years, although slight and non-specific lenticular changes have been seen at the age of 10 (Klein, 1958) or 13 years (de Jong, 1955), but after the age of 20 it is the rule and the vision is generally disturbed before the age of 40. The degree of cataract is not correlated with the severity of the disease (Sautter, 1941; Thomasen, 1948; Kuhn and Piesbergen, 1957): a patient in the terminal stages of myotonia has shown no lenticular opacities and, conversely, the classical type of cataract has been seen in a patient in whom the presence of the illness was denoted only by myotonia in the thenar eminence (Vogt, 1924). It is also possible that the changes in the lens may be the only evidence of the disease in the absence of all symptoms of myotonia (Thomasen, 1948; de Jong, 1955; Klein, 1958; Jéquier and Todorov, 1967).

Heredity. Since Greenfield (1911) first described its familial occurrence and a full study of its incidence was made by Fleischer (1916–22), the

hereditary nature of myotonic dystrophy has been accepted.[1] The disease
is transmitted as a dominant trait by a polyphenous gene with very complete
penetrance but varying considerably in expressivity (Fig. 202).   The
history of many families has shown an interesting sequence. In the earlier
generations the malady remains latent but a high frequency of senile cataract
may be seen; in a subsequent generation the signs become more pronounced
and the disease appears in several members, as it were in an explosion, when
the complete picture is patently evident of cataractous, myotonic and general
symptoms, whereafter it disappears owing to the lack of offspring. As a rule
the fully developed disease is confined to one generation of which some
members may remain healthy, some may have premature cataract, others may

FIGS. 203 and 204.—CATARACT IN MYOTONIC DYSTROPHY.

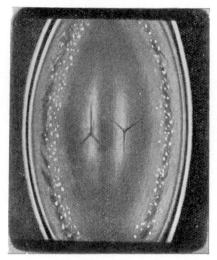
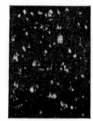

FIG. 203.   FIG. 204.

Fig. 203, optical section.   Fig. 204, surface view of the anterior cortex
(J. E. Caughey).

have some muscular defect in an incomplete form, and yet others present the
full syndrome of muscular atrophy with myotonia and extra-muscular
symptoms including cataract.

   Clinically, the characteristic type of cataract originally noted by
Greenfield (1911) and confirmed by Ormond (1911), Hirschfeld (1911),
Hoffmann (1912), Löhlein (1914) and Fleischer (1918), has now become well

   [1] Curschmann (1912), Hoffmann (1912), Wilson (1918), Kyrieleis (1925), Scheffels (1925),
Heine (1925), Berg (1927), Henke and Seeger (1927), Gifford *et al.* (1929), Waardenburg (1932),
Caughey (1933), Souter (1933), Huber (1935), Vos (1936–38), Waring *et al.* (1940), Allen and
Barer (1940), Maas and Paterson (1943–50), Franceschetti and Mach (1944), Franceschetti
et al. (1947–48), Thomasen (1948) (21 families), Girardet and Ott (1948), Farber (1949), Boersner
(1952), Forster and Barth (1954), Klingler and Brückner (1954), Klein (1958) (100 families),
de Jong (1955), Appelmans *et al.* (1956), Waardenburg *et al.* (1961), Caughey and Myrianthopoulos (1963), Junge (1966), and many others.

recognized.[1] In its early stages the cataract can be seen only with the slit-lamp and does not cause any disturbance of vision. Its pathognomonic feature is the bilateral appearance of a carpet of dust-like and punctate opacities intermingled with larger angulated flakes giving an iridescent display of scintillating colours, mainly red and green; these opacities are sharply localized in a thin zone of cortex just underneath the anterior and posterior capsules, particularly the latter, leaving the anterior and posterior zones of discontinuity and the nucleus free (Figs. 203–4). This stage is frequently described as the *Vogt-type cataract* (1922).

The first stage may persist for some years without change, but it tends to develop into the second stage which can be recognized without the slit-lamp when the changes become more diffuse (the *Fleischer-type cataract*,

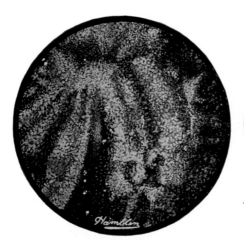
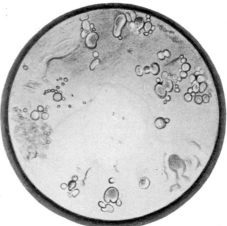

Fig. 205.—Cataract in Myotonic Dystrophy.

The posterior cortex in a woman aged 45, showing well-marked changes (Leslie Paton).

Fig. 206.—Cataract in Myotonic Dystrophy.

Advanced stage (W. C. Souter).

1921) (Fig. 205). It is typically associated with a stellate grouping of opacities at the posterior pole due to a progressive opacification of the lens fibres along the lines of the sutures. The sharp localization of the initial lesions to one cortical layer is presumably due to the involvement of the single stratum of the newest fibres of the lens at the time when the disease has progressed to a certain point; the subsequent stellate appearances at the posterior pole indicate a more diffuse and widespread involvement of

[1] Hauptmann (1918), Vogt (1921–24), Lüssi (1922), Scheffels (1925), Foix and Lagrange (1925), Kyrieleis (1925), Goulden (1928), Gifford *et al.* (1929), Bencini (1929), Nordmann (1931), Caughey (1933), Vos (1933–61), Waring *et al.* (1940), Allen and Barer (1940), Sautter (1941), Franceschetti and Mach (1944), Thomasen (1948), Barth (1954), de Jong (1955), Koch *et al.* (1956), Lynas (1957), Kuhn and Piesbergen (1957), Klein (1958), Goldmann and Favre (1961), Simon (1962), Pendefunda *et al.* (1964), Burian and Burns (1966), Oniki and Mukuno (1966), Bayülkem *et al.* (1966), P. François *et al.* (1967), Van Dyke and Swan (1967).

the fibres. The condition may remain stationary in this stage for several years with little alteration in vision (Bencini, 1929), but gradually evolves into a third and final stage with the development of water-fissures and a slow opacification of the entire lens so that the cataract eventually becomes mature after the manner of the senile type (Fig. 206). This final development may be rapid.

The *differential diagnosis*, apart from the presence of systemic signs of the disease, depends on the topography and nature of the lenticular opacities, particularly on their great number, their smallness and discreteness and their hue, some being white and others being highly coloured, together with the clarity of the anterior and posterior zones of discontinuity. It is distinguished from a hypocalcæmic cataract by the presence of opacities in the zones of discontinuity and their fibrinoid character in this condition, but the punctate lenticular involvement in cretinism, mongolian idiocy, and diabetes should be remembered.

Pathological examinations of the lens have been undertaken by a number of investigators.[1] In the early stages separated from the capsule by a thin lenticular layer there is a zone in which several nucleated fibres are seen together with spherical and fissural vacuoles and small opacities. The origin of the coloured iridescence has been disputed. On the basis of finding an increased content of cholesterol in the lens, Vogt (1921) concluded that this appearance was due to the presence of crystals of this substance, a view supported by Bunge (1938) and Sautter (1941); with this Waring and his colleagues (1940) disagreed and van den Heuvel (1961) considered that droplets of lipids released from disintegrating fibres could account for the phenomenon.

For the general disease no effective *treatment* is known. For the cataract the results of surgical removal are good, the incidence of complications being no greater than those found in cases of senile cataract; and in the absence of retinal changes or optic atrophy the visual results are equally satisfactory.

Two diseases are frequently associated with myotonic dystrophy— congenital myotonia and congenital paramyotonia; by some they are considered to be different manifestations of the same malady, but most authorities share the view of Curschmann (1912) that they are separate entities.

THE CONGENITAL MYOTONIA OF THOMSEN

This disease was first described as *ataxia muscularis* by Julius Thomsen (1876) of Schleswig, a physician who was himself a victim of it and published his paper on the refusal of the Prussian medical authorities to exempt one of his similarly affected sons from military service; he described its occurrence in 20 members of his family in 4 generations from 1742, and his great-nephew, K. Nissen (1923), continued the record to 35 cases in 7 generations. It is thus a hereditary condition, transmitted as a dominant

[1] Vogt (1921), Gil and Querol (1931), Vos (1936), Sautter (1941), Trelles *et al.* (1956).

trait, although often occurring sporadically (Becker, 1963). Congenital in its onset or appearing in early childhood, it is characterized by the generalized signs of myotonia without muscular atrophy; on the contrary, the patient appears robust in sharp contrast to the emaciated, sad and decayed appearance of the sufferer from myotonic dystrophy. Again in contrast to the latter, the congenital condition affects the entire striated muscular system and is not localized, there are no other systemic manifestations and it persists unchanged throughout life. The difficulty of relaxing the muscles may, however, be marked; a hand-shake becomes a prolonged embarrassment, to rise quickly from a sitting position is impossible, and on stumbling the patient may fall down and remain on the floor with all his muscles tensed.

From the ocular point of view the myotonia affects the extra-ocular and palpebral muscles, but the ocular tension remains normal and although cataractous changes have occasionally been reported,[1] it would appear that the lenticular changes are not specific to myotonia (Thomasen, 1948; Klein, 1958).

Treatment is usually unnecessary. Cold, prolonged rest or excitement aggravates the symptoms, warmth and alcohol alleviate them, and relief may be obtained on occasions when they are particularly embarrassing by quinine (0·3 to 0·6 G. t.i.d.) which is also a useful pre-operative measure if surgery is required.

THE CONGENITAL PARAMYOTONIA OF EULENBURG

This rare congenital disease described by Albert Eulenburg (1886) is transmitted as a dominant trait and is characterized by the occurrence of a myotonic phase and a myasthenic phase; in the first the patient becomes rigid, sometimes so markedly that movements are difficult or impossible, while in the second the muscles become so flaccid that again most activities are impossible. The first usually occurs under the influence of cold or emotional stress and the second when the patient is warm.

From the ocular aspect the myotonia may affect the palpebral and extra-ocular muscles and cataract is very rare; only one case has been reported as being specific to paramyotonia (de Jong, 1955).

Allen and Barer. *Arch. Ophthal.*, **24**, 867 (1940).
Appelmans, Michiels and Françoisse. *Bull. Soc. belge Ophtal.*, No. 113, 372 (1956).
Barth. *Ophthalmologica*, **128**, 288 (1954).
Batten and Gibb. *Brain*, **33**, 187 (1909).
Bayülkem, Aydinei and Sirin. *Tip Dünyasi*, **39**, 389 (1966).
Becker. *Proc. 2nd int. Cong. hum. Genet.*, Rome (1961), 1547 (1963).
Bencini. *Boll. Oculist.*, **8**, 575 (1929).
Berg. *Dtsch. Z. Nervenheilk.*, **98**, 29 (1927).
Boersner. *Confin. neurol.* (Basel), **12**, 1 (1952).
Bunge. *v. Graefes Arch. Ophthal.*, **139**, 50 (1938).

Burian and Burns. *Trans. Amer. ophthal. Soc.*, **64**, 250 (1966).
Caughey. *Trans. ophthal. Soc. U.K.*, **53**, 60 (1933).
Neurology (Minneap.), **8**, 469 (1958).
Caughey and Myrianthopoulos. *Dystrophia Myotonica and Related Disorders*, Springfield (1963).
Curschmann. *Dtsch. Z. Nervenheilk.*, **45**, 161 (1912).
Eulenburg. *Neurol. Zbl.*, **5**, 265 (1886).
Farber. *Arch. Ophthal.*, **41**, 450 (1949).
Fleischer. *Ber. dtsch. ophthal. Ges.*, **40**, 441 (1916).
v. Graefes Arch. Ophthal., **96**, 91 (1918).
Klin. Mbl. Augenheilk., **67**, 306 (1921).

[1] Yealland (1923), Heine (1925), Grönholm (1927), Knaur (1936), Focosi (1941), Walton and Nattrass (1954), Caughey (1958).

Fleischer. *Arch. Rassen- u. Gesellsch.-Biol.*, **14**, 13 (1922).

Focosi. *Boll. Oculist.*, **20**, 249 (1941).

Foix and Lagrange. *Ann. Oculist.* (Paris), **162**, 637 (1925).

Forster and Barth. *Helv. med. Acta*, **21**, 99 (1954).

Franceschetti, Klein and Walthard. *Schw. Arch. Neurol.*, **60**, 48 (1947); **61**, 152 (1948).

Franceschetti and Mach. *Helv. med. Acta*, **11**, 887 (1944).

François, P., Asseman, Blervacque and Constantinides. *Bull. Soc. franç. Ophtal.*, **80**, 475 (1967).

Gifford, Bennett and Fairchild. *Arch. Ophthal.*, **1**, 335 (1929).

Gil and Querol. *Arch. Oftal. B. Aires*, **6**, 527 (1931).

Girardet and Ott. *Confin. neurol.* (Basel), **8**, 336 (1948).

Goldmann and Favre. *Ophthalmologica*, **141**, 418 (1961).

Goulden. *Trans. ophthal. Soc. U.K.*, **48**, 97 (1928).

Greenfield. *Rev. Neurol. Psychiat.*, **9**, 169 (1911).

Grönholm. *Acta ophthal.* (Kbh.), **5**, 166 (1927).

Hauptmann. *Klin. Mbl. Augenheilk.*, **60**, 576 (1918).

Heine. *Z. Augenheilk.*, **55**, 1 (1925).

Henke and Seeger. *Biol. Zbl.*, **47**, 727 (1927).

van den Heuvel. *Ophthalmologica*, **141**, 44 (1961).

Hirschfeld. *Z. ges. Neurol. Psychiat.*, **5**, 682 (1911).

Hoffmann. *v. Graefes Arch. Ophthal.*, **81**, 512 (1912).

Huber. *Z. Augenheilk.*, **85**, 310 (1935).

Jéquier and Todorov. *Rev. Oto-neuro-ophtal.*, **39**, 317 (1967).

de Jong. *Dystrophia Myotonica, Paramyotonia and Myotonia Congenita* (Thesis), Utrecht (1955).

Junge. *Docum. ophthal.*, **21**, 1 (1966).

Klein. *J. Génét. hum.*, Suppl. 7 (1958).

Klingler and Brückner. *Schw. Arch. Neurol. Psychiat.*, **73**, 475 (1954).

Knaur. *Arch. Psychiat. Nervenkr.*, **105**, 226 (1936).

Koch, Taubert and Wachtel. *Medizinische*, **40**, 1421 (1956).

Kuhn and Piesbergen. *Klin. Mbl. Augenheilk.*, **130**, 329 (1957).

Kyrieleis. *Klin. Mbl. Augenheilk.*, **74**, 404 (1925).
Z. Augenheilk., **54**, 185 (1925).

Ladekarl and Stürup. *Nord. Med.*, **7**, 1376 (1940).

Leyden. *Klinik. d. Rückenmarkskrankheiten*, Berlin, **1** (1874).

Löhlein. *Klin. Mbl. Augenheilk.*, **52**, 453 (1914).

Lüssi. *Schw. med. Wschr.*, **52**, 796 (1922).

Lynas. *Ann. hum. Genet.*, **21**, 318 (1957).

Maas and Paterson. *Brain*, **66**, 55 (1943); **73**, 318 (1950).

Nissen. *Z. klin. Med.*, **97**, 58 (1923).

Nordmann. *Ann. Oculist.* (Paris), **168**, 438 (1931).

Oniki and Mukuno. *Rinsho Ganka*, **20**, 1315 (1966).

Ormond. *Trans. ophthal. Soc. U.K.*, **31**, 214 (1911).

Paulian and Tudor. *Spitalul* (Buc.), **59**, 131 (1939). See *Zbl. ges. Neurol. Psychiat.*, **95**, 521 (1940).

Pendefunda, Cernea and Dobrescu. *Oftalmologia* (Buc.), **8**, 219 (1964).

Sautter. *v. Graefes Arch. Ophthal.*, **143**, 1 (1941).

Scheffels. *Klin. Mbl. Augenheilk.*, **74**, 512 (1925).

Simon. *Arch. Ophthal.*, **67**, 312 (1962).

Souter. *Trans. ophthal. Soc. U.K.*, **53**, 73 (1933).

Steinert. *Dtsch. Z. Nervenheilk.*, **37**, 38 (1909); **39**, 168 (1910).

Thomasen. *Myotonia. Thomsen's Disease. Paramyotonia. Dystrophia. Myotonica* (Thesis), Aarhus (1948).

Thomsen. *Arch. Psychiat. Nervenkrankh.*, **6**, 706 (1876).

Trelles, Gutierrez, Aranibar and Palomino. *Rev. neuro-psiquiat.*, **19**, 139 (1956).

Van Dyke and Swan. *Trans. Amer. Acad. Ophthal.*, **71**, 838 (1967).

Vogt. *Schw. med. Wschr.*, **51**, 669 (1921).
Klin. Mbl. Augenheilk., **67**, 330 (1921); **69**, 120 (1922); **72**, 421 (1924).
v. Graefes Arch. Ophthal., **108**, 192, 212 (1922).

Vos. *Ned. T. Geneesk.*, **77**, 1930 (1933); **80**, 2399 (1936).
Klin. Mbl. Augenheilk., **91**, 187 (1933).
Cataracta myotonica (Diss.), Groningen (1936).
Ann. Oculist. (Paris), **175**, 641 (1938).
Ophthalmologica, **141**, 37 (1961).

Waardenburg. *Das menschl. Auge u. seine Erbanlagen*, Haag (1932).

Waardenburg, Franceschetti and Klein. *Genetics and Ophthalmology*, Oxon., **1**, 923 (1961).

Walton and Nattrass. *Brain*, **77**, 169 (1954).

Waring, Ravin and Walker. *Arch. intern. Med.*, **65**, 763 (1940).

Wilson, Kinnier. *Trans. ophthal. Soc. U.K.*, **38**, 183 (1918).

Wochner, Drews, Srober and Wallmann. *J. clin. Invest.*, **45**, 321 (1966).

Yealland. *Proc. roy. Soc. Med.*, **16**, Sect. Neurol., 45 (1923).

DEFICIENCY CATARACT

Despite its ready occurrence in experimental animals fed on a diet deficient in certain amino acids or vitamins,[1] cataract is not a common feature in deficiency disease in man; indeed, the evidence is inconclusive that such a sequence occurs. It is true that the frequency of cataract

FIGS. 207 and 208.—ANOREXIA NERVOSA (Dorothy Miller).

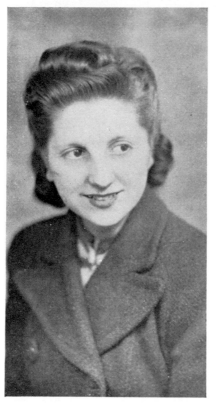

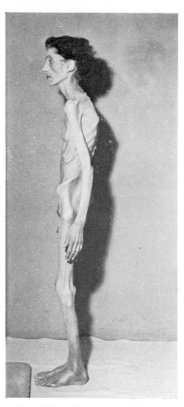

FIG. 207.—The patient aged 18 at the happy stage of life.

FIG. 208.—Two years after marriage at the age of 19. Weight approximately 3 stone.

occurring at an early age in many underdeveloped countries has given rise to the theory that malnutrition is an ætiological factor. It is equally true that suggestions have been made that lenticular opacities may be due to a deficiency in protein (Zuidema, 1955–59) or the specific deficiency of vitamins such as vitamin A (Pillat, 1929), riboflavine (Torokhova, 1947; Falcone, 1952) or nicotinic acid in pellagra (Barthélemy and Onfray, 1931; Barthélemy

[1] p. 95.

1933; Spillane, 1947; Djacos, 1949; Bouzas, 1956); but in no case has the evidence been conclusive. Interesting cases have been reported by Miller (1958) and Stigmar (1965) of young women with anorexia nervosa who

FIGS. 209 to 211.—CATARACT DUE TO ANOREXIA NERVOSA (Dorothy Miller).
The lens of the patient seen in Figs. 207 and 208.

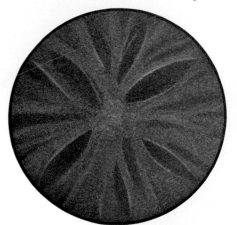 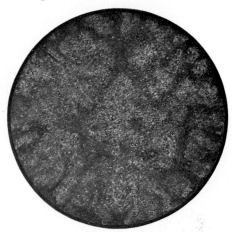

FIG. 209.—The anterior lens cortex.   FIG. 210.—The posterior lens cortex.

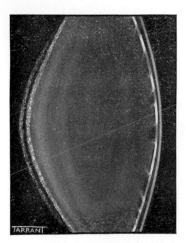

FIG. 211.—Optical section. The anterior cortex is to the right.

developed bilateral rapidly progressive cataracts starting subcapsularly and ultimately requiring surgery (Figs. 207–211); but this is exceptional.

In this connection the rare occurrence may be mentioned of the development of a congenital zonular cataract presumably due to *hypervitaminosis-D* in an infant whose mother had received large doses of this vitamin (Gérard-Lefebvre, 1947).

Barthélemy. *Bull. Soc. franç. Derm.*, **40**, 582 (1933).

Barthélemy and Onfray. *Bull. Soc. Ophtal. Paris*, 135 (1931).

Bouzas. *Bull. Soc. franç. Ophtal.*, **69**, 124 (1956).

Djacos. *Ann. Oculist.* (Paris), **182**, 279 (1949).

Falcone. *Arch. ital. Sci. Med. trop.*, **33**, 619 (1952).

Gérard-Lefebvre. *Arch. franç. Pédiat.*, **4**, 193 (1947).

Miller. *Trans. ophthal. Soc. U.K.*, **78**, 217 (1958).

Pillat. *Arch. Ophthal.*, **2**, 56, 399 (1929).

Spillane. *Nutritional Disorders of the Nervous System*, Edinb. (1947).

Stigmar. *Acta ophthal.* (Kbh.), **43**, 787 (1965).

Torokhova. *Vestn. oftal.*, **26**, 33 (1947).

Zuidema. *Docum. Med. geogr. trop.* (Amst.), **7**, 229 (1955); **11**, 70 (1959).

ORGANIC ACIDURIA

The blood contains some twenty amino acids which are filtrable at the renal glomeruli but are largely absorbed by the tubules so that they appear in the urine only in minute amounts. An excess may be present in the urine in two circumstances. An *overflow aminoaciduria* may occur when an excessive quantity of one or more amino acids is present in the plasma as may occur in hepatic insufficiency or when the metabolism of a particular acid is blocked as in phenylketonuria. Alternatively a *renal aminoketonuria* may develop when tubular absorption is defective, either as an inborn anomaly affecting one (glycinuria) or a group of amino acids (cystinuria) or many metabolites (Fanconi's syndrome),[1] or is acquired in states of deficiency of vitamins C or D.

Systematic chromatographic studies in cases of congenital cataract have revealed the presence of aminoaciduria in a significant number, mainly in males (47%, Franceschetti and Avanza, 1957; 28%, François, 1959; Isola *et al.*, 1960; Franceschetti, 1962). Some of the amino acids may be considered normal but others are abnormal (threonine, histidine, valine, leucine, tyrosine, proline, arginine and others); in many cases the same defect was found in the parents and siblings, suggesting a recessive sex-linked heredity. Infantile glaucoma is also a relatively common ocular complication (Franceschetti, 1962). The metabolic significance of this finding, however, is not yet clear.

Aminoaciduria is also found in association with cataract in several other conditions wherein its presence may be of significance. It is present, for example, in GALACTOSÆMIA (Bickel and Hickmans, 1952; Holzel *et al.*, 1952), disappearing on a galactose-free diet (Hsia *et al.*, 1954)[2] and in HEPATO-LENTICULAR DEGENERATION.[3]

Finally, aminoaciduria may be encountered in several syndromes with varying systemic manifestations accompanied by cataract. This association has been seen in PHENYLKETONURIA (Parks and Schwilk, 1963), HOMO-CYSTINURIA (Gerritsen and Waisman, 1964; Presley and Sidbury, 1967), a

[1] Vol. III, p. 1127.
[2] p. 174.
[3] p. 195.

condition more usually accompanied by dislocation of the lens,[1] FANCONI'S SYNDROME[2] (Worthen and Good, 1955), and in association with dwarfism and external ophthalmoplegia (Avanza and Balavoine, 1959), but Lowe's syndrome is typically linked with lenticular opacities.

THE OCULO-CEREBRO-RENAL SYNDROME (*Lowe's syndrome*), described by Lowe and his colleagues (1952), characterized by renal dwarfism, muscular hypotonia and hyporeflexia, aminoaciduria with a renal defect in the production of ammonia, and mental retardation, is frequently associated with cataract and congenital glaucoma.[3] The condition generally occurs in males as a recessive sex-linked trait and the close relatives especially on the maternal side may show punctate lenticular opacities suggesting that they were carriers (Terslev, 1960; Wilson *et al.*, 1963; Fisher *et al.*, 1967). As a rule the disease is fatal; it is usually explained as due to a defect in the renal tubules. Surgical treatment of the cataract has rarely been successful.

Appelmans, Michiels, Walravens and Doyen. *Bull. Soc. belge Ophtal.*, No. 116, 311 (1957).

Avanza and Balavoine. *Bull. Soc. franç. Ophtal.*, **72,** 331 (1959).

Bickel and Hickmans. *Arch. Dis. Childh.*, **27,** 348 (1952).

Bickel and Thursby-Pelham. *Arch. Dis. Childh.*, **29,** 224 (1954).

Breton, Gaudier, Ponte and Walbaum. *Pédiatrie,* **14,** 908 (1959).

Debré, Royer, Lestradet and Straub. *Arch. franç. Pédiat.,* **12,** 337 (1955).

Dent and Smellie. *Proc. roy. Soc. Med.,* **54,** 335 (1961).

Denys and Corbeel. *Bull. Acad. roy. Méd. belg.,* **9,** 485 (1964).

Denys, Corbeel, Eggermont and Malbrain. *Pédiatrie,* **13,** 636 (1958).

Falls. *Arch. Ophthal.,* **62,** 188 (1959).

Fisher, Hallett and Carpenter. *Arch. Ophthal.,* **77,** 642 (1967).

Franceschetti. *Bull. Schweiz. Acad. Med. Wiss.,* **17,** 414 (1962).

Franceschetti and Avanza. *Atti Soc. oftal. ital.,* **17,** 530 (1957).

François. *Les cataractes congénitales,* Paris, 331 (1959).

François, Woillez, Wannebroucq and Guyon. *Bull. Soc. Ophtal. Fr.,* **64,** 570 (1964).

Gérard-Lebèbvre, Biserte, Woillez *et al. Pédiatrie,* **12,** 527 (1957).

Gerritsen and Waisman. *Pediatrics,* **33,** 413 (1964).

Greaves. *Proc. roy. Soc. Med.,* **56,** 25 (1963).

Grislain. *Rev. port. Pediat.,* **21,** 359 (1958).

Haut and Joannides. *Arch. Ophtal.,* **26,** 21 (1966).

Holzel, Komrower and Wilson. *Brit. med. J.,* **1,** 194 (1952).

Hooft, Valcke and Herpol. *Acta pœdiat. belge,* **18,** 197 (1964).

Hsia, D. and H., Green, Kay and Gellis. *Amer. J. Dis. Child.,* **88,** 458 (1954).

Isola, Bauza, Ferrer *et al. Arch. Pediat. Uruguay,* **31,** 144, 228 (1960).

Jacobi and Tympner. *Klin. Mbl. Augenheilk.,* **149,** 867 (1966).

Johnson. *N.Z. med. J.,* **65,** 243 (1966).

Kühnhardt. *Klin. Mbl. Augenheilk.,* **145,** 893 (1964).

Lovrincevic and Cristaldi. *Sem. Med.* (B. Aires), **121,** 1520 (1962).

Lowe, Terry and MacLachlan. *Amer. J. Dis. Child.,* **83,** 164 (1952).

Matteini and Cotrozzi. *Rass. Neurol. veg.,* **18,** 285 (1964).

Monnet, Matray and Etienne. *Pédiatrie,* **10,** 617 (1955).

Parks and Schwilk. *Amer. J. Ophthal.,* **56,** 140 (1963).

Presley and Sidbury. *Amer. J. Ophthal.,* **63,** 1723 (1967).

Richards, Donnell, Wilson *et al. Amer. J. Dis. Child.,* **109,** 185 (1965).

Sacrez, Juif, Kuetgens *et al. Arch. franç. Pédiat.,* **17,** 815 (1960).

Schaper and Horstmann. *Mschr. Kinderheilk.,* **111,** 17 (1963).

Schoen and Young. *Amer. J. Med.,* **27,** 781 (1959).

---

[1] p. 298.   [2] Vol. III, p. 1127.

[3] Bickel and Thursby-Pelham (1954), Monnet *et al.* (1955), Debré *et al.* (1955), Gérard-Lefèbvre *et al.* (1957), Appelmans *et al.* (1957), Denys *et al.* (1958), Grislain (1958), Breton *et al.* (1959), Schoen and Young (1959), Falls (1959), Sacrez *et al.* (1960), Dent and Smellie (1961), Franceschetti (1962), Lovrincevic and Cristaldi (1962), Greaves (1963), Schaper and Horstmann (1963), Steidl (1963), Wilson *et al.* (1963), Schwartz *et al.* (1964), Trautmann (1964), François *et al.* (1964), Hooft *et al.* (1964), Denys and Corbeel (1964), Matteini and Cotrozzi (1964), Kühnhardt (1964), Richards *et al.* (1965), Haut and Joannides (1966), Johnson (1966), Jacobi and Tympner (1966), and others.

Schwartz, Hall and Gabuzda. *Amer. J. Med.*, **36**, 778 (1964).
Steidl. *Un. méd. Canada*, **92**, 462 (1963).
Terslev. *Acta pædiat.*(Uppsala), **49**, 635 (1960).
Trautmann. *Klin. Mbl. Augenheilk.*, **145**, 60 (1964).

Wilson, Richards and Donnell. *Arch. Ophthal.*, **70**, 5 (1963).
Worthen and Good. In *Essays on Pediatrics* (Ed. Good and Platou), Minneapolis, 305 (1955).

In other metabolic anomalies cataract is an occasional complication.

MUCOPOLYSACCHARIDOSIS I (GARGOYLISM: HURLER'S DISEASE: DYSOSTOSIS MULTIPLEX),[1] a congenital disturbance of the metabolism of carbohydrates usually associated with a cloudy cornea,[2] has been found to be accompanied by congenital cataract (Cavallotti, 1952; Hatt, 1952).

The disturbances of lipid metabolism sometimes associated with lenticular opacities include REFSUM'S SYNDROME (1945–46), a condition described in a previous Volume.[3] Among the other ocular manifestations, the most dramatic of which is an atypical pigmentary degeneration of the retina, cataract, usually posterior and subcapsular in type, is a relatively frequent occurrence.[4]

ANGIOKERATOMA CORPORIS DIFFUSUM (*Fabry's disease*, 1898), a sex-linked recessive condition showing multiple lipid depositions (Rahman, 1962–63), has already been described in a previous Volume[5] where the retinal complications were described. Corneal opacities are frequently found in the deeper layers of the epithelium, often arranged in whorls, but involvement of the lens has rarely been mentioned. In 50% of their cases, however, Spaeth and Frost (1965) noted fine feathery opacities radiating subcapsularly from the posterior pole along the lines of the posterior sutures. The changes were subtle and the opacities asymptomatic.

In ESSENTIAL HYPERCHOLESTEROLÆMIC XANTHOMATOSIS,[6] the cerebral type of the disease described by van Bogaert and his colleagues (1937) which is associated with retardation of development, imbecility, hypogenitalism and cerebellar ataxia, bilateral juvenile coronary cataracts may occur.

HYPOPHOSPHATASIA, a metabolic anomaly described by Rathbun (1948), characterized by a diminution of alkaline phosphatase in the serum and hypercalcæmia with skeletal anomalies and nephrocalcæmia, may be associated with ocular anomalies such as keratopathy[7] and occasionally cataract (Bethune and Dent, 1960).

---

[1] Vol. III, p. 1155.   [2] Vol. VIII, p. 1071.   [3] Vol. X, p. 488.
[4] Kjellson (1953), Fleming (1957), Billings *et al.* (1957), Ashenhurst *et al.* (1958), Gordon and Hudson (1959), Toussaint *et al.* (1959), Veltema and Verjaal (1961), Richterich *et al.* (1963), Harders and Dieckmann (1964).
[5] Vol. X, p. 459.   [6] Vol. VIII, p. 1084.   [7] Vol. VIII, p. 1090.

HEPATO-LENTICULAR DEGENERATION (*Wilson's disease*) is a hereditary disease with a recessive transmission, characterized by a coarse nodular cirrhosis of the liver often associated with progressive damage to the central nervous system, particularly the cortex, the basal ganglia and the putamen of the lenticular nucleus resulting in tremors and rigidity. It may appear acutely in childhood or early adolescence (the *progressive hepato-lenticular degeneration* of Wilson, 1912) or as a slowly evolving disease in the 3rd and 4th decades (the *pseudo-sclerosis* of Westphal-Strümpell, 1883/1898). It is associated with an inborn error in the synthesis of cerulo-plasmin resulting in an excessive absorption of copper and other metals from the intestine and their deposition in various organs where they are bound to proteins. Ocularly the most common feature is the Kayser-Fleischer ring in the cornea[1] composed of copper and other metals, but involvement of the lens is not very uncommon,[2] probably occurring in 1 in 8 cases. The typical lesion is a *sunflower cataract*. It is invisible by transmitted light and is thus not seen with the ophthalmoscope, nor does it seriously impair vision; for this reason it has been termed a *pseudo-cataract*. By focal illumination, however, it presents one of the most beautiful pictures in ophthalmology. There is a thick, powdery deposit located in and under-neath the anterior capsule of a delicate and brilliant colour varying from green to brown or red which gives a lively display of variegated and shimmer-ing hues. The pupillary area is especially involved so that a disc-shaped deposit accumulates here from which spokes run outwards towards the periphery resembling the petals of a sunflower, a configuration probably determined by the movements of the folds on the posterior surface of the iris (Vogt, 1923). If mydriasis is maintained, the peripheral rays are replaced by an extension of the central disc (Jess, 1929–30). Treatment of the disease by BAL or D-penicillamine occasionally improves the lenticular deposit, but this is by no means invariable.

Ashenhurst, Millar and Milliken. *Brit. med. J.*, **2**, 415 (1958).

Bethune and Dent. *Amer. J. Med.*, **28**, 615 (1960).

Billings, O'Callaghan and O'Day. *Trans. ophthal. Soc. Aust.*, **17**, 131 (1957).

van Bogaert, Scherer and Epstein. *Une forme cérébrale de la cholestérinose généralisée*, Paris (1937).

Bonnet, P., Moreau and Bonnet, I. *Rev. oto-neuro-ophtal.*, **27**, 477 (1955).

Cavallotti. *Pediatria* (Napoli), **60**, 357 (1952).

Fabry. *Arch. Derm. Syph.* (Wien), **43**, 187 (1898).

Fleischer. *Ber. dtsch. ophthal. Ges.*, **36**, 128 (1910).
Klin. Mbl. Augenheilk., **68**, 41 (1922).

Fleming. *Neurology* (Balt.), **7**, 476 (1957).

Funder. *Klin. Mbl. Augenheilk.*, **125**, 472 (1954).

Goldberg and von Noorden. *Arch. Ophthal.*, **75**, 162 (1966).

Gordon and Hudson. *Brain*, **82**, 41 (1959).

Harders and Dieckmann. *Dtsch. med. Wschr.*, **89**, 248 (1964).

Hatt. *Strasbourg méd.*, **3**, 893 (1952).

Jess. *Klin. Mbl. Augenheilk.*, **79**, 145 (1927).
Z. Augenheilk., **69**, 59 (1929).
Kurzes Hb. d. Ophthalmologie, Berlin, **5**, 170 (1930).

[1] Vol. VIII, p. 986.

[2] Fleischer (1910–22), Vogt (1921–29), Siemerling and Oloff (1922), Jess (1927), Thiel (1934), Rohrschneider (1934), Funder (1954), P. Bonnet *et al.* (1955), Moreau and Mugneret (1961), Moreau and Semonin (1963), Stucchi and Tissieres (1963), Rix (1965), Goldberg and von Noorden (1966).

Kjellson. *Nord. Med.*, **49**, 460 (1953).
Moreau and Mugneret. *Bull. Soc. Ophtal. Fr.*, **61**, 41 (1961).
Moreau and Semonin. *Bull. Soc. Ophtal. Fr.*, **63**, 282 (1963).
Rahman. *Clin. Res.*, **10**, 393 (1962). *Arch. Ophthal.*, **69**, 708 (1963).
Rathbun. *Amer. J. Dis. Child.*, **75**, 822 (1948).
Refsum. *Nord. Med.*, **28**, 2682 (1945). *Acta psychiat. scand.*, Suppl. 38, 1 (1946).
Richterich, Kahlke, van Mechelen and Rossi. *Klin. Wschr.*, **41**, 800 (1963).
Rix. *Klin. Mbl. Augenheilk.*, **146**, 695 (1965).
Rohrschneider. *Arch. Augenheilk.*, **108**, 391 (1934).
Siemerling and Oloff. *Klin. Wschr.*, **1**, 1087 (1922).

Spaeth and Frost. *Arch. Ophthal.*, **74**, 760 (1965).
Strümpell. *Dtsch. Z. Nervenheilk.*, **12**, 115 (1898).
Stucchi and Tissieres. *Confin. neurol.* (Basel), **23**, 165 (1963).
Thiel. *Klin. Mbl. Augenheilk.*, **93**, 12 (1934).
Toussaint, Coers and Toppet. *Bull. Soc. belge Ophtal.*, No. 122, 383 (1959).
Veltema and Verjaal. *Rev. neurol.* (Paris), **104**, 15 (1961).
Vogt. *Klin. Mbl. Augenheilk.*, **66**, 277 (1921); **83**, 417 (1929). *v. Graefes Arch. Ophthal.*, **112**, 122 (1923).
Westphal. *Arch. Psychiat.* (Berl.), **14**, 87, 767 (1883).
Wilson. *Brain*, **34**, 295 (1912).

Syndermatotic Cataract

Certain types of cutaneous disease have been associated with cataract since the time of Rothmund (1868). Clinically such cataracts occur in young persons, are of bilateral incidence and are typically composed of discrete opacities, and since the diseases in which they occur used to be ascribed to endocrine insufficiency the lenticular changes were often attributed to a primarily endocrine origin. That this is the case is not proven; they are best considered together not as *cataracta dermatogenes* but as *cataracta syndermatotica* (Kugelberg, 1934) since the two lesions are not cause-and-effect but parallel symptoms. It is not surprising, however, that the lens and the skin should tend to act in consort in view of their common ectodermal nature.

In most of these dermatoses the occurrence of cataract is rare and incidental so that an association may even be questioned (Lyevre and Lévy, 1966); in three, however, it occurs so frequently as to constitute an integral part of a syndrome—atopic dermatitis and Rothmund's and Werner's syndromes; in anhidrotic dysplasia it is less common.

ATOPIC DERMATITIS

ATOPIC DERMATITIS (ECZEMA) is the commonest cutaneous disease associated with cataract. This chronic dermatitis has a constitutional allergic basis, in which there is usually a hereditary tendency whether it occurs in infants (infantile eczema), in adolescence or persists into adult life. The allergic nature of the condition is now generally recognized (Coca, 1934; Hill and Sulzberger, 1935; Hill, 1955); most of the patients have a family history of and themselves share in other allergies with eosinophilia (Daniel, 1935; Brunsting, 1936; Hampton and Cooke, 1941; Simon, 1944). Other ætiological views which are now outdated are that its origin is essentially psychogenic (Vidal, 1889), endocrine (Löwenstein, 1934), metabolic (Buschke, 1943) or that it is due to a vitamin deficiency.

In the infant the eczema is acute, vesicular and papular, usually appearing about the age of 3 months; in the chronic forms which occur in youth and adult life (*Besnier's prurigo*) (frequently termed *neurodermatitis*), the most prominent features are an erythematous thickening of the skin which,

FIGS. 212 to 215.—SYNDERMATOTIC CATARACT.

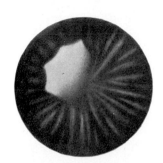

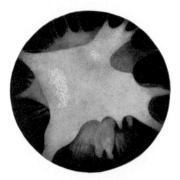

FIG. 212.—In a child with infantile eczema (A. Löwenstein).

FIG. 213.—In a 35-year-old patient (A. Löwenstein).

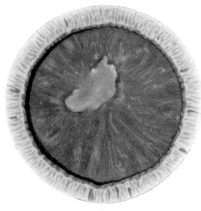

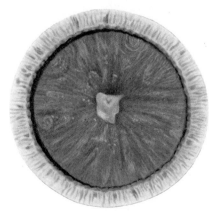

FIG. 214.

FIG. 215.

FIGS. 214 and 215.—Atopic cataract in neurodermatitis. Fig. 214, right lens; Fig. 215, left lens.

with intermittent exacerbations, becomes papular, scaly, thickened and hyperpigmented in lichenified patches with considerable oozing, crusting and pruritus, particularly in the antecubital and popliteal fossæ, the wrists, the neck and sometimes the forehead and around the eyes.

As was first described by N. Andogsky (1914) in St. Petersburg, cataract occurs in association with this type of dermatitis (*Andogsky's syndrome*) in from 8 to 10% of cases.[1]   The involvement of the lens is usually bilateral, although one eye only may be affected (8 out of 58 cases, Sack, 1947), and the opacification usually develops in the third decade although it may be delayed until the fifth. Two types occur. The typical variety, first described by Vogt (1922), takes the form of a dense subcapsular plaque with radiating out-riders in the anterior or posterior cortex, at first in the pupillary area until in the course of time the entire lens becomes opaque (Figs. 212–5). In the histological examination of such a lens, Vail (1966) found a localized degeneration and proliferation of the subcapsular epithelium into the under-lying cortex where widespread degenerative changes constituted the typical plaque or shield.   Alternatively, an opacity resembling a complicated cataract starts subcapsularly at the posterior pole, sending out striæ which also involve the anterior cortex (Beetham, 1940).   In both types complete opacification of the lens eventually develops.   Other ocular complications may occur, such as an atopic kerato-conjunctivitis,[2] a uveitis,[3] conical cornea along with the cataract,[4] and a retinal detachment both before and after surgical extraction of the cataract[5] and even in the absence of cataract (Balyeat, 1937).

In the *treatment* of such a cataract every effort should be made to minimize the allergy before surgery by systemic steroids.   If this is impossible, surgery should at least be postponed until a period when the allergy is quiet, and the extraction should, if possible, be intracapsular.   It may well happen if this cannot be done that the occurrence of vitreous opacities in quantity or the development of an atopic keratitis after surgery may render the operation useless.

Algan. *Bull. Soc. belge Ophtal.*, No. 124, 887 (1960).

Andogsky. *Klin. Mbl. Augenheilk.*, **52**, 824 (1914).

Baer. *Arch. Derm.* (Chic.), **35**, 368 (1937).

Balyeat. *Amer. J. Ophthal.*, **20**, 580 (1937).

Beetham. *Arch. Ophthal.*, **24**, 21 (1940).

Bernard, Bénard, Lacourt and de Rollat. *Ann. Oculist.* (Paris), **199**, 1068 (1966).

Brunsting. *Arch. Derm.* (Chic.), **34**, 935 (1936); **47**, 713 (1943).

Brunsting, Reed and Bair. *Arch. Derm.* (Chic.), **72**, 237 (1955).

Buschke. *Arch. Ophthal.*, **30**, 751 (1943).

Carleton. *Brit. J. Derm.*, **55**, 83 (1943).

Charleux and Paufique. *Bull. Soc. Ophtal. Fr.*, 61 (1957).

Coca. *J. Amer. med. Ass.*, **103**, 1275 (1934).

Coles and Laval. *Arch. Ophthal.*, **48**, 30 (1952).

Cordes and Cordero-Moreno. *Amer. J. Ophthal.*, **29**, 402 (1946).

[1] Davis (1921), Vogt (1922), Siegrist (1928), Ollendorff and Levy (1932), Metzger (1932), Löwenstein (1934), Kugelberg (1934), Daniel (1935–54), Sulzberger (1936), Brunsting (1936–43), Baer (1937), Beetham (1940), Milner (1941), Schönfeld (1941), Carleton (1943) (46 reported cases), McDannald (1943), Cordes and Cordero-Moreno (1946), Sack (1947), Katavisto (1949), Cowan and Klauder (1950), Sprafke (1950), Thompson (1950), Coles and Laval (1952), Dubois-Poulsen and François (1953), Hertzberg (1954), Hurlbut and Domonkos (1954), Gilkes (1955), Brunsting et al. (1955) (136 cases out of 1,158), Ingram (1955), Krogh (1957), Charleux and Paufique (1957), Ring (1958), Pommier and Magnard (1958), Rougier et al. (1958), Kornerup and Lodin (1959), François (1960), Algan (1960), Karel et al. (1963), Bernard et al. (1966), Nordmann (1966).

[2] Vol. VIII, p. 446.   [3] Vol. IX, p. 699.

[4] Hurlbut and Domonkos (1954), Brunsting et al. (1955), Ring (1958), Spencer and Fisher (1959), Franceschetti and Carones (1960), François (1960), Jütte and Lemke (1965), Koźmińska and Filipowicz-Banachowa (1965), Lemke and Jütte (1966), Singh and Mathur (1968).

[5] Cordes and Cordero-Moreno (1946), Mylius (1949), Coles and Laval (1952), Vetter (1957), Klemens (1962).

Cowan and Klauder. *Arch. Ophthal.*, **43**, 759 (1950).

Daniel. *J. Amer. med. Ass.*, **105**, 481 (1935). *Acta XVII int. Cong. Ophthal.*, Montreal-N.Y., **2**, 616 (1954).

Davis. *Sth. med. J.*, **14**, 237 (1921).

Dubois-Poulsen and François, P. *Bull. Soc. Ophtal. Fr.*, 255 (1953).

Franceschetti and Carones. *G. ital. Oftal.*, **13**, 143 (1960).

François. *Bull. Soc. belge Ophtal.*, No. 124, 890 (1960).

Gilkes. *Proc. roy. Soc. Med.*, **48**, 1041 (1955). *Trans. ophthal. Soc. U.K.*, **75**, 301 (1955).

Hampton and Cooke. *J. Allergy*, **13**, 63 (1941).

Hertzberg. *Med. J. Aust.*, **1**, 36 (1954).

Hill. *J. Pediat.*, **47**, 648, 752 (1955).

Hill and Sulzberger. *Arch. Derm.* (Chic.), **32**, 451 (1935).

Hurlbut and Domonkos. *Arch. Ophthal.*, **52**, 852 (1954).

Ingram. *Brit. J. Derm.*, **67**, 43 (1955).

Jütte and Lemke. *Klin. Mbl. Augenheilk.*, **147**, 12 (1965).

Karel, Myska and Kvicalová. *Csl. Ofthal.*, **19**, 130 (1963).

Katavisto. *Acta ophthal.* (Kbh.), **27**, 581 (1949).

Klemens. *Klin. Mbl. Augenheilk.*, **140**, 657 (1962).

Kornerup and Lodin. *Acta ophthal.* (Kbh.), **37**, 508 (1959).

Koźmińska and Filipowicz-Banachowa. *Przegl. derm.*, **52**, 589 (1965).

Krogh. *Nord. Med.*, **58**, 1085 (1957).

Kugelberg. *Klin. Mbl. Augenheilk.*, **92**, 484 (1934).

Lemke and Jütte. *Derm. Wschr.*, **152**, 921 (1966).

Löwenstein. *v. Graefes Arch. Ophthal.*, **132**, 224 (1934).

Lyevre and Lévy. *Arch. Ophtal.*, **26**, 545 (1966).

McDannald. *Arch. Ophthal.*, **30**, 767 (1943).

Metzger. *Klin. Mbl. Augenheilk.*, **89**, 821 (1932).

Milner. *Brit. med. J.*, **1**, 356 (1941).

Mylius. *Klin. Mbl. Augenheilk.*, **115**, 247 (1949).

Nordmann. *Arch. port. Oftal.*, **18**, Suppl., 267 (1966).

Ollendorff and Levy. *Arch. Derm. Syph.* (Wien), **164**, 683 (1932).

Pommier and Magnard. *J. Méd. Lyon*, **39**, 555 (1958).

Ring. *N.Z. med. J.*, **10**, 41 (1958).

Rothmund. *v. Graefes Arch. Ophthal.*, **14** (1), 159 (1868).

Rougier, Colomb and Magnard. *Bull. Soc. Ophtal. Fr.*, 402 (1958).

Sack. *Ann. Allergy*, **5**, 353 (1947).

Schönfeld. *Klin. Mbl. Augenheilk.*, **107**, 589 (1941).

Siegrist. *Der graue Altersstar*, Berlin (1928).

Simon. *J. Amer. med. Ass.*, **125**, 350 (1944).

Singh and Mathur. *Brit. J. Ophthal.*, **52**, 61 (1968).

Spencer and Fisher. *Amer. J. Ophthal.*, **47**, 332 (1959).

Sprafke. *Z. Haut- u. Geschl.-Krankh.*, **9**, 98 (1950).

Sulzberger. *Arch. Derm.* (Chic.), **34**, 328 (1936).

Thompson. *Arch. Derm.* (Chic.), **61**, 433 (1950).

Vail. *Travaux d'ophtalmologie modern* (dedicated to J. Mawas), Paris, 343 (1966).

Vetter. *Klin. Mbl. Augenheilk.*, **130**, 264 (1957).

Vidal. *Traité descriptif des maladies de la peau*, Paris (1889).

Vogt. *v. Graefes Arch. Ophthal.*, **109**, 154, 197 (1922).

THE ROTHMUND SYNDROME

This syndrome, first described by August Rothmund (1868) of Munich, is a relatively rare disease occurring mainly in females and transmitted as a recessive trait, frequently with consanguinity in the parents[1] (Fig. 216). The dermatosis takes on the form of *poikiloderma atrophicans vasculare*; it develops with eruptive and exudative lesions which progress towards atrophy, cicatrization and sclerosis of the skin accompanied by telangiectasia, areas of depigmentation and hyperpigmentation, dystrophies of the nails and the teeth, and frequently hypogenitalism as well as cataract. The lesions of the skin usually appear during the first year of life, and the cataract, which may be congenital and zonular in type (Cole *et al.*, 1945), is habitually

[1] Rothmund (1868), Siegrist (1928), Seefelder (1935), Carleton (1943), Maeder (1949), Habermann and Fleck (1955), and others.

Flandin, Poumeau-Delille and Olivier. *Bull. Soc. méd. Hôp. Paris*, **52**, 1181 (1936).

Franceschetti. *Dermatologica*, **106**, 129 (1953).

Franceschetti and Maeder. *Ophthalmologica*, **117**, 196 (1949).

Georgiadès. *Bull. Soc. hellén. Ophtal.*, **20**, 479 (1952).

Gregersen. *Acta ophthal.* (Kbh.), **34**, 347 (1956).

Gregory. *Brit. J. Ophthal.*, **39**, 44 (1955).

Guillaumat and Maeder. *Bull. Soc. Ophtal. Fr.*, 411 (1949).

Habermann and Fleck. *Z. Kinderheilk.*, **77**, 306 (1955).

Hernández-Benito and García Pérez. *Arch. Soc. oftal. hisp.-amer.*, **25**, 507 (1965).

Jílek and Kúta. *Sborn. lék.*, **66**, 55 (1964).

Kansky and Franzot. *Acta derm. venereol.* (Stockh.), **43**, 441 (1963).

Kleeberg. *Acta med. orient.*, **8**, 145 (1949).

Kleiber. *Klin. Mbl. Augenheilk.*, **65**, 923 (1920).

Knoth, Baethke and Hoffmann. *Hautarzt*, **14**, 145 (1963).

Louw. *Acta med. scand.*, **121**, 333 (1945).

Maeder. *Ann. Oculist.* (Paris), **182**, 809 (1949).

Mannkopf and Hanney. *v. Graefes Arch. Ophthal.*, **159**, 643 (1958).

Marshall. *Amer. J. Ophthal.*, **45** (2), 143 (1958).

Merz, Tausk and Dukes. *Amer. J. Ophthal.*, **55**, 488 (1963).

Moehlig. *J. Amer. med. Ass.*, **132**, 640 (1946).

Müller and Andersson. *Acta med. scand.*, **146**, Suppl. 283, 1 (1953).

Oppenheimer and Kugel. *Amer. J. med. Sci.*, **202**, 629 (1941).

Páez Allende and Fabiano. *Rev. Asoc. Méd. argent.*, **79**, 293 (1965).

Paufique, Rougier and Colomb. *Bull. Soc. Ophtal. Fr.*, 238 (1958).

Perloff and Phelps. *Ann. intern. Med.*, **48**, 1205 (1958).

Petrohelos. *Amer. J. Ophthal.*, **56**, 941 (1963).

Rigg. *Digest Ophthal. Otolaryng.*, **20**, 735 (1958).

Riley, Wieland, Markis and Hamwi. *Ann. intern. Med.*, **63**, 285 (1965).

Rothmund. *v. Graefes Arch. Ophthal.*, **14** (1), 159 (1868).

Rud. *Acta ophthal.* (Kbh.), **34**, 255 (1956).

Schnyder. *Schweiz. med. Wschr.*, **65**, 719 (1935).

Seefelder. *Z. Augenheilk.*, **86**, 81 (1935).

Segal. *Oftalmologia* (Buc.), **3**, 135 (1959).

Siegrist. *Der graue Altersstar*, Berlin, 239 (1928).

Silver. *Amer. J. Dis. Child.*, **111**, 182 (1966).

Suri, Lal, Chatterjee and Sagoraya. *J. Indian med. Ass.*, **47**, 34 (1966).

Szafran. *Klin. oczna*, **31**, 267 (1961).

Thannhauser. *Ann. intern. Med.*, **23**, 559 (1945).

J. Amer. med. Ass., **130**, 238 (1946).

Thomson. *Brit. J. Derm.*, **48**, 221 (1936).

Valero and Gellei. *Brit. med. J.*, **2**, 351 (1960).

Voisin. *Ann. méd.-psychol.*, **1**, 228 (1950).

Werner. *Ueber Katarakt in Verbindung mit Sclerodermie* (Diss.), Kiel (1904).

Wortzel, Newman and Toczek. *J. Newark Beth Israel Hosp.*, **15**, 40 (1964).

In certain other diseases of the skin cataract occurs more rarely and is possibly an incidental accompaniment—focal dermal hypoplasia, congenital dyskeratosis, congenital ichthyosis, psoriasis and incontinentia pigmenti.

FOCAL DERMAL HYPOPLASIA

In this condition, possibly transmitted as a recessive trait, a congenital hypoplasia or atrophy of the skin wherein it becomes fine, fragile and transparent is sometimes accompanied by congenital cataract (Siemens, 1929).

CONGENITAL DYSKERATOSIS

This condition, which is transmitted as a sex-linked recessive trait and is characterized by a reticulate pigmentation of the skin often accompanied by leucoplakia of the mucous membranes and a palmo-plantar dyskeratosis and occasionally by widespread anomalies such as alopœcia, pachyonychia, dwarfism, hypogenitalism and oligophrenia, has been associated with a bilateral congenital cataract (Schäfer, 1925; de Graciansky and Boulle, 1952).

CONGENITAL ICHTHYOSIS

In this disease a diffuse patchy erythema develops into a hyperkeratosis; it may be associated with congenital cataract, but the association is a rarity (Siemens, 1929,

1 in 242 cases; Jancke, 1950; Pinkerton, 1958; Paufique *et al.*, 1963). The occurrence of lenticular opacities in elderly patients is probably fortuitous (Jay *et al.*, 1968).

PSORIASIS

Only a few cases of cataract have been associated with psoriasis and these are probably incidental (Manna and Jankowski, 1966); Trovati (1937) found cataract in 6 children, and Collier (1962) minor lenticular opacities in 9 out of 13 patients with the disease.

INCONTINENTIA PIGMENTI (*the Bloch-Sulzberger syndrome*, 1926/1928)

This condition which is usually seen in females consists of a patchy pigmentation which occurs congenitally. In addition to other ocular defects,[1] congenital cataract commonly develops often associated with uveitis of which it may be a sequel (Sulzberger *et al.*, 1938; Jaramillo *et al.*, 1948; Curth, 1949; Gasteiger, 1951; Ito, 1951; Guillaumat, 1964).

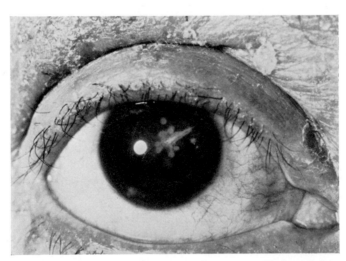

FIG. 217.—CATARACT IN FOLIACEOUS PEMPHIGUS (F. Amendola).

Cataract has been observed in other diseases of the skin but the reported occurrence has been so rare as to indicate an incidental and exceptional association—alopœcia areata (Muller and Winkelmann, 1963; Muller and Brunsting, 1963), total alopœcia (Papastratigakis, 1922; von Bahr, 1967), dermatitis herpetiformis (Kobbert, 1951), lichen follicularis (Zoldan, 1962), keratosis follicularis (Darier's disease) (Gjessing, 1922; Buschke, 1943), vitiligo (Renard *et al.*, 1955), koilonychia (Heidensleben, 1960), foliaceous pemphigus (Amendola, 1949–63, 12 in 240 cases) (Fig. 217), epidermolysis bullosa (Vlad *et al.*, 1965), hydroa vacciniforme (Molnár, 1966), xeroderma pigmentosum (Trematore, 1936; Mehregan, 1963; Gloria, 1966; Ostfeld *et al.*, 1968), and prurigo æstivalis (Blodi, 1948).

Amendola. *Amer. J. Ophthal.*, **32**, 35 (1949).   Bloch. *Schweiz. med. Wschr.*, **7**, 404 (1926).
   Arq. bras. Oftal., **26**, 29 (1963).   Blodi. *Acta ophthal.* (Kbh.), **26**, 279 (1948).
von Bahr. *Trans. ophthal. Soc. U.K.*, **87**, 811   Buschke. *Arch. Ophthal.*, **30**, 751 (1943).
   (1967).   Collier. *Bull. Soc. Oftal. Fr.*, **62**, 59 (1962).

[1] Vol. III, p. 1131.

Curth. *J. invest. Derm.*, **13**, 233 (1949).
Gasteiger. *Ber. dtsch. ophthal. Ges.*, **57**, 292 (1951).
Gjessing. *T. norske Lœgeforen.*, **42**, 411 (1922).
Gloria. *Ann. Ottal.*, **92**, 436 (1966).
de Graciansky and Boulle. *Atlas de dermatologie*, Paris (1952).
Guillaumat. *Bull. Soc. franç. Ophtal.*, **67**, 195 (1964).
Heidensleben. *Acta ophthal.* (Kbh.), **38**, 1 (1960).
Ito. *Tohoku J. exp. Med.*, **54**, 67 (1951).
Jancke. *Klin. Mbl. Augenheilk.*, **117**, 286 (1950).
Jaramillo, Manterola and Rosselot. *Rev. chil. pediat.*, **19**, 654 (1948).
Jay, Blach and Wells. *Brit. J. Ophthal.*, **52**, 217 (1968).
Kobbert. *Z. Haut- u. Geschl.-Kr.*, **10**, 494 (1951).
Manna and Jankowski. *Klin. oczna*, **36**, 371 (1966).
Mehregan. *Arch. Derm.*, **87**, 469 (1963).
Molnár. *Klin. Mbl. Augenheilk.*, **148**, 390 (1966).
Muller and Brunsting. *Arch. Derm.*, **88**, 330 (1963).

Muller and Winkelmann. *Arch. Derm.*, **88**, 202 (1963).
Ostfeld, Mitrea and Achim. *Oftalmologia* (Buc.), **12**, 153 (1968).
Papastratigakis. *Paris Méd.*, **45**, 475 (1922).
Paufique, Ravault, Moulin and Bonnet-Géhin. *Bull. Soc. Ophtal. Fr.*, **63**, 240 (1963).
Pinkerton. *Arch. Ophthal.*, **60**, 393 (1958).
Renard, Puech and Saraux. *Bull. Soc. Ophtal. Fr.*, 257 (1955).
Rudd. *Hospitalstid.*, **70**, 525 (1927).
Schäfer. *Arch. Derm. Syph.* (Berl.), **148**, 425 (1925).
Siemens. *Arch. Derm. Syph.* (Berl.), **157**, 382; **158**, 111 (1929).
Sjögren. *Acta genet.* (Basel), **6**, 80 (1956).
Sjögren and Larsson. *Acta psychiat. neurol. scand.*, Suppl. 113 (1957).
Sulzberger. *Arch. Derm. Syph.* (Berl.), **154**, 19 (1928).
Sulzberger, Fraser and Hunter. *Arch. Derm. Syph.* (Chic.), **38**, 57 (1938).
Trematore. *Lett. oftal.*, **13**, 103 (1936).
Trovati. *Ann. Ottal.*, **65**, 256 (1937).
Vlad, Mirodon and Mitrea. *Oftalmologia* (Buc.), **9**, 335 (1965).
Zoldan. *Boll. Oculist.*, **41**, 613 (1962).

Cataract in Osseous Disease

Cataract is associated with several deformities and diseases of bone but in many cases this may well be incidental.

The CRANIO-FACIAL DYSOSTOSES may be accompanied by cataract in addition to the other ocular anomalies that may appear, such as optic atrophy and exophthalmos.[1]

In *oxycephaly*, congenital cataract has occasionally been found[2]; it may also occur in *plagiocephaly* (Renard and Laporte, 1951) and in the hereditary *cranio-facial dysostosis* of Crouzon (1912–29)[3] (Debré and Pétot, 1927), but cannot be said to be an essential complication of the deformity.

In the FACIAL DYSTROPHIES, *oto-mandibular dysostosis*[4] may be associated with lenticular opacities (François and Haustrate, 1953–54), as well as the *Pierre-Robin syndrome* of *microgenia and glossoptosis* (Lawton Smith and Stowe, 1961).

In a case showing internal frontal hyperostosis, widening of the orbito-sellar angle and fusion of the 2nd and 3rd vertebræ, Collier (1961) observed a unilateral coralliform and cuneiform cataract.

OSTEITIS DEFORMANS (*Paget's disease*), a condition of unknown origin characterized by an increase in the destruction and formation of bone, has occasionally been associated with the development of punctate lenticular opacities of the "endocrine" type (Vergne, 1908; Dreyfus and Mamou,

---

[1] Vol. III, p. 1038.
[2] Kraus (1902), Alexander (1903), Patry (1905), Aubaret and Guillot (1934), Lartigue (1939), Sourdille *et al.* (1939), Gänsslen (1940), Falls (1943), Vest (1955), and others.
[3] Vol. III, p. 1048.　　　　　　　　　　　　[4] Vol. III, p. 1025.

1947; Boltansky, 1947; d'Ermo, 1951). Whether this is incidental is not yet clear; both the calcium and phosphorus in the serum are normal, but the serum alkaline phosphatase is unusually high.

Alexander. *Münch. med. Wschr.*, **50,** 1534 (1903).

Aubaret and Guillot. *Rev. oto-neuro-ophtal.*, **12,** 279 (1934).

Boltansky. *Bull. Soc. Méd. Hôp. Paris*, **63,** 1054 (1947).

Collier. *Arch. Ophtal.*, **21,** 253 (1961).

Crouzon. *Bull. Soc. Méd. Hôp. Paris*, **33,** 545 (1912).
Ann. Méd., **25,** 184 (1929).

Debré and Pétot. *Arch. Méd. Enf.*, **30,** 274 (1927).

Dreyfus and Mamou. *Bull. Soc. Méd. Hôp. Paris*, **63,** 1112 (1947).

d'Ermo. *Boll. Oculist.*, **30,** 477 (1951).

Falls. *Arch. Ophthal.*, **29,** 210 (1943).

François and Haustrate. *Bull. Soc. belge Ophtal.*, No. 104, 356 (1953).
Ann. Oculist. (Paris), **187,** 340 (1954).

Gänsslen. Just's *Hb. d. Erbbiologie d. Menschen*, Berlin, **4** (1), 415 (1940).

Kraus. *Zur Kasuistik d. Sehnervenleiden bei Schädelmissbildungen* (Diss.), Giessen (1902).

Lartigue. *Contribution a l'étude de la cataracte dans l'oxycéphalie* (Thèse), Paris (1939).

Patry. *Contribution à l'étude des lésions oculaires dans les malformations crâniennes, spécialement dans l'oxycéphalie* (Thèse), Paris (1905).

Renard and Laporte. *Arch. Ophtal.*, **11,** 739 (1951).
Bull. Soc. franç. Ophtal., **64,** 176 (1951).

Smith, J. L., and Stowe. *Pediatrics*, **27,** 128 (1961).

Sourdille, Eoche-Duval and Gendron. *Bull. Soc. Ophtal. Paris*, 186 (1939).

Streiff. *Ophthalmologica*, **120,** 79 (1950).

Vergne. *Ann. Oculist.* (Paris), **140,** 321 (1908).

Vest. *Ann. pœdiat.* (Basel), **184,** 14 (1955).

Osmotic Cataract

We have seen that an upset of the osmolarity of the serum is probably a factor of importance in the early intumescent stages of diabetic cataract. The same basis may account for the onset of the total cataract which may develop suddenly in the extreme stages of *cholera*, the osmotic dilution of the blood owing to loss of salts leading to a diminished osmolarity of the body-fluids and thus to a transference of fluid from the aqueous into the lens. A similar origin might have caused the sudden appearance of a reversible stellate subcapsular cataract in a patient described by Junceda Avelló (1963); he was given renal dialysis for acute renal failure due to a congenital anomaly of the kidney; the lenticular opacities rapidly progressed until the fundus was obscured and 12 hours later the lens again became clear with the return of normal vision.

Junceda Avelló. *Arch. Soc. oftal. hisp.-amer.*, **23,** 817 (1963).

Multiple Syndromes with Cataract

The composite clinical pictures formed by many of those conditions conveniently termed syndromes are frequently associated with lenticular opacities, sometimes appearing congenitally and sometimes developing at a later stage. Although many of these have already been discussed, several deserve mention in this connection.

THE SYNDROME OF BRITTLE BONES, BLUE SCLERÆ AND DEAFNESS (*van der Hoeve's syndrome*) is described in a previous Volume.[1] Cataract, either of the zonular or cortical type, has been reported on several occasions particularly in the variety characterized by osteopsathyrosis and macular atrophy of the skin (Voorhoeve, 1918; Blegvad and Haxthausen, 1921; Wenda, 1949).

[1] Vol. III, p. 1098.

CHONDRODYSTROPHIA CALCIFICANS CONGENITA PUNCTATA (CONGENITAL STIPPLED EPIPHYSES) (*Conradi's syndrome*, 1914) involving widespread ectodermal and meso-dermal anomalies with mental retardation, has also been described elsewhere.[1] It is characteristically complicated by a bilateral cataract, particularly in girls. The cataract is usually total but sometimes nuclear, appearing congenitally or within the first year of life (Fig. 218). With two exceptions (Jeune *et al.*, 1953; Armaly, 1957), all the patients recorded with cataract died before the age of two years, signifying a severe form of the condition.[2]

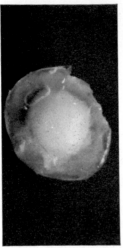

FIG. 218.—CHONDRO-DYSTROPHIA CALCIFI-CANS CONGENITA PUNCTATA.

The cataractous lens (N. Ashton).

MANDIBULO-OCULO-FACIAL DYSCEPHALY has also been described elsewhere.[3] In the localized type associated with the names of Hallermann and Streiff wherein the most pro-minent feature is a "bird-face", congenital cataract frequently with microphthalmos and microcornea is a common feature.[4] Spontaneous absorption of the lens may occur after rupture of the capsule.[5] In the more generalized type wherein the bird-face is combined with nanism and other widespread anomalies, bilateral congenital cataracts, complete or incom-plete, have been described in all but one of the 26 reported cases. The cataract rapidly develops into the morgagnian state releasing milky fluid on discission.[6]

In this connection HYPERPLASTIC CONGENITAL MESO-DERMAL DYSTROPHY (ARACHNODACTYLY : *Marfan's syndrome*) should be mentioned.[7] The striking lenticular feature is spherophakia often with dislocation of the lens, but localized lenticular opacities may be present.[8]

In ARTHROGRYPOSIS MULTIPLEX, with its characteristic fibrotic ankylosis of the joints, congenital bilateral cataract has been observed in an infant who also had pterygium coli (Beyer *et al.*, 1956).

TURNER'S SYNDROME, the " symmetrical form " of the status Bonnevie-Ullrich,[9] has been associated with congenital cataract (De la Chapelle, 1962; Lessel and Forbes, 1966). In the case reported by Khodadoust and Paton (1967), a male aged 13, the cataract was probably secondary to a long-standing retinal detachment in a highly myopic eye. The syndrome in females is associated with anomalies in the sex-chromosomes, but the males who have a similar phenotypical appearance show a normal karyotype as far as can be detected by present methods of investigation, but cataract cannot be said to be an essential accompaniment.

[1] Vol. III, p. 1118.
[2] Conradi (1914), Lightwood (1930), Bateman (1936), Bloxsom and Johnston (1938), Maitland (1939), Lund (1943), Ford *et al.* (1951), Scott (1952), Paufique and Étienne (1954), Forni (1960), Defauw and Massa (1962), Nordmann (1966), and others.
[3] Vol. III, p. 1023.
[4] Hallermann (1948), Pau (1950), Ponte (1958), Falls and Schull (1960), van Balen (1961), Guyard *et al.* (1962), Ardouin *et al.* (1962), Roth (1962).
[5] Blodi (1957), François (1958–59), Wolter and Jones (1965).
[6] Bergmeister (1912), Ullrich and Fremerey-Dohna (1953), Leffertstra (1956), François (1958).
[7] Vol III, p. 1102.
[8] Weve (1931), Franceschetti (1932), King (1934), François (1935), Bakker (1936), Kilgore (1939), Wagner (1952), and others.
[9] Vol. III, p. 1113.

In a modified form of the STATUS DYSRAPHICUS involving the maxilla, a zonular cataract was noted by Fonseca (1938). In certain cases of *Duane's retraction syndrome*, multiple ocular defects including congenital cataract have been associated with widespread systemic anomalies which have suggested that the clinical picture thus presented is a manifestation of the status dysraphicus.[1]

In MAURIAC'S SYNDROME (1930), characterized by juvenile diabetes, hepatomegaly, osteoporosis and retardation of growth, Rosselet and Beck (1958) observed the development of a typical diabetic cataract.

The RUBINSTEIN-TAYBI SYNDROME (1963), a congenital condition of unknown ætiology characterized by motor anomalies and mental retardation, deformities of the extremities and palate and frequently by epicanthus and strabismus, is occasionally complicated by cataract (Roy *et al.*, 1968; Padfield *et al.*, 1968).

In certain ANOMALIES OF THE BRAIN, cataract is an occasional feature: *micrencephaly*,[2] *lissencephaly*,[3] and *congenital spastic paraplegia (Little's disease)*[4] (2 cases of cataract in 100 cerebral palsies, Breakey, 1955; 4 cases of cataract in 86 cerebral palsies, Yannet, 1944; 1 case in 98, Schachat *et al.*, 1957; Blumel *et al.*, 1960).

PROGRESSIVE MYOCLONIC CEREBELLAR DYSSYNERGY is a rare hereditary cerebellar ataxia transmitted in some families as a dominant trait, first described by James Ramsay Hunt (1914–21), the New York neurologist. It is characterized by an intention tremor appearing about the age of 7 years in the hands and gradually becoming generalized to involve particularly the head and limbs associated with irregular myoclonic spasms until it becomes difficult to maintain the equilibrium and impossible to coordinate ordinary activities such as walking. The causal lesion is an atrophy of the dentate nucleus and the superior cerebellar peduncle. In a Swiss family of this type Franceschetti and his colleagues (1954) observed 3 members in 3 generations with the complete syndrome and 8 others who were affected by tremors; 6 individuals developed bilateral pre-senile cataracts either as a single lesion or associated with the neurological disease.

PIGMENTARY DYSTROPHY of the retina is commonly associated with the development of cataract of a complicated type in later life.[5] So also are other tapeto-retinal dystrophies in which systemic anomalies occur: the *Laurence-Moon-Biedl syndrome*[6] wherein the retinal dystrophy is combined with obesity and polydactyly, *Hallgren's syndrome* (1959)[7] wherein deafness, vestibulo-cerebellar ataxia and psychiatric disturbances occur and cataract usually appears before the age of 40 years; and the *segmentary ectodermal syndrome* of Sanchez Salorio (1955) wherein oligophrenia, retarded development and frequently muscular dystrophy occur.[8]

OLIGOPHRENIA is frequently associated with cataract. In the *Torsten Sjögren syndrome* (1935) wherein oligophrenia is transmitted as a recessive trait with cataract, the lenticular opacities are usually congenital, typically zonular or total, sometimes anterior polar or posterior cortical, but they may develop during the first months or years of life.[9]

---

[1] Vol. III, p. 994.   [2] Vol. III, p. 1073.   [3] Vol. III, p. 1077.
[4] Vol. III, p. 1091.   [5] p. 225.   [6] Vol. X, p. 610.
[7] Vol. X, p. 614.   [8] Vol. III, p. 1150.
[9] Forty-four cases, Sjögren (1935); 18 cases, Franceschetti and Brugger (1944); Heuyer *et al.* (1947), Guillaumat *et al.* (1948), Schachter (1950–59), Kirman (1952), Dufour *et al.* (1954), Toselli and Volpi (1961), Warburg (1963).

The *syndrome of Marinesco-Sjögren*[1] (Marinesco *et al.*, 1927–31; Sjögren, 1947–50) is characterized by congenital spino-cerebellar ataxia in addition to congenital cataract and oligophrenia.[2]

Other associations have been noted, such as the occurrence of oligophrenia with congenital cataract, keratoconus, ectopia of the vitreous and optic atrophy (Pfändler, 1950) or with marked microphthalmos and disorganization of the globe (Whitnall and Norman, 1940; Andersen and Warburg, 1961). These have been described elsewhere.[3]

MONGOLISM, a syndrome in which mental retardation is associated with widespread anomalies, is typically associated with punctate, arcuate and sutural lenticular opacities. These have been fully described in a previous Volume.[4]

DEAFNESS is a further association with cataract. Its occurrence with pigmentary dystrophy of the retina is well-known.[5] Nerve-deafness due to anomalies in the inner ear associated with renal disease and anterior polar cataract as a heredo-familial anomaly (*Alport's syndrome*, 1927) has been described in children.[6] In the case reported by Grimaud and his colleagues (1962) the child was deaf and dumb. The anterior polar cataract may be associated with an anterior lenticonus (Fig. 77).

A case of congenital cataract associated with deafness and cardiac anomalies, resembling in many respects the complications of maternal rubella in the child but without a history of this infection in the mother, was reported by Ramón Guerra (1950).

NIEDEN'S SYNDROME (1887) of multiple telangiectases with congenital cataract is a rarity wherein lenticular opacities may appear in youth (Terrien and Prélat, 1959) or adult life (Petersen, 1954); aortic stenosis and organic disease of the heart develop at an early stage.

HÆMOLYTIC ANÆMIA. *Congenital hœmolytic jaundice*, characterized by the destruction of the erythrocytes during hæmolytic crises with icterus and splenomegaly accompanied by microspherocytosis, reticulosis and multiple skeletal anomalies, has been noted to be associated with cataract (François, 1961).

In the *hœmolytic anœmia*, due to a deficiency of glucose-6-phosphate dehydrogenase in the erythrocytes, a cataract may occur which may be due to the effect of a similar lack of this enzyme in the lens itself (Zinkham, 1961; Westring and Pisciotta, 1966).

Alport. *Brit. med. J.*, **1**, 504 (1927).
Alter, Talbert and Croffead. *Neurology* (Minneap.), **12**, 836 (1962).
Andersen and Warburg. *Arch. Ophthal.*, **66**, 614 (1961).
Ardouin, Urvoy and Bezier. *Bull. Soc. Ophtal. Fr.*, **62**, 438 (1962).
Armaly. *Arch. Ophthal.*, **57**, 491 (1957).
Bakker. *Arch. Augenheilk.*, **109**, 353 (1936).
van Balen. *Ophthalmologica*, **141**, 53 (1961).
Bateman. *Proc. roy. Soc. Med.*, **29**, 745 (1936).
Bergmeister. *Beitr. Augenheilk.*, **8** (79), 537 (1912).

Beyer, Lausecker, Levy and Bartolo. *Arch· franç. Pédiat.*, **13**, 286 (1956).
Blegvad and Haxthausen. *Brit. med. J.*, **2**, 1071 (1921).
Blodi. *Arch. Ophthal.*, **57**, 593 (1957).
Bloxsom and Johnson. *Amer. J. Dis. Child.*, **56**, 103 (1938).
Blumel, Evans and Eggers. *Arch. Ophthal.*, **63**, 246 (1960).
Breakey. *Arch. Ophthal.*, **53**, 852 (1955).
Brownell and Wolter. *Arch. Ophthal.*, **71**, 481 (1964).
Conradi. *Jb. Kinderheilk.*, **80**, 86 (1914).

---

[1] Vol. III, p. 1147.

[2] Richards (1950), Hagen *et al.* (1951), Garland and Moorhouse (1953), Franceschetti *et al.* (1956), Dureux *et al.* (1958), Müller (1962), Alter *et al.* (1962), Prot and Zielinska (1962).

[3] Vol. III, p. 1148.　　　　[4] Vol. III, p. 1137.　　　　[5] Vol. X, p. 609.

[6] Sohar (1954), Reyersbach and Butler (1954), Goldbloom *et al.* (1957), Grimaud *et al.* (1962), Dubach and Gsell (1962), Gregg and Becker (1963), Merz *et al.* (1963), Brownell and Wolter (1964), Perrin (1964).

Defauw and Massa. *Bull. Soc. belge Ophtal.*, No. 131, 411 (1962).

De la Chapelle. *Acta endocr.* (Kbh.), Suppl. 65 (1962).

Dubach and Gsell. *Lancet*, **1**, 159 (1962).

Dufour, Jéquier, Cuendet and Michels. *Bull. Soc. franç. Ophtal.*, **67**, 318 (1954).

Dureux, Cordier, Ziza and Tridon. *Rev. neurol.* (Paris), **98**, 777 (1958).

Falls and Schull. *Arch. Ophthal.*, **63**, 409 (1960).

Fonseca. *Arch. Clin. oftal.* (Lisbon), **5**, 23 (1938).

Ford, Schneider and Brandon. *Pediatrics*, **8**, 380 (1951).

Forni. *Ophthalmologica*, **139**, 322 (1960).

Franceschetti. *Klin. Mbl. Augenheilk.*, **88**, 686 (1932).

Franceschetti and Brugger. *Schweiz. med. Wschr.*, **74**, 255 (1944).

Franceschetti, Klein and Willener. *Schweiz. Arch. Neurol. Psychiat.*, **74**, 419 (1954).

Franceschetti, Marty and Klein. *Confin. neurol.* (Basel), **16**, 271 (1956).

François. *Bull. Soc. franç. Ophtal.*, **48**, 157 (1935).

Boll. Oculist., **37**, 161 (1958).

Les cataractes congénitales, Paris, 367 (1959).

Amer. J. Ophthal., **52**, 207 (1961).

Garland and Moorhouse. *J. Neurol. Neurosurg. Psychiat.*, **16**, 110 (1953).

Goldbloom, Fraser, Waugh *et al.* *Pediatrics*, **20**, 421 (1957).

Gregg and Becker. *Arch. Ophthal.*, **69**, 293 (1963).

Grimaud, Cordier, Dureux *et al.* *Rev. Oto-neuro-ophtal.*, **34**, 59 (1962).

Guillaumat, Surugue and Chabat. *Bull. Soc. Ophtal. Paris*, 244 (1948).

Guyard, Perdriel and Ceruti. *Bull. Soc. Ophtal. Fr.*, **62**, 442 (1962).

Hagen, Noad and Latham. *Med. J. Aust.*, **1**, 217 (1951).

Hallermann. *Klin. Mbl. Augenheilk.*, **113**, 315 (1948).

Hallgren. *Acta psychiat. scand.*, **34**, Suppl. 138 (1959).

Heuyer, Lebovici, Leroy *et al.* *Arch. franç. Pédiat.*, **4**, 638 (1947).

Hunt. *Brain*, **37**, 247 (1914); **44**, 490 (1921).

Jeune, Larbre, Carron and Couette. *Arch. franç. Pédiat.*, **10**, 914 (1953).

Khodadoust and Paton. *Arch. Ophthal.*, **77**, 630 (1967).

Kilgore. *Trans. Pac. Cst. oto-ophthal. Soc.*, **24**, 223 (1939).

King. *Proc. roy. Soc. Med.*, **27**, 298 (1934).

Kirman. *Lancet*, **1**, 694 (1952).

Leffertstra. *Ophthalmologica*, **132**, 204 (1956).

Lessel and Forbes. *Arch. Ophthal.*, **76**, 211 (1966).

Lightwood. *Proc. roy. Soc. Med.*, **24**, 564 (1930).

Lund. *Proc. roy. Soc. Med.*, **36**, 381 (1943).

Maitland. *Brit. J. Radiol.*, **12**, 91 (1939).

Marinesco, Draganesco and Vasiliu. *Bull. Soc. roum. Neurol.*, **4**, 16 (1927).

Encéphale, **26**, 97 (1931).

Mauriac. *Gaz. Sci. Méd. Bordeaux*, **51**, 402 (1930).

Merz, Tausk and Dukes. *S. Dak. J. Med. Pharm.*, **16**, 23 (1963).

Müller, K. *Z. Kinderheilk.*, **87**, 348 (1962).

Nieden. *Zbl. prakt. Augenheilk.*, **11**, 353 (1887).

Nordmann. *Amer. J. Ophthal.*, **61**, 1256 (1966).

Padfield, Partington and Simpson. *Arch. Dis. Childh.*, **43**, 94 (1968).

Pau. *Klin. Mbl. Augenheilk.*, **117**, 529 (1950).

Paufique and Étienne. *Bull. Soc. franç. Ophtal.*, **67**, 42 (1954).

Perrin. *Ann. Oculist.* (Paris), **197**, 329 (1964).

Petersen. *Acta ophthal.* (Kbh.), **32**, 565 (1954).

Pfändler. *Ophthalmologica*, **119**, 103 (1950).

Ponte. *G. ital. Oftal.*, **11**, 401 (1958).

Prot and Zielinska. *Neurol. Neurochir. Psychiat. pol.*, **12**, 479 (1962).

Ramón Guerra. *Arch. Pediat.* (Uruguay), **21**, 153 (1950).

Reyersbach and Butler. *New Engl. J. Med.*, **251**, 377 (1954).

Richards. *J. ment. Sci.*, **96**, 537 (1950).

Rosselet and Beck. *Ophthalmologica*, **135**, 533 (1958).

Roth. *Bull. Soc. Ophtal. Fr.*, **62**, 500 (1962).

Roy, Summitt, Hiatt and Hughes. *Arch. Ophthal.*, **79**, 272 (1968).

Rubinstein and Taybi. *Amer. J. Dis. Child.*, **105**, 588 (1963).

Sanchez Salorio. *Arch. Soc. oftal. hisp.-amer.*, **15**, 496 (1955).

Schachat, Wallace, Palmer and Slater. *Pediatrics*, **19**, 623 (1957).

Schachter. *Pédiatrie*, **39**, 885 (1950).

Aggiorn. pediat., **10**, 1 (1959).

Scott. *Proc. roy. Soc. Med.*, **45**, 452 (1952).

Sjögren. *Z. ges. Neurol. Psychiat.*, **152**, 263 (1935).

Acta psychiat. neurol., **46**, Suppl., 286 (1947).

Confin. neurol. (Basel), **10**, 293 (1950).

Sohar. *Harefuah*, **47**, 161 (1954).

Terrien and Prélat. *Bull. Soc. Pédiat. Paris*, **11**, 370 (1959).

Toselli and Volpi. *Ann. Ottal.*, **87**, 111 (1961).

Ullrich and Fremerey-Dohna. *Ophthalmologica*, **125**, 73, 144 (1953).

Voorhoeve. *Lancet*, **2**, 740 (1918).

Wagner. *Klin. Mbl. Augenheilk.*, **120**, 640 (1952).

Warburg. *Acta ophthal.* (Kbh.), **41**, 157 (1963).

Wenda. *Arch. Ophtal.*, **9**, 44 (1949).

Westring and Pisciotta. *Arch. intern. Med.*, **118**, 385 (1966).

Weve. *Arch. Augenheilk.*, **104**, 1 (1931).

Whitnall and Norman. *Brit. J. Ophthal.*, **24**, 229 (1940).

Wolter and Jones. *Ophthalmologica*, **150**, 401 (1965).

Yannet. *J. Pediat.*, **24**, 38 (1944).

Zinkham. *Bull. Johns Hopk. Hosp.*, **109**, 206 (1961).

Complicated Cataract

CATARACTA COMPLICATA was a concept introduced by Otto Becker (1876) to embrace the lenticular changes which frequently appear in various intra-ocular diseases such as " retinal detachment, intra-ocular tumours, cysticercus, absolute glaucoma, cyclitis, iridocyclitis, and the unknown processes which result in buphthalmos and other ectatic processes in the eyes "; his concept still holds although its basis has been broadened. The essential clinical features of such cataracts were detailed with great exactitude by Ernst Fuchs (1910). Clinically they assume many forms but in general they start in the superficial cortex; the opacities may be punctate, striate or diffuse and they often give rise to a characteristic polychromatic lustre.

In the majority of cases such cataracts are presumably due to a derangement of the metabolism of the lens by an interference with its permeability or the diffusion into it of toxins either from the inflammatory focus or from the products of degeneration caused by disease; and owing to the thinness of the posterior capsule and its lack of a supporting epithelial barrier, the earliest clinical changes are typically seen in the region of the posterior pole (Pau, 1950). They occur in three circumstances: in inflammations of the globe, in widespread degenerative states, and when the ocular circulation is gravely impaired.

INFLAMMATORY COMPLICATED CATARACT

This type of complicated cataract assumes two different forms depending on whether the exciting inflammation is a severe anterior uveitis or a long-standing posterior uveitis.

CATARACTS IN INFLAMMATIONS OF THE ANTERIOR SEGMENT

IRIDOCYCLITIS is the most common cause of such a cataract, a sequence already described in a previous Volume.[1] The opacities have no characteristic feature whether the uveitis is exudative or granulomatous in type, is due to organismal infection or to bacterial allergy, or is caused by sarcoidosis or sympathetic ophthalmitis. In the earlier stages they may be accentuated in the region nearest to the most acute inflammation. This is seen in the development of subcapsular opacities beneath posterior synechiæ (Fig. 45) in which case they are usually situated eccentrically; over them epithelial proliferation is usually active but opacification of the lens tends to spread. In the later stages of a chronic anterior uveitis a complete cataract tends to develop slowly, usually after the inflammation

[1] Vol. IX, p. 88.

has existed for some years, and is frequently preceded by a plastering of the lens by cyclitic exudates. This exudative material may make observation of the lens difficult or impossible, and its extent can sometimes be gauged clinically only after an iridectomy has been performed. The evolution of the cataract is usually gradual, and if the uveal inflammation is brought under control, its progress may stop; but with a persistence of the cyclitis, opacification of the entire lens proceeds until it finally assumes a densely white, mother-of-pearl appearance showing crystalline and calcareous deposits and is frequently covered with new blood vessels from the iris (Figs. 219–20).

FIGS. 219 and 220.—COMPLICATED CATARACT.

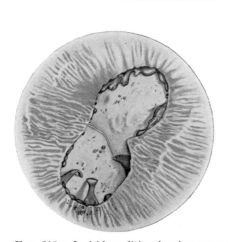 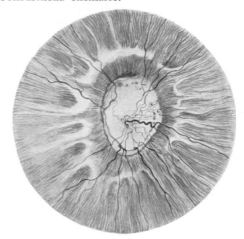

FIG. 219.—In iridocyclitis, showing many synechiæ.

FIG. 220.—In an old case of iridocyclitis with a profuse growth of new vessels from the iris.

Pathologically[1] the lens usually shows more profound degenerative changes than are evident in a simple senile cataract, and in the later stages liquefaction, cholesterol deposition and calcification are prominent while the capsule becomes thickened and the whole lens becomes shrunken, distorted and tremulous (Fig. 221). The most characteristic feature, however, is the thickening of the capsule associated with a proliferation of the epithelium which almost invariably multiplies to cover the entire posterior surface so that a continuous layer lines the capsule without interruption, a process which is most evident when the lens has become embedded in a mass of organized cyclitic tissue. The new epithelium on the posterior surface continues to grow, suffering vesicular enlargement into Wedl's cells[2]; these migrate into the cortex and form a characteristic feature

[1] Wagenmann (1891), Treacher Collins (1896), Fuchs (1906–17), Burchart (1910), Schlippe (1910), Schall (1921), von Szily (1938), Samuels (1943), Davids (1949), and others.
[2] p. 26.

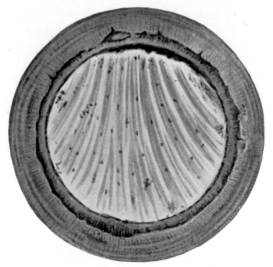

Fig. 221.—Complicated Cararact.

Shrunken lens with plicated capsule after iridocyclitis (T. Harrison Butler).

of such cataracts (Fig. 222). In those cases, however, in which the lens is surrounded by granulation tissue or becomes embedded in pus as in a panophthalmitis, this proliferative activity does not appear, and the capsule itself may become completely absorbed. In this event the barrier to the entrance of inflammatory tissue into the lens is broken, and vas-

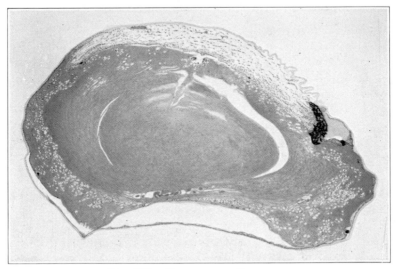

Fig. 222.—Complicated Cataract.

Advanced stage. Flattened anterior capsular cataract. Wandering of epithelial cells to the posterior surface. Wedl's cells and calcification (A. von Szily).

cularized fibrous tissue may form and ossification may ultimately develop (Fig. 223).

It is interesting that biochemical changes have been observed in cases of experimental uveitis in animals, some of them being apparent before the lenticular opacities develop; these include a diminution of the consumption of glucose and of pyruvic and lactic acids, a decrease in the alkaline reserve and changes in the permeability of the lens (Auricchio, 1949–56; Auricchio and Ambrosio, 1953).

Treatment is frequently difficult and depends on the activity of the uveal inflammation. A considerable amount of vision can sometimes be

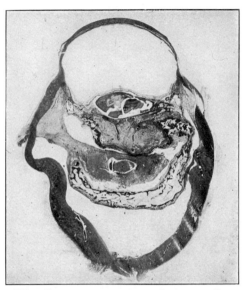

FIG. 223.—CALCIFICATION OF THE LENS AND CHOROID.

From a man aged 28 who had acute cyclitis following measles at the age of 5. Note the dome-shaped cornea resembling buphthalmos, retracted iris, calcareous lens, cyclitic membrane, detached retina and bone in the choroid showing true medullary spaces (× 3) (J. H. Parsons).

attained by an iridectomy at the stage when the lenticular opacities are mainly central in position, but surgical extraction should seldom be undertaken while active cyclitis is present or fresh keratic precipitates are in evidence lest a recrudescence of the inflammation supervene and vision be ultimately lost from phthisis bulbi. The prognosis may, however, be good in carefully selected cases provided the eye has remained quiet for some time, the tension is normal, and the operation is performed under an umbrella of corticosteroids. A preliminary iridectomy may sometimes be of value as an indication of how the eye may be expected to stand up to major operative procedures, and by breaking down adhesions it prepares the way for the subsequent extraction, but it is rarely necessary; in all cases an intracapsular extraction should be attempted lest the uveitis be activated by phacolytic products.

In this connection mention should be made of the complicated cataracts which may be associated with the collagen diseases. The most typical is that occurring in *chronic polyarthritis in children (Still's disease)*,[1] in rheumatoid arthritis[2] (Fig. 224) and in *polyarteritis nodosa*.[3] In *diffuse scleroderma* the occurrence of bilateral cataract has also been noted (Aguilera Maruri and del Cerro, 1937; Bovi, 1958; Mihail, 1958).

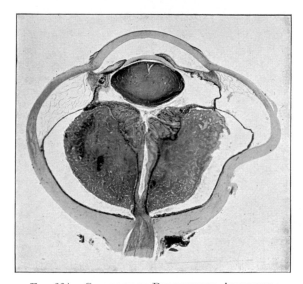

FIG. 224.—CATARACT IN RHEUMATOID ARTHRITIS.
Chronic iridocyclitis with secondary cataract (M. J. Hogan, S. J. Kimura and P. Thygeson).

KERATITIS of a severe degree is frequently complicated by the development of cataract. We have seen elsewhere[4] that a pyramidal, subcapsular or total cataract may follow the perforation of an ulcer in infancy, and in adult life it is a common sequel to a serpiginous ulcer.[5] In these cases the damage to the lens may be due to the diffusion of toxins from the cornea, and after perforation of the cornea when the lens comes into direct contact with it the result may be more dramatic. The portion of the lens most gravely affected is within the pupillary area where the protection of the iris is lacking and here in mild cases the subcapsular epithelium tends to proliferate but in severe cases to necrose, thus facilitating the entry of toxins (von Hippel, 1896; Samuels, 1942). Eventually the same pathological changes occur as are observed in cataracts secondary to uveitis: calcareous degeneration, shrinkage into a membranous cataract or liquefaction and morgagnian degeneration.

[1] Vol. IX, p. 537.
[2] Vol. IX, p. 535.
[3] Vol. IX, p. 548.
[4] Vol. VIII, p. 122.
[5] Vol. VIII, p. 780.

CATARACT IN INFLAMMATIONS OF THE POSTERIOR SEGMENT

The lenticular opacities complicating a posterior uveitis, sometimes called CHOROIDAL CATARACT, present typical features differentiating this from all other types of cataract; these were first fully described by Vogt (1919). The first sign seen with the slit-lamp is a subcapsular iridescence of brilliant colours, particularly red and blue, at the posterior pole, giving rise to a *polychromatic lustre*. This is rapidly followed by the appearance of dot-like opacities with a similar polychromatic lustre in the posterior cortex. These gradually become denser and spread until they congregate into a conglomerate mass increasing in extent and thickness which now appears yellow by focal illumination (Figs. 225–6). The histological changes are

FIGS. 225 and 226.—POSTERIOR CATARACT (T. Harrison Butler).

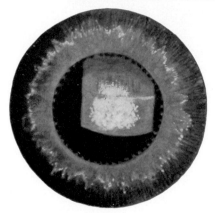 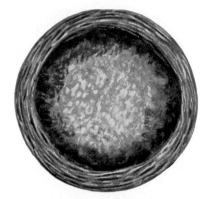

FIG. 225.—Posterior cortical and capsular cataract. Seen with the loupe : early stage.

FIG. 226.—Posterior cortical cataract. Seen with the loupe : advanced stage.

confined to this region (Fig. 227). The plaque has a loose and porous consistency containing dense opacities and vacuoles so that it has a tufted or breadcrumb appearance, frequently interspersed with densely white areas of calcification occurring at a relatively early stage (Figs. 228–9). As it increases in size the opacity usually takes the form of a rosette, an appearance caused by a delay in the involvement of the fibres between the sutures (Fig. 230). At this stage in the thicker central region the polychromatic lustre is lost and remains only in the attenuated peripheral parts of the rosette. As opacification proceeds, it usually progresses in two directions by sudden leaps; the opacities spread axially towards the centre of the lens and also peripherally in concentric layers parallel to the posterior surface. As they develop these become larger, denser and more yellow, and are always preceded by a whitish cloudy haze so that there is no sharp separation between the opaque area and the clear cortex. Frequently a new plaque

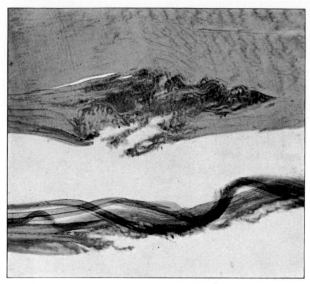

FIG. 227.—POSTERIOR CORTICAL CATARACT ($\times$ 60) (J. H. Parsons).

FIGS. 228 and 229.—COMPLICATED CATARACT.

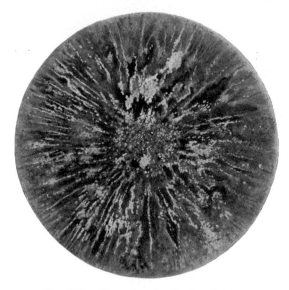

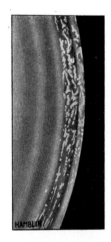

FIG. 228.—Secondary to chorioretinitis.

FIG. 229. — Secondary to chorioretinitis; optical section of the posterior pole.

appears behind the posterior border of the adult nucleus which acts as a
second centre of opacification and spreads in a manner similar to the first.
Thereafter the same changes, preceded by the typical polychromatic lustre
and developing into the formation of a rosette, commence in the superficial
cortex at the anterior pole; here the opacities are less distinct than in the
posterior cortex and appear white rather than yellow. They also extend
axially as well as peripherally and gradually the entire lens becomes opaque.
Eventually, often after a very slow evolution, the cataract reaches the
stage of maturity in which the lens appears shrunken with a thickened
and wrinkled capsule showing cretaceous deposits, and may even become
tremulous and dislocated.

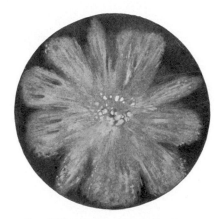

FIG. 230.—COMPLICATED CATARACT.
Following choroiditis, showing typical rosette formation.

The *diagnosis* of a choroidal cataract is of importance since the
question of its operability opens up considerations wider than the state of
the lens itself; but fortunately its recognition is rendered easy by the two
characteristics which distinguish it from all other types—*the presence of a
polychromatic lustre in the early stages, and the fact that the opacities are never
clearly demarcated from the surrounding tissue but are submerged in a cloudy
haze.* It is of great importance also that the slit-lamp reveals the characteristic lustre before any opacities are visible with the ophthalmoscope so
that a certain diagnosis can be made from the earliest stages.

The two most important points in differential diagnosis are a *cupuliform senile
cataract* and a *traumatic cataract.* In the former the opacities are dome-shaped and not
arranged in a rosette, the thickness is uniform throughout and is not increased in the
axial region, there is no polychromatic lustre, and there is no enveloping cloudy haze.
Traumatic cataract, instead of assuming a rosette-form, follows the design of the lens
fibres in a feathery pattern and here, too, the pathognomonic lustre is absent. It
must be remembered, of course, that in old people a complicated cataract is usually

FIGS. 231 to 233.—TREMATODE LARVÆ IN THE LENSES OF FISH.

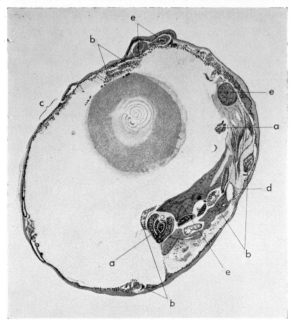

FIG. 231.—*a*, living larvæ; *b*, dead larvæ; *c*, a rupture in the capsule healed by overgrowth of epithelium; *d*, degenerative lens tissue resembling an after-cataract; *e*, transformed cortical tissue (F. Salzer).

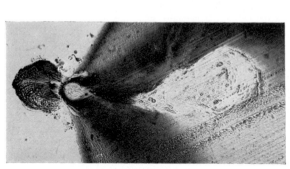 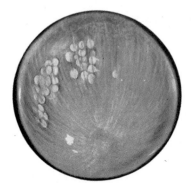

FIG. 232.   FIG. 233.

FIGS. 232 and 233.—The fluke, *Diplostomum*, in the lens of a trout (N. Ashton).

FIG. 232.—The entry of the fluke into the lens showing a herniation of the lens material at the point of perforation of the capsule.

FIG. 233.—Drawing of the lens containing many larvæ.

associated with pre-existing senile opacities in the lens which may to some extent obscure the characteristic picture.

PARASITIC INVASION of the lens is rare. The presence of filaria-like *threadworms* in the lens itself giving rise to cataract has exceptionally been reported.[1] Most of the

[1] Vol. IX, p. 456.

observations have been by early investigators (von Nordmann, 1832; Gescheidt, 1833; Schöler, 1875), but more recent reports have appeared (Salzer, 1924–25; Mickiewicz and Leontjewa, 1962). The phenomenon is undoubtedly extremely rare. However that may be, the presence of trematodes is relatively common in the lenses of fish both in Europe and America (von Nordmann, 1832; Hofer, 1904; Greeff, 1907; Salzer, 1907; Lewis, 1931) (Figs. 231–3). The *cysticercus* can invade every tissue of the eye[1] but a resting place in the lens is exceptional (von Graefe, 1866; 2 out of 1,216 cases, Talkovskey, 1951). A secondary cataract may, of course, develop if the globe is disorganized by the invasion of parasites.

Aguilera Maruri and del Cerro. *Act. dermo-sifilogr.* (Madrid), **48**, 303 (1957).
Auricchio. *Ann. Ottal.*, **75**, 89 (1949).
  G. ital. Oftal., **8**, 242, 251 (1955).
  Boll. Oculist., **35**, 217 (1956).
Auricchio and Ambrosio. *G. ital. Oftal.*, **6**, 489 (1953).
Becker. *Graefe-Saemisch Hb. d. ges. Augenheilk.*, 1st ed., Leipzig, **5**, 227 (1876).
  Zur Anatomie d. gesunden u. kranken Linse, Wiesbaden (1883).
Bovi. *di Clinica* (Bologna), **18**, 99 (1958).
Burchart. *Die Histologie d. Katarakt bei chronischer Uveitis* (Diss.), Freiburg (1910).
Collins, Treacher. *Researches*, London (1896).
Davids. *v. Graefes Arch. Ophthal.*, **149**, 156 (1949).
Fuchs. *Z. Augenheilk.*, **15**, 191 (1906).
  Lhb. d. Augenheilk., Wien (1910).
  v. Graefes Arch. Ophthal., **93**, 381 (1917).
Gescheidt. *v. Ammons Z. Ophthal.*, **3**, 405 (1833).
von Graefe. *v. Graefes Arch. Ophthal.*, **12** (2), 174 (1866).
Greeff. *Arch. Augenheilk.*, **56**, 330 (1907).
von Hippel. *v. Graefes Arch. Ophthal.*, **42** (2), 194 (1896).

Hofer. *Hb. d. Fischkrankheiten*, Munich (1904).
Lewis. *Arch. Ophtal.*, **48**, 801 (1931).
Mickiewicz and Leontjewa. *Klin. oczna*, **32**, 59 (1962).
Mihail. *Oftalmologia* (Buc.), **3**, 153 (1958).
von Nordmann. *Mikrographische Beitr. z. Naturges. d. Wirbellosen Thiere*, Berlin (1832).
Pau. *Ber. dtsch. ophthal. Ges.*, **56**, 240 (1950).
Salzer. *Arch. Augenheilk.*, **58**, 19 (1907).
  Ber. dtsch. ophthal. Ges., **44**, 278 (1924).
  v. Graefes Arch. Ophthal., **115**, 515 (1925).
Samuels. *Arch. Ophthal.*, **27**, 345 (1942); **29**, 583 (1943).
Schall. *Klin. Mbl. Augenheilk.*, **67**, 584 (1921).
Schlippe. *Arch. Augenheilk.*, **67**, 97 (1910).
Schöler. *Berl. klin. Wschr.*, **12**, 682 (1875).
von Szily. *Trans. ophthal. Soc. U.K.*, **58**, 595 (1938).
Talkovskey. *Sov. Med.*, No. 12, 17 (1951).
Vogt. *Klin. Mbl. Augenheilk.*, **62**, 582, 593 (1919).
Wagenmann. *v. Graefes Arch. Ophthal.*, **37** (2), 21 (1891).

EMBRYOPATHIC CATARACT

Special interest attaches to a type of secondary cataract which appears in the offspring owing to the trans-placental transmission of an infection from the mother usually acquired during the first three months of pregnancy.[2] The occurrence of such a phenomenon was first established in Sydney by Sir Norman Gregg (1941–45) in the case of rubella, and lesions of this type were termed *embryopathies* by Töndury (1951–62). Apart from rubella, the most common maternal infections liable to cause such a lesion are syphilis and toxoplasmosis; the influence of other infections is more questionable. The occurrence of a secondary cataract due to a systemic infection after birth without other ocular involvement is exceptional.[3]

CONGENITAL SYPHILIS is the only instance of bacterial infection which gives rise to a characteristic type of cataract. A typical complicated cataract

[1] Vol. IX, p. 478.   [2] Vol. III, p. 391.   [3] p. 224.

may, of course, occur as a result of a severe intra-uterine syphilitic irido-cyclitis (Igersheimer, 1928), as well as a nondescript bilateral total cataract in patients infected before birth (Desvignes, 1947; Gözberk, 1953; Sédan and Sédan-Bauby, 1953). A peculiar lesion, however, is the BROWN SAUCER-SHAPED CATARACT of Vogt (1931) which is seen in later life in eyes which had been affected by interstitial keratitis and syphilitic choroiditis[1] (Fig. 234); it is of congenital origin affecting a zone around the posterior aspect of the embryonic nucleus and is usually noticed in the fifth decade of life. Histologically the affected area has been found to contain a deposit of muco-polysaccharides (Dubler, 1960). Although it is usually bilateral, a unilateral

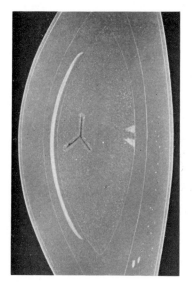

FIG. 234.—SYPHILITIC BROWN SAUCER-SHAPED CATARACT OF VOGT (H. Dubler).

case has been reported (Hallermann, 1952), and a similar morphological appearance has been seen in non-syphilitic patients (10 out of 22 cases, Remler, 1952).

SCARLATINA in the mother due to a hæmolytic streptococcal infection about the second month of pregnancy has been associated with congenital cataract in the infant, a sequence which may have been incidental (Clapp, 1945).

Viral infections in the mother during the second month of pregnancy are the most frequent cause of a complicated embryopathic cataract.

RUBELLA is the commonest maternal infection to produce such a lesion. It is to be remembered that intra-uterine rubella is biologically and clinically a very different disease from the acquired infection. In the latter a transient

[1] Rosen (1949), Hallermann (1952), Remler (1952), Forni (1953), Dubler (1960).

mild illness results wherein the virus is present in the pharyngeal secretions and the blood for only 48 hours until the specific neutralizing antibody (which gives permanent immunity) makes its appearance; in the former the virus arrives before the fœtus has developed an immunological defence so that extensive cellular parasitism occurs wherein the virus probably becomes incorporated into the DNA of the infected cells, replicates as the cells divide and may persist for a period of 18 months or more after birth (Rawls *et al.*, 1965–67; Cooper and Krugman, 1967). In the fœtal infection the lenticular opacities are thus frequently associated with widespread anomalies such as microphthalmos, deafness, and anomalies of the heart and central nervous

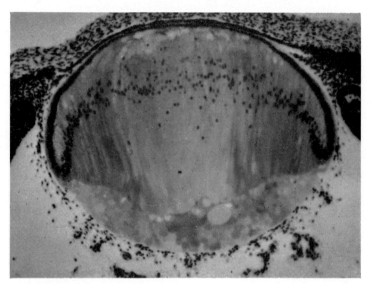

FIG. 235.—TOTAL CATARACT.
In a young child, due to maternal rubella (N. Ashton).

system. This sequence was first noted by Gregg (1941) and subsequently by Swan and others (1943–46) in Australia, whereafter its occurrence was verified in most countries of the world and the literature is now very extensive[1]; over 1,000 cases were collected by Günther (1953), and Hertzberg (1968), examining 50 patients with congenital rubella born after the 1940–1 epidemic, found that 10 were surgically aphakic, 7 of them in both eyes. In some 60% of these cataract occurs while other ocular anomalies may be present such as a secondary pigmentary retinal degeneration,[2] atrophy of the iris, mesodermal dysgenesis, corneal opacities, congenital glaucoma, strabismus or nystagmus and microphthalmos. The cataract is usually but by no means invariably bilateral; it may be nuclear, atypical or total, and may progress after birth to complete opacification of the lens which eventually

[1] See Vol. III, p. 393.　　　　　[2] Vol. X, p. 530.

may become shrunken and membranous (Ehrlich, 1948) or may even be spontaneously absorbed (P. and S. Delthil, 1951). As a rarity the infant may be born with clear lenses and develop bilateral cataracts after some months (Menser *et al.*, 1966). The visual results after surgery are not good, usually 6/60 ; the best vision found by Hertzberg (1968) was 6/24.

FIGS. 236 to 238.—CATARACT IN MATERNAL RUBELLA (J. R. Wolter *et al.*).

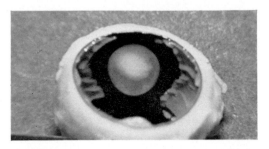

FIG. 236.—In a 56-day-old male infant. Gross view of the left microphthalmic eye, showing the lamellar cataract.

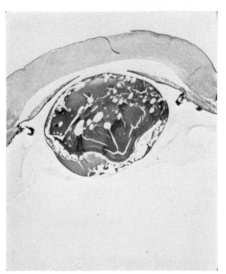

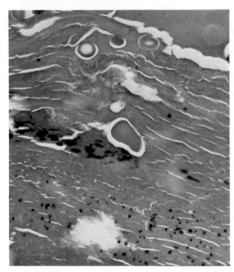

FIG. 237.—In an 8-day-old male infant, showing the shallow anterior chamber and a small cataractous lens.

FIG. 238.—From the same case as Fig. 236, showing, superiorly, morgagnian globules, and granular accumulations of calcium crystals (below).

Histological examination[1] has shown that the posterior epithelial cells are completely destroyed about one month after the mother has acquired the infection but the subcapsular and equatorial cells are relatively un-

[1] Swan (1944), Cordes and Barber (1946), Helweg-Larsen and Nielsen (1948), Bourquin (1948), Cordes (1949), Töndury (1951–55), Babel (1954–59), Roy *et al.* (1966), Wolter *et al.* (1966), Scheie *et al.* (1967), Zimmerman (1968), and others.

affected and continue to develop into fibres which later tend, however, to degenerate and may also suffer complete destruction (Figs. 235–8). In the case reported by Wolter and his colleagues (1964) there was a congenital unilateral aphakia together with an absence of the anterior chamber and iris so that the ciliary processes were adherent to the cornea (Fig. 239). These changes start in intra-uterine life and proceed after birth due, in Töndury's (1952–55) view, to the persistence of the virus in the epithelial cells; in fact, the virus has been recovered from such lenses after birth

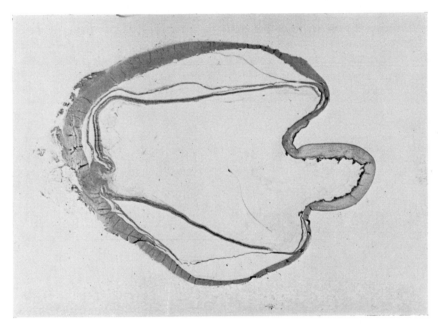

FIG. 239.—APHAKIA AFTER MATERNAL RUBELLA.

The infection occurred during the first trimester of pregnancy. The microphthalmic eye shows an absence of the anterior chamber, of the iris and of the lens; the ciliary processes are on the back of the cornea. On the temporal side of the optic disc there is excessive glial formation and a retinal fold (J. R. Wolter).

(Cotlier et al., 1966; Hambidge et al., 1966; Reid et al., 1966; Murphy et al., 1967) and in the developing lens fibres of experimentally infected rats (Bohigian et al., 1968).

Congenital cataract has followed other maternal viral infections in the early months of pregnancy but these are of less importance, being sporadic in their incidence with little proved causal relationship: measles (Ellett, 1945; Schachter, 1949; Guzzinati, 1954), poliomyelitis (Töndury, 1952), influenza (Lefebvre and Merlen, 1948; Gregg, 1956), epidemic hepatitis (Töndury, 1954; Gregg, 1956), zoster (Duehr, 1955), and epidemic parotitis (Ellett, 1945; di Ferdinando, 1952; Agarwal and Raizada, 1954).

CONGENITAL TOXOPLASMOSIS[1] is the only important parasitic infection which gives rise to an embryopathic cataract. In this infestation an ordinary complicated cataract may occur, associated with a severe uveitis or choroiditis sometimes with microphthalmos, but opacification of the lens may appear as a primary event without other discernible ocular lesions.[2] The cataract is sometimes unilateral but usually affects both eyes; it may involve the posterior cortex, the anterior subcapsular region or the entire lens.

The *treatment* of this type of cataract is often difficult, sometimes because of the presence of other ocular anomalies, the frequent smallness of the pupil and shallowness of the anterior chamber, or the density of the embryonic nucleus which makes absorption difficult. Nevertheless, although the resultant vision is frequently poor, in bilateral cases a discission operation should be undertaken as early as is reasonably possible; repetitions are usually necessary. Unilateral cases, however, are probably best left undisturbed.

Agarwal and Raizada. *Brit. J. Ophthal.*, **38**, 383 (1954).

Babel. *Ophthalmologica*, **127**, 333 (1954); **137**, 183 (1959).

Bohigian, Fox and Cotlier. *Amer. J. Ophthal.*, **65**, 196 (1968).

Bourquin. *Les malformations du nouveau-né*, Paris (1948).

Clapp. *Trans. Amer. ophthal. Soc.*, **43**, 147 (1945).

Cooper and Krugman. *Arch. Ophthal.*, **77**, 434 (1967).

Cordes. *Arch. Ophthal.*, **42**, 596 (1949).

Cordes and Barber. *Arch. Ophthal.*, **36**, 135 (1946).

Cotlier, Fox and Smith. *Amer. J. Ophthal.*, **62**, 233 (1966).

Danis. *Bull. Soc. belge Ophtal.*, No. 95, 501 (1950).

Dekking. *Ophthalmologica*, **117**, 1 (1949).

Delthil, P. and S. *Arch. franç. Pédiat.*, **8**, 47 (1951).

Desvignes. *Arch. Ophtal.*, **7**, 174 (1947).

Dubler. *Arch. Ophtal.*, **20**, 389 (1960).

Duehr. *Amer. J. Ophthal.*, **39**, 157 (1955).

Ehrlich. *Amer. J. Ophthal.*, **31**, 224 (1948).

Ellett. *Trans. Amer. ophthal. Soc.*, **43**, 144 (1945).

di Ferdinando. *Boll. Oculist.*, **31**, 427 (1952).

Fisher and Wilson. *Amer. J. Roentgenol.*, **59**, 816 (1948).

Forni. *Ophthalmologica*, **125**, 343 (1953).

François. *Schweiz. Arch. Neurol. Psychiat.*, **78**, 87 (1956).

François. *Les cataractes congénitales*, Paris, 535 (1959).

Glees. *Ophthalmologica*, **126**, 361 (1953).

Gözberk. *Ann. Oculist.* (Paris), **186**, 141 (1953).

Gregg. *Trans. ophthal. Soc. Aust.*, **3**, 35 (1941); **4**, 119 (1944).
Med. J. Aust., **1**, 313 (1945).
Trans. Amer. Acad. Ophthal., **60**, 199 (1956).

Günther. *Mschr. Kinderheilk.*, **101**, 385 (1953).

Guzzinati. *Boll. Oculist.*, **33**, 833 (1954).

Hallermann. *Klin. Mbl. Augenheilk.*, **121**, 641 (1952).

Hambidge, Shaffer, Marshall and Hayes. *Brit. med. J.*, **1**, 650 (1966).

Helweg-Larsen and Nielsen. *Ugeskr. f. Læger*, **110**, 1394 (1948).

Hertzberg. *Amer. J. Ophthal.*, **66**, 269 (1968).

Igersheimer. *Syphilis u. Auge*, Berlin (1928).

Kaufman. *Amer. J. Ophthal.*, **34**, 1611 (1951).

Koch, Wolf, Cowen and Paige. *Arch. Ophthal.*, **29**, 1 (1943).

Lavat. *Arch. Ophtal.*, **13**, 252 (1953).

Lefebvre and Merlen. *Sem. Hôp. Paris*, **24**, 2541 (1948).

Magnusson and Wahlgren. *Acta path. microbiol. scand.*, **25**, 215 (1948).

Menser, Harley, Housego and Murphy. *Lancet*, **2**, 771 (1966).

Murphy, Reid, Pollard et al. *Amer. J. Ophthal.*, **64**, 1109 (1967).

[1] Vol. IX, p. 413.

[2] Koch *et al.* (1943), Fisher and Wilson (1948), Schwarz *et al.* (1948), Magnusson and Wahlgren (1948), Dekking (1949), Ridley (1949), Danis (1950), Kaufman (1951), Rabkin and Javett (1952), Glees (1953), Lavat (1953), François (1956–59).

Rabkin and Javett. *S. Afr. med. J.*, **26**, 41 (1952).

Rawls, Melnick, Rosenber *et al.* *Proc. Soc. exp. Biol.* (N.Y.), **120**, 623 (1965).

Rawls, Phillips, Melnick and Desmond. *Arch. Ophthal.*, **77**, 430 (1967).

Reid, Murphy, Gillespie *et al.* *Med. J. Aust.*, **1**, 540 (1966).

Remler. *Klin. Mbl. Augenheilk.*, **121**, 647 (1952).

Ridley. *Brit. J. Ophthal.*, **33**, 397 (1949).

Rosen. *Arch. Ophthal.*, **42**, 749 (1949).

Roy, Fuste, Hiatt *et al.* *Amer. J. Ophthal.*, **62**, 222 (1966).

Schachter. *Praxis*, **38**, 421 (1949).

Scheie, Plotkin and Kertesz. *Arch. Ophthal.*, **77**, 440 (1967).

Schwarz, Rose and Fry. *Pediatrics*, **1**, 478 (1948).

Sédan and Sédan-Bauby. *Bull. Soc. Ophtal. Fr.*, 38 (1953).

Swan. *J. Path. Bact.*, **56**, 289 (1944).
Trans. ophthal. Soc. Aust., **4**, 132 (1944).

Swan, Tostevin and Black. *Med. J. Aust.*, **2**, 889 (1946).

Swan, Tostevin, Moore *et al.* *Med. J. Aust.*, **2**, 201 (1943).

Töndury. *Klin. Mbl. Augenheilk.*, **119**, 449 (1951).
Helv. pœdiat. Acta, **7**, 105 (1952).
CIBA-Symp., Basel, **2**, 138 (1954).
Münch. med. Wschr., **97**, 1009 (1955).
Embryopathien, Berlin (1962).

Vogt. *Lhb. u. Atlas. d. Spaltlampenmikroskopie d. lebenden Auges*, Berlin, **2**, 434 (1931).

Wolter, Hall and Mason. *Amer. J. Ophthal.*, **58**, 1011 (1964).

Wolter, Insel, Willey and Brittain. *J. pediat. Ophthal.*, **3**, 29 (1966).

Zimmerman. *Amer. J. Ophthal.*, **65**, 837 (1968).

DEGENERATIVE COMPLICATED CATARACT

A complicated cataract may accompany several degenerative conditions affecting the globe; the most common of these are high myopia, retinal dystrophies, essential iris atrophy, vitreo-retinal dystrophy, heterochromia, retinal detachments, absolute glaucoma and intra-ocular neoplasms.

HIGH MYOPIA. Cataract frequently develops in highly myopic eyes about or after mid-life. It usually occurs in the posterior cortex somewhat resembling the senile type of cupuliform opacity (Fig. 240); it is of very insidious onset and slow evolution, and it is often problematical to decide how far the loss of visual acuity is due to lenticular and how far to retinal changes.

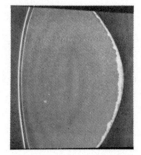

FIG. 240.—MYOPIC CATARACT.

Complicated cataract in the posterior pole in degenerative myopia (M. Berliner).

PIGMENTARY RETINAL DYSTROPHY is so frequently associated with a complicated cataract as almost to be expected in the later stages of the disease.[1] The opacity occurs in the posterior cortex, appearing more often and earlier in those cases with a dominant than with a recessive transmission (Sorsby, 1951) and, although its progression is usually extremely slow, it causes a considerable degree of visual disability owing to the smallness of the visual field usually present in long-standing cases (Fig. 241). Histologically the subcapsular epithelium has been found to extend almost to the posterior pole and the underlying cortex contains numerous clefts and vacuoles filled with fluid and the debris of degenerated fibres (Wagenmann,

[1] Vol. X, p. 608.

1891; Knapp, 1918; Verhoeff, 1931). It is interesting that in the homologous disease transmitted hereditarily in rats the same type of cataract may occur (Bourne *et al.*, 1938). A similar posterior cortical cataract may appear in RETINAL APLASIA (LEBER'S AMAUROSIS)[1] (Gillespie, 1966).

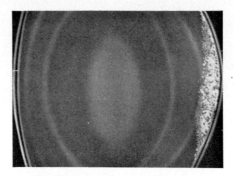

FIG. 241.—DYSTROPHIC CATARACT.
Complicated cataract located in the posterior cortex occurring with pigmentary retinal dystrophy (M. Berliner).

ESSENTIAL ATROPHY OF THE IRIS[2] is rarely complicated by cataract (Tribin-Piedrahita and Barbosa, 1963).

The DOMINANT VITREO-RETINAL DYSTROPHY of Wagner is typically associated with the development of cataract.[3] Punctate opacities appear in the posterior and anterior cortex at puberty and usually during the fourth decade the cataract has become total and requires extraction, a somewhat difficult procedure owing to the fluidity of the vitreous.

HETEROCHROMIC CATARACT is a typical feature of the condition often known as the heterochromic cyclitis of Fuchs (1906), but this is probably a degenerative or circulatory anomaly depending on a disturbance of the sympathetic rather than an inflammatory state.[4] The opacities, which eventually develop in a majority of cases (70%, Perkins, 1961), begin as fine dots in the posterior cortex frequently accompanied by striæ in the periphery, which spread until the entire lens rapidly becomes opaque (Fig. 242). Surgical extraction is easy and the operative prognosis is usually good, particularly if the intracapsular technique is possible (Huber, 1961; Coles, 1964); but complications may develop. It has been pointed out that a filiform hyphæma frequently follows paracentesis of the anterior chamber in this type of heterochromia and is, indeed, pathognomonic of the condition (Amsler and Verrey, 1946; François, 1954; Franceschetti, 1955; Goldberg *et al.*, 1965); fine new vessels may be present in the angle of the

[1] Vol. X, p. 653. [2] Vol IX, p. 686.
[3] Vol. X, p. 662. [4] Vol. IX, p. 816.

anterior chamber, and a post-operative hyphæma may occur after cataract surgery, sometimes associated with a vitreous hæmorrhage (Stallard, 1965; Ward and Hart, 1967; Norn, 1968). Simple glaucoma is a second complication of this type of heterochromia[1] which may disappear after removal of the cataract (Coles, 1964); ocular hypertension after an operation for cataract may occur and, although it may well be controlled by medical treatment, surgery may again be necessary (Ward and Hart, 1967).

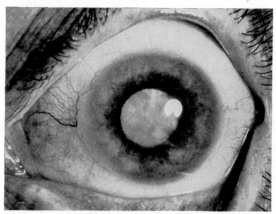

FIG. 242.—HETEROCHROMIC CYCLITIS OF FUCHS.
A typical case showing a mature cataract (Inst. Ophthal.).

Interesting cases were recorded by Marchesani and Koch (1950) wherein a rapidly developing cataract with other ocular signs developed in patients with long-standing disease of the middle ear. The resemblance of the condition to heterochromic cataract suggested to these authors that both lesions were due to a simultaneous disturbance of the sympathetic supply to the eye and ear.

RETINAL DETACHMENT is accompanied by a complicated cataract usually after the detachment has been present for a considerable time but also occasionally in the relatively early stages (Yoshioka et al., 1965). The cataract usually starts subcapsularly in the posterior cortex but the same course of events may occur as in senile cataract; in either case a diffuse opacification of the lens matures rapidly and usually suffers calcareous degeneration. Not infrequently the lens ultimately shrinks, becomes tremulous, and may eventually become dislocated. Extraction is rarely indicated unless for cosmetic reasons.

GLAUCOMATOUS CATARACT is a nuclear opacity which usually develops in cases of absolute glaucoma when the eye is blind. Starting in the nucleus and progressing slowly, the entire lens becomes involved, eventually assuming a yellow or white appearance (Priestley Smith, 1879; Zubareva,

[1] p. 649.

1967) ; finally, the lens may shrink and suffer calcareous degeneration (Thiel, 1931). The opacification of the lens is presumably due to the raised tension and the disturbance of nutrition caused by degenerative changes in the eye. In these blind eyes surgical extraction is not indicated.

The punctate subcapsular opacities left as evidence of an acute glaucomatous attack have already been noted.[1] The annoying development of lenticular opacities in patients with glaucoma after surgical relief of the tension especially by trephining will be noted later.[2]

OCULAR NEOPLASMS are sometimes associated with the development of opacities. Those due to mechanical pressure of the tumour itself on the lens as well as those which follow actual rupture of the capsule have already been noted.[3] A complicated cataract which rapidly becomes total, however, commonly arises presumably due to the absorption of toxic degenerative products from the tumour. Indeed, this complication of an intra-ocular neoplasm is so common that the presence of a complete unilateral cataract without obvious cause should always excite suspicion of the existence of a neoplasm, and suggests the advisability of the excision of a blind cataractous eye when other evidences of infective iridocyclitis are not present.[4]

Amsler and Verrey. *Ophthalmologica*, **111**, 177 (1946).
Bourne, Campbell and Pyke. *Brit. J. Ophthal.*, **22**, 608 (1938).
Coles. Sorsby's *Modern Ophthalmology*, London, **4**, 636 (1964).
Franceschetti. *Amer. J. Ophthal.*, **39** (2), 50 (1955).
François. *Ann. Oculist.* (Paris), **187**, 255 (1954).
Fuchs. *Z. Augenheilk.*, **15**, 191 (1906).
Gillespie. *Amer. J. Ophthal.*, **61**, 874 (1966).
Goldberg, Erozan, Duke and Frost. *Arch. Ophthal.*, **74**, 604 (1965).
Huber. *Ophthalmologica*, **141**, 122 ; **142**, 66 (1961).
Knapp. *Trans. Amer. ophthal. Soc.*, **16**, 59 (1918).
Marchesani and Koch. *v. Graefes Arch. Ophthal.*, **150**, 329 (1950).

Norn. *Acta ophthal.* (Kbh.), **46**, 685 (1968).
Perkins. *Uveitis and Toxoplasmosis*, London, 42 (1961).
Smith, Priestley. *Glaucoma*, London (1879).
Sorsby. *Genetics in Ophthalmology*, London, 168 (1951).
Stallard. *Eye Surgery*, 4th ed., Bristol (1965).
Thiel. Schieck-Bruckner's *Kurzes Hb. d. Ophthalmologie*, Berlin, **4**, 700 (1931).
Tribin-Piedrahita and Barbosa. *Arch. Soc. oftal. hisp.-amer.*, **23**, 609 (1963).
Verhoeff. *Arch. Ophthal.*, **5**, 392 (1931).
Wagenmann. *v. Graefes Arch. Ophthal.*, **37** (1), 230 (1891).
Ward and Hart. *Brit. J. Ophthal.*, **51**, 530 (1967).
Yoshioka, Tejima and Endo. *Acta Soc. ophthal. jap.*, **69**, 545 (1965).
Zubareva. *Oftal. Zh.*, **22**, 15 (1967).

ANOXIC CATARACT

A failure of the vascular circulation in the eye commonly leads to the production of a complicated cataract.

PULSELESS DISEASE, due to an obliteration of the great vessels arising from the aorta resulting in arterial hypotension in the area of their supply has been described in a previous Volume[5] where it was pointed out that the development of cataract at a late stage is a relatively common event (Skipper and Flint, 1952; Hedges, 1964). The lenticular opacities are at

[1] p. 40.   [2] p. 536.   [3] p. 59.
[4] Vol. IX, p. 894.   [5] Vol. X, p. 367.

first subcapsular and cortical but eventually the lens becomes completely opaque.

In THROMBO-ANGIITIS OBLITERANS (*Buerger's disease*), an inflammatory type of obliterative vascular disease of obscure origin described elsewhere,[1] the retinal vessels may be affected and a rapidly maturing complicated cataract may result (Hager, 1950). Extraction should be undertaken in the knowledge that surgery may result in phthisis of the globe.

Cataract has also been reported in RAYNAUD'S DISEASE[2] (Cattaneo, 1931; Romagnoli, 1957).

In NECROSIS OF THE ANTERIOR SEGMENT after surgery for a retinal detachment a cataract is a relatively common complication (O'Day *et al.*, 1966; Crock, 1967).

Cattaneo. *Arch. Ottal.*, **38**, 684 (1931).

Crock. *Trans. ophthal. Soc. U.K.*, **87**, 513 (1967).

Hager. *Ber. dtsch. ophthal. Ges.*, **56**, 355 (1950).

Hedges. *Arch. Ophthal.*, **71**, 28 (1964).

O'Day, Galbraith, Crock and Cairns. *Lancet*, **2**, 401 (1966).

Romagnoli. *Atti Soc. oftal. Lomb.*, **12**, 244 (1957).

Skipper and Flint. *Brit. med. J.*, **2**, 9 (1952).

CATARACT COMPLICATING SYSTEMIC DISEASE

Bilateral cataract, sometimes called *cataracta cachectica*, usually of uniform distribution in the lens cortex and maturing rapidly, is occasionally seen in acute toxic illnesses. The most typical are infective fevers—diphtheria, malaria, typhus, cholera, smallpox, scarlatina, typhoid fever; but cataract may occur in similarly severe toxic states, such as extreme cachexia, nephritis, pernicious anæmia, or after a massive loss of blood. Other less authentic types, some of which may have been incidental, have been described in tuberculous subjects (Legrand, 1950; Simonelli and Azzolini, 1950), in cases of ornithosis (17 in 21 infected patients, Schubert, 1961), Cooley's anæmia (thalassæmia major) (Panzardi, 1947), and the profound anæmia following ankylostomiasis (El-Naggar, 1961). An exceptional case of the occurrence in an infant of a post-natal cataract without other ocular involvement which appeared after a severe attack of meningo-encephalitis was reported by Babel (1960). The prognosis of these cataracts is secondary to that of the exciting illness, for they are usually operable if the patient recovers.

POST-NATAL CATARACT IN PREMATURITY

The development of post-natal cataracts has been observed in premature infants on several occasions.[3] The cataract commences in the nucleus and may remain zonular but usually develops rapidly to become total and mature in a few months. The reason for the development of the lenticular opacities is unknown, but in most cases the general condition of the child and often of the mother has been poor; it will be remembered that retrolental fibroplasia is not associated with lenticular opacities.[4]

[1] Vol. X, p. 237.   [2] Vol. X, p. 81.

[3] Guy (1954), Liebman (1955), Castrén (1955), Ryan (1956), François (1959), Ziegler (1960), Babel (1960), Brown (1963), McDonald (1964), Nordmann (1965–66), McCormick (1968).

[4] Vol. X, p. 187.

Babel. *Arch. Ophtal.*, **20**, 146 (1960).

Brown. *Trans. ophthal. Soc. U.K.*, **83**, 493 (1963).

Castrén. *Acta ophthal.* (Kbh.), Suppl. 44 (1955).

El-Naggar. *Bull. ophthal. Soc. Egypt*, **54**, 223 (1961).

François. *Les cataractes congénitales*, Paris (1959).

Guy. *Amer. J. Ophthal.*, **38**, 65 (1954).

Legrand. *Ann. Oculist.* (Paris), **183**, 58 (1950).

Liebman. *Arch. Ophthal.*, **54**, 257 (1955).

McCormick. *Canad. J. Ophthal.*, **3**, 202 (1968).

McDonald. *Guy's Hosp. Rep.*, **113**, 296 (1964).

Nordmann. *Arch. Ophtal.*, **25**, 43 (1965).
Amer. J. Ophthal., **61**, 1256 (1966).

Panzardi. *Boll. Oculist.*, **26**, 189 (1947).

Ryan. *Amer. J. Ophthal.*, **41**, 310 (1956).

Schubert. *Klin. Mbl. Augenheilk.*, **138**, 394 (1961).

Simonelli and Azzolini. *G. ital. Oftal.*, **3**, 401 (1950).
Atti Soc. oftal. ital., **12**, 235 (1950).

Ziegler. *Ann. Pœdiat.* (Basel), **194**, 76 (1960).

Toxic Cataract

Several chemicals, some used therapeutically as drugs, others in industry, have been shown to give rise to cataract. The effects of some of these on animals have already been noted in the section on experimental cataract; their clinical effects will be fully discussed in the Volume which deals with toxicology where the literature will be cited[1]; but for the sake of completeness it is useful to summarize the most important here.

Among the *substituted hydrocarbons* should be mentioned NAPHTHALENE,[2] DINITROPHENOL[3] which used to be a common agent for the reduction of weight, and PARADICHLOROBENZENE, used as an insecticide which may be inhaled. Another drug with similar implications is CHLORPROMAZINE.

Among the *nitro compounds*, cataract may be caused by DINITRO-O-CRESOL, also a reducing agent and an insecticide, and TRINITROTOLUENE, used in the manufacture of explosives and liable to be inhaled in the factory.

CARBROMAL (monobromodiethyl acetylurea), used as a sedative and a component of several of such drugs, has been said to cause opacification of the lens after prolonged administration.

TRIPARANOL, a drug used to reduce the cholesterol in the serum, among its many systemic effects has been found to give rise to cataract.[4]

ERGOT has given rise to the development of cataract following convulsive ergotism.

PANTOCAINE, administered topically over a long period, has been recorded as causing the development of numerous opaque subcapsular flecks (Schrader, 1962).

THALLIUM has been reported to give rise to cortical opacities in the lens.

Other metals used therapeutically either topically or systemically, sometimes penetrating the globe as foreign bodies or absorbed by workers in industry, give rise to a characteristic pigmentation of the anterior capsule occasionally associated with disseminated punctiform subcapsular opacities. The most typical of these are SILVER (argyrolentis), MERCURY (mercurialentis), COPPER (the sunflower cataract of chalcosis, also seen in hepato-lenticular degeneration[5]), and IRON (the cataract of siderosis).

The CORTICOSTEROIDS when given systemically for periods longer than a year have been found in a significant number of cases to produce posterior cortical opacities in the lens somewhat resembling the cataract caused by

----

[1] Vol. XIV. [2] p. 106. [3] p. 109.
[4] p. 116. [5] p. 195.

radiation.[1] Similarly, the topical use of these drugs over many months has been observed to result in the development of posterior subcapsular opacities of the same type[2] (Figs. 243–5); the sequence is by no means invariable (Williamson and Jasani, 1967), but the changes in the lens may be associated

FIGS. 243 to 245.—CORTICOSTEROID CATARACT (S. Younessian).

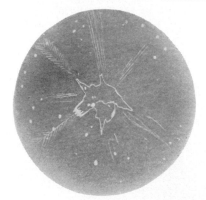 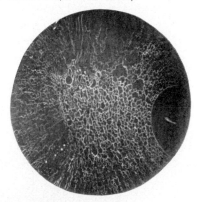

FIG. 243.—The anterior cortex.   FIG. 244.—The posterior cortex.

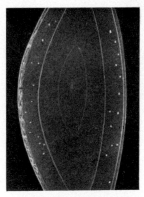

FIG. 245.—Optical section; the anterior surface is to the right.

with a steroid-induced glaucoma.[3] It is interesting that although the administration of corticosteroids does not lead to the formation of cataract in rats, it tends to hasten the development of this lesion after feeding galactose.[4]

[1] Black *et al.* (1960), Gordon *et al.* (1961), I. A. and I. A. Abrahamson (1961), Oglesby *et al.* (1961), Giles *et al.* (1962), Toogood *et al.* (1962), Crews (1963), Lindholm *et al.* (1965), Havre (1965), Spencer and Andelman (1965), Sundmark (1966), Williamson and Dalakos (1967), and others.
[2] Valerio (1963), Cronin (1964), Streiff (1964), Becker (1964), Crews (1965), Valerio *et al.* (1965), Frandsen (1966), Younessian (1967).
[3] p. 701.   [4] p. 89.

MIOTIC CATARACT. That the prolonged topical administration of strong miotics, particularly of the *anticholinesterase group* (DFP, echothiophate, demecarium bromide, diethyl-*p*-nitrophenyl phosphate (Mintacol)) can cause lenticular opacities was first noticed by Harrison (1960) in a young girl on treatment with DFP for esotropia. The opacities were feathery and rosette-like, situated subcapsularly in the anterior cortex; they did not interfere with vision and faded away on cessation of the treatment. Subsequent reports have been in glaucomatous patients similarly treated, particularly in those over 60 years of age, in whom specific lens changes may appear, sometimes after a few months' use of the drug.[1]

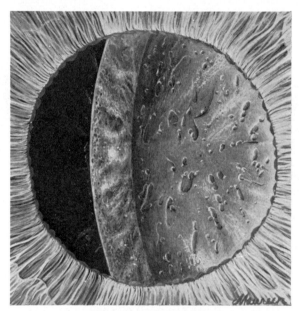

FIG. 246.—CATARACT FROM PHOSPHOLINE IODIDE.

Composite drawing of the lens showing patchy superficial opacification; the vacuoles and irregular streaks are more clearly seen by retro-illumination at the right of the lens (R. N. Shaffer and J. Hetherington).

Axelsson and Holmberg (1966), for example, observed lenticular changes in 50% of 78 eyes treated with echothiophate for a mean period of 12 months, while they found similar changes in 10% of glaucomatous patients treated with pilocarpine for an average of 22 months. Shaffer and Hetherington (1966) noted such changes in 38% of 60 patients treated with DFP, demecarium bromide or echothiophate, and de Roetth (1966) confirmed these observations, finding them in 51% of patients treated with echothiophate and in 16% treated with pilocarpine. Similar observations have been

[1] Axelsson and Holmberg (1966), de Roetth (1966), Shaffer and Hetherington (1966), Tarkkanen and Karjalainen (1966), Shaffer (1967), Axelsson (1968), Leopold (1968).

reported by Tarkkanen and Karjalainen (1966) with demecarium bromide and echothiophate, and by Axelsson (1968) with echothiophate and Mintacol.

The cataract starts as tiny vacuoles in and below the anterior capsular epithelium which multiply to give a mossy appearance, while iridescent opacities may also be present (Fig. 246); at a later stage posterior cortical and nuclear changes develop together with myopia. It is said that cessation of the drug stays the progress of the lesion. The specific appearance of the cataract and its occurrence in only the treated eye of patients with uni-lateral glaucoma suggest a causal sequence but this has been questioned (Cinotti and Patti, 1968; Thoft, 1968). We have seen[1] that experimental cataract can be produced by these drugs in the incubated lenses of animals associated with a reduction in the respiration and a disturbance of ionic transport.

Abrahamson, I. A. and I. A. *Eye, Ear, Nose and Thr. Mthly.*, **40**, 266 (1961).
Axelsson. *Acta ophthal.* (Kbh.), **46**, 83, 99 (1968).
Axelsson and Holmberg. *Acta ophthal.* (Kbh.), **44**, 421 (1966).
Becker. *Invest. Ophthal.*, **3**, 492 (1964).
Black, Oglesby, von Sallmann and Bunim. *J. Amer. med. Ass.*, **174**, 166 (1960).
Cinotti and Patti. *Amer. J. Ophthal.*, **65**, 25 (1968).
Crews. *Brit. med. J.*, **1**, 1644 (1963).
   Proc. roy. Soc. Med., **58**, 533 (1965).
Cronin. *Arch. Ophthal.*, **72**, 198 (1964).
Frandsen. *Acta ophthal.* (Kbh.), **44**, 307 (1966).
Giles, Mason, Duff and McLean. *J. Amer. med. Ass.*, **182**, 719 (1962).
Gordon, Kammerer and Freyberg. *J. Amer. med. Ass.*, **175**, 127 (1961).
Harrison. *Amer. J. Ophthal.*, **50**, 153 (1960).
Havre. *Arch. Ophthal.*, **73**, 818 (1965).
Leopold. *Amer. J. Ophthal.*, **65**, 297 (1968).
Lindholm, Linnér and Tengroth. *Acta ophthal.* (Kbh.), **43**, 120 (1965).
Oglesby, Black, von Sallmann and Bunim. *Arch. Ophthal.*, **66**, 519, 625 (1961).
de Roetth. *Trans. ophthal. Soc. U.K.*, **86**, 89 (1966).

Amer. J. Ophthal., **62**, 619 (1966).
Schrader. *Klin. Mbl. Augenheilk.*, **140**, 287 (1962).
Shaffer. *Symp. on Glaucoma* (Trans. N. Orleans Acad. Ophthal., ed. Becker), St. Louis (1967).
Shaffer and Hetherington. *Trans. Amer. ophthal. Soc.*, **64**, 204 (1966).
Spencer and Andelman. *Arch. Ophthal.*, **74**, 38 (1965).
Streiff. *Ophthalmologica*, **147**, 143 (1964).
Sundmark. *Acta ophthal.* (Kbh.), **44**, 291 (1966).
Tarkkanen and Karjalainen. *Acta ophthal.* (Kbh.), **44**, 932 (1966).
Thoft. *Arch. Ophthal.*, **80**, 317 (1968).
Toogood, Dyson, Thompson and Mularchyk. *Canad. med. Ass. J.*, **86**, 52 (1962).
Valerio. *Bull. Soc. franç. Ophtal.*, **76**, 572 (1963).
Valerio, Carones and de Poli. *Boll. Oculist.*, **44**, 127 (1965).
Williamson and Dalakos. *Brit. J. Ophthal.*, **51**, 839 (1967).
Williamson and Jasani. *Brit. J. Ophthal.*, **51**, 554 (1967).
Younessian. *Ophthalmologica*, **154**, 350 (1967).

After-cataract

No consideration of after-cataract would be complete without a note of DETMAR WILHELM SOEMMERRING [1793–1871] (Fig. 247) of Göttingen, after whom the remnants of the peripheral part of an incompletely removed lens have been eponymously called. He was an investigator of wide interests and it will be remembered[2] that his main work was the study of the structure of the eyes of vertebrates of many types.

AFTER-CATARACT (sometimes called SECONDARY CATARACT[3]) is the term applied to the remnants of the lens left behind after its discission or operative

[1] p. 119.   [2] Vol. I, p. 259.
[3] Secondary cataract is more frequently used to describe a cataract secondary to ocular disease.

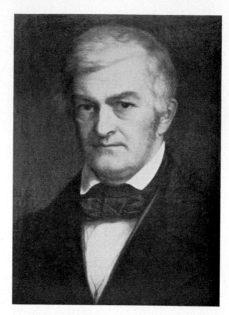

FIG. 247.—DETMAR WILHELM SOEMMERRING
[1793–1871].

removal by the extracapsular method or after its destruction by trauma. These remnants may comprise the following elements:

1. *Capsular remains*, particularly of the posterior capsule, which may be diaphanous and thin. Associated with the capsule is the subcapsular epithelium which almost always shows some proliferation and may occasionally give rise to the large globular bladder cells of Elschnig (1911).

2. *Capsulo-lenticular remains* in which a mass of lenticular fibres is associated with the capsule. These may be arranged irregularly, or may be amassed in the periphery, where they form a ring enclosed between the anterior and posterior capsules leaving the pupillary area relatively free (the *ring of Soemmerring*, 1828).

3. *Pigmentary, hæmorrhagic or inflammatory fibrous elements* may form organized masses in addition to the capsular and lenticular remains, in which the iris may become incorporated.

In their slighter degrees capsular remains may be invisible with the ophthalmoscope and may not interfere with vision, but they are always distinguishable with the slit-lamp (Fig. 248). The pupil may remain active and regular, and the capsule appears as a fine veil-like curtain separated by a clear space from the iris in front and again from the anterior face of the vitreous behind. It always exhibits numerous crinkles and folds and often a polychromatic lustre. In the more marked degrees there may be a considerable amount of the remains of the cortical fibres of the lens, usually arranged in bundles of a snowy colour with a frayed appearance, and such remnants, sometimes enclosed between folds of the anterior and posterior capsules, may form bands of considerable thickness and strength (Fig. 249).

Associated with these passive remnants there is considerable proliferative activity of the epithelium, sufficient, indeed, to suggest to the older writers the concept of a " regeneration of the lens " (Textor, 1842; Milliot, 1872; Baas, 1899). This phenomenon occurs preferentially, but by no means exclusively, in younger patients and concerns the subcapsular epithelium which in time may line the entire posterior capsule (Becker, 1883; Wagenmann, 1889–91; and others) and, turning round the torn margins, may cover both sides of the anterior capsule (Cowan and Fry, 1937);

FIGS. 248 and 249.—AFTER-CATARACT.

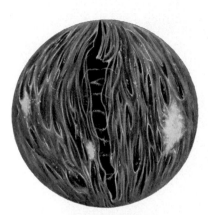

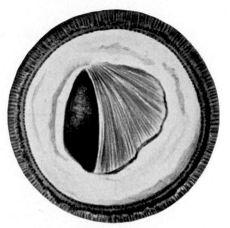

FIG. 248.—The posterior capsule after a vertical discission. The vitreous is seen behind.

FIG. 249.—The two capsules after extracapsular removal of the lens (T. Harrison Butler).

this is the same process that occurs in the regeneration of the lens after its substance has been removed from the capsule in certain animals.[1] This activity may be associated with the deposition of hyaline capsular material forming irregular masses and membrane-like strata (Wagenmann, 1889; Hocquard, 1902); while in other localities the cells may be several layers thick, in which case each layer may be separated by loose interlacing bands of hyaline tissue similar to that of the capsule (Figs. 250–1).

Frequently the individual cells become swollen and vacuolated, and eventually may attain considerable dimensions (Hirschberg, 1901; Elschnig, 1911); Cowan and McDonald (1939) noted their presence in some 25% of cases. Such cells, sometimes termed the GLOBULAR or BLADDER-CELLS OF ELSCHNIG, are reminiscent of the vesicular cells of Wedl[2] and probably

[1] Vol. III, p. 71.   [2] p. 26.

FIGS. 250 and 251.—AFTER-CATARACT (F. Tooke).

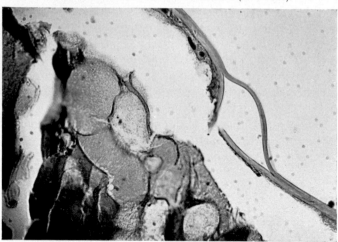

FIG. 250.—Cortical remains consisting of lens fibres, some of which are intact but many of which form tumescent spaces filled with amorphous debris. Note the separation of the zonular lamella.

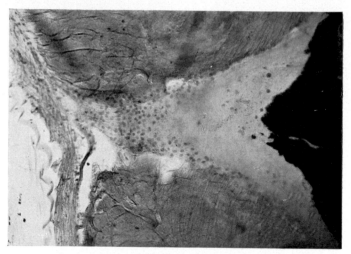

FIG. 251.—Showing proliferation of cuboidal epithelial cells.

represent aberrant attempts of the epithelium to form new fibres. They are rounded or oval and transparent, like toy balloons or soap bubbles (ELSCHNIG'S PEARLS) (Fig. 252); they may be single or arranged in clumps like bunches of grapes or masses of frog's spawn, sometimes protruding into the anterior chamber (Djacos, 1954) and, particularly in young patients on whom a discission or linear extraction of a cataract has been performed, may eventually occlude the entire pupillary aperture. Single cells may

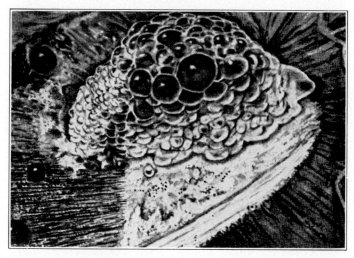

FIG. 252.—ELSCHNIG'S PEARLS (T. Harrison Butler).

attain a considerable size (2 mm., Cowan and Fry, 1937). The picture they produce may vary from time to time; sometimes they appear a few days after operation and they may continue to form and vanish over a period of years. Pathological examination shows them to be large vesicle-like structures enclosed by an extremely attenuated wall. At other times much more solid opaque cysts of capsular material are formed which may eventually burst (Fig. 253).

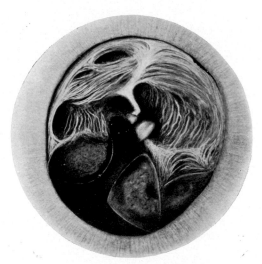

FIG. 253.—AFTER-CATARACT.
Cystic proliferation of the epithelium.

Free *lentoid bodies*, measuring 40 to 240 μ and consisting of parallel lenticular fibres coursing in a single direction with vacuoles, may arise from the subcapsular epithelium, and may be found not only in the after-cataract but adhering to the iris or the cornea or in the vitreous (Thiel, 1926); they represent another abortive type of lenticular regeneration.

Pigmentary remains in the form of a fine, brown, powdery deposit from the iris on the membrane formed by an after-cataract are a commonplace, even although the extraction has been uncomplicated and has been followed by little or no post-operative reaction; the deposition is due to a dispersion of the pigment following a traumatic disintegration of the pigmentary epithelium lining the posterior surface of the iris and the ciliary body. An extremely interesting phenomenon, however, is the occasional active and abundant proliferation of the pigmented cells which may become inter-mingled with the lenticular remains sometimes forming large pigmented plaques, an occurrence often particularly evident in diabetic cataract (Brückner, 1919; Fuchs, 1920; Sgrosso, 1932; Mans, 1933).

A more serious occurrence is the incorporation of *organizing material from post-operative hæmorrhage or cyclitic exudates* into the after-cataract. In the latter event especially, if the cyclitic process remains active, increasing amounts of plastic exudate and cellular infiltration occur, to be followed by fibroblastic invasion and cicatrization so that a dense opaque mass occupies the entire pupillary area. In such cases, of course, the functional value of the eye may well be lost owing to the general disintegration of the globe in phthisis bulbi.

THE RING (OR CUSHION) OF SOEMMERRING is a relatively common feature occurring particularly in young people after an operation of discission or the extracapsular extraction of cataract or a penetrating trauma to the lens; it is thus a typical sequel of the discission of a congenital cataract or Fukala's operation for myopia. It was first described clinically by Detmar Wilhelm Soemmerring (1828) and shortly thereafter by Werneck (1833) and Textor (1842); it had already been recognized in experiments on animals by Dietrich (1824) and Cocteau and Leroy-d'Étiolle (1827) and in these its formation was subsequently studied by Gonin (1896) and Wessely (1910). It evolves when the torn anterior capsule becomes retracted and its edges become adherent to the posterior capsule so that a ring of folded capsule containing a varying quantity of lens substance forms and persists behind the iris. The central part in the pupillary area is usually occupied by a thin membrane consisting essentially of the posterior capsule to which may be added fibrous tissue laid down by fibroblasts from the iris. As a rule there are large numbers of lenticular fibres enclosed in the folded capsule behind the iris and, particularly in young subjects, this mass is increased by the proliferation of epithelial cells and the regeneration of new fibres protected from the lytic action of the aqueous by the capsule. Clinically the ring is not seen behind the iris unless an iridectomy has been performed (Fig. 254) or occasionally if the pupil has been very widely dilated; an exceptional case was described by Lijó Pavía (1931) wherein a traumatic aniridia had occurred. The ring may be complete, incomplete, or segmented like a string of sausages (Fig. 255). Pathological examinations have shown that the epithelium grows to line both the posterior and anterior capsules; it forms new fibres entrapped within the ring so that it grows in dimensions while layers of hyaline material may be added; at the same time gross degenerative changes are common, resulting in the formation of amorphous debris, morgagnian globules and calcareous degeneration (Figs. 256–7).

FIGS. 254 and 255.—SOEMMERRING'S RING

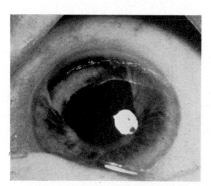 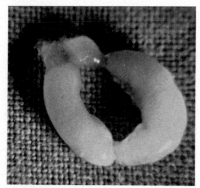

FIG. 254. In a man aged 90. Part of the lens is visible within the site of an iridectomy above following extra-capsular extraction of the lens (N. L. Stokoe).

FIG. 255.—A ring after its surgical removal, in a woman aged 40. A discission was made for a traumatic cataract at the age of 19. The ring had been posteriorly dislocated in front of an intact hyaloid face of the vitreous (P. R. Laibson and P. S. McDonald).

So long as the ring remains *in situ*, no symptoms arise and vision is maintained through the axial aperture but, particularly in myopic eyes in which the zonule is stretched and degenerated and the vitreous is fluid, it may break loose. This complication may occur, usually with but some-times without a history of trauma which may be minor in degree. The subluxation may be into the pupillary aperture (Lijó Pavía, 1931; Tooke, 1933; Stokoe, 1957), anteriorly into the anterior chamber (Adam, 1911; Schneider, 1927; Jess, 1931; Nègre, 1933; Jacoby and Wolpaw, 1935; Guha, 1938–62; Arruga, 1953), or into the vitreous (Wessely, 1910; Poos, 1931; Rizzini, 1955; Laibson and McDonald, 1965). In an anterior dislocation the ring is seen in the anterior chamber like a small white pessary (Fig. 258) and the accident is usually followed by a sharp inflammatory reaction with raised ocular tension; excision of the eye for absolute glaucoma has followed (Jess, 1931), but successful removal of the ring by forceps through a corneal

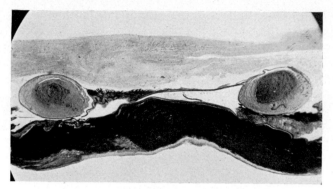

FIG. 256.—SOEMMERRING'S RING.

In its normal position behind the iris after extracapsular cataract extraction (after F. Tooke).

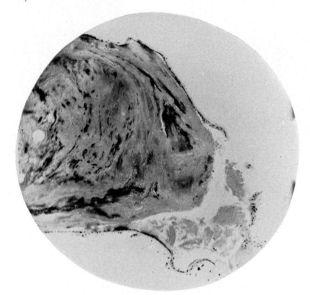

FIG. 257.—SOEMMERRING'S RING.

Section of the edge of a ring removed from the anterior chamber in a woman aged 78 who had a discission operation in youth. The subcapsular epithelium covers the posterior as well as the anterior surface; it has been torn at the equator (N. L. Stokoe).

section may be followed by an excellent result (Jess, 1931; Tooke, 1933), although if much degeneration has occurred, it may behave on manipulation much as a morgagnian cataract and melt away in milky fluid. A dislocation posteriorly, on the other hand, may be associated with no symptoms or impairment of vision (Poos, 1931), unless by chance the ring floats behind the pupillary aperture. Because of this complication Laibson and McDonald (1965) succeeded in removing such a ring by first transfixing it with a needle passed through the pars plana behind the plane of the iris when the patient was in the prone position, and thereafter removing it through an anterior incision with an iris hook.

The prevention of an after-cataract is of the greatest importance, an ideal which, of course, is most readily attained by an intracapsular extraction. It is to be remembered, however, that even when the lens is removed completely in its capsule, some degree of condensation and clouding of the anterior face of the vitreous may eventually occur. If an extracapsular operation is contemplated, the amount of lenticular remains is minimized if the operation is postponed until the cataract is mature, a consideration, however, which cannot override economic necessities or the unhappiness of a long period of virtual blindness. During the operation a free incision of the

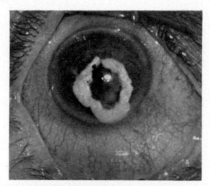

FIG. 258.—SOEMMERRING'S RING.

In a woman aged 58 who had suffered a traumatic cataract from a perforating injury. The ring is dislocated into the anterior chamber (A. Arruga).

anterior capsule or the removal of a central portion of it by forceps lessens the tendency to secondary complications, as also does the assiduous removal of soft cortical material by lavage. The avoidance of post-operative hæmorrhage or inflammation is of the greatest importance, as well as prolonged post-operative atropinization.

The *treatment* of an after-cataract is entirely surgical—the division of the membrane or of bands by a knife, a knife-needle or scissors, or their complete excision. Sobansky and Goetz (1963) removed the remnants after twisting them around an iris-hook introduced in the anterior chamber. In all cases it is important that the manipulations should be as delicate as possible, to avoid both a subsequent retinal detachment and a post-operative inflammatory reaction with the reformation of plastic exudates. The division of an elastic or leathery membrane may be a difficult and tricky proceeding with a discission knife; rather than using unjustifiable force it may be wise to use two discission knives, one with the edge facing upwards,

FIGS. 259 to 262.—ELSCHNIG'S CAPSULO-IRIDECTOMY (S. J. H. Miller).

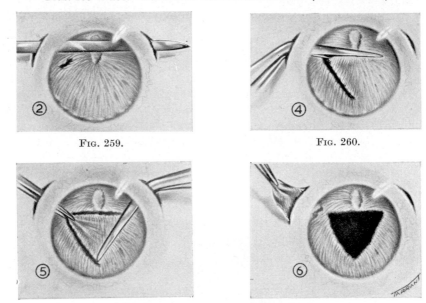

FIG. 259.   FIG. 260.

FIG. 261.   FIG. 262.

FIG. 259.—The iris is incised before the two concentric incisions have been made.
FIG. 260.—The de Wecker's scissors cut a large V-shaped incision in the iris-capsule diaphragm, which is completed by excising the triangle thus formed (Fig. 261) and removing it, leaving the appearance seen in Fig. 262.

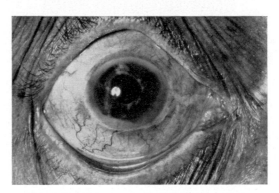

FIG. 263.—ELSCHNIG'S CAPSULO-IRIDECTOMY.
To show the structure of the new pupil (S. J. H. Miller).

the other downwards, manipulating them as scissors (Kleberger, 1960), or to open the eye and excise the membrane or, if the pupil is drawn peripherally, to perform an iridotomy or, when the capsule is also involved, the capsulo-iridectomy of Elschnig (1912) (Figs. 259–63). The time of intervention is also of importance. A discission should not be done until all post-operative reaction or inflammation has completely disappeared, the eye shows no congestion and the aqueous is clear from excess protein, cells and debris. These considerations become more important in the case of complicated cataracts, for a premature attempt to create a gap in the pupil in such cases will almost certainly be followed by its reclosure by plastic exudate so that the last condition is worse than the first.

The continued formation of bladder cells may constitute an annoying therapeutic problem, for repeated attempts at discission almost invariably fail to maintain a pupillary aperture. They can, however, frequently be removed by irrigation of the anterior chamber assisted, if necessary, by dislodging them with the tip of the irrigator or a cyclodialysis spatula (Chandler, 1954; Hofmann, 1961; Gundersen, 1966; and others). Alternatively, their growth may be inhibited by intermittent short exposures to x-rays (Clark, 1966)[1]; epithelial cysts may be destroyed by light-coagulation (Charamis, 1964).

Adam. *Zbl. prakt. Augenheilk.*, **35**, 67 (1911).

Arruga. *Amer. J. Ophthal.*, **36**, 1727 (1953).

Baas. *Münch. med. Wschr.*, **46**, 1609 (1899).

Becker. *Zur Anatomie d. gesunden u. kranken Linse*, Wiesbaden (1883).

Brückner. *Klin. Mbl. Augenheilk.*, **62**, 461 (1919).

Chandler. *Trans. Amer. Acad. Ophthal.*, **58**, 382 (1954).

Charamis. *Bull. Soc. franç. Ophtal.*, **77**, 449 (1964).

Clark. *Amer. J. Ophthal.*, **61**, 1081 (1966).

Cocteau and Leroy-d'Étiolle. *J. Physiol.* (Paris), **7**, 30 (1827).

Cowan and Fry. *Arch. Ophthal.*, **18**, 12 (1937).

Cowan and McDonald. *Arch. Ophthal.*, **22**, 1074 (1939).

Dietrich. *Ueber die Verwundungen des Linsensystems*, Tübingen (1824).

Djacos. *Bull. Soc. hellén. Ophtal.*, **22**, 136 (1954).

Elschnig. *Klin. Mbl. Augenheilk.*, **49** (1), 444 (1911); **50** (1), 538 (1912).

Fuchs. *Klin. Mbl. Augenheilk.*, **64**, 1 (1920).

Gonin. *Beitr. path. Anat.*, **19**, 497 (1896).

Guha. *Ueber den Soemmering'schen Kristallwulst* (Diss.), Berlin (1938).
Brit. J. Ophthal., **35**, 226 (1951).
J. All-India ophthal. Soc., **10**, 39 (1962).

Gundersen. *Amer. J. Ophthal.*, **61**, 1124 (1966).

Hirschberg. *Einführung in d. Augenheilkunde*, Leipzig, **2**, 159 (1901).

Hocquard. *Arch. Ophtal.*, **22**, 435 (1902).

Hofmann. *Wien. klin. Wschr.*, **73**, 859 (1961).

Jacoby and Wolpaw. *Arch. Ophthal.*, **13**, 634 (1935).

Jess. *Kurzes Hb. d. Ophthal.*, Berlin, **5**, 248 (1930).
Klin. Mbl. Augenheilk., **86**, 98 (1931).

Kleberger. *Ber. dtsch. ophthal. Ges.*, **63**, 445 (1960).

Laibson and McDonald. *Arch. Ophthal.*, **73**, 643 (1965).

Lijó Pavía. *Arch. Oftal. hisp.-amer.*, **31**, 295 (1931).

Mans. *Klin. Mbl. Augenheilk.*, **90**, 650 (1933).

Milliot. *J. Anat. Physiol.*, **8**, 1 (1872).

Nègre. *Bull. Soc. Ophtal. Paris*, 388 (1933).

Poos. *Klin. Mbl. Augenheilk.*, **86**, 449 (1931).

Rizzini. *G. ital. Oftal.*, **8**, 505 (1955).

Schneider. *Amer. J. Ophthal.*, **10**, 273 (1927).

Sgrosso. *Boll. Oculist.*, **11**, 737 (1932).

Sobansky and Goetz. *Klin. Mbl. Augenheilk.*, **142**, 892 (1963).

Soemmerring. *Beobachtungen u. d. organischen Veränderungen im Auge nach Staaroperationen*, Frankfurt (1828).

Stokoe. *Brit. J. Ophthal.*, **41**, 348 (1957).

Textor. *Ueber d. Wiedererzeugung d. Kristallinse*, Würzburg (1842).

Thiel. *Z. Augenheilk.*, **58**, 86 (1926).

Tooke. *Brit. J. Ophthal.*, **17**, 466 (1933).

Wagenmann. *v. Graefes Arch. Ophthal.*, **35** (1), 172 (1889); **37** (2), 21 (1891).

Werneck. *v. Ammons Z. Ophthal.*, **3**, 473 (1833).

Wessely. *Arch. Augenheilk.*, **66**, 277 (1910).

[1] Vol. VII, p. 764.

THE TREATMENT OF CATARACT
Medical Treatment

Bearing a name associated in the popular mind with the catastrophe of blindness or alternatively with the ordeal of an operation, with a symptomatology characterized by a slowly progressive and apparently inevitable diminution of vision at a time when physical disabilities make the patient depend necessarily more and more upon reading for his happiness, and having a course which no palliative treatment can appreciably alter, cataract presents a therapeutic problem with all the characteristics necessary to stimulate the exploitation of more or less illegitimate " cures." To a large extent the reputation which temporarily attaches to such cures is due to the fact that many cataracts independently of any treatment progress exceedingly slowly, and in their evolution many of them show periods of visual betterment owing to refractive changes in the lens; the delay and the improvement are readily attributed to the nostrum. The point of view of the patient in submitting to such exploitation is understandable; the healer may derive comfort from the hope that he is allaying the anxieties of his patient and saving him from more flagrant exploitation by others; but psychological motives apart, from the time of Celsus (" when recent a cataract is often removed by medicine ") and Galen (" a cataract at the beginning can be dispersed, but not later "), the history of the therapeutics of cataract presents a unique display of what can most charitably be called extreme credulity in unsupported theories or wishful interpretation of clinical results. It is true that in certain forms of cataract in the early stages, if the exciting conditions are controlled, the opacities may clear so long as irreversible changes have not taken place in the lens; but it is also true that once an organic opacity is formed it is immutable. The coagulation of protein is an irreversible chemical change. It seems not unreasonable to hope that in the future, when our knowledge of these changes and the factors causing them is more fully developed, it may be possible to prevent the incidence of cataract or delay its development; but at the present time, while it is certainly legitimate and incumbent upon the physician to attack or eliminate any exciting cause or predisposition that is known or suspected, this is as far as honesty can go.

The methods which have been advised for the treatment of cataract are legion. They may be considered under two headings—treatment designed to delay the development or cause the absorption of the opacities, and treatment designed to improve nutritional and metabolic disturbances or deficiencies which may play some determining part in the opacification of the lens. There remain the provision of optical expedients to aid the patient when the diminution of vision becomes embarrassing, and finally the removal of the opaque lens by operative measures.

The first category can be rapidly dismissed, for local treatment designed
to cause delay in the formation of the opacities or to promote their absorption
when formed has little basis in reason and as little justification in results.
It is to be remembered, however, that when the independence and isolation
of the lens are recalled, it is by no means impossible that future progress in
knowledge may indicate local measures which may so maintain or stimulate
its metabolism that opacification may be prevented.   In the meantime, it
may be of interest from the historical point of view to summarize the views
advanced.   Unfortunately, the four basic necessities for scientific investigation have invariably been wanting: that the observations should be
conducted under strictly controlled conditions, that a sufficient number of
cases with controls should be studied from which significant statistics can
be deduced, that psychological factors should be eliminated concerning both
the physician and the patient, and that the results should be repeatable in
other clinics.   Again unfortunately, most observations have been conducted
by ophthalmologists lacking a basic scientific training, and at least one by a
convicted criminal.[1]

The *administration of drugs* has been the most common expedient, and one of the
oldest remedies proposed was *iodine* which, with a view to aiding absorption, has been
given in every conceivable form, mainly as iodide—by mouth, as drops, in an eyebath,
as a salve, in subconjunctival injections and by iontophoresis or as an aerosol.[2]   It is
true that iodine does enter the lens from the conjunctival sac (Daniels, 1931), although
with difficulty and in small quantity (Löhlein, 1910), but no basis exists for the
extravagant claims put forward with regard to its therapeutic efficacy in this and other
conditions presumed to be of a " sclerotic " nature.   *Calcium* was frequently advised
with the iodide, either by mouth or as a salve (Treu, 1907; Taylor, 1924; Hildesheimer,
1929; Burdon-Cooper, 1933) and, owing to its diminution in the cataractous lens,
potassium either by mouth as the iodide or locally by iontophoresis (Mackay *et al.*,
1932; Burdon-Cooper, 1933; Salit, 1938).   It is true that the maintenance of a high
serum calcium level by the administration of the metal or of irradiated ergosterol
(Rauh, 1936) may prevent the development of cataract when the calcium/phosphorus
ratio is unbalanced.   Meesmann (1938), on the other hand, advocated dihydrotachysterol, a calcium-mobilizer useful in the cataract of tetany, for cases of senile
cataract, but it is of value only in this particular type of cataract and in senile cases
the serum calcium is normal.   *Cysteine* introduced by electrophoresis was advocated
by Tcherictchy (1964).   *Homeopathic remedies*, such as infinitesimal doses of naphthalene or secale have, of course, had their advocates (Tischner, 1914; and others).

The production of a *local hyperæmia* has been claimed to be useful owing to its
supposedly beneficial effect on the nutrition of the lens.   Various methods have been
enthusiastically practised: the instillation of dionine (Connor, 1909; Jones, 1913;
Pollock, 1923; Greenwood, 1924; Blake, 1949), or boracic and glycerin (Kalish, 1890;
Weeks, 1930), subconjunctival injections of cyanide of mercury (Smith, 1912–28;
Dean, 1924–27), injections of lactogenin (a milk preparation) (Harkness, 1925), and so on.

Physical methods of treatment have also received a trial: radium, even although

---

[1] See Report of the National Research Council of America, *J. Amer. med. Ass.*, **152**, 707
(1953).

[2] Badal (1902), Verderau (1904), von Pflugk (1906), Pick (1909), Dor (1911), Meyer-
Steineg (1913–24), Walter (1914), Gilbert (1924), Gallois (1951), Misar (1967), and many
others.

it causes cataract (Cohen and Levin, 1920; Levin, 1920; Franklin and Cordes, 1920), pneumo-massage and electrotherapy (Campbell, 1917; Harris, 1924).

The systemic administration of compounds of the *sulphonamide* group has been said to improve the vision in patients with senile cataract and has also been said to be useless (H. and C. Hackmann, 1958; Müller and Kleifeld, 1960; Voisin and Paquelin, 1960–62). *Acetazolamide* has been similarly recommended (Carballo, 1957).

With a view to stimulating the metabolism of the lens, an additional supply of active substances lacking in the cataractous lens has been given with the diet (sulphydryl compounds, Kögel, 1931) or they have been topically administered by iontophoresis (ascorbic acid, Alexeev, 1960; cysteine, Doskach, 1960; Pletneva et al., 1962).

As in most conditions of a degenerative nature, treatment by *tissue therapy* as advocated by Filatov[1] has been said to give good results (Szymanski, 1952).

Immunological therapeutics have had their place. Römer (1907–10) was the pioneer in this line of thought: he claimed that specific toxins for lens substance (phakolysins) are formed in the body owing to faulty metabolism against which immunity could be acquired by immunization. Lentocalin, a preparation of lenticular protein, was employed for this purpose. Salus (1926) used a subconjunctival injection of an emulsion of cataractous lenses (Cataractolysin); and others have tried beef lens extract for systemic immunization (Selinger, 1935). Davis (1932) employed lens protein in the hope that it would produce specific lysins which will absorb the lenticular opacities; but any treatment based on the use of lens antigen has yielded no results which can be substantiated (Ellis, 1928; Biffis and Quaglio, 1933; Selinger, 1935; and others). The use of an extract of fish lenses, an extraordinary and completely illusory technique initiated on no scientific basis by Shropshire (1937), received support (Shropshire et al., 1952; da Silveira, 1953), but has been found to be not only useless but dangerous because of the production of anaphylactic reactions (Breinin, 1953).

Finally, the prevention or retardation of the opacities has been claimed by those who have seen in the activity of the ciliary muscle an ætiological factor in cataract by the constant employment of spectacles to ease accommodative strain (Schoen, 1887–89; and others).

The second line of approach—the rectification of the metabolic failures which are responsible for cataract—has more to recommend it. In those few cases wherein the ætiology is clear and simple, the results may be good and the progress of opacification may cease or in early cases be reversed. Thus typical diabetic or galactosæmic cataract may be arrested by adequate control of the systemic disease, as well as the type of cataract due to hypocalcæmia; but when these principles have been stretched and applied to more debatable problems, the results have been more than disappointing.

Thus senile cataract has been attributed to a pluri-glandular failure, particularly of the gonads, and hence treatment has been advocated by ovarian extracts (Gallus, 1923), the male sex hormones (Keyton, 1950; Davids, 1953) or a mixture of thyroid, parathyroid and gonad extracts (Euphakin, Siegrist, 1928) together with vasotomy; here again the results have been less than inconclusive. A curious application of this concept said to give favourable results has been the use of parotin, the hormone of the salivary gland (Tsuchiya, 1962; Tennichi, 1964).

Similarly, in view of the possibility of inducing cataract experimentally by the deprivation of certain vitamins, the lavish use of these substances has been recom-

[1] Vol. VII, p. 725.

mended, particularly vitamins B, C and D; but such treatment has been found to be valueless (Urbanek, 1938; Malling, 1938; Wagner *et al.*, 1938; and others).

Whatever the ætiology of senile cataract may be, it is usual that its development is associated with the onset of senile changes generally throughout the body, and its presence should serve as an indication for reviewing the general life and habits of the patient. Herein lies the importance of examining the eyes of all patients over middle age under a mydriatic, for the state of the lens is the one sign of senescence which can be diagnosed in its earliest microscopic stage with certainty. A complete systemic examination should exclude gross foci of infection or detect any constitutional disease (diabetic, hypertensive and so on). Work, rest and recreation should also be reviewed and the stresses of living should be so adjusted that they become compatible as far as possible both with physical limitations and with the full realization of life.

The third problem in the treatment of cataract is to mitigate as far as possible the optical disadvantages under which the patient may be labouring. Repeated and careful tests of the refraction every six months or so are essential, since progressive myopia and changes both in the strength and axis of cylinders are the rule owing to refractive changes occurring in the lens. Dazzling by bright light can be relieved by tinted glasses, and when the maximum acuity is required at the same time, a tinting of the periphery of the lens frequently gives considerable relief. Amber-tinted glasses which cut the readily diffused short rays are perhaps the most generally useful. Moreover, for close work the efficient arrangement of the illumination is of the utmost value; it should be brilliant if the pupillary area is free, duller and placed to the side and behind if the opacities are central. The contrast obtained by using a sheet of dark paper so cut that it isolates a few lines of print at a time may also be of considerable assistance in reading. Telescopic spectacles will allow some people to read who would otherwise be unable to do so; and a magnifying glass held in the hand or supported on the page will give similar aid to those in whom it seems desirable to postpone an operation.[1] In cases of axial cataract, dilatation of the pupil by a weak solution of atropine (1/12%) is safe even in elderly people provided the angle of the anterior chamber is open, but it is well to exclude the development of glaucoma by periodic examinations; if there is any doubt on this question an optical iridectomy is a safer procedure in patients on whom the major operation of extraction may not be advisable.

At the same time it is desirable to sustain by every means the patient's morale and dispel his anxieties. The term " cataract " has an unfortunate connotation, and while it should not be used by the ophthalmologist in the many cases of stationary opacities, and rarely in the case of progressive opacities until they begin to embarrass vision, when it is used stress should

---

[1] See Vol. V.

be laid on the fact that the condition is curable, that blindness will not ensue, that the ordeal of an operation is much less in realization than in anticipation, and that, allowing for certain optical disadvantages, the operative results are good.

Alexeev. *Oftal. Zh.*, No. 2, 85 (1960).
Badal. *Bull. Soc. franç. Ophtal.*, **19**, 422 (1902).
Biffis and Quaglio. *Ann. Ottal.*, **61**, 641 (1933).
Blake. *N. Carolina med. J.*, **10**, 309 (1949).
Breinin. *J. Amer. med. Ass.*, **152**, 698 (1953).
Burdon-Cooper. *Trans. ophthal. Soc. U.K.*, **53**, 401 (1933).
Campbell. *Amer. J. Electrother.*, **35**, 357 (1917).
Carballo. *Arch. Oftal. B. Aires*, **32**, 227 (1957).
Cohen and Levin. *Rev. cub. Oftal.*, **2**, 457 (1920).
Connor. *Ophthal. Rec.*, **18**, 10 (1909).
Daniels. *Z. Augenheilk.*, **75**, 129 (1931).
Davids. *Klin. Mbl. Augenheilk.*, **122**, 296 (1953).
Davis. *Amer. Med.*, **27**, 1 (1932).
Dean. *Trans. Amer. Acad. Ophthal.*, **29**, 131 (1924); **32**, 231 (1927).
Dor. *Clin. Ophtal.*, **3**, 11 (1911).
Doskach. *Indian med. Forum*, **11**, 184 (1960).
Ellis. *Arch. Ophthal.*, **57**, 46 (1928).
Franklin and Cordes. *Amer. J. Ophthal.*, **3**, 643 (1920).
Gallois. *Bull. Soc. franç. Ophtal.*, **64**, 89 (1951).
Gallus. *Arch. Augenheilk.*, **92**, 34 (1923).
Gilbert. *Z. Augenheilk.*, **53**, 343 (1924).
Greenwood. *Trans. Amer. Acad. Ophthal.*, **29**, 125 (1924).
Hackmann, H. and C. *Münch. med. Wschr.*, **100**, 1817 (1958).
Harkness. *Amer. J. Ophthal.*, **8**, 132 (1925).
Harris. *Amer. J. Electrother.*, **42**, 226 (1924).
Hildesheimer. *XIII int. Cong. Ophthal.*, Amsterdam, **1**, 216 (1929).
Jones. *Ann. Ophthal.*, **22**, 659 (1913).
Kalish. *Med. Rec.*, **37**, 341 (1890).
Keyton. *J. med. Ass. Ala.*, **19**, 198 (1950).
Kögel. *v. Graefes Arch. Ophthal.*, **126**, 502 (1931).
Levin. *Amer. J. Roentgenol.*, **7**, 107 (1920).
Löhlein. *Arch. Augenheilk.*, **65**, 417 (1910).
Mackay, Stewart and Robertson. *Brit. J. Ophthal.*, **16**, 193 (1932).
Malling. *Med. Rev.* (Bergen), **55**, 280 (1938).
Meesmann. *Klin. Mbl. Augenheilk.*, **101**, Suppl. 1 (1938).
Meyer-Steineg. *Wschr. Ther. Hyg. Auges*, **16**, 377 (1913); **17**, 221, 229 (1914); **19**, 153 (1916).
Meyer-Steineg. *Dtsch. med. Wschr.*, **50**, 111 (1924).
Misar. *Wien. klin. Wschr.*, **79**, 707 (1967).
Müller and Kleifeld. *Klin. Mbl. Augenheilk.*, **137**, 25 (1960).
von Pflugk. *Klin. Mbl. Augenheilk.*, **44** (2), 400 (1906).
Pick. *Z. Augenheilk.*, **21**, 302 (1909).
Pletneva, Jartseva and Burdyanskaya. *Helmholtz ophthal. Inst.*, *Sci. Notes*, **7**, 313 (1962).
Pollock. *Glasg. med. J.*, **99**, 32 (1923).
Rauh. *Ber. dtsch. ophthal. Ges.*, **51**, 357 (1936).
Römer. *Arch. Augenheilk.*, **56**, Erg., 150 (1907).
Ber. dtsch. ophthal. Ges., **35**, 195 (1908); **36**, 97 (1910).
Salit. *v. Graefes Arch. Ophthal.*, **139**, 654 (1938).
Salus. *Med. Klin.*, **22**, 1787 (1926).
Schoen. *Arch. Augenheilk.*, **17**, 1 (1887); **19**, 77 (1889).
Ber. dtsch. ophthal. Ges., **20**, 170 (1889).
Selinger. *Arch. Ophthal.*, **14**, 244 (1935).
Shropshire. *Arch. Ophthal.*, **17**, 505, 508 (1937).
Shropshire, Ginsburg and Jacobi. *Science*, **116**, 276 (1952).
Siegrist. *Der graue Altersstar*, Berlin (1928).
da Silveira. *Arch. bras. Oftal.*, **16**, 34 (1953).
Smith. *Clin. Ophtal.*, **4**, 234 (1912).
Trans. ophthal. Soc. U.K., **48**, 89 (1928).
Szymanski. *Arch. bras. Oftal.*, **15**, 40 (1952).
Tcherictchy. *Oftal. Zh.*, No. 4, 278 (1964).
Taylor. *Lancet*, **2**, 700 (1924).
Tennichi. *Med. J. mutual Aid Ass.*, **13**, 6 (1964).
Tischner. *Wschr. Ther. Hyg. Auges*, **17**, 301 (1914).
Treu. *Arch. Augenheilk.*, **57**, 56 (1907).
Tsuchiya. *Rinsho-Ganka*, **16**, 19 (1962).
Urbanek. *Klin. Mbl. Augenheilk.*, **101**, 670 (1938).
Verderau. *Clin. Ophtal.*, **10**, 358 (1904).
Voisin and Paquelin. *Ann. Oculist.* (Paris), **193**, 768 (1960); **195**, 504 (1962).
Wagner, Richner and Karbacher. *Klin. Mbl. Augenheilk.*, **101**, 543 (1938).
Walter. *Wschr. Ther. Hyg. Auges*, **17**, 306, 313 (1914).
Weeks. *J. Amer. med. Ass.*, **94**, 403 (1930).

Surgical Treatment

History

The story of the evolution of the surgical relief of cataract is long and full of interest. The earliest authentic records come from ancient Hindu medicine long before the Christian era. In this amazingly advanced community the occurrence of cataract was recognized as an opacity developing in the " eye-apple " long before the acceptance of this view in Europe in the second half of the 18th century, and its treatment by couching the lens was widely practised. The greatest exponent of this school was Suśruta,[1] who taught the foundations of surgery based on anatomical dissections, practised aseptic surgery (advising that the operating room be fumigated with sweet vapours and that the surgeon keep his hair and beard short, his nails and hands clean and wear a sweet-smelling dress) and apparently used some kind of inhalation anæsthetic. In the wealth of his teaching on general surgery, he dealt systematically and elaborately with the anatomy, physiology and pathology of the eye, and he described several different varieties of cataract, giving an admirable account of the technique of its treatment by couching and the post-operative care which he successfully practised. It would seem obvious that this extremely detailed account, probably written before the Hippocratic era, was the outcome of previous knowledge and experience accumulated over a long period in the rich civilization of early Hindustan.

This operation of *couching* or *reclination* was widely employed in India in those early times and has been continued until our present century (Plate III), but there is no record of the surgical relief of cataract in the extant literature of Babylonian, ancient Egyptian or classical Greek medicine although bronze instruments suggesting their use for this purpose have been found in the islands of Cos and Samos. In the Hippocratic writings cataract had no remedy. It is possible, however, that Suśruta's teaching reached Alexandria during or after the Indian expedition of Alexander the Great. However that may be, the Roman writers—Celsus [*c.* 25 B.C.–A.D. 50] who lived in the reign of the Emperor Tiberius, and Galen [*c.* A.D. 131–201] in the time of the Emperor Marcus Aurelius—indicated that surgery for cataract was practised in the Alexandrian School probably as an outcome of Hindustan medicine, the names of Herophilos [*c.* 344–280 B.C.] and Philoxenes [*c.* 250 B.C.] being mentioned. Celsus himself in his *De medicina*, the oldest classical medical treatise to survive to our day, gave a detailed account of the operation of couching, believing that the material dispersed was not the lens but an inspissated humour lying in an empty space between the centrally placed lens and the pupil.[2] It is interesting that the Hindus practised a safer method of couching than the Alexandrian Greeks and Romans; the former pierced the sclera with a sharp lancet and then inserted a blunt instrument the side of which could be used to depress the lens, while Celsus used one sharp instrument whereby the capsule was often ruptured and complications subsequently developed. The later Arabs, however, went back to the safer Hindu technique with two instruments, a method still used by the native Indian coucher (Elliot, 1917).

[1] *Suśruta Samhita*, Vol. 7, chap. 17, verses 59–73. (See Vol. II, p. 18.)   [2] p. 3,

This tradition was maintained in Arabian ophthalmology which was essentially an interpretation of Alexandrian and Roman teaching; but there were two exceptions. Rhazes [*c.* 865–925] in his *Content of Medicine* attributed, without proof, an extraction of the opacity to Antyllos, a famous surgical contemporary of Galen, who advised needling of the cataract with

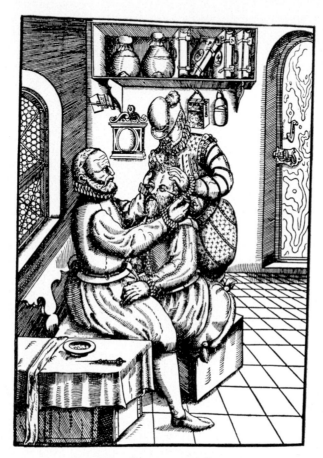

Fig. 264.—Couching for Cataract.

The operation of couching for cataract as performed in mediæval Europe and practised by Bartisch (from Bartisch's 'Οφθαλμοδουλεία, *das ist Augendienst*, 1583).

subsequent evacuation through a glass tube; but Ammar [996–1020], the most original of the Arabian School, inserted a hollow needle and sucked out the opaque material of a soft cataract. Nevertheless, Avenzoar [*c.* 1109–62] of Seville, one of the greatest of the later Spanish-Arabian writers summed up the position in his *Theisir* by writing that the treatment of cataract by extraction is impossible and reclination only is permissible.

PLATE III
Couching for Cataract in India

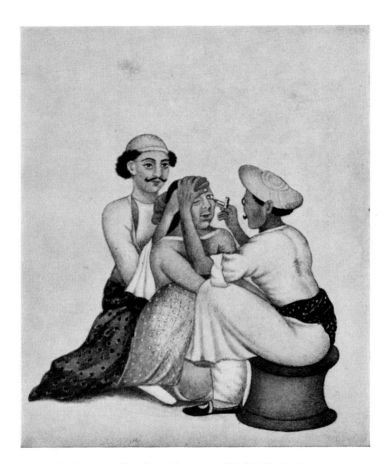

A picture dating from the siege of Delhi (R. R. James).

In mediæval Europe the same tradition prevailed until the middle of the 17th century (Figs. 264–5). It is said that Stephan Blaukaart, one of the Dutch disciples of the great Franciscus Sylvius at Leyden, removed a cataract through a corneal incision in 1668,[1] but a new interest arose after the demonstration by Michel Pierre Brisseau to the *Académie Royale des Sciences* in Paris in 1705 that cataract was an opacity of the lens and not a coagulated humour in front of it.[2] Shortly thereafter an opaque lens was delivered from a living eye in 1707 after its accidental anterior dislocation

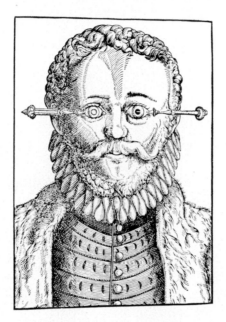

FIG. 265.—COUCHING FOR CATARACT.

Bartisch's illustration of the operation for couching. The cataract is seen in the pupil of the right eye while the pupil of the left eye has been cleared (from Bartisch's Ὀφθαλμοδουλεία, *das ist Augendienst*, 1583).

during the operation of couching by one of the greatest of French ophthalmologists, Charles Saint-Yves, who published his feat in 1708. Similarly, cataractous lenses dislocated into the anterior chamber were extracted through a corneal incision by Jean Louis Petit in 1708 in Paris; a membranous cataract was removed with a hook on three occasions by Johann Conrad Freytag[3] of Zürich, while the English surgeon, Benedict Duddell in 1736, by inserting through the capsule a lancet concealed in a cannula, extracted cases of soft cataract which could not be couched into the vitreous but had been dislocated into the anterior chamber. The first, however, to

---

[1] See Atkinson, *J. Ophthal. Otol. Laryng.*, **30**, 322 (1926). [2] p. 65.
[3] See J. H. Freytag (the son of J. C. Freytag), *Dissert. medica de cataracta*, Strasburg (1721).

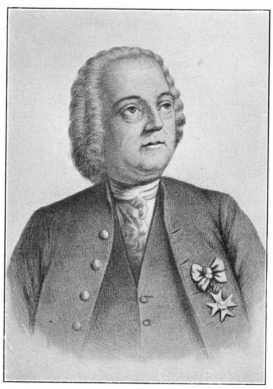

FIG. 266.—JACQUES DAVIEL
[1696–1762].

make a planned extraction of cataract from its natural position behind the iris was Jacques Daviel who made known his technique in 1748[1]; thereby he inaugurated a revolution in ophthalmic surgery.

JACQUES DAVIEL [1696–1762] (Fig. 266) is thus one of the most important figures in the entire history of ophthalmology. His life was colourful. Born in La Barre in Normandy in poor circumstances, he became an apprentice in surgery to his uncle in Rouen and in 1713 became a student-surgeon in the Army. When plague, brought to Marseilles in a ship from the Orient, developed as an epidemic in the south of France, he volunteered in 1719 to go to Marseilles and took his newly married wife with him to a

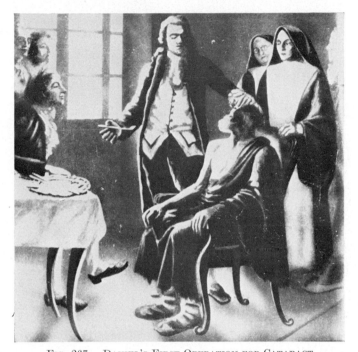

FIG. 267.—DAVIEL'S FIRST OPERATION FOR CATARACT.
Daviel is seen about to operate on Brother Felix, the hermit of Aiguill en Provence, on April 8th, 1745 (courtesy of G. E. Jayle).

city where 50,000 out of the 100,000 inhabitants died from this devastating disease; for this he received from the French King the Cross of the Knight of St. Roch and was made a master-surgeon by the aldermen of Marseilles (1722) and surgeon to the Hôtel Dieu of that city (1723). In 1740 he was elected a corresponding member of the Royal Academy of Surgery. In 1746 he settled in Paris where he prospered and in 1749 was appointed surgeon-oculist to Louis XV. Full of honours (Fig. 1) he died in the Hotel Balance in Geneva in 1762. Over his grave in the cemetery of the Grand Saxonix Church, two miles north of Geneva, the ophthalmologists of Switzerland in 1885 fittingly erected a marble headstone with the inscription " Post Tenebras Lux ".

Daviel had performed many operations for couching but, like all his contemporaries, not always with success. When operating on a wig-maker called Farian, he

[1] Lettre sur les maladies des yeux. *Mercure de France*, Paris, 198 (1748).

failed to couch the lens; basing his next action on the knowledge he had gained from extensive dissections of cadavers at Marseilles, he incised the lower segment of the cornea, lifted the flap with forceps and, inserting a needle behind the lens, brought it out together with some vitreous (Fig. 267). By 1750 he was convinced he would do

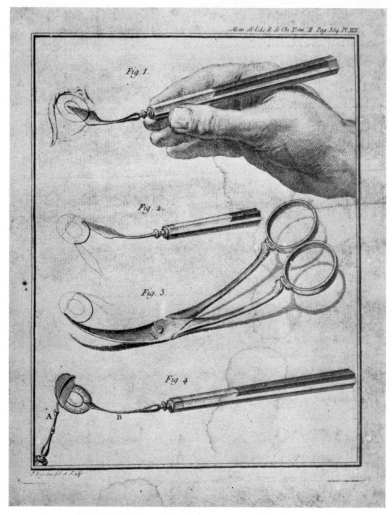

FIG. 268.—DAVIEL'S EXTRACTION OF CATARACT.

Daviel's original illustration published in *Mém. Acad. roy. Chir.*, Paris, **2**, 337 (1753), showing the instruments and the use to which they were put.

no more couching; in 1753 he sent to the Royal Academy of Surgery one of the most important papers ever contributed to ophthalmic literature wherein he reported 115 extractions of cataract with 100 successes[1] and in 1756 his statistics were 434

[1] Sur une nouvelle méthode de guérir la cataracte par l'extraction du crystallin: *Mém. Acad. roy. Chir.*, Paris, **2**, 337 (1753).

extractions with only 50 failures[1]—a very satisfactory outcome in comparison with couching.

Daviel's operation (1753) was complicated (Figs. 268–9). He first made an incision at the lower limbus with a triangular knife and this was enlarged on either

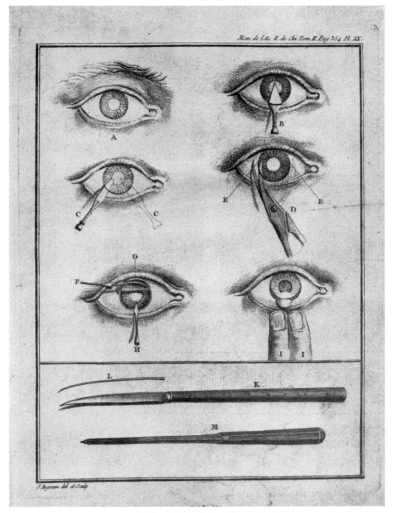

FIG. 269.—DAVIEL'S EXTRACTION OF CATARACT.
From the same paper as Fig. 268, indicating the steps of Daviel's operation.

side with a blunt-pointed, double-edged knife; thereafter he enlarged the incision on both sides with two suitably curved scissors designed to correspond to the configuration of the limbus so that the incision extended above the level of the pupil. A spatula was then introduced into the eye and while it raised the cornea from the lens the capsule was incised with a sharp needle, the spatula was inserted between the

[1] *Journal de Médecine*, Paris, 124 (1756).

Figs. 270 to 282.—The Development of Cataract Knives
(after J. Hirschberg).

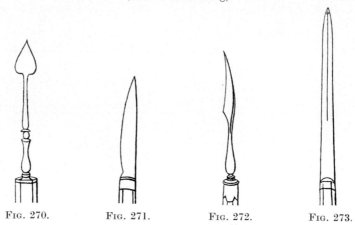

FIG. 270.   FIG. 271.   FIG. 272.   FIG. 273.

FIG. 270.—Daviel, Paris (1752).   FIG. 271.—de la Faye, Paris (1753).
FIG. 272.—Sharp, London (1753).   FIG. 273.—Poyet, Paris (1753).

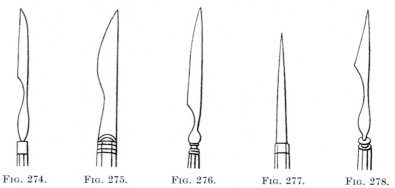

FIG. 274.   FIG. 275.   FIG. 276.   FIG. 277.   FIG. 278.

FIG. 274.—Warner, London (1754).   FIG. 275.—Bérenger, Paris (1755).
FIG. 276.—Young, Edinburgh (1756).   FIG. 277.—Tenon, Paris (1757).   FIG. 278.—
ten Haaf, Rotterdam (1761).

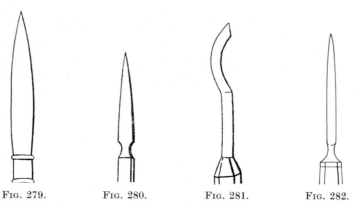

FIG. 279.   FIG. 280.   FIG. 281.   FIG. 282.

FIG. 279.—Pamard, Avignon (1769).   FIG. 280.—Bell, London (1785).
FIG. 281.—Pellier de Quengsy, Paris (1789).   FIG. 282.—A modern Graefe knife.

iris and the lens to loosen the latter and the cataract was expressed by gentle pressure. If the cataract were soft, lens matter was removed by a curette, the pupil was re-adjusted, the cornea replaced and a bandage applied.

Daviel's technique was by no means easy and for some considerable time couching remained the standard method of treatment. The greatest surgical authorities such as Percival Pott [1714–88] in England (1775), Antonio Scarpa [1747–1832] in Italy (1801), and Guillaume Dupuytren [1777–1835] in France (1832) continued to use and advocate the old procedure of couching which, indeed, died hard, but improvements and simplifications to Daviel's procedure rapidly appeared. In 1752 George de la Faye [1699–1781], the distinguished ophthalmologist who became Vice-Director of the Royal Academy of Surgery in Paris, greatly simplified the operation and made it more practical by using two instruments only, a single knife (bistoury) to make the incision and a cystitome to incise the lens capsule, the whole procedure lasting " no longer than a minute " (Fig. 271). de la Faye practised this on cadavers but was anticipated in its clinical application by Samuel Sharp [?1700–1778] of London who, in 1753, made a puncture and counter-puncture and cut downwards through the lower limbus. de la Faye also advocated extraction with the capsule intact when that was possible. New and improved types of knife were introduced by Poyet of Paris (1753), Joseph Warner of London (1754), Louis Bérenger of Bordeaux (1755), Thomas Young of Edinburgh (1756), and Jacques René Tenon of Paris (1757) (Figs. 272–7), while Gerhard ten Haaf of Rotterdam (1761), and after him Guillaume Pellier de Quengsy, the itinerant oculist of Montpellier (1789–90), simplified the procedure by incising the capsule with the point of the knife between the puncture and counter-puncture (Figs. 278, 281). The next three dramatic advances were made by Pierre-François-Bénézet Pamard of Avignon (Fig. 283) who, between 1759 and 1784, advised that the patient lie on his back instead of being seated as had hitherto been the practice as for couching, used an instrument (a " trèfle ") to fixate the eye, and made an incision with a specially designed broad knife in the upper part of the cornea instead of the lower (Fig. 279), the last innovation being heartily welcomed by Benjamin Bell (1785) in Edinburgh (Fig. 280) ; it is interesting that Wenzel (1786) made an incision in the upper part of the cornea with a keratome instead of a knife, a method now frequently employed. A further advance was made at the beginning of the following century by Carl Himly of Göttingen who, in 1801, introduced mydriasis before the operation, while a preliminary iridectomy was practised in 1862 by Albert Mooren of Düsseldorf.[1]

Originally the section used was corneal in location ; Julius Jacobson in 1863 had practised a limbal incision which reduced complications to 2%, and finally, in 1866, Albrecht von Graefe introduced his technique of combined " linear extraction ". Herein an iridectomy was performed at the time of operation and the " linear incision " was through the sclera in the plane of the largest possible circle of the limbus, whereupon after discission of the capsule the lens was expelled ; the occurrence, however, of irido-cyclitis and sympathetic ophthalmitis led to the adoption of a more anterior incision but otherwise von Graefe's method became generally adopted, sometimes as a " simple" extraction without iridectomy (H. Knapp, 1887). The idea of a peripheral iridectomy with its optical and cosmetic advantages was advanced by Bajardi (1895) in Torino and enthusiastically advocated by Elschnig (1911–12).

Intracapsular extraction, whereby the lens is extracted entire with its capsule leaving no remnants behind, is obviously the method of choice, but it has only recently become universally popular. It was first deliberately planned by Samuel Sharp (1753) of London who expelled the lens from the eye by the pressure of his thumb, a method used by several subsequent

[1] Vol. IX, p. 914.

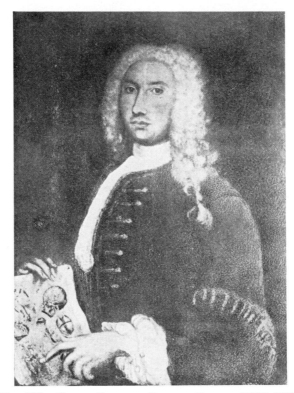

FIG. 283.—PIERRE-FRANÇOIS-BENEZET PAMARD [1728–1793].
Taken from *Les Œuvres de P.-F.-B. Pamard* by A. Pamard and P. Pansier, 1900.

The Pamards were indeed a distinguished family, containing a succession of seven generations of surgeons dating from the middle of the 17th century to the 20th: Pierre Pamard [1669–1728], Nicolas-Dominique Pamard [1702–1783], Pierre-François-Bénézet Pamard [1728–1793], Jean Baptiste-Antoine-Bénézet Pamard [1763–1827], Paul-Antoine-Marie Pamard [1802–1872], Alfred Pamard [1837–1920] who wrote the book about P.-F.-B. Pamard in 1900 and was in turn succeeded by his son, Paul.

surgeons. Pressure on the globe by instruments was an alternative technique, such as by a curette (Christiaen, 1845), a spoon (Reuling, 1879) or a strabismus hook, a method popularized particularly by Colonel Henry Smith (1900–26) on incredible numbers of patients in India following the technique devised by Malronez of Amritsar.[1] Contemporaneously with Sharp, the more direct technique of pushing the lens out after impaling its posterior pole with a needle thrust through the sclera was adopted by Richter (1773), a method also employed by Beer (1799) and von Canstatt (1871). The alternative expedient of lifting it out with a spoon or a loop (vectis) (Reuling, 1879) was introduced by A. and H. Pagenstecher (1866–71), a dangerous technique but sometimes of great value today in cases of subluxation. All these procedures involving pressure on the globe tend to cause a loss of vitreous so that the method which forms the basis of modern practice is to extract the lens by traction. The first to do so was Terson (1870) who grasped the capsule with toothed forceps; he was followed by Landesberg (1878) using iris forceps, and finally by Eugene Kalt (1894–1925) of Paris (Fig. 284) who devised a smooth forceps specially for the purpose. This type of instrument with its many modifications has been widely exploited most particularly by such surgeons as Stanculeanu (1912) of Bucharest, Arnold Knapp (1914–47) of New York, Anton Elschnig (1922–32) of Prague (Fig. 25), and Arthur Sinclair (1925) of Edinburgh.

Three other methods have been introduced to remove the lens intracapsularly. A suction cup was used originally by Stoewer (1902) and Hulen (1910) and popularized by Ignacio Barraquer (1917–24) of Barcelona, who designed an erisophake controlled by an electric pump; Dimitry (1933) used the more simple method of suction by a syringe, and A. E. Bell (1948) by a stiff rubber bulb. A second suggestion was made by Lacarrère of Madrid (1932) who used diathermo-coagulation with a double-pronged needle; and more recently a cryosurgical probe was first similarly employed by T. Krwawicz (1961) of Lublin in Poland.

Zonular destruction is obviously an aid to the intracapsular extraction of cataract for thereby less force is required to free and expel the lens. This was first done mechanically by di Luca (1866) who slipped a curved probe around the lens, and at a later date by Andrew (1883) with a bent needle, and has now become more practicable by dissolving it with a solution of α-chymotrypsin (J. Barraquer, 1958).

Sutures as a safety measure to close the section after surgery were introduced by Henry W. Williams (1867) of New England (Fig. 285) who first inserted a single corneo-scleral suture and later (1869) conjunctival sutures; he used a shortened and freshly pointed sewing needle threaded with a strand of fine glover's silk. The technique stimulated few followers but 30 years later corneo-scleral sutures were introduced into Europe by

[1] Unpublished. See paper read by his assistant, Chaud, at the Indian Medical Congress, Calcutta, 1894.

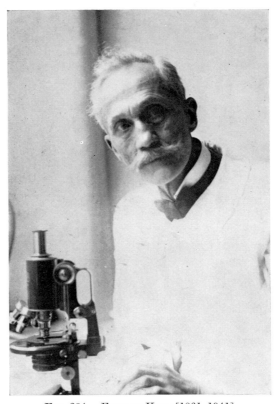

FIG. 284.—EUGENE KALT [1861–1941]

He devised the first forceps specifically for intracapsular extraction. This photograph was taken by himself in his laboratory at the Quinze-Vingts Hospital, Paris.

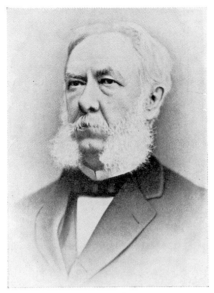

FIG. 285.—HENRY WILLARD WILLIAMS
[1821–1895].

Kalt (1894) and the first conjunctivo-scleral suture was described by Verhoeff (1916); preplaced sutures were employed by Suarez de Mendosa (1891). Their value in assisting rapid and firm healing is great; and during this century the number of types introduced and their variety—and the time sometimes spent in inserting them by enthusiasts—are extraordinary (see Hudson, 1951).

Two further advances of historical interest were the introduction of local anæsthesia and akinesia. To Karl Koller (1884) of Vienna we owe the immense advantage of operating under topical *analgesia* by the instillation of drops of cocaine, and the extension of this to regional anæsthesia by retrobulbar injection was suggested by Elschnig (1928). Motor *akinesia* was initially introduced by van Lint (1914) of Brussels; he paralysed the orbicularis muscle, a technique modified by R. E. Wright (1921–26) of Madras who injected the trunk of the facial nerve as it emerged from the stylomastoid foramen, and simplified by O'Brien (1929) of Iowa who injected the temporo-facial division of the nerve as it crossed over the condyle of the mandible.

The OPERATION OF DISCISSION for a soft cataract also traces its origin to early times. Both Celsus and Galen in describing the operation for the relief of cataract advised that, if depression were impossible, the cataract should be cut in pieces by the needle and " dissipated in many parts ", and the latter recounted that the knowledge of the relief of cataract among the

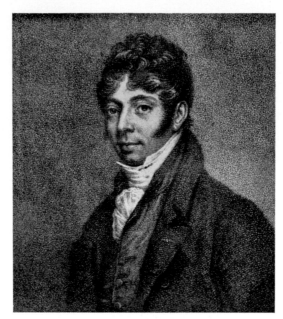

FIG. 286.—JOHN CUNNINGHAM SAUNDERS
[1773–1810].

ancients derived from the fable that wild goats with this disease practised self-surgery by charging into a thorny bush and puncturing the eye. In Arabian ophthalmology such writers as Rhazes and Ammar advised " tearing the cataract to pieces " by a needle and, if it were possible, sucking out the soft lens matter through a hollow needle. In the Middle Ages in Europe, however, only couching was performed although in the Renaissance the highly original French surgeon, Ambroise Paré (1575) (who introduced the ocular speculum) favoured discission but dismissed suction as impracticable. Jacques Guillemeau (1585) was the first to recognize that the disintegration and dissolution of a soft cataract (" cataracta lacta ", because " the colour and substance resembled milk ") could occur and he and Richard Banister (1622) deliberately practised the operation of discission, a technique advocated by Paul Barbette (1672) in children and used by such surgeons as Sir William Read (1706), Maître-Jan (1711) and particularly Percival Pott (1772–78) who did much to popularize the procedure. These authorities introduced the needle posteriorly through the sclera; the first to use the anterior approach through the cornea was Georg Conradi (1797). Discission as an operation for cataract in children was finally established as a routine by John Cunningham Saunders at Moorfields Eye Hospital in London (1811) (Fig. 286), while Benjamin Travers (1814) at the same hospital introduced the technique of the removal of the soft lens-matter by curette evacuation.

It is true that the aspiration method, resembling the suction technique of the Arabian surgeons, had been intermittently practised by such writers as Galeazzo (1533),[1] Borri (1669)[2] and Pecchioli (1838),[3] and was reintroduced by Blanchet (1847) and Laugier (1847–48) in Paris and Teale (1864) in London, but it was regarded as an accessory procedure and not adopted into general practice; only recently has it been revived. The only decisive innovation which has since been made has been the concept of S. Lewis Ziegler (1921) of Boston who practised a " complete discission " wherein a V-shaped incision is made deeply into the lens. While to France must go the credit of introducing and standardizing the operation for the extraction of cataract in the adult, to London must go the credit for the deliberate practice of intracapsular extraction, as also for the surgical development of the treatment of cataract in children.

It is interesting that *convex spectacles* for use in aphakic eyes were first mentioned by Benito Daza de Valdés of Seville in 1623, although his recommendation was not practised until a century had passed.

Andrew. *Brit. med. J.*, **1**, 41 (1883).

Bajardi. *G. Accad. Med. Torino*, 251 (1895).

Banister. *Treatise of 113 Diseases of the Eyes and Eyeliddes*, London (1622).

Barbette. *Opera chirurgico-anatomica*, Lugdoni, Pt. 1, chap. 16, 61 (1672).

Barraquer, I. *Clin. Ophtal.*, **8**, 387 (1917); **10**, 167 (1920).
Ann. Oculist. (Paris), **157**, 328 (1920); **158**, 429 (1921).
Amer. J. Ophthal., **3**, 721 (1920).
Arch. Ophthal., **51**, 448, 501 (1922).
Brit. med. J., **2**, 660 (1924).

Barraquer, J. *An. Med. Cir.* (Barcelona), **34**, 148 (1958).

Beer. *Methode den grauen Staar samt der Kapsel Auszuziehen*, Wien (1799).

Bell, A. E. *Amer. J. Ophthal.*, **31**, 610 (1948).

Bell, B. *A System of Surgery*, 2nd ed., Edinb. (1785).

Bérenger. *Mém. Acad. Sci.*, Paris, **3**, 29 (1755).

Blanchet. *Ann. Oculist.* (Paris), **18**, 38 (1847).

von Canstatt. *Klin. Mbl. Augenheilk.*, **9**, 131 (1871).

Christiaen. *Ann. Oculist.* (Paris), **13**, 181 (1845).

Conradi. Arneman's *Mag. f. Wundarzneiwiss.*, Göttingen, **1**, 59 (1797).

Daza de Valdés. *Uso de los antojos para todo genero de vista*, Seville (1623).

Daviel. *Mercure de France*, 198 (1748); 172 (1760).
Mém. Acad. roy. Chir., Paris, **2**, 337 (1753).
J. Méd., Paris, 124 (1756).

Dimitry. *Arch. Ophthal.*, **9**, 261 (1933).

Duddell. *A Supplement to the Treatise of the Diseases of the Horny-Coat and Cataract of the Eye*, London (1736).

Dupuytren. v. Ammons *Z. Ophthal.*, **2**, 460 (1832).

Elliot. *Indian Operation of Couching for Cataract*, London (1917).

Elschnig. *Arch. Augenheilk.*, **69**, 319 (1911); **98**, 300 (1928).
Ann. Ophthal., **21**, 447 (1912).
Klin. Mbl. Augenheilk., **52**, 262 (1914).
Ber. dtsch. ophthal. Ges., **43**, 168 (1922); **44**, 145 (1924).
Amer. J. Ophthal., **8**, 355 (1925).
Schmerz, **1**, 114 (1928).
Z. Augenheilk., **75**, 1 (1931).
Die intrakapsulare Starextraktion, Berlin (1932).

de la Faye. *Mém. Acad. roy. Chir.*, Paris, **2**, 563 (1753).

von Graefe. v. *Graefes Arch. Ophthal.*, **5** (1), 158 (1859); **12** (1), 150 (1866); **13** (2), 549 (1867); **14** (3), 106 (1868).
Brit. med. J., **1**, 379 (1867).

Guillemeau. *Traité des maladies de l'œil, qui sont en nombre de cent treize*, Paris (1585).

ten Haaf. *Korte Verhandeling nopens de nieuwe wyze om de cataracta te genezen*, Rotterdam (1761).

Himly. *Ophthalmologische Beobachtungen u. Untersuchungen*, Bremen (1801).

Hudson. *Ophthal. Lit.*, **5**, 3 (1951).

Hulen. *Ophthal. Rec.*, **19**, 651 (1910).

Jacobson. *Ein neues u. gefahrloses Operationsverfahren z. Heilung d. grauen Staares*, Berlin (1863).

[1] Galeatius di Sancta Sophia. See *Opus medicinæ in nonum tractatum libri Rhasis*, Hagenoae (1533).

[2] Francisci Josephi Burrhus, *Epistolæ duæ ad Th. Bartholinum, II*, Hafniae (1669).

[3] See Sichel (1847).

Kalt. *Arch. Ophtal.*, **14,** 639 (1894).
  Ann. Oculist. (Paris), **143,** 41 (1910); **162,** 489 (1925).
Knapp, A. *Trans. Amer. ophthal. Soc.*, **13,** 666 (1914).
  Arch. Ophthal., **46,** 27 (1917); **50,** 115, 426 (1921); **38,** 1 (1947).
  Trans. ophthal. Soc. U.K., **45,** 117 (1925); **66,** 133 (1946).
Knapp, H. *Arch. Ophthal.*, **16,** 54 (1887).
Koller. *Ber. dtsch. ophthal. Ges.*, **16,** 60 (1884).
Krwawicz. *Brit. J. Ophthal.*, **45,** 279 (1961); **47,** 36 (1963); **49,** 37 (1965).
Lacarrère. *Klin. Mbl. Augenheilk.*, **88,** 778 (1932).
Landesberg. *v. Graefes Arch. Ophthal.*, **24** (3), 59 (1878).
Laugier. *Ann. Oculist.* (Paris), **17,** 29 (1847); **20,** 28 (1848).
van Lint. *Ann. Oculist.* (Paris), **151,** 420 (1914).
di Luca. *Il Morgagni*, Naples, Nos. 2 and 3 (1866). Quoted by Kirby, *Surgery of Cataract*, Phila. (1950).
Maître-Jan. *Traité des maladies de l'œil*, Troyes, 186 (1711).
Mooren. *Die verminderten Gefahren einer Hornhautvereiterung bei der Staar-extraction*, Berlin (1862).
O'Brien. *Arch. Ophthal.*, **1,** 447 (1929).
Pagenstecher, A. *Klinische Beobachtungen a. d. Augenheilanstalt zu Wiesbaden*, **3,** 1 (1866).
Pagenstecher, H. *Ann. Oculist.* (Paris), **66,** 126 (1871).
  Die Extraction des grauen Staares bei geschlossener Kapsel, Wiesbaden (1877).
Pamard. *Mém. Acad. roy. Chir.*, Paris (1759–84).
  See *Les œuvres de P.-F.-B. Pamard* (by A. Pamard and P. Pansier, Paris, 81, 119, 127 (1900).
Paré (1575). See *Œuvres complètes* (ed. Malgaigne), Paris (1840–1).
Pecchioli. *Gaz. méd. Paris*, 3 (1838).
Pellier de Quengsy. *Précis au cours d'opérations sur les yeux*, Paris (1789–90).
Petit, J. L. *Hist. Acad. roy. Sci.*, Paris, 501 (1708).
Pott. *Chirurgical Observations relative to the Cataract*, etc., London (1772).
  Chirurgical Works, London (1778).

Poyet. *Mém. Acad. roy. Chir.*, Paris, **2,** 353, 578 (1753).
Read. *A Treatise of the Eyes*, London (1706).
Reuling. *N.Y. med. J.*, **29,** 1 (1879).
Richter. *Abhdl. vom der Ausziehung des grauen Staars*, Göttingen (1773).
Saint-Yves. *Hist. Acad. roy. Sci.*, Paris, 501 (1708).
  Nouveau traité des maladies des yeux, Paris (1722).
Saunders. *A Treatise on some Practical Points relating to the Diseases of the Eye*, London (1811). (Published posthumously.)
Scarpa. *Saggio di osservazioni e d'esperienze sulle principali malattie degli occhi*, Pavia (1801).
Sharp. *Phil. Trans.*, **48,** 161, 322 (1753).
Sichel. *Ann. Oculist.* (Paris), **17,** 104 (1847).
Sinclair. *Trans. ophthal. Soc. U.K.*, **45,** 127 (1925).
Smith, H. *Ind. med. Gaz.*, **35,** 241 (1900); **36,** 220 (1901); **40,** 327 (1905).
  Brit. med. J., **2,** 719 (1903).
  The Treatment of Cataract, Calcutta (1910).
  Ophthal. Rec., **24,** 449 (1915).
  Arch. Ophthal., **50,** 515 (1921); **55,** 213 (1926).
Stanculeanu. *Klin. Mbl. Augenheilk.*, **50** (1), 527 (1912).
Stoewer. *Ber. dtsch. ophthal. Ges.*, **30,** 296 (1902).
Suarez de Mendoza. *Bull. Soc. franç. Ophtal.*, **9,** 64 (1891).
Teale. *Roy. Lond. ophthal. Hosp. Rep.*, **4,** 197 (1864).
Tenon. *De cataracta*, Paris (1757).
Terson. *Rev. méd. Toulouse*, **6,** 76 (1870).
Travers. *Med.-Chir. Trans.* (Lond.), **5,** 391, 405 (1814).
Verhoeff. *Arch. Ophthal.*, **45,** 479 (1916).
Warner. *Cases in Surgery*, 2nd ed., London, 30 (1754).
Wenzel. *Traité de la cataracte*, Paris (1786).
Williams. *Roy. Lond. ophthal. Hosp. Rep.*, **6,** 28 (1867).
  Arch. Ophthal., **1,** 98 (1869).
Wright. *Amer. J. Ophthal.*, **4,** 445 (1921).
  Arch. Ophthal., **52,** 166 (1923); **55,** 555 (1926).
Young, Thomas. *Essays and Observations Physical and Literary on the Extraction of Cataract*, Edinb., **2,** 324 (1756). See Hubbell, *Ophthal. Rec.*, **9,** 547 (1900).
Ziegler. *J. Amer. med. Ass.*, **77,** 1100 (1921).

Contemporary Surgery

Written in Collaboration with Mr. James R. Hudson

SURGERY IN CHILDREN

The indications and surgical techniques applicable to the treatment of congenital cataract or of an acquired cataract, traumatic or otherwise, in young children have been considered in a previous Volume.[1] These may be briefly summarized by stating that if the visual acuity of one eye is 6/18 or better, aided if necessary by pupillary

[1] Vol. III, p. 757.

dilatation or even an iridectomy, operation on the lens should be postponed for some years. In bilateral cases one eye may well be subjected to operation at the age of 6 months and the second during the third year, but complications are less common if surgery can be postponed until the second and preferably the fourth year. The most applicable technique in very young children is discission which usually requires repetition unless it is combined with suction, and over the age of 2 years discission may be followed after a few days by a linear extraction. In very young children, provided a large portion of the anterior capsule is removed and a sector iridectomy is performed, most of the lens can be irrigated away if the lavage is conducted with sufficient thoroughness (Roy, 1968). In making a decision whether surgery is advisable, it should be remembered that the post-operative visual prognosis in cases of congenital cataract is on the whole disappointing, often because of the presence of other mal-formations of the eye (including macular aplasia); statistics show that 40% of patients acquire vision of 6/18 or over, 25% of 6/60 or less, while a percentage of from 6 to 10 becomes blind.

THE EXTRACTION OF CATARACT

INDICATIONS FOR SURGERY

The indications for the surgical treatment of cataract in adults are related to the visual acuity, the occupational needs of the patient, the stage of development of the cataract, and any special circumstances related to the nature of the cataract or to any associated ocular disease. Although the theoretically ideal time for operation is probably when a cataract has reached maturity, an immature cataract presents no difficulty with modern surgical methods taking advantage of zonulysis, cryosurgical instruments, systemic agents for the reduction of the intra-ocular pressure, reliable techniques of general anaesthesia, and advances in premedication, local analgesia and akinesia.

The level of vision at which cataract extraction should be considered is a matter affecting the individual patient himself. In an aged patient with bilateral cataract one eye should be operated on when he can no longer get about comfortably or read; he should not be allowed without some special reason to abandon his usual activities and sink into listlessness. In such cases, also, provided the patient has stood the first operation well and unless he is frail and inactive, it is usually advisable to operate on the second eye at a later date, both to obtain the advantages of binocular vision and to insure against the possibility of damage by injury or disease to the first eye, a relatively common occurrence in the aged which would necessitate an operation in less advantageous circumstances at a still more advanced age if visual efficiency is to be maintained. A myopic individual, however, with only 6/36 or even 6/60 vision may be happy as long as he can continue to read because of the degree of his myopia. A patient, on the other hand, whose livelihood demands a high standard of vision such as the driver of a vehicle or one whose work (or pleasure) depends on concentrated reading, may wish to have his visual acuity improved when it is still as good as 6/18 or even 6/12 in each eye. The surgeon, therefore, has the task of making his decision not in relation to the level of the visual acuity but to the degree of the visual handicap, the patient's personal needs and, indeed, his personal make-up. Should surgery be deemed advisable, in bilateral cases operative treatment should usually be advised for the worse eye.

In cases of uniocular cataract when the visual acuity falls below 6/36, some judgment is required. The restoration of binocular function after surgery by the use of contact lenses or even an intra-ocular lens-implant is not invariably certain; although in elderly patients the gradual development of lenticular opacities is generally followed by a post-operative resumption of binocular function with the aid of contact lenses, this is not the invariable experience of younger patients when a sudden loss of vision results from a traumatic cataract. The visual demands of younger patients are generally more exacting than those in the later age-groups, but the advantages of better vision after operation must be weighed against the relatively higher risks of cataract surgery in the young and the increased risk of a subsequent retinal detachment or an aphakic glaucoma. There are many occupations in which accurate vision and binocular function are advantageous or even essential; the advisability of operating when there is still a reasonable standard of vision in one eye must be considered if the patient finds that he has lost the advantages of binocularity which he may require so that he will necessarily be compelled to give up his occupation or abandon any of his usual important activities. At the same time, in every case the visual disabilities of an aphakic eye—of which more anon—should be clearly pointed out and the preliminary period of difficulty in optical adjustment should be stressed; without such a warning many patients, particularly the aged, are otherwise disappointed with the functional result of surgery no matter how technically perfect it may have been.

The maturity of a cataract is an indication for its surgical removal lest the complications of hypermaturity develop, including glaucoma due to the intumescence of a hypermature lens, phacolytic glaucoma, and phacotoxic uveitis with secondary glaucoma.[1] Even in an elderly person with good corrected vision in one eye the extraction of a mature cataract is advisable unless the patient elects to risk these complications or unless he is so frail that further surgical treatment would be a menace to his general health. The possibility of visual failure in the better eye should also be taken into account, and operative treatment should be considered if there is reason to believe that the vision of the good eye may not outlast the patient. In these circumstances the possible risk to the patient's general health should be explained both to him and to his immediate relatives.

Phacotoxic glaucoma[2] is always an indication for the extraction of a cataract, although topical treatment with steroids and mydriatics aided by systemic treatment with acetazolamide to bring the ocular tension under control by medical means may relieve the surgeon of the disadvantages of

[1] Vol. IX, p. 500.   [2] p. 663.

urgent surgery. Phacolytic glaucoma and glaucoma secondary to intumescence of the lens, however, frequently require urgent surgical intervention. A dislocated lens presents a much more difficult problem which is considered elsewhere.[1]

If retinal disease has been observed prior to the development of a cataract so that the standard of visual recovery can be anticipated, it may be advisable to delay surgery until it can be established that the changes in the lens are at least partly responsible for the increasing visual failure. If cataract is not the sole cause, the degree to which it is responsible should be carefully assessed; when there is a reasonable doubt, the patient should be taken into the surgeon's confidence and a mutual decision reached if it is thought that at least some improvement will reward operative intervention. The assessment of macular function may be made clinically[2] even if the central area cannot be clearly seen, but visible macular changes are not always a sign of reduced macular vision, while the additional magnification of the aphakic correction must be borne in mind when considering the advantages of surgical treatment. In patients with known retinal disease, such as cases of pigmentary retinal dystrophy wherein the visual field is markedly restricted, cataract extraction can be of benefit when the lenticular opacities are sufficiently advanced to add significantly to the visual disability. In cases of suspected retinal detachment with complicated cataract, electro-oculography and electroretinography may confirm the presence or absence of retinal function, but unless the history is well known, extraction may be worthwhile and should be undertaken in doubtful situations.

Although diabetes is not an absolute contra-indication to cataract surgery, many young diabetics with cataract have also advanced retinopathy and may also have signs of impending obstruction of the central retinal vein. Such cases are unlikely to benefit from surgery and, unless the cataract is mature, operation is better avoided. Such a policy will probably leave the patient with some residual vision for a longer period than would be expected to follow operative intervention. Elderly patients with diabetes of relatively recent onset do not usually suffer from retinopathy, certainly not of any severity, and apart from ensuring reasonable control of the disease during the operative and post-operative periods, they do not require any unusual steps on the part of the surgeon except, perhaps, to take special care that the capsule is not ruptured.[3]

Systemic diseases other than diabetes need no more than their usual medical management. Severe hypertension increases the risk of expulsive hæmorrhage during or after surgery and both pre-operative and post-operative measures to minimize this risk are fully justified. Blood diseases associated with bleeding tendencies should be identified and, where possible, controlled; for hæmophiliacs, an infusion of porcine anti-hæmophiliac

[1] p. 659.   [2] p. 146.   [3] p. 62.

globulin has been successfully employed (Strauss and Ramsell, 1968). Patients receiving anticoagulant treatment following cardiac infarcts are best managed with the co-operation of a physician. The physical ability of the patient to remain reasonably quiet, as from difficulty in breathing, should also receive consideration; but in this connection efficient suturing abolishes the necessity for recumbency and complete immobility, for the patient can safely sit up in a chair on the first post-operative day. Finally, the mental capacity to withstand the anxiety of the surgical ordeal is also of importance, but it is to be remembered that binocular bandaging which some aged people cannot easily tolerate is unnecessary.

PRE-OPERATIVE MANAGEMENT

Apart from the question of ocular or systemic disease, many authors in the past have emphasized the necessity for a detailed examination of the patient to eliminate any inflammatory or infective focus which may give rise to an endogenous post-operative infection. While the wholesale removal of such foci is unlikely to reduce significantly the incidence of post-operative complications, it is certainly worthwhile to deal with obvious dental infection, since the bacteræmia induced by dental sepsis of any degree is acknowledged. The presence of aural infection also requires attention, and bacteriological control of chronic suppurative otitis media is essential in view of the possible presence of *Ps. pyocyanea*.

Local preparation of the eye and the surrounding field for the operation is to some extent a matter for the surgeon's own choice. The establishment of patency of the lacrimal passages or at least the absence of evidence of infection of the sac is a sensible precaution, and dacryocystorhinostomy or dacryocystectomy should be considered in cases wherein any doubt arises. The value of conjunctival cultures, while necessary when infection seems possible, is very much a matter of opinion in clinically clean cases. Many surgeons claim that this is unnecessary, but there is something to be said for this practice since it provides the patient and the surgeon with the assurance that every possible and reasonable precaution is being taken for the security of the eye. Alternatively, the use of topical antibiotics as a preparatory measure is the routine practice of a number of surgeons, but is advocated by others only when there are special indications.

PRE-OPERATIVE MEDICATION has undergone striking changes during the past two decades, and the ambulant patient who was virtually unprepared for the considerable mental trauma of intra-ocular surgery has been succeeded by the properly prepared patient, adequately premedicated, who reaches the operating theatre relaxed and often asleep under the effects of the appropriate analgesic and hypnotic drugs. If general anæsthesia is preferred either by the patient or by the surgeon, the responsibility rests on the anæsthetist, who should be familiar with the requirements of ophthalmic surgery, to provide a quiet subject with an ocular tension adequately lowered by a halothane gas or other anæsthetic agent, and a post-operative recovery-period free from nausea or sickness.[1] Facial akinesia is a wise precaution even with general anæsthesia, and a retro-ocular injection is always advisable with a topical analgesic and also assists in lowering the intra-ocular pressure and attaining a laxity of the orbital contents which contribute to the successful and uncomplicated completion of the operation.

It is generally agreed that lowering the ocular tension prior to extraction of the lens decreases any tendency for the loss of vitreous. The most simple way to achieve this is by a retrobulbar injection of an analgesic which itself reduces the tension after one or two minutes, followed by simple digital massage of the globe, a technique first described by Atkinson (1955) and fully reviewed by Kirsch and Steinman (1955) and now widely followed (Hildreth, 1961; and others); this can usually reduce the tension to about 10 mm. Hg. Others have adopted the (perhaps unnecessary) procedure of hypotensive osmotic therapy (Friedman *et al.*, 1962) or acetazolamide (Agarwal and Malik, 1957; Gundzik and Mayer, 1963). It should be remembered, however, that this manœuvre cannot be accepted as eliminating the possibility of a loss of vitreous; indeed, Metz (1967) found in a series of 289 patients subjected to a retrobulbar injection and digital massage that the tension in 275 who had no loss of vitreous averaged 10·3 mm. Hg while in the 14 who suffered this complication the tension was 9·5 mm. Hg. It must be remembered, however, that excessive reduction of the ocular tension may add to the difficulty of making the incision. Finally, a further measure for the control of vitreous loss is the use of the Flieringa-Bonaccolto ring to support the globe during surgery in cases wherein this event is anticipated.

THE CHOICE OF OPERATION

In outlining the principles by which the method of treatment is determined in a particular case it must be acknowledged that the best technique is that which produces the most consistent results in the hands of an individual surgeon. In this review no attempt will be made to dogmatize, but general consideration will be given to the different surgical techniques and the indications for each.

In younger patients, up to 20 years of age, a primary discission followed if necessary by curette evacuation provides a safe, if sometimes tedious method of treatment; alternatively a suction procedure may be preferred which has the advantage of removing some if not most of the lens matter at a single operation. Intracapsular extraction became transiently popular in this age-group with the advent of alpha-chymotrypsin, but was soon abandoned when the danger of extracting a cataract in the presence of

[1] Moore (1955), Failing (1955), Atkinson (1955), Condon (1956), Mietus *et al.* (1959), Anderson (1959), Fasanella (1963–65), Esposito (1965), and others. See Vol. VII, p. 603.

vitreo-lental adhesions became evident; the same considerations, of course, apply more emphatically to congenital cataract.

In the third decade curette evacuation (linear extraction) and extra-capsular extraction are both practicable methods with no undue attendant risk. The latter method remains a satisfactory operation for patients in their fourth decade, but above this age intracapsular extraction with the aid of alpha-chymotrypsin is safe and if undertaken with suitable pre-cautions it achieves a satisfactory result without undue danger. In the fifth and sixth decades intracapsular extraction is indicated, and the old view that myopia, previous inflammation, a fluid vitreous or other patho-logical changes contra-indicate total extraction has been disproved. Zonulysis[1] as a routine is frequently employed in patients between the ages of 40 and 60 years; indeed, the availability of this adjunct to cataract surgery has played a considerable part in the increased popularity of intra-capsular extraction in patients in the fourth and fifth decades.

Over the age of 60 years intracapsular extraction is a fully established technique, and the use of alpha-chymotrypsin remains a matter of opinion, for at least a proportion of surgeons do not think any additional aid is required to rupture the zonule mechanically in such patients, and certain complications have been reported from its routine use[2]; these, however, are rare if the enzyme has been thoroughly washed out of the eye after 2 or 3 minutes. Zonulysis can well be used in selected cases in this group in which experience with the first eye has indicated the possibility of an abnormal risk attendant upon the routine intracapsular procedure, either because of associated vitreous loss or the early or late post-operative development of a retinal detachment.

CATARACT EXTRACTION IN ADULTS

So much has been written about the details of operative technique in cataract surgery during the past twenty years that it would be difficult to mention, let alone summarize, the extensive literature; for this purpose text-books on ophthalmic surgery should be consulted.

Whereas the use of a simple lid-speculum gives rise to few problems with extra-capsular extraction, its use in intracapsular surgery presents the difficulty that pressure on the globe will almost certainly cause vitreous loss. To safeguard against this, special specula have been devised modifying the original instrument of Arruga (1930) in which adjustable arms are supported by the bony prominences around the orbit. A more effective method which relieves all pressure on the globe is to employ lid-sutures passed through the skin near the lid-margins (2 in the upper and 1 in the lower) (Horner, 1935) or attached to the mosquito lid-clamps introduced by Castroviejo (1939) and later simplified (1965), the sutures in either case being held or fixed to the surgical drapes by hæmostatic forceps.

Fixation of the globe, in addition to the use of fixation forceps when making the section, is advisable with any type of anæsthesia and is necessary with general

_____

[1] Vol. VII, p. 714.   [2] p. 286.

anæsthesia; it is most conveniently attained by a fixation (bridle) suture through the tendon of the superior rectus muscle and fixed to the head-towel by hæmostatic forceps (Elschnig, 1914–31).

Wound-closure, at one time completely neglected and then usually achieved with one or two conjunctival sutures, has now become increasingly (and often unnecessarily) complicated. There is no doubt that the rapid healing of the wound depends both upon the cleanness of the incision and its adequate closure. The latter implies the use of sutures; their main advantages are that the incidence of post-operative hyphæmata, prolapse of the iris or epithelial ingrowth is reduced, while the added security makes prolonged immobility after surgery unnecessary. In this connection, however, it should be remembered that the rapid and uncomplicated healing of the eye and the comfort of the patient depend to a considerable extent on the rapidity of the operation and a minimum of traumatic interference; an elaborate system of sutures which may require up to half-an-hour for their insertion and tying is therefore bad surgery.

An almost innumerable number of sutures of different type and complexity has been suggested[1]; in nature they may be conjunctival, corneal, conjunctivo-scleral, corneo-scleral or corneo-conjunctivo-scleral. To a certain extent the individual type used depends on the incision employed, but at least one corneo-scleral suture is advisable which is preferably inserted before the incision is made to avoid mis-alignment and subsequent distortion of the wound and unnecessary manipulation of the globe after the eye has been opened; at the least, a post-sectional suture should be introduced through a track marked before the cornea and sclera have been separated. Whether the sutures are of silk and are subsequently removed (not always an easy procedure) or are allowed to remain subconjunctivally, or are of absorbable catgut so that no subsequent manipulations are required, as well as the number employed, are matters of choice for the individual surgeon. In all circumstances, however, and particularly in the case of corneal sutures, these should penetrate only the outer half of the tissue lest epithelialization occur along their tracks; non-absorbable sutures are most safely removed by the 7th post-operative day to forestall infiltration and necrosis along their tracks with the subsequent hindrance to rapid fibroblastic repair (Dunnington and Regan, 1950–52).

A conjunctival flap adequately covering the complete length of the incision is a further necessity for satisfactory closure of the wound unless a corneal incision is particularly indicated (as when a filtering scar for an operation for glaucoma is already present). Such a flap ensures rapid sealing of the wound and is the most effective measure against an epithelial downgrowth (Dunnington, 1951). When the incision is made with a keratome or a knife *ab externo* and completed with scissors, it must be fashioned and temporarily reflected over the cornea before the incision is made.

Ideal closure of the wound therefore entails a cleanly cut incision, the presence of an adequate conjunctival flap, firm approximation of the lips of the wound by sutures without distortion, and these ends should be effected by a technique as rapid, non-traumatic and uncomplicated as possible; to this end the incision itself, the preparation of the conjunctival flap and the use of sutures should all be designed.

The making of the corneo-scleral incision has been extensively discussed in the literature, the relative merits of vertical, sloping, and stepped incisions all having their supporters.[2] Undoubtedly, the classical simple incision with a Graefe knife involving at the same time the fashioning of a conjunctival flap is the most elegant, most rapid and atraumatic technique, but many surgeons have abandoned it for other methods partly because of the desire to insert several appositional sutures before the incision

[1] For reviews, see Spratt (1928), O. R. Wolfe and McLeod (1932), Ellett (1937), J. M. McLean (1940), Hughes and Owens (1945), D. P. Bell (1949), Hudson (1951), Pape (1967), and many others.
[2] See Dobree (1959).

is completed and partly because its successful accomplishment demands a high degree
of operative skill and more constant practice than is often available. Alternative
methods are the use of a keratome or of an *ab externo* incision with either a scalpel-
handle and disposable blade or one of a number of instruments in which the cutting
agent is a segment of a razor blade; in either case, the wound is enlarged by corneal
scissors. Whatever technique is used the incision must be adequate to enable the lens
to be extracted without the use of unnecessary force to deliver it through the wound,
but not of greater size than is necessary for its easy removal. An inadequate wound will
increase the risk of rupture of the capsule and of endothelial damage due to the manipulation of instruments over the inner surface of the cornea.

The relative merits of an extraction leaving a round pupil or an enlarged aperture
with a full iridectomy have been widely discussed in the literature, the reasons given by
the proponents of one or other technique varying to some extent with their own special
interests. In cases of complicated cataract wherein the iris is heavily bound down to
the lens with posterior synechiæ, a complete iridectomy may be desirable, and this is
necessary when vitreous presents at or through the wound immediately the incision
is completed so that an extraction by a vectis may be required. Incidentally, in order
to avoid a post-operative iridocyclitis, every endeavour should be made to deliver a
complicated cataract by the intracapsular technique. The possibility of post-operative
closed-angle glaucoma is also advanced as a reason for a complete iridectomy, as also
is the difficulty of making an adequate examination of an aphakic detachment of the
retina through a round pupil after the extraction. The main objects of iridectomy
in intracapsular extraction are to prevent post-operative pupillary blockage and
prolapse of the iris; these complications can be prevented by one or two small basal
iridectomies leaving the pupillary margin untouched, with the optical and cosmetic
advantages that this entails. Whereas it is probably true to say that there is no
established place for a simple extraction without any iridectomy, too much prominence
is given to the controversy concerning operations leaving a round pupil and those
involving a complete iridectomy. In general, an intact pupil is desirable when it can
be obtained at no extra risk and is usually to be preferred, although no great disability
follows a sector iridectomy.

In the extraction of the lens, as we have seen in the preceding section,
two main techniques are available. In the EXTRACAPSULAR OPERATION the
two important factors are to use an instrument which will remove an adequate area of the anterior lens capsule to allow the easy delivery of the
nucleus, and the removal of as much soft lens matter as possible at the time
of surgery. These principles have led to a preference for the use of toothed
capsule forceps as a means of opening and removing the capsule rather than
the classical and simpler method of incising it with a cystitome (Figs. 287–8).
Subsequent irrigation of the anterior chamber is generally carried out and,
in addition to ensuring the absolute sterility of the solution employed,
attention to its temperature and constitution is important to minimize
endothelial damage. Finally, the wound should be carefully freed from
iris and capsule and atropine instilled.

Kelman (1967) has found that a senile cataract may be aspirated satisfactorily
after emulsification by ultrasonic radiation.

The subsequent CAPSULOTOMY which is required if the posterior capsule
remains intact should be undertaken soon after the eye has become quiet

lest its subsequent consolidation make the needling unnecessarily difficult and traumatic. At this stage the operation is easy while the posterior capsule is still elastic, and a small opening some 3 or 4 mm. in diameter made with a needle-knife is all that is required, for a larger rent may allow a herniation of the vitreous. If stout bands exist which cannot be left untouched, these are most safely severed by dividing a few fibres at a time, or the strand is fixated with the aid of a second needle lest forceful and repeated traction lead to the development of a hyphæma or a traumatic iridocyclitis or result in a dislocation of the lens capsule or detachment of the retina. When an organized membrane exists or considerable proliferation of the epithelium of the anterior capsule has occurred, a CAPSULECTOMY may be

FIGS. 287 and 288.—EXTRACAPSULAR CATARACT EXTRACTION.
(H. B. Stallard, *Eye Surgery*, John Wright & Sons, Bristol.)

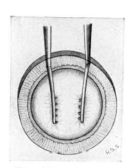

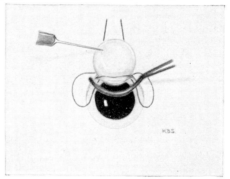

FIG. 287.—A wide anterior capsulectomy is made with toothed capsular forceps.

FIG. 288.—The extraction of a cataract from the right eye, showing the delivery of the lens by Arruga's expressor aided by a cystitome.

desirable through a keratome incision. The problems presented by an aftercataract of this type have already been noted.[1]

INTRACAPSULAR EXTRACTION is now undoubtedly accepted as the method of most general application, and for this procedure each surgeon has his own technique. It is difficult to assess the relative merits of the several methods which have been and are still being described in the literature. Generally, there are three principles underlying the operation: (1) the freeing of the lens by rupture or solution of the zonule, (2) the expression or extraction of the lens within its intact capsule and with minimal endothelial damage to the cornea, and (3) the closure of the wound without the loss of vitreous (Figs. 289–91). Rupture of the zonule was originally achieved mechanically by traction on the lens with counter-pressure below over the zonular fibres, using either the classical tumbling method (Knapp, 1915;

[1] p. 233.

FIGS. 289 to 291.—INTRACAPSULAR CATARACT EXTRACTION.

(H. B. Stallard, *Eye Surgery*, John Wright & Sons, Bristol.)

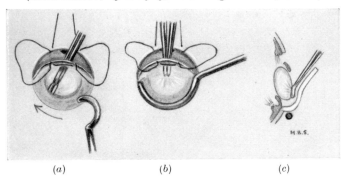

(a)   (b)   (c)

FIG. 289—*a*. Rotation of the lens by the capsular forceps from the 6 to the 8 o'clock position with counter-pressure at the limbus at 4 o'clock. *b*. The lens is lifted forward and is separated by Arruga's expressor below. *c*. Section to show the forward lift of the lens.

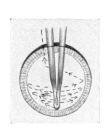

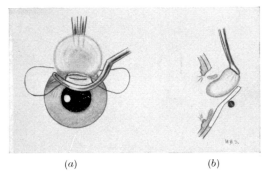

(a)   (b)

FIG. 290.   FIG. 291.

FIG. 290.—Diagrammatic representation of the approximate extent of the rotation of the lens with the capsular forceps before the suspensory ligament is adequately ruptured as indicated by the dotted line.

FIG. 291.—*a*. Delivery of the tumbled lens by gentle forceps traction followed by the expressor. *b*. Section to show the position of the forceps, the lens and the expressor.

Elschnig, 1932; H. Arruga, 1933; and many others) or by sliding the lens (Verhoeff, 1927; Kirby, 1949). More recently the introduction of zonulysis by J. Barraquer (1958) using alpha-chymotrypsin has greatly facilitated the successful practice of intracapsular surgery, certainly after the age of 40 years. Direct mechanical separation of the zonule was described by Kirby (1949) as a safe, conservative and valuable technique which facilitates its delivery in difficult cases and has been practised by others (Callahan, 1967).

Several methods of removal and delivery of the lens have been practised. The most simple is by direct external pressure (as by a strabismus hook) at the lower part of the limbus as was widely practised in India by H. Smith (1910–26); this, however, was not generally employed owing to the danger of the loss of vitreous until the use of zonulysis has made it again safe and easy (Ellis, 1961; and many others). The alternative method is by traction aided by a less degree of pressure. This has usually been done by specially designed forceps, either by direct action as initially used by Kalt (1894) and modified by many others such as Knapp (1914), Elschnig (1922) or H. Arruga (1933), or cross-action forceps (Sinclair, 1932; Castroviejo, 1939), many types of which have been developed. Extraction by a loop (or vectis) as practised by Pagenstecher (1865) is now used only when a viscid vitreous appears anterior to the lens after the incision is made or in cases of displacement of the lens. Suction devices were successfully developed for clinical use such as the erisophake of Ignacio Barraquer (1917) and have been subsequently improved in simplicity and reliability, as by the simple stiff rubber bulb introduced by A. E. Bell (1948) (Fig. 292). This technique is particularly valuable in the extraction of hypermature cataracts with tense capsules, but several surgeons have used the method as a routine. Similarly, the two-pronged electro-diaphake of Lacarrère (1932) has occasionally been employed. Finally, the cryo-extraction introduced by Krwawicz (1960) has impressed many surgeons by its ease and by the advantage that the grip on the capsule

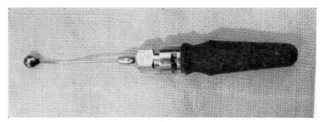

FIG. 292.—ERISOPHAKE
Modified from the original instrument of A. E. Bell with a cup on the left and a stout rubber bulb on the right (A. C. Esposito).

is reinforced by the freezing of a small area of lens substance immediately under it so that little or no external pressure is required[1] (Fig. 293). The number of useful and sophisticated cryosurgical instruments available is continuing to increase, using such agents as liquid or other forms of carbon dioxide, liquid nitrogen or the Peltier effect due to the passage of a direct current through two dissimilar metals and, as with the erisophake, their reliability and ease of manipulation are improving.[2] The practical use of such instruments, involving traction rather than pressure from below in the extraction of the lens, makes it necessary that the surgeon should acquire a new technique, and an adequate exposure is necessary to allow the introduction of the instrument without the possibility of its adhesion to the cornea or iris during its manipulation; damage to the corneal endothelium is particularly to be avoided (Taylor and Dalburg, 1968) (Figs. 294–5). If in any of these techniques the capsule is ruptured, the operation is continued as an extracapsular extraction.

[1] Goleminova (1962), Paramei and Kozlov (1963), Wilczek (1963), Conway (1965), Krwawicz (1965–67), Algan (1967), Wilczek and Kahl (1967), Metz (1967), Busti (1967), Rubinstein (1967–68), Penner and Holland (1968), Taylor and Dalburg (1968), Worthen and Brubaker (1968), and many others.
[2] Kelman (1965), Amoils (1965–67), Rubinstein (1965), Fodor (1967), du Toit (1967), Sanders (1967), Worthen and Brubaker (1967), Edwards et al. (1967), Shea (1967), Worst (1968), and others.

The difficult problem of the combined treatment of cataract and glaucoma when both occur together in the same eye and require surgery will be discussed at a later stage.[1]

When the lens is extracted intracapsularly, miosis should be induced to prevent a herniation of the vitreous with the use of 2% pilocarpine or intracameral acetyl-choline (Amsler and Verrey, 1949; J. Barraquer, 1964; Catford and Millis, 1967), or intracameral carbamylcholine chloride (carbachol) (Beasley *et al.*, 1968). As a final step it is a wise procedure to fill the anterior chamber with air or saline in order to push the iris backwards from the wound to restore to some extent the intra-ocular pressure and

FIG. 293.—A CRYOPROBE.
As used for cataract extraction (K. Rubinstein).

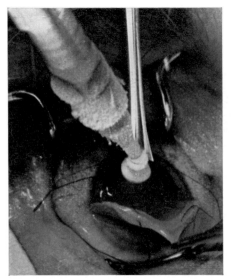 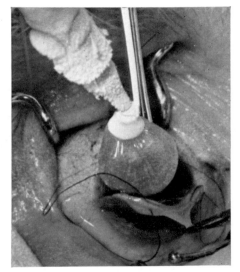

FIG. 294.   FIG. 295.
FIGS. 294 and 295.—CRYO-EXTRACTION OF THE LENS (K. Rubinstein).

to minimize the likelihood of a prolapse of the vitreous into the anterior chamber. Finally, the root of the iris should be freed from the wound leaving a central and symmetrical miotic pupil.

The post-operative care after the extraction of a cataract does not involve the prolonged immobilization of the patient that was common practice before effective sutures were employed. In the absence of complications, only the eye which was operated on requires protection by a pad covered by a cartella or aluminium shield fixed to the forehead and cheek by adhesive strapping; particularly if the anterior chamber has been

[1] p. 555.

filled with air a semi-Fowler position with a back-rest is the safest; and if his general health requires it, the patient can be allowed to sit in a chair and use a commode the day following the operation. The wound is rapidly healed[1]; the epithelium and endothelium have usually coapted by the second day and the conjunctival flap is usually sealed down after 24 hours; stromal healing, commencing anteriorly, is firm in 10 days and is complete after 3 weeks. Dark glasses may be substituted for the dressing in 7 days although it is wise to cover the eye with a shield during the night for a further week lest the patient inadvertently rub his eyes during sleep. It is usually safe to send the patient home on the 10th day. If the eye remains congested and shows signs of iridocyclitic irritation, atropine may be administered on the 4th or 5th day and topical corticosteroids somewhat later.

While this may be taken as a safe routine, many surgeons advise more lax measures. Some avoid a pad and bandage and rely only on a shield. Others would shorten the period in hospital to 8 or 6 days. Indeed, extraction has been conducted as an " office procedure " and the patient sent home or to a hotel with instructions to " take it easy " after secure suturing and with the protection of a metal shield over the dressing; no significant difference has been claimed between the prognosis in these cases and those which have been in hospital (Ching, 1958; Jervey and Brown, 1963; Beard, 1967). This may be so, but most surgeons would be more conservative.

The Complications of Cataract Extraction

The complications which may follow an operation for the extraction of cataract seem to comprise a formidable list, but their incidence is relatively rare and serious eventualities need only be expected in less than 4% of cases. Most of these are described in other Volumes of this *System* so that a brief mention is all that is required in this connection.

1. An EXPULSIVE HÆMORRHAGE is a rare but disastrous event which usually occurs in aged patients with vascular disease and hypertension immediately after the intra-ocular pressure has been lowered on completing the incision, or occasionally some hours or days after surgery. It may be expected to occur in some 0·2% (Vail, 1965) or 0·36% of cases (Müller, 1966). The symptoms and pathology of the condition have already been described[2] as well as the fact that, apart from exceptional cases wherein an immediate sclerotomy has given relief, the only expedient usually available is evisceration of the globe.

2. PROLAPSE OF THE VITREOUS in any quantity during the operation is an unpleasant complication, particularly if the gel is formed and not fluid and degenerated; if it is (as in a highly myopic eye), it is rapidly replaced by intra-ocular fluid with little untoward effects. Before operation on an eye wherein this accident is to be expected (as after its previous occurrence in the fellow eye) several precautionary measures may be taken—the production of absolute akinesia, including the extra-ocular muscles by a retrobulbar injection of anæsthetic, the absence of all pressure on the globe, the previous use of hypotensive agents such as acetazolamide or oral glycerol combined with digital pressure on the globe and, if necessary, the use of Flieringa's ring. With modern surgery the incidence should not be higher than 3%

[1] Vol. VIII, p. 604.   [2] Vol. IX, p. 29.

(Vail, 1965; Müller, 1966; Kettesy, 1967). If the prolapse occurs immediately after the section is made, a complete iridectomy and extraction by a vectis is usually necessary, at the same time making sure that all pressure is taken off the globe. If it accompanies or follows extraction of the lens, a corneo-scleral suture should be immediately tightened, the prolapsed knuckle of vitreous excised flush with the incision, the wound freed from vitreous as much as possible by an iris repositor or cyclodialysis spatula, a miotic instilled and the anterior chamber filled with air after the remaining sutures have been tied to remove the gel as much as possible from the wound. The sequels which may follow such a prolapse may be serious: defective coaptation of the lips of the wound into which the iris and pupil may be drawn (a deformity which may be prevented by a sphincterotomy diametrically opposite at 6 o'clock), a high degree of astigmatism, retinal detachment, bullous keratopathy and corneal opacities, œdema of the optic disc and macula, and iridocyclitis which may progress to shrinkage of the globe. In general, statistics show that approximately 6% of such eyes are lost within a year and usually within two months, and of the remainder 18% have no useful vision after a year and only 20% have vision better than 6/18 after 3 years; after 3 years, however, the chances of retaining this vision are high (Vail, 1965).

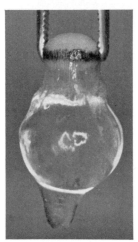

FIG. 296.—ADHESION OF THE HYALOID LAYER OF THE VITREOUS TO THE LENS CAPSULE.

The preparation was kept in formalin before the photograph was taken, after removal of the cornea from an excised eye. The intact vitreous body could be pulled out of the globe by pulling only on the lens (R. J. Wolter).

After an uncomplicated intracapsular extraction some prolapse of the vitreous into the anterior chamber is the rule which may be considerable if the hyaloid face has ruptured.[1] A post-operative rupture of the hyaloid face may occur usually between 14 and 28 days after operation with a prolapse of vitreous often accompanied by some temporary pain and circumcorneal injection. Jaffe and Light (1966) found that this occurred in 32% of round-pupil extractions and in 38% when a sector iridectomy had been made. In some cases wherein the prolapse is considerable, the vitreous may adhere to the wound, a complication which may occur up to 3 months after surgery; while in many cases the prolapse is associated with a posterior detachment of the vitreous,[2] in which case vitreous adhesions to the macular region may result in the development of macular œdema and even of cystoid macular degeneration with the loss of central vision. The types of prolapse which may occur will be discussed at a later stage.[3]

An adhesion of the hyaloid layer of the vitreous to the capsule of the lens, usually associated with a persistent hyaloid artery, a condition relatively common in early life,[4] may result in the unfortunate complication of the loss of a considerable amount of vitreous during an intracapsular extraction (Fig. 296) (Vail, 1954; Reese and Wadsworth, 1958; Wolter, 1961).

3. A PROLAPSE OF THE IRIS usually occurs within 48 hours after the operation but may be a late event appearing 10 to 15 days later when this tissue becomes incarcerated between the lips of the wound or even protrudes beneath the conjunctival flap or escapes from beneath it. In the first case, in the early stages the iris may be freed by the use of strong miotics, but if this is unsuccessful it should be stroked back

into the anterior chamber provided it has remained under the conjunctival flap; if it has escaped beyond it the prolapsed tissue should be excised. A late prolapse has a tendency to increase progressively since the section tends gradually to open; in this event it should be removed. An *ab externo* incision is made and pre-placed sutures inserted when it is half-way through the limbus, the iris should be freely abscised and the wound covered with a pre-formed conjunctival hood-flap.

4. A HYPHÆMA is a relatively frequent post-operative occurrence, usually appearing in a small percentage of patients between the 3rd and 5th days but sometimes up to the 7th day. Its incidence is not affected by systemic disease except that it is more common in diabetes and blood dyscrasias. It probably arises from tearing of the new-formed vessels bridging the corneo-scleral wound and is therefore less common with efficient suturing, and is generally caused by a sudden movement or inadvertent interference with the eye usually during sleep; in this event the sudden pain awakens the patient who, in his immediate confused anxiety, may interfere further with the eye. In the vast majority of cases the blood absorbs within 7 days only occasionally leaving some staining of the corneal endothelium or a vitreous haze which may diminish the vision for some months; significant permanent damage, however, is rare (Spencer, 1967). In a few cases a total hyphæma, particularly if the ocular tension is raised, requires paracentesis and washing out with urokinase.[1]

Cyclonamine (Dicynone; Ethamsylate; diethylammonium 1,4-dihydroxy-3-benzenesulphonate), a synthetic hæmostatic drug, has been favourably reported to prevent or diminish post-operative hæmorrhage, given the day before and 2 to 3 hours before surgery either intramuscularly (500 mg. each time) or by mouth (Stucchi and Nouri, 1962; Vicari, 1963–64; Hypher and Carpenter, 1968).

5. DELAYED HEALING with re-opening of the incision is a rare event characterized by a loss of aqueous usually causing a shallow anterior chamber some days after the operation and the possible development of a cystoid cicatrix. It tends to occur after a corneal incision and may be associated with the incarceration of the capsule, iris or vitreous in the wound, or with the presence of tight and deep corneo-scleral sutures giving rise to necrosis and fistulization. Re-suturing of the wound may be necessary followed by the formation of a conjunctival hood-flap, and usually an injection of air into the anterior chamber.

6. A CILIO-CHOROIDAL DETACHMENT, as we have seen,[2] is very common indeed immediately after an extraction operation, and a clinically observable detachment occurs some days after surgery in 10 to 15% of cases. This is associated with a shallowness or absence of the anterior chamber and usually with a delayed closure of the surgical wound. Most cases resolve without sequel within 2 to 3 weeks; if the detachment persists for a long period, atrophic and pigmentary changes may appear in the fundus and corneal opacities and an iridocyclitis may develop, but the greatest danger lies in the formation of peripheral anterior synechiæ owing to the collapse of the anterior chamber with the consequent development of a secondary glaucoma. This danger becomes acute if the anterior chamber does not show signs of re-forming before 2 weeks. In such cases the incision should be carefully searched for leakage, a procedure aided by the instillation of fluorescein, and any fistula closed by cauterization and a conjunctival hood-flap. Further persistence may require to be dealt with by aspiration of the suprachoroidal fluid and filling the anterior chamber with air.

7. A DELAYED RE-FORMATION OF THE ANTERIOR CHAMBER arises when the pressure behind the iris-diaphragm is greater than that in the anterior chamber (Christensen, 1967); this is sometimes but not invariably associated with a cilio-choroidal detachment. As we have seen, this complication is usually the result of a leaking wound; if present this should be treated as already indicated, and after the re-suturing of the

[1] Vol. IX, p. 23. [2] Vol. IX, p. 952.

wound an injection of air into the anterior chamber is usually advisable. Alternatively, the condition may be due to pupillary blockage (Etienne, 1967); this may be combatted by mydriasis, or by a large peripheral iridectomy and the injection of air into the anterior chamber to separate the vitreous and iris from the cornea, if necessary through the approach of a cyclodialysis.[1] A deepening of the chamber may be induced by the use of hypotensive agents such as acetazolamide (Rettinger and Meyer-Schwickerath, 1967) or osmotic therapy such as oral glycerol (A. B. and A. L. Radian, 1967; Bucci and Neuschüler, 1967; Leone and Callahan, 1967). In all cases it is unwise to leave the chamber collapsed for more than a few days lest extensive peripheral synechiæ develop. A final resort, particularly in cases of persistent cilio-choroidal detachment, is aspiration of the vitreous cavity, particularly of any aqueous pooled at the posterior pole.[2]

8. An ŒDEMA OF THE POSTERIOR POLE, sometimes involving a papillœdema and usually a macular œdema, is a not uncommon event after an uncomplicated cataract extraction, occurring in perhaps 2% of cases. The latter lesion is the more serious since it may eventually lead to cystoid degeneration and permanent impairment of central vision. This sequence has been described by a number of authors[3] and the leak of œdematous fluid into the optic disc and the central area of the retina has been demonstrated by fluorescein angiography[4] (Figs. 297–300). Most authors have concluded that the œdema is due to the mechanical traction of vitreo-retinal adhesions (Tolentino and Schepens, 1965); but the impossibility of demonstrating these by biomicroscopy of the vitreous as well as the occurrence of exudative vitreous opacities led Gass and Norton (1966) to conclude that some cases are inflammatory in origin. However that may be, the condition is a serious and a potentially disappointing sequel to a technically good operation (Fig. 369).

9. CORNEAL CHANGES following cataract surgery are infrequent, but are of great importance as they tend to cause persistent irritability of the eye in addition to their severe effect on the visual results. Changes in the corneal curvature are almost constant; they have been studied with ophthalmometric methods which have demonstrated a reduction in curvature of both the anterior and posterior surfaces (Alajmo, 1950; Floyd, 1951; Franco Lara, 1958). The resulting corneal astigmatism can be considerably minimized if the lips of the wound are accurately aligned and their subsequent slight separation is prevented by accurate suturing. Giardini and Cambiaggi (1956) found a post-operative increase in corneal thickness which they thought was related to a hyperhydration of the cornea accentuated by excessive manipulation within the anterior chamber; on the other hand, Lange (1954) found no outstanding factor as a cause of such corneal swelling other than a predisposition in glaucomatous eyes. The most common corneal complication is *striate keratopathy* due to rucking of Descemet's membrane[5]; this is a temporary phenomenon of little importance. A marked *corneal œdema* may follow a split in or a detachment of Descemet's membrane, usually as a result of damage from instruments introduced into the eye; in such cases the corneal opacity tends to clear after several months (Sugar, 1967), but an extensive stripping of this membrane may be treated by the injection of air into the anterior chamber and replacing it with a cyclodialysis spatula (Sparks, 1967). Corneal anæsthesia with a dystrophic keratopathy leading to the development of bullous keratopathy[6] is an intractable condition, the treatment of which has been frequently disappointing[7]; the use of Gundersen's flaps (Sugar, 1964) and of puncture of Bowman's membrane with diathermy (Salleras's method) has recently been described (Accinelli, 1964). The management of a corneal endothelial dystrophy with acrylic corneal inlays has been

[1] p. 544.　　　　　　　　[2] p. 370.
[3] Irvine (1953), Nicholls (1954–56), Chandler (1954), Welch and Cooper (1958), Reese and Carroll (1958), Tolentino and Schepens (1965), Reese *et al.* (1966), Gehring (1968).
[4] Novotny and Alvis (1961), Justice and Sever (1965), Gass and Norton (1966).
[5] Vol. VIII, p. 705.　　　　[6] Vol. VIII, pp. 669, 671.　　　　[7] Vol. VIII, p. 674.

FIGS. 297 to 300.—MACULAR ŒDEMA AND PAPILLITIS FOLLOWING
CATARACT EXTRACTION (J. D. M. Gass and E. W. D. Norton).

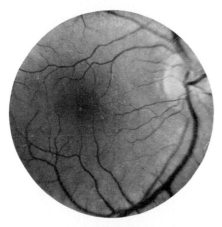

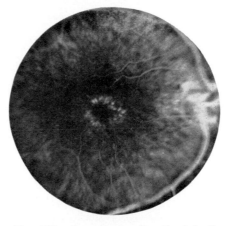

FIG. 297.—The fundus showing slight and hardly visible stellate changes indicative of cystoid œdema of the macula.

FIG. 298.—One minute after the injection of fluorescein showing leakage of the dye into the macular area.

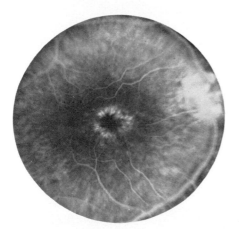

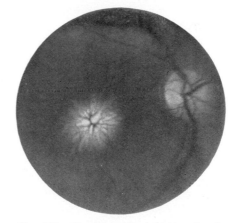

FIG. 299.—Progressive leakage of the dye around the macula.

FIG. 300.—One hour after injection showing a stellate figure surrounded by fluorescein pooled within intraretinal cystoid spaces.

described by Choyce (1965–66) and the results appear to be more encouraging than those of previously described methods of treatment. In the presence of this condition, intracameral manipulations should be reduced to a minimum and alpha-chymotrypsin should, if possible, not be used. *Corneal opacities* sometimes associated with a bullous keratopathy, as we have seen, may develop as a result of prolonged contact with vitreous prolapsed into the anterior chamber or with the iris and vitreous resulting from a failure in the re-formation of the anterior chamber, while very occasionally a dystrophic condition may develop for no apparent reason some months after an uncomplicated extraction.

10. An EPITHELIAL INGROWTH is a serious condition unusually difficult to treat.

FIGS. 301 and 302.—EPITHELIAL INGROWTHS (N. Ashton).

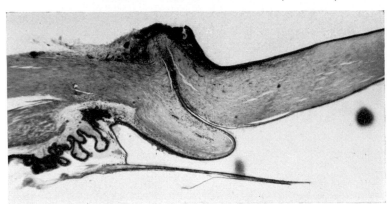

FIG. 301.—Epithelialization of the anterior chamber following cataract extraction. The corneal section has healed only superficially and the deeper portion of the wound, the corneal endothelium and the posterior surface of the iris stump are completely lined with squamous epithelium (H. &. E.; × 30).

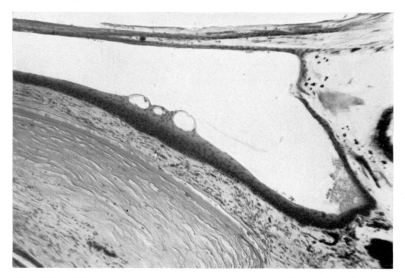

FIG. 302.—High-power view showing the squamous epithelium on the posterior aspect of the iris which is adherent to the cornea. The epithelium can be traced round the surface of the ciliary body and over a fine cyclitic membrane. Bullous formation is present in the epithelium (H. & E.; × 135).

It is generally caused by a delayed closure of the wound, particularly if any ocular tissue is incarcerated in it. In this event the vigour of the regeneration of the epithelium enables it rapidly to line the lips of the wound and spread down the inner surface of the cornea, over the trabeculæ, the anterior surface of the iris and the vitreous in several stratified layers of cells (Figs. 301–2); occasionally localized epithelial cysts are formed which may attain a considerable size (Wheeler, 1956) (Fig. 303). This epithelial ingrowth has been produced experimentally by D. R. Smith and his colleagues (1967) by reversing a disc of the cornea so that the epithelium faced inwards. With the slit-lamp the ingrowth appears as a characteristic thin grey veil on the inner surface of the cornea spreading downwards from the wound, and over the iris as a film frequently spotted with pigment granules and swollen goblet cells. The results are usually disastrous: a dystrophic keratitis is accompanied by an irritative iritis, and a recalcitrant secondary glaucoma tends to follow the blockage of the drainage channels, a complication which usually requires the ultimate excision of the globe unless the epithelialization ceases in the upper segment of the eye. The frequency of this type of secondary glaucoma will be discussed at a later stage.[1]

Treatment is difficult. If a fistulous wound is eliminated, surgical removal of the epithelium from the inner surface of the cornea has been attempted (Long and Tyner, 1957) or its destruction by alcohol and curetting (Maumenee, 1957; Sullivan, 1967), but a more effective procedure for this aspect of epithelial invasion is cryosurgery, a procedure which may also be used to destroy a localized cyst (Ferry and Naghdi,

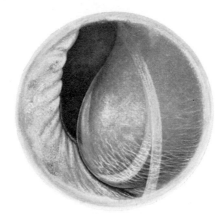

Fig. 303.—Traumatic Implantation Cyst after a Cataract Extraction.

In a patient aged 74, two years after surgery. There was a deep striate keratitis and a large transparent cyst arising from the limbal area at 2 o'clock, filling half the anterior chamber and extending into the pupillary area (J. R. Wheeler).

1967), while photocoagulation of the growth over the anterior surface of the iris is sometimes successful (Maumenee, 1964). These measures are probably more promising than irradiation either by x-rays or such agents as strontium-90, as has frequently been attempted (Anton, 1967).

11. UVEITIS. A post-operative iridocyclitis may develop on the 3rd or 4th post-operative day, usually mild and irritative in nature in intracapsular extractions and readily controlled by atropine and steroids unless there has been a loss of vitreous. In extracapsular extractions, however, it may be more severe, particularly when much soft matter remains behind mixed with vitreous. When this occurs in an eye sensitized to lenticular protein, the resulting phaco-anaphylactic uveitis may be severe and may become disastrous when a second extracapsular extraction or a discission is performed after sensitization has been acquired by a similar operation on its fellow. Such a lens-induced uveitis and its treatment are described elsewhere,[2] as well as the occasional occurrence some weeks after a uniocular extracapsular extraction of a similar inflammation in the fellow eye if it also harbours a cataract.[3] A sympathetic uveitis is a

[1] p. 719.

[2] Vol. IX, p. 500.   [3] Vol. IX, p. 506.

FIGS. 304 and 305.—POST-OPERATIVE MYCOTIC ENDOPHTHALMITIS
(B. S. Fine and L. E. Zimmerman).

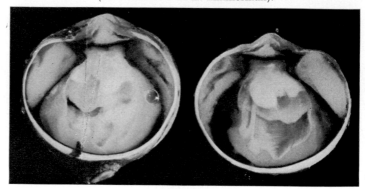

FIG. 304.—Enucleated eye opened in the vertical plane showing the purulent exudate in the vitreous cavity and the anterior chamber. A serous exudate fills the suprachoroidea detaching the ciliary body and the peripheral choroid and also occupies the subretinal space beneath the detached retina.

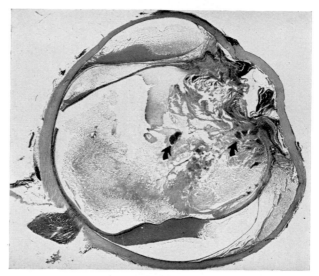

FIG. 305.—The dense infiltration of the ciliary body and the iris with acute and chronic inflammatory cells. The anterior vitreous is infiltrated diffusely with polymorphonuclear leucocytes and there are several micro-abscesses indicated by arrows. The scar of the surgical incision is seen on the upper limbus.

rare sequel of an extraction unless it has been complicated by loss of vitreous or the incarceration of the ocular tissues in the wound.[1]

12. OCULAR INFECTIONS used to be a very serious complication of cataract extractions but since the use of antibiotic drugs this menace has become much less serious, for the incidence of bacterial infection has been more effectively prevented and when it does occur its course more adequately controlled. This subject has already been

[1] Vol. IX, p. 564.

discussed[1] when it was pointed out that statistics show that prior to 1945 such infections occurred in some 1% of extractions and since that time have been reduced to 0·1%. Most of these are immediate infections due to contamination at the time of surgery either from the patient's ocular adnexa or the appurtenances of the theatre including eyedrops and solutions used for washing out the anterior chamber. Some are still serious; thus Allen and Mangiaracine (1964) reported 26 such cases of which 10 eyes had to be eviscerated and 7 developed phthisis. As a prophylactic measure, subconjunctival injections of an antibiotic have mainly been advocated.[2] Unfortunately, the widespread use of antibiotics and steroids has been accompanied by an increase in fungal infections,[3] the infection being derived either from the patient's conjunctival sac or through spores in the theatre; these are more difficult to treat than bacterial infections and may well be destructive[4] (Figs. 304–5).

Late infections, however, may occur some months or years after the operation usually associated with a badly healed or fistulous wound with the incarceration of uveal tissue in it (Fig. 306). These cases are less virulent than immediately post-

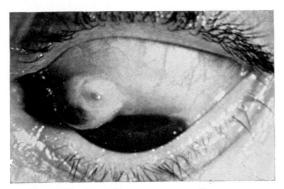

FIG. 306.—LATE POST-OPERATIVE INFECTION.

After a cataract operation a prolapse occurred; 3 years later the bleb became exogenously infected: its appearance one day after the infection was noted. The eye settled after topical treatment with polymyxin B and scopolamine (H. S. Sugar and T. Zekman).

operative infections and may resolve with rapid and effective treatment, but if the vitreous has become infected the visual results are poor (Sugar and Zekman, 1958).

13. A SECONDARY GLAUCOMA following a cataract extraction is a not unusual event occurring in some 1 to 7% of cases after an extracapsular extraction with a further similar figure after capsulotomy, and in about 2% after an intracapsular operation. The rise in tension may result from several causes, such as pupillary blockage by vitreous or (in extracapsular operations) by lens substance or exudates from a postoperative iridocyclitis, delayed re-formation of the anterior chamber (12% of cases after 8 days; 44% of cases after 10 to 12 days), iridocyclitis, loss of vitreous, hyphæma or hæmorrhage into the vitreous, while a phacogenic glaucoma may result from an anaphylactic reaction, or a recalcitrant glaucoma may develop one or more years after surgery owing to an epithelial ingrowth. The characteristics of these types of glaucoma

[1] Vol. IX, p. 49.
[2] Pearlman (1956), Cassady (1967), Chalkley and Shoch (1967).
[3] Vol. IX, p. 383.
[4] Greetham and Makley (1957), Foster et al. (1958), Fine and Zimmerman (1959), Posner (1959), Theodore et al. (1961–62), Küper (1962), Diamond and Kirk (1962), de Almeida (1963).

and their treatment are discussed elsewhere.[1] It is interesting that after an uncomplicated operation the eye is usually hypotensive for some weeks (Roberts, 1968).

14. A RETINAL DETACHMENT is a relatively rare sequel of a cataract extraction which has been discussed in a previous Volume.[2] This unfortunate accident occurs most frequently in myopic eyes and statistics show that it may be expected in some 2% of operations whether extra- or intra-capsular, although this figure is considerably increased in the first case by a somewhat higher figure following capsulotomy, particularly when the capsule has been tough and repeated needlings have been required. In both types of extraction a post-operative detachment usually occurs within the first four post-operative years, often before the first, and it usually follows a loss of vitreous particularly when this has become incarcerated in the wound along with capsular remnants.[3] The advisability of prophylactic treatment for such eyes by photocoagulation or cryosurgery has been discussed elsewhere.[4]

15. A PROLIFERATION OF THE CAPSULAR EPITHELIUM is an unpleasant sequel of an extracapsular extraction; when much of the anterior capsule remains a Soemmerring's ring may form. The prevention of these manifestations of an after-cataract, their clinical characteristics and treatment are discussed elsewhere.[5]

16. COMPLICATIONS ARISING FROM ZONULYSIS deserve a short note, but there are few if the enzyme is thoroughly washed out of the anterior chamber within 2 or 3 minutes. It has been said that healing of the wound is retarded (Townes, 1960; Radnót and Pajor, 1960; McWilliam, 1961), while on histological examination of patients who died soon after an operation, an absence of reparative activity was claimed by Landolt and Heinzen (1960); in their large controlled series of cases, however, neither Remky (1962) nor Tokunaga (1966) could find any significant signs of this complication. A delayed re-formation of the anterior chamber was found by Verdi and his colleagues (1960) and Radnót and Pajor (1960) but not by Paliaga and Cornelio (1960), while Matteucci (1959) and Leydhecker (1961) concluded that herniation of the vitreous was accentuated. Endothelial damage to the cornea was reported by Orlowski (1960) and Honegger (1963) and corneal vascularization by Hill (1959). Degenerative changes visible with the electron microscope were produced by Tokunaga (1966) in the eye of the rabbit only if the enzyme were injected in high concentration and allowed to remain for a long period (4 to 20 minutes). If the enzyme is introduced experimentally into the vitreous of this animal, degenerative changes may similarly appear in the retina (Vail *et al.*, 1960), but this has been recorded clinically only exceptionally and if the vitreous itself were degenerate (Radnót and Pajor, 1960). The occurrence of a secondary glaucoma will be noted elsewhere.[6] In general, it would therefore appear that complications need not be feared if the enzyme is used with caution in patients over the age of 30 or preferably 40 years provided the wound is adequately sutured, there is no evidence of a dystrophy of the corneal endothelium, and the enzyme is washed away sufficiently soon. This should be done even although there is some evidence that the enzyme may be inactivated to some extent by the anti-chymotrypsin activity of the eye (Lee and Lam, 1968).

DISCISSION AND EVACUATION

In young patients the abundance of soluble and relative scarcity of insoluble protein in the lens as well as the smallness of the nucleus make surgical treatment of a cataract by discission and evacuation a suitable procedure; in very young eyes a discission, which may have to be repeated, may suffice, but over the age of two years evacuation of the lens material is

[1] Chapter IX. [2] Vol. X, p. 786. [3] pp. 370, 374.
[4] Vol. X, p. 824. [5] p. 233. [6] p. 720.

usually advisable. Any such operation should be done only under full mydriasis which should be maintained post-operatively for several weeks or months; alternatively, a sector iridectomy should be performed as a prophylactic measure against post-operative pupillary blockage.

In DISCISSION the cortex and nucleus of the lens are broken up by a knife-needle in cross-shaped incisions or by multiple incisions, but the through-and-through V-shaped discission advocated by Ziegler (1921) may involve complications owing to the mixing of vitreous with lens material and the onset of glaucoma. If the ocular tension rises some days after the discission, an evacuation of the lens substance should be undertaken.

EVACUATION may be practised at the same time as the discission in a single procedure in children under the age of 6 years. Moncreiff (1946–59) frequently succeeded in obtaining a clear pupil in an operation wherein the needling was immediately followed by irrigation by a fine irrigator introduced through the needle-puncture so that the soft lens material was washed out of the capsular sac into the anterior chamber. Following the initial procedure of the Arabian surgeons, Rhazes and Ammar, re-introduced in the middle of last century by French and English surgeons, the discission may be combined with aspiration through a syringe or a tube, sometimes combined with lavage with a needle-cannula.[1]

A LINEAR EXTRACTION wherein the opaque lens substance is expressed with the aid of a curette introduced through a keratome incision followed by irrigation is perhaps the most commonly employed technique. It is often undertaken some days after a discission but may be performed in very young children as an initial procedure if the lavage is sufficiently thorough (Roy, 1968).

Complications unfortunately follow these procedures in a considerable number of cases and for this reason a single surgical interference is preferable to multiple operations. These include a secondary glaucoma usually as a result of pupillary blockage, prolapse of the iris or incarceration of tags of capsule, prolapse of the vitreous, iridocyclitis, a phaco-anaphylactic reaction when the fellow eye is operated on in bilateral cases and, at a later stage, detachment of the retina. The last is relatively common particularly after multiple operations and may be expected in some 10% of cases,[2] a circumstance which should contra-indicate such a procedure when it is unnecessary, as in the treatment of myopia in young patients. Finally, as complete an evacuation as is possible of the lens substance should be achieved to avoid the formation of an excessive after-cataract with the difficulties which its treatment may entail.[3]

In young children the most common complication is the development of secondary glaucoma due to pupillary blockage and resulting in the formation of peripheral anterior synechiæ. To prevent this unfortunate sequel which may end disastrously, Chandler (1968) recommended the performance of a sector iridectomy together with two peripheral iridectomies and three sphincterotomies.

[1] Dean (1926), Wilder (1928), Blaess (1938), Wolfe (1955), Scheie (1960), Carbajal (1961), Fasanella (1963), Allen (1966), Girard (1967), Scheie *et al.* (1967), Hogan (1967), Parks and Hiles (1967), Rice (1967), and others.
[2] Vol. X, p. 787.   [3] p. 233.

The historical operation of RECLINATION or DEPRESSION of a cataract as practised in ancient or mediæval times is most safely undertaken with Lang's twin-knives, one of which has a sharp tip, the other a blunt. The first is introduced into the anterior chamber and then rapidly withdrawn without the loss of aqueous; the second is inserted through the corneal puncture and used to force the lens backwards and downwards until it lies on the retina anterior to the equator. Thereafter the patient is nursed sitting up in bed or in an easy chair. Such an operation is now rarely performed but may occasionally be legitimate in dealing with a dislocated lens occupying the pupillary area[1] or a cataract in an old and frail patient whose life-expectancy is not sufficiently long to allow time for the development of a phacolytic uveitis, a glaucoma or a retinal degeneration or detachment.

THE VISUAL CORRECTION OF AN APHAKIC EYE

Although the results of cataract surgery are usually technically excellent in uncomplicated cases with a reasonably tractable patient, the functional results are not so favourable particularly in the case of the nervous or aged. With the simple method of correction by *aphakic spectacles*, the loss of accommodation, the restriction of the visual field, the concentric scotoma in the near periphery and the distortion of contours outside the visual axis together constitute a formidable problem which is usually resolved in a relatively short time by an intelligent and adaptable patient but may remain indefinitely incapacitating with the anxious and unadaptable type. To these are added the difficulty of diplopia in uniocular cases with some vision in the fellow eye, for the image of an aphakic eye corrected by spectacles is one-third larger than that of a normal eye, a degree of aniseikonia which cannot be resolved and necessitates the occlusion of the fellow eye or the blurring of its image by an equally strong lens. These difficulties are fully discussed in the Volume on Optics[2]; but their seriousness has led to the use of contact lenses or intra-ocular implants in an endeavour to restore to the aphakic eye some of the advantages and adaptability of natural vision.

CONTACT LENSES[3]

A contact lens reduces the size-difference in an aphakic eye to between 4% and 10% so that binocular vision is usually possible although the aniseikonia is almost at the limit of toleration for the maintenance of binocular single vision[4]; moreover, the visual field is enlarged, the prismatic distortion caused by aphakic spectacles is abolished and the annoying circular scotoma

---

[1] See Rambo (1955), Good and Ratnaraj (1968).
[2] Vol. V.   [3] See Vol. V.
[4] Williamson-Noble (1938), Mann (1938–47), Town (1939), von Györffy (1940), Jaensch (1942), Neill (1946), and many others.

is absent, while the loss of accommodation is easily overcome by the use of presbyopic spectacles. The development of corneal lenses in place of the older haptic corneo-scleral lenses has greatly increased their use and although some disappointing results have been reported most surgeons have obtained excellent results in suitable patients.[1] It is interesting that suppression of the vision may develop following a traumatic cataract, and in this respect F. Ridley (1953) found that the important time-interval is between the damage to the lens and the operation, rather than between the latter and the fitting of the contact lens. The patients thus treated, however, must be carefully chosen; such lenses have the disadvantages of being expensive, time-absorbing in their fitting and re-fitting, frequently uncomfortable to wear although this is considerably diminished with the semi-anæsthetic cornea following the surgical incision, and may occasionally damage the cornea; moreover, to the aged and incoordinate type of patient who is so frequently affected by senile cataract, their insertion and removal is often impossible, an objection, however, to some extent overcome by the use of the corneal rather than the haptic type of lens.

INTRA-OCULAR IMPLANTS

An intra-ocular lenticulus produces a smaller image than a contact lens thus facilitating binocular vision in uniocular aphakia and results in the best type of optical correction, provided complications do not occur; in eyes thus treated, binocular vision is frequently attained with ease (Hirtenstein, 1961). The pioneer in the development of this technique was H. Ridley (1951–57) who implanted an acrylic lenticulus with the appropriate optical correction within the lens capsule behind the iris some time after an extracapsular extraction wherein all soft lens substance had been removed at the time of operation and the posterior capsule remained intact. The novelty and difficulty of the technique stimulated few surgeons to exploit it.[2] Although Ridley himself at first obtained a considerable proportion of good visual results, these could not be compared with those obtained by the classical methods of surgery and aphakic spectacle correction, while a high proportion of complications occurred such as dislocation of the lenticulus, the profuse deposition of pigment, and the development of an exudative uveitis, sometimes necessitating the removal of the lens or even of the eye. Several pathological examinations from such eyes have confirmed these findings (R. Smith, 1956; François et al., 1956; Rintelen and Saubermann, 1956; Ashton and Choyce, 1959).

These results led to the abandonment of this type of operation but

[1] Hirtenstein (1950), F. Ridley (1953), Rosenbloom (1953), Dyer and Ogle (1960), Neill (1962), Figueroa and Barreau (1963), Abel (1963), Torres (1964), Riehm and Thiel (1965), and many others.
[2] A. Arruga (1951), Charamis (1952), de Roetth (1953), J. A. McLean (1953), Anton (1953), Gupta (1953), H. and A. Arruga (1954), Barraquer-Moner (1955), François et al. (1956), and others.

they stimulated the use of *anterior chamber implants*, a technique introduced by Strampelli (1953–55). Several modifications of the mode of fixation have been introduced, the optical portion being always in the anterior chamber (Figs. 307–12). Strampelli's (1953) original implant was steadied by a rigid frame resting in the angle of the anterior chamber, an elastic frame similarly placed was used by Dannheim (1957–62), while its flanges may be made to penetrate into the limbus (Strampelli, 1954). An alternative is fixation onto the iris or (in extracapsular extractions) onto the iris and the lens capsule (Binkhorst, 1959–67; Binkhorst and Leonard, 1967). To these original suggestions other surgeons have introduced modifications (J. Barraquer, 1956; Choyce, 1958–66; Epstein, 1959; Boberg-Ans, 1961; and

FIGS. 307 to 312.—LENS IMPLANTS (C. D. Binkhorst).

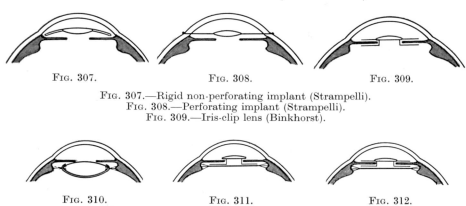

FIG. 307.   FIG. 308.   FIG. 309.

FIG. 307.—Rigid non-perforating implant (Strampelli).
FIG. 308.—Perforating implant (Strampelli).
FIG. 309.—Iris-clip lens (Binkhorst).

FIG. 310.   FIG. 311.   FIG. 312.

FIG. 310.—The original posterior chamber lens of Ridley.
FIG. 311.—Irido-capsular lens (Binkhorst).
FIG. 312.—Iris-clip and irido-capsular lens (Binkhorst).

others), but the technique is not altogether free from complications such as corneal dystrophies or uveitis (Zorab, 1962).

In an eye into which the original type of implant introduced by Strampelli had been inserted 6 weeks previously, Ashton and Choyce (1959) found some distortion of the corneo-iridic angle with ciliary atrophy, a localized inflammatory reaction and macular œdema. Somewhat similar results were obtained histologically by Ashton and Boberg-Ans (1961) in the examination of an eye into which a Boberg-type implant had been inserted (Figs. 313–5). To some extent the intense uveitis which sometimes occurs with any type of implant may be due to the method of storage and sterilization. Acrylic material, for example, adsorbs cetrimide to a sufficient extent to act as an irritant when introduced into the eye (F. Ridley, 1957). Binkhorst and Flu (1956) described a method of sterilization using ultra-violet light, but this is associated with changes in the surface layer of the plastic; implants are now usually stored in a weak solution of caustic soda.

In general, while the use of implants in the anterior chamber can produce the best post-operative optical results and is the safer of the two

FIGS. 313 to 315.—ANTERIOR CHAMBER IMPLANTS.

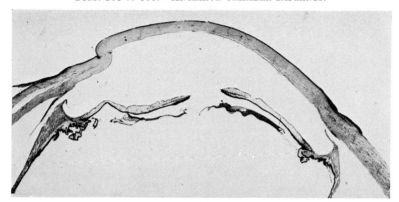

FIG. 313.—Histology of the anterior segment in an eye which received an anterior chamber implant of the Strampelli type. The corneo-iridic angles are distorted to form cups of dystrophic tissue extending outwards and backwards into the ciliary body. Remnants of the lens are seen behind the iris (N. Ashton and D. P. Choyce).

FIGS. 314 and 315.—THE ANGLE OF THE ANTERIOR CHAMBER IN AN EYE WHICH RECEIVED AN ANTERIOR CHAMBER IMPLANT OF THE BOBERG-ANS TYPE (N. Ashton and J. Boberg-Ans).

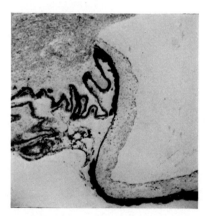

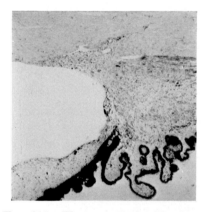

FIG. 314.—The angulation and retroversion of the iris are well seen but the trabeculæ and Schlemm's canal are normal. There are delicate adhesions between the iris and the ciliary body (× 34).

FIG. 315.—The root of the iris showing atrophy and a mild inflammatory reaction in the neighbouring tissues (× 34).

techniques, most surgeons are disinclined to use them as a routine. It can well be argued that while the results of a cataract extraction are usually so good and the use of contact lenses so safe and easy (in selected cases) it is perhaps unwise to gamble on further surgical procedures which require considerable specialized technical skill and a healthy eye on which to operate, the results of which in the absence (at present) of long-term observations are somewhat problematical.

It may be noted that Cavka (1956) made the unique suggestion of substituting the lens of a cadaver for a cataractous lens; in the case reported the transplanted lens was clear after six months.

Abel. *Optom. Wkly.*, **54**, 1647 (1963).
Accinelli. *Arch. Oftal. B. Aires*, **39**, 123 (1964).
Agarwal and Malik. *Ophthalmologica*, **133**, 153 (1957).
Alajmo. *G. ital. Oftal.*, **3**, 439 (1950).
Algan. *Canad. J. Ophthal.*, **2**, 169 (1967).
Allen, H. F., and Mangiaracine. *Arch. Ophthal.*, **72**, 454 (1964).
Allen, J. C. *Amer. J. Ophthal.*, **62**, 1141 (1966).
de Almeida. *Rev. bras. Oftal.*, **22**, 53 (1963).
Arnoils. *Trans. ophthal. Soc. U.K.*, **85**, 577 (1965).
    Arch. Ophthal., **78**, 201 (1967).
Amsler and Verrey. *Ann. Oculist.* (Paris), **182**, 936 (1949).
Anderson. *General Anœsthesia* (Ed. Evans and Gray), London, **2**, 264 (1959).
Anton. *Arch. Soc. cubana Oftal.*, **3**, 93 (1953).
    Klin. Mbl. Augenheilk., **150**, 675 (1967).
Arruga, A. *Arch. Soc. oftal. hisp.-amer.*, **11**, 1490 (1951).
Arruga, H. *Arch. Oftal. hisp.-amer.*, **30**, 593 (1930).
    Bull. Soc. franç. Ophtal., **46**, 270 (1933).
    Cirurgia ocular, Barcelona (1945).
Arruga, H. and A. *Rev. esp. Oto-neuro-oftal.*, **13**, 1 (1954).
Ashton and Boberg-Ans. *Brit. J. Ophthal.*, **45**, 543 (1961).
Ashton and Choyce. *Brit. J. Ophthal.*, **43**, 577 (1959).
Atkinson. *Anesthesia in Ophthalmology*, Springfield (1955).
Barraquer, I. *An. Med. Cir.*, **2**, 57 (1917).
Barraquer, J. *Trans. ophthal. Soc. U.K.*, **76**, 537 (1956); **79**, 393 (1959).
    Klin. Mbl. Augenheilk., **133**, 609 (1958).
    Amer. J. Ophthal., **57**, 406 (1964).
Barraquer, J., and Bailbé. *Bull. Scc. Ophtal. Fr.*, 567 (1958).
Barraquer-Moner. *Ann. Oculist.* (Paris), **188**, 364 (1955).
Beard. *Eye, Ear, Nose, Thr. Mthly.*, **46**, 989 (1967).
    Arch. Ophthal., **77**, 577 (1967).
Beasley, Borgmann, McDonald and Belluscio. *Arch. Ophthal.*, **80**, 39 (1968).
Bell, A. E. *Amer. J. Ophthal.*, **31**, 610 (1948).
Bell, D. P. *Amer. J. Ophthal.*, **32**, 639 (1949).
Binkhorst. *Trans. ophthal. Soc. U.K.*, **79**, 569 (1959).
    Ophthalmologica, **139**, 500 (1960).
    Brit. J. Ophthal., **46**, 343 (1962); **51**, 767, 772 (1967).
    Klin. Mbl. Augenheilk., **151**, 21 (1967).
Binkhorst and Flu. *Brit. J. Ophthal.*, **40**, 665 (1956).
Binkhorst and Leonard. *Amer. J. Ophthal.*, **64**, 947 (1967).

Blaess. *Arch. Ophthal.*, **19**, 902 (1938).
Boberg-Ans. *Brit. J. Ophthal.*, **45**, 37 (1961).
Bucci and Neuschüler. *Boll. Oculist.*, **46**, 116 (1967).
Busti. *Ann. Ottal.*, **93**, 44 (1967).
Callahan. *Amer. J. Ophthal.*, **63**, 316 (1967).
Carbajal. *Amer. J. Ophthal.*, **52**, 361 (1961).
Cassady. *Amer. J. Ophthal.*, **64**, 1081 (1967).
Castroviejo. *Amer. J. Ophthal.*, **22**, 1018 (1939).
    Trans. Amer. ophthal. Soc., **63**, 355, 358 (1965).
Catford and Millis. *Brit. J. Ophthal.*, **51**, 183 (1967).
Cavka. *Docum. ophthal.*, **10**, 373 (1956).
Chalkley and Shoch. *Amer. J. Ophthal.*, **64**, 1084 (1967).
Chandler. *Trans. Amer. Acad. Ophthal.*, **58**, 382 (1954).
    Amer. J. Ophthal., **65**, 663 (1968).
Charamis. *Bull. Soc. hellen Ophtal.*, **20**, 155, 183, 340 (1952).
Ching. *J. int. Coll. Surg.*, **29**, 429 (1958).
Choyce. *Trans. ophthal. Soc. U.K.*, **78**, 459 (1958); **80**, 201 (1960); **86**, 507 (1966).
    Brit. med. J., **2**, 609 (1959).
    Lancet, **1**, 90 (1960).
    Brit. J. Ophthal., **49**, 432 (1965).
Christensen. *Amer. J. Ophthal.*, **64**, 600 (1967).
Condon. *Brit. J. Anœsth.*, **28**, 80 (1956).
Conway. *Brit. J. Ophthal.*, **49**, 141 (1965).
Dannheim. *Ber. dtsch. ophthal. Ges.*, **60**, 267 (1957).
    An. Inst. Barraquer, **3**, 570 (1962).
Dean. *Trans. Amer. Acad. Ophthal.*, **31**, 261 (1926).
Diamond and Kirk. *Amer. J. Ophthal.*, **51**, 1124 (1962).
Dobree. *Brit. J. Ophthal.*, **43**, 513 (1959).
Dunnington. *Amer. J. Ophthal.*, **34**, 36 (1951).
Dunnington and Regan. *Arch. Ophthal.*, **43**, 407 (1950).
    Amer. J. Ophthal., **35**, 167 (1952).
Dyer and Ogle. *Amer. J. Ophthal.*, **50**, 11 (1960).
Edwards, Woodget, Mueller and Ludek. *Brit. J. Ophthal.*, **51**, 415 (1967).
Ellett. *Arch. Ophthal.*, **17**, 523 (1937).
Ellis. *Amer. J. Ophthal.*, **51**, 26 (1961).
Elschnig. *Klin. Mbl. Augenheilk.*, **52**, 262 (1914).
    Ber. dtsch. ophthal. Ges., **43**, 168 (1922).
    Z. Augenheilk., **75**, 1 (1931).
    Die intrakapsulare Starextraktion, Berlin (1932).
Epstein. *Brit. J. Ophthal.*, **43**, 29 (1959).
Esposito. *Brit. J. Ophthal.*, **37**, 61 (1953); **46**, 697 (1962).
    Sth. med. J. (Bgham, Ala.), **58**, 992 (1965).

Etienne. *Ann. Oculist.* (Paris), **200,** 729 (1967).
Failing. *Calif. Med.,* **82,** 32 (1955).
Fasanella. *Complications in Eye Surgery,* Phila. (1957 ; 1965).
 Modern Advances in Cataract Surgery, Phila. (1963).
Ferry and Naghdi. *Arch. Ophthal.,* **77,** 86 (1967).
Figueroa and Barreau. *Arch. chil. oftal.,* **20,** 58 (1963).
Fine and Zimmerman. *Amer. J. Ophthal.,* **48,** 151 (1959).
 Brit. J. Ophthal., **43,** 753 (1959).
Floyd. *Amer. J. Ophthal.,* **34,** 1525 (1951).
Fodor. *Cs. oftal.,* **23,** 207 (1967).
Foster, Almeda and Littman. *Arch. Ophthal.,* **60,** 555 (1958).
Franco Lara. *Arch. Asoc. evit. Ceg. Mex.,* **1,** 417 (1958).
François, Rabaey and Evens. *Ann. Oculist.* (Paris), **189,** 923 (1956).
Friedman, Byron and Turtz. *Arch. Ophthal.,* **67,** 421 (1962).
Gass and Norton. *Trans. Amer. ophthal. Soc.,* **64,** 232 (1966).
Gehring. *Arch. Ophthal.,* **80,** 626 (1968).
Giardini and Cambiaggi. *Ophthalmologica,* **131,** 41 (1956).
Girard. *Arch. Ophthal.,* **77,** 387 (1967).
Goleminova. *Vestn. oftal.,* **75** (5), 74 (1962).
Greaves. *Trans. ophthal. Soc. U.K.,* **75,** 121 (1955).
Greetham and Makley. *Arch. Ophthal.,* **58,** 558 (1957).
Gundzik and Mayer. *Amer. J. Ophthal.,* **56,** 933 (1963).
Gupta. *Ophthal. J. Gandhi Eye Hosp.,* **3,** 13 (1953).
von Györffy. *Klin. Mbl. Augenheilk.,* **104,** 81 (1940).
Hildreth. *Amer. J. Ophthal.,* **51,** 1237 (1961).
Hill. *Brit. J. Ophthal.,* **43,** 325 (1959).
Hirtenstein. *Brit. J. Ophthal.,* **34,** 668 (1950).
 Trans. ophthal. Soc. U.K., **81,** 631 (1961).
Hogan. *Amer. J. Ophthal.,* **63,** 821 (1967).
Honegger. *Klin. Mbl. Augenheilk.,* **143,** 75 (1963).
Horner. *Amer. J. Ophthal.,* **18,** 33 (1935).
Hudson. *Ophthal. Lit.,* **5,** 3 (1951).
Hughes and Owens. *Amer. J. Ophthal.,* **28,** 40 (1945).
Hypher and Carpenter. *Brit. J. Ophthal.,* **52,** 375 (1968).
Irvine. *Amer. J. Ophthal.,* **36,** 599 (1953).
Jaensch. *Med. Klin.,* **38,** 131 (1942).
Jaffe and Light. *Arch. Ophthal.,* **76,** 541 (1966).
Jervey and Brown. *Amer. J. Ophthal.,* **56,** 58 (1963).
Justice and Sever. *Univ. of Miami neuro-ophthal. Symp.* (Ed. J. L. Smith), St. Louis, **2,** 82 (1965).
Kalt. *Arch. Ophtal.,* **14,** 639 (1894).
Kelman. *Trans. Amer. Acad. Ophthal.,* **69,** 353 (1965).

Kelman. *Amer. J. Ophthal.,* **64,** 23 (1967).
Kettesy. *Klin. Mbl. Augenheilk.,* **150,** 785 (1967).
Kirby. *Brit. J. Ophthal.,* **33,** 3 (1949).
Kirsch and Steinman. *Arch. Ophthal.,* **54,** 697 (1955).
Knapp, A. *Trans. Amer. ophthal. Soc.,* **13,** 666 (1914).
 Arch. Ophthal., **44,** 1 (1915).
Krwawicz. 28 *Cong. Pol. ophthal. Soc.,* Poznań (1960).
 Brit. J. Ophthal., **45,** 279 (1961).
 Trans. ophthal. Soc. U.K., **85,** 545 (1965).
 Klin. oczna, **37,** 801, 931 (1967).
Küper. *Klin. Mbl. Augenheilk.,* **140,** 827 (1962).
Lacarrère. *Klin. Mbl. Augenheilk.,* **88,** 778 (1932).
Landolt and Heinzen. *Ophthalmologica,* **139,** 313 (1960).
Lange. *Klin. Mbl. Augenheilk.,* **125,** 583 (1954).
Lee and Lam. *Amer. J. Ophthal.,* **66,** 528 (1968).
Long and Tyner. *Arch. Ophthal.,* **58,** 396 (1957).
Leone and Callahan. *Amer. J. Ophthal.,* **63,** 1686 (1967).
Leydhecker. *Klin. Mbl. Augenheilk.,* **138,** 381 (1961).
McLean, J. A. *Trans. canad. ophthal. Soc.,* **6,** 119 (1953).
McLean, J. M. *Arch. Ophthal.,* **23,** 554 (1940).
McWilliam. *Trans. ophthal. Soc. U.K.,* **81,** 105 (1961).
Mann. *Trans. ophthal. Soc. U.K.,* **58,** 109 (1938).
 Brit. J. Ophthal., **31,** 565 (1947).
Matteucci. *Ann. Ottal.,* **85,** 489 (1959).
Maumenee. *Trans. Amer. Acad. Ophthal.,* **61,** 51 (1957).
 Trans. Amer. ophthal. Soc., **62,** 153 (1964).
Metz. *Amer. J. Ophthal.,* **64,** 309 (1967).
 N.Y. St. J. Med., **67,** 3247 (1967).
Mietus, Hague and Carbone. *Amer. J. Ophthal.,* **47,** 487 (1959).
Moncreiff. *Amer. J. Ophthal.,* **29,** 1513 (1946).
 Wien. klin. Wschr., **71,** 902 (1959).
Moore. *Brit. J. Ophthal.,* **39,** 109 (1955).
Müller, H. *Wiss. Z. Univ. Greifswald,* **15,** 507 (1966).
Neill. *Amer. J. Optom.,* **23,** 399 (1946) ; **39,** 169 (1962).
Nicholls. *Amer. J. Ophthal.,* **37,** 665 (1954).
 Arch. Ophthal., **55,** 595 (1956).
Novotny and Alvis. *Circulation,* **24,** 82 (1961).
Orlowski. *Klin. oczna,* **20,** 365 (1960).
Pagenstecher. *Klin. Mbl. Augenheilk.,* **3,** 316 (1865).
Paliaga and Cornelio. *Ann. Ottal.,* **86,** 333 (1960).
Pape. *v. Graefes Arch. Ophthal.,* **173,** 199 (1967).

Paramei and Kozlov. *Vestn. oftal.*, **76** (3), 66 (1963).
Parks and Hiles. *Amer. J. Ophthal.*, **63**, 10 (1967).
Pearlman. *Arch. Ophthal.*, **55**, 516 (1956).
Penner and Holland. *Brit. J. Ophthal.*, **52**, 498 (1968).
Posner. *Eye, Ear, Nose, Thr. Mthly.*, **38**, 1051 (1959).
Radian, A. B. and A. L. *Ophthalmologica*, **153**, 277 (1967).
Radnót and Pajor. *Klin. Mbl. Augenheilk.*, **136**, 370 (1960).
Rambo. *Arch. Ophthal.*, **54**, 471 (1955).
Reese and Carroll. *Trans. Amer. Acad. Ophthal.*, **62**, 765 (1958).
  Amer. J. Ophthal., **45**, 659 (1958).
Reese, Jones and Cooper. *Trans. Amer. ophthal. Soc.*, **64**, 123 (1966).
Reese and Wadsworth. *Amer. J. Ophthal.*, **46**, 495 (1958).
Remky. *An. Inst. Barraquer*, **3**, 209 (1962).
Rettinger and Meyer-Schwickerath. *Klin. Mbl. Augenheilk.*, **150**, 665 (1967).
Rice. *Trans. ophthal. Soc. U.K.*, **87**, 491 (1967).
Ridley, F. *Trans. ophthal. Soc. U.K.*, **73**, 373 (1953).
  Brit. J. Ophthal., **41**, 359 (1957).
Ridley, H. *Trans. ophthal. Soc. U.K.*, **71**, 617 (1951).
  Brit. J. Ophthal., **36**, 113 (1952); **38**, 156 (1954); **41**, 355 (1957).
  J. int. Coll. Surg., **26**, 335 (1956).
Riehm and Thiel. *Klin. Mbl. Augenheilk.*, **146**, 589 (1965).
Rintelen and Saubermann. *Ophthalmologica*, **131**, 369 (1956).
Roberts. *Amer. J. Ophthal.*, **66**, 520 (1968).
de Roetth. *Amer. J. Ophthal.*, **36**, 1568 (1953).
Rosenbloom. *Amer. J. Optom.*, **30**, 536 (1953).
Roy. *Amer. J. Ophthal.*, **65**, 81 (1968).
Rubinstein. *Trans. ophthal. Soc. U.K.*, **85**, 555 (1965).
  Brit. J. Ophthal., **51**, 178 (1967).
  Adv. in Ophthal., **19**, 1 (1968).
Sanders. *Amer. J. Ophthal.*, **64**, 160 (1967).
Scheie. *Amer. J. Ophthal.*, **50**, 1048 (1960).
Scheie, Rubenstein and Kent. *Amer. J. Ophthal.*, **63**, 3 (1967).
Shea. *Canad. J. Ophthal.*, **2**, 163 (1967).
Sinclair. *Trans. ophthal. Soc. U.K.*, **52**, lvii (1932).
Smith, D. R., Somerville and Shea. *Canad. J. Ophthal.*, **2**, 158 (1967).
Smith, H. *The Treatment of Cataract*, Calcutta (1910).
  Arch. Ophthal., **55**, 213 (1926).
Smith, R. *Brit. J. Ophthal.*, **40**, 473 (1956).
Sood and Ratnaraj. *Amer J. Ophthal.*, **66**, 687 (1968).
Sparks. *Arch. Ophthal.*, **78**, 31 (1967).
Spencer. *Canad. J. Ophthal.*, **2**, 203 (1967).

Spratt. *Amer. J. Ophthal.*, **11**, 347 (1928).
Strampelli. *Atti Soc. oftal. Lombarda*, **8**, 292 (1953).
  Ann. Ottal., **80**, 75 (1954).
  Atti Cong. Soc. oftal. ital., **15**, 427 (1955).
Strauss and Ramsell. *Brit. J. Ophthal.*, **52**, 242 (1968).
Stucchi and Nouri. *Ther. Umschau*, **19**, 481 (1962).
Sugar. *Amer. J. Ophthal.*, **57**, 977 (1964); **63**, 140 (1967).
Sugar and Zekman. *Amer. J. Ophthal.*, **46**, 155 (1958).
Sullivan. *Trans. ophthal. Soc. U.K.*, **87**, 835 (1967).
Taylor and Dalburg. *Arch. Ophthal.*, **79**, 3 (1968).
Theodore, Littman and Almeda. *Arch. Ophthal.*, **66**, 163 (1961).
  Amer. J. Ophthal., **53**, 35 (1962).
du Toit. *Brit. J. Ophthal.*, **51**, 496, 500 (1967).
Tokunaga. *Folia ophthal. jap.*, **17**, 948 (1966).
Tolentino and Schepens. *Arch. Ophthal.*, **74**, 781 (1965).
Torres. *Arch. port. Oftal.*, **16**, 137 (1964).
Town. *Arch. Ophthal.*, **21**, 1021 (1939).
Townes. *Arch. Ophthal.*, **64**, 108 (1960).
Vail. *Trans. Amer. Acad. Ophthal.*, **58**, 367 (1954).
  Amer. J. Ophthal., **59**, 573 (1965).
Vail, Schwartz, B. and J. B., von Sallmann et al. *Trans. Amer. Acad. Ophthal.*, **64**, 16 (1960).
Verdi, Lasagni and Ranieri. *Ann. Ottal.*, **86**, 473 (1960).
Verhoeff. *Trans. Amer. ophthal. Soc.*, **25**, 54 (1927).
Vicari. *Praxis*, **52**, 124 (1963).
  Méd. et Hyg., **22**, 1072 (1964).
Welch and Cooper. *Arch. Ophthal.*, **59**, 665 (1958).
Wheeler. *Brit. J. Ophthal.*, **40**, 245 (1956).
Wilczek. *Klin. oczna*, **33**, 391 (1963).
Wilczek and Kahl. *Klin. oczna*, **37**, 949 (1967).
Wilder. *Trans. Amer. Acad. Ophthal.*, **33**, 113 (1928).
Williams. *Recent Advances in Ophthalmic Science*, Boston (1866).
  Arch. Ophthal. Otol., **1**, 98 (1869).
Williamson-Noble. *Trans. ophthal. Soc. U.K.*, **58**, 535 (1938).
Wolfe. *J. int. Coll. Surg.*, **23**, 739 (1955).
Wolfe and McLeod. *Arch. Ophthal.*, **8**, 238 (1932).
Wolter. *Amer. J. Ophthal.*, **51**, 511 (1961).
Worst. *Amer. J. Ophthal.*, **65**, 587 (1968).
Worthen and Brubaker. *Arch. Ophthal.*, **78**, 451 (1967); **79**, 8 (1968).
Ziegler. *J. Amer. med. Ass.*, **77**, 1100 (1921).
Zorab. *Trans. ophthal. Soc. U.K.*, **82**, 705 (1962).

CHAPTER IV

DISPLACEMENTS OF THE LENS

CORNELIUS REA AGNEW [1830–1888] (Fig. 316) is a suitable introduction to this Chapter inasmuch as he inaugurated a method for the surgical treatment of a posteriorly dislocated lens with the aid of a " bident " or twin-pronged needle (1885). It is interesting that the technique excited little attention at the time, comments being almost as frequently unfavourable as favourable, but almost a century later it has been revived and is the most popular method in use today. His other original advances in surgery included a new operation for divergent squint and a technique for dealing with a thickened capsule in secondary cataract. His greatest contributions to ophthalmology in America, however, were professional and social. He qualified at Columbia University in New York and was appointed surgeon to the New York Eye and Ear Infirmary (1855). As was usual in America at the time, he studied abroad—in Dublin under Sir William Wilde, in London under Sir William Bowman and George Critchett, and in Paris under Sichel and Desmarres. After his return he was made Surgeon-General to the State of New York (1858) and on the outbreak of the Civil War he became medical director of the New York Volunteer Hospital; thereafter he established the Brooklyn Eye and Ear Hospital (1868), the Manhattan Eye and Ear Hospital (1869), and at the request of the Faculty he established an ophthalmic clinic in the College of Physicians and Surgeons of New York (1866), becoming professor of ophthalmology and otology at Columbia College. He was the first President of the New York Ophthalmological Society (1864), and was one of the founder members of the American Ophthalmological Society and its President from 1873 to 1878. Intensely religious and greatly beloved, he spent much time in social and charitable activities and did most in his generation to establish ophthalmology, then just emergent in America, in the position it has still retained.

Normally the lens remains suspended by the fibres of the suspensory ligament so that its axis corresponds approximately to the visual line; it may become displaced owing to a congenital defect in the zonule or through disease or trauma whereby the suspensory apparatus is weakened so that the lens becomes tremulous or subluxated, or it is ruptured so that a complete dislocation occurs. The latter is a serious condition too frequently resulting in grave complications, particularly uveitis and glaucoma, which are unusually difficult to treat. For this reason the literature on the subject is large.[1]

A *hereditary* influence has been noted in the literature of the occurrence in adult life of a " spontaneous " dislocation of the lens, an accident possibly determined on a congenital basis. The longest pedigree of this type started by Vogt (1905) and completed by Wallmann and Ammann (1964) traced a family over 6 generations from

[1] For large series of cases, see Dorsch (1900), Stoewer (1901), Grob (1901), Hegner (1915), Ringelhan and Elschnig (1931), Knobloch (1931), McDonald and Purnell (1951), Nirankari and Chaddah (1967).

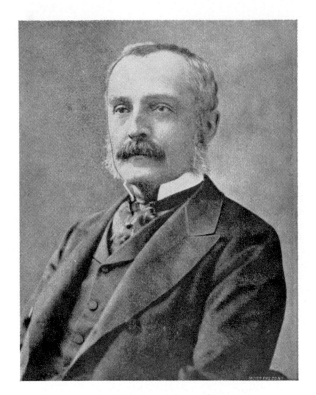

FIG. 316.—CORNELIUS REA AGNEW [1830–88].

1770, wherein a backward and downward dislocation occurred. In the pedigree studied by Falls and Cotterman (1943) dislocation occurred in 24 members between the ages of 3 and 70 years, 13 of them developing glaucoma. Harshman (1948) reported a family in which 10 out of 20 members in 3 generations had glaucoma, 6 of them having dislocated lenses, usually into the anterior chamber (Fig. 317). Anterior and posterior dislocations occurred in a mother and 4 children during the 4th decade of life in a family reported by Holtermann and Schmidt (1963).

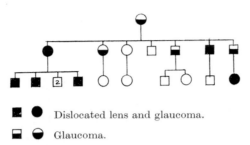

■ ● Dislocated lens and glaucoma.

▣ ◒ Glaucoma.

FIG. 317.—DISLOCATION OF THE LENS WITH GLAUCOMA.
(After J. P. Harshman, 1948.)

Displacements of the lens may be classified ætiologically into three types:

(a) congenital;

(b) traumatic;

(c) consecutive or spontaneous, resulting from intra-ocular disease giving rise to mechanical stretching, inflammatory disintegration or degeneration of the zonule.

The incidence of these three types varies in the statistics given by different authors, probably depending on the importance given to minor trauma: Table II gives some estimates from the literature. In general, the congenital cases are bilateral, the acquired unilateral, and in the latter the usual age for its occurrence is during the fifth and sixth decades.

TABLE II
THE TYPES OF DISPLACEMENT OF THE LENS

	Congenital %	Traumatic %	Consecutive or Spontaneous %
Mooren (1894)	10·8	31·9	57·3
Grob (1901)	14·4	56·8	28·8
Ringelhan and Elschnig (1931) .	12·9	56·2	30·9
Knobloch (1931)	17·1	62·3	20·6
McDonald and Purnell (1951) .	35	47	18
Nirankari and Chaddah (1967) .	18	22	60

CONGENITAL ECTOPIA of the lens, almost invariably a bilateral subluxation associated with defective fibrogenesis of the zonule, has already been described in a previous

Volume.[1] It is to be noted that in these cases a late dislocation of the lens may occur in adult life sometimes apparently spontaneously, sometimes after trauma, involving the same disabilities and liable to give rise to the same complications as those occurring without a congenital origin.   The ectopia is usually associated with the congenital mesodermal dystrophies (the syndromes of Marfan and less frequently of Marchesani[2]) or with homocystinuria,[3] less commonly with other systemic anomalies particularly affecting mesodermal tissues such as cutis hyperelastica (the Ehlers-Danlos syndrome),[4] proportional dwarfism, oxycephaly,[5] Crouzon's disease,[6] Sprengel's deformity,[7] or the Sturge-Weber syndrome.[8]

TRAUMATIC DISPLACEMENTS will be considered in a subsequent volume.[9]

CONSECUTIVE OR SPONTANEOUS DISPLACEMENTS

Displacements owing to mechanical stretching of the zonule are seen most commonly in conditions such as buphthalmos (von Hippel, 1897; Hegner, 1915), staphylomata or ectasias of the globe (Panas, 1894), or in high myopia (von Hippel, 1874; Hirschberg, 1876; Wagenmann, 1889; Halben, 1897; Ringelhan and Elschnig, 1931; and others). A similar accident may also follow the sudden strain resulting from the perforation of a large central corneal ulcer when, indeed, the lens may be completely extruded from the eye.   Cyclitic inflammatory adhesions may also pull the lens out of position, as may also the scar-tissue in Eales's disease (Cross and Choyce, 1953) or traction bands in the vitreous following the treatment of a retinal detachment by diathermy (Richards and Ellis, 1958); while intra-ocular tumours may push it out of place. Inflammatory destruction of the zonule occurs in panophthalmitis, when it may be completely disorganized; moreover, the same process is seen less dramatically in chronic inflammations when the zonule is invaded by cyclitic granulation tissue (von Michel, 1906; Ringelhan and Elschnig, 1931).   More usually, however, the cause is a degenerative or atrophic condition of the zonular fibres, a circumstance which, in view of the common origin of the two structures, is usually accompanied by degeneration and liquefaction of the vitreous gel.   This occurs particularly in high myopia, old choroiditis or cyclitis, in detachments of the retina, in the degenerative chemical changes associated with chalcosis (Goondorova, 1956), or merely as part of gradually increasing senile degeneration which involves fragility in the suspensory apparatus.   Finally, one of the most common causes is the development of hypermaturity in a cataract in which case the degenerative changes affect the zonule also, while at the same time it is stretched by shrinkage of the lens; the fact that dislocation of such lenses frequently occurs spontaneously or with great readiness in the manipulations during their removal, constitutes an argument of some weight against leaving a hypermature cataract to reach the shrunken stage.

Once the degeneration of the zonule has occurred, the actual dislocation of the lens may occur spontaneously by its own weight, or by some trauma,

[1] Vol. III, p. 710.   [2] Vol. III, p. 1102.   [3] Vol. IX, p. 646.
[4] Vol. III, p. 1111.   [5] Vol. III, p. 1040.   [6] Vol. III, p. 1048.
[7] Vol. III, p. 1060.   [8] Vol. III, p. 1124.   [9] Vol. XIV.

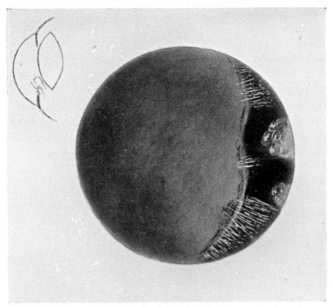

FIG. 318.—SPONTANEOUS SUBLUXATION OF THE LENS.
Showing two areas of vitreous prolapse (A. J. Bedell.)

frequently quite insignificant in degree, such as a strain or a cough. On dislocation the zonule may remain attached to the lens, in which case the fibres undergo a degeneration which renders them progressively more opaque (Fig. 318). A detachment at the ciliary insertion, however, is rare; more usually it occurs at the zonular lamella and the edge of the lens shows no

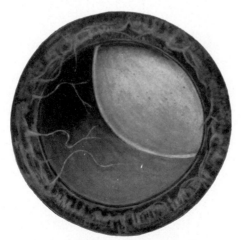

FIG. 319.—SUBLUXATION OF THE LENS.
There is no trace of a zonule; vestigial remains of the pupillary membrane are evident
(T. Harrison Butler).

fringe of fibres (Fig. 319).   In this event the whole suspensory apparatus is drawn behind the iris, although occasionally a portion of the suspensory ligament, having lost its ciliary attachment, is seen floating about associated with a fine pellucid membrane (the zonular lamella) (Fig. 59) (Meesmann, 1922; Maggiore, 1924; Jess, 1926; Stein, 1926; Busacca, 1927).

TREMULOUSNESS OF THE LENS on movements of the eye without its actual displacement is a rarity, but has been observed in anterior megalophthalmos and in a hypermature cataract (d'Ombrain, 1936); the phenomenon is probably due to a degenerated suspensory ligament and the presence of a fluid vitreous.

Displacements of the lens may be classified topographically as in the following scheme:

A. SUBLUXATION, the displaced lens remaining in the plane behind the iris in the patellar fossa.

B. LUXATION or DISLOCATION, when the lens is completely displaced from the patellar fossa, in which case it may appear:

  (i) incarcerated in the pupil;
  (ii) in the anterior chamber;
  (iii) in the vitreous, when it may either
      (a) float about—*lens natans*, or
      (b) become anchored—*lens fixata*;
  (iv) in the subretinal space, passing through a retinal tear, or in the subscleral space;
  (v) it may wander from one locality to the other (WANDERING LENS);
  (vi) it may be extruded out of the globe, either partially (PHACOCELE or LENTICELE), or completely, either through a perforating corneal ulcer, or through a traumatic rupture of the sclera, in which case it may rest subconjunctivally or under Tenon's capsule.

SUBLUXATION gives rise to visual symptoms varying in degree depending on the position occupied by the lens.   If it remains in its primary axis, the sole result may be the development of a lenticular myopia, since the curvature increases owing to relaxation of the suspensory apparatus.   Alternatively, however, it may be tilted on a vertical, horizontal or oblique axis, resulting in a marked astigmatism, which is always difficult and usually impossible to correct adequately with spectacles or contact lenses.   More usually, however, the lens becomes longitudinally displaced so that it almost fills the pupillary aperture, in which event the images are completely distorted by the myopic astigmatism of the equatorial region.   If the displacement is sufficient to become apparent in the pupil so that the lens occupies part of the pupillary aperture while the other part is aphakic, such a subluxation is accompanied by uniocular diplopia, an indistinct image being seen through the aphakic, and a distorted image through the phakic part.   The condition may be rendered still more difficult optically if the lens moves with alterations in the position of the head, for varying confusion images are then produced.

The objective signs accompanying such a subluxation are usually obvious. The anterior chamber is deep, and if some rotation of the lens has occurred the depth may vary in different sectors. Owing to the lack of its usual support, any movement of the eyes gives a readily marked tremulousness to the iris (*iridodonesis*). In focal illumination the lens appears grey, particularly in the equatorial region, owing to the increased internal reflection of light, and by ophthalmoscopic examination its edge, if it lies in the pupillary aperture, appears as a black crescent owing to the total reflection of the light coming from the fundus. The slit-lamp may show the reflex line running circumferentially around the posterior surface of the lens marking the attachment of the hyaloideo-capsular ligament and indicating that the anterior face of the vitreous is subluxated with the lens (Slezak, 1963); this attachment explains the frequent loss of vitreous which accompanies the extraction of such a lens. With the slit-lamp the zonular fibres may also be seen, sometimes stretched and sometimes torn, and in the aphakic area the anterior face of the vitreous may herniate forwards. Ophthalmoscopically a double image of the fundus may be seen, one through the phakic and the other through the aphakic area of the pupil.

Such a subluxated lens may remain in the pupillary aperture indefinitely, giving rise to no symptoms other than the optical disability. Occasionally, although relatively rarely, it eventually turns opaque, but alternatively, it may give rise to a uveitis or a secondary glaucoma.[1] A further complication is its complete dislocation, an event which may occur after remaining for many years in the patellar fossa.

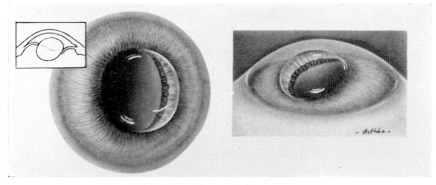

FIG. 320.—MARFAN'S SYNDROME.
Showing a dislocated lens blocking the pupillary aperture (A. C. Hilding).

DISLOCATION OF THE LENS is a more serious matter than its subluxation. It may be dislocated into the pupillary aperture where it becomes incarcerated (Fig. 320). This is a rare event usually occurring after trauma, when the lens may suffer an axial rotation through 90° so that its equator

----
[1] p. 659.

presents through the pupil, or even a complete version so that the anterior surface faces the vitreous (Figs. 321–2). It is possible that in these cases a complete dislocation may have been prevented by the spasmodic contraction of the pupil (Veasey, 1901; Ask, 1913).

In a complete dislocation out of the pupillary area the vision corresponds to that of an aphakic eye, and the absence of the lens from the pupillary aperture is recognized by the deep anterior chamber, the tremulousness of the iris, the absence of lenticular reflexes on focal illumination, and the direct observation of the anterior face of the vitreous by the slit-lamp.

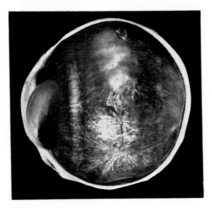

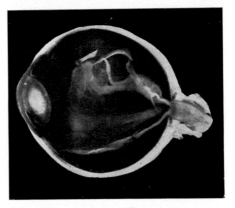

FIG. 321.—SUBLUXATION OF THE LENS AFTER A CONTUSION.

The lens has suffered a complete version, the anterior surface being turned towards the vitreous; it is partially dislocated into the anterior chamber. There is no trace of the suspensory ligament. The iris is also retroverted, forming a collar round the equator of the lens (Museum, Inst. Ophthal.).

FIG. 322.—ANTERIOR DISLOCATION OF THE LENS AFTER A CONTUSION.

The lens is dislocated forwards into the anterior chamber, the iris is seen behind it above but in front of it below. There is a large retinal detachment (Museum, Inst. Ophthal.).

If the lens is *dislocated into the anterior chamber* it can be recognized initially as a clear body in the deepened chamber appearing more convex and smaller than is usual. Sometimes it almost fills the chamber and sometimes it lies in its lower part; occasionally it is reversed so that its posterior surface is next to the cornea (Saunders, 1889; Ask, 1913; Stein, 1926). If the lens is clear it looks like a drop of oil with its rim showing a golden lustre (Figs. 323–4), and through its substance the iris is seen with the pupil spasmodically contracted; if it is opaque it appears as a white disc (Fig. 325). Occasionally the condition is well tolerated with the retention of good (aphakic) vision for long periods if the pupillary aperture is clear (Rampoldi, 1882–86; 25 years, Ayberk, 1939), a happy course of events which may even follow the dislocation of a hypermature lens (Batra *et al.*, 1966); at other times the lens may disintegrate or even become absorbed (Fig. 326); an

FIGS. 323 to 326.—DISLOCATION OF THE LENS INTO THE ANTERIOR CHAMBER.

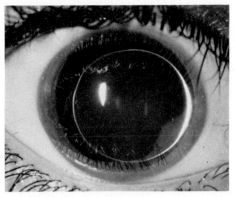

FIG. 323.—In a girl aged 6 with Marchesani's syndrome (R. F. Jones).

FIGS. 324 and 325.—In a girl aged 15 with Marfan's syndrome (B. K. Das Gupta and R. K. Basu).

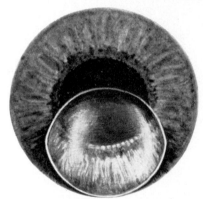

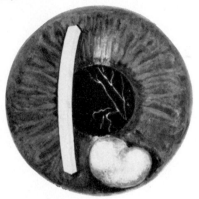

FIG. 324.—In the left eye there is a dislocated clear lens, ovoid in shape, showing a brilliant gold and yellow reflex from its margin.

FIG. 325.—The right eye (seen with the slit-lamp) shows zonular remnants in the pupil and a shrunken cataractous lens in the lower part of the anterior chamber.

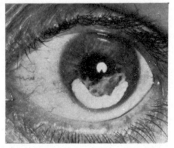

FIG. 326.—The remains of the lens in the anterior chamber after traumatic dislocation (Inst. Ophthal.).

exceptional event is the development of a " massage " cataract appearing after the lens comes repeatedly into contact with the cornea (Schmid, 1946). Too frequently, however, complications arise, the most prominent of which are a severe iridocyclitis, a corneal dystrophy resulting in an opacity probably from damage to the endothelium, and most commonly an acute and intractable secondary glaucoma (Burk, 1912; Wagenhäuser, 1912; 14 out of 15 cases, Hegner, 1915; 90% of cases, Maggiore, 1924; and others).

A *posterior dislocation* is a more common event and is usually tolerated better than an anterior displacement, but the ultimate prognosis is again problematical (Figs. 327–8). Clinically the same appearance of an aphakic

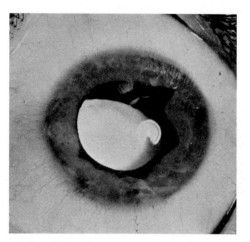

Fig. 327.—Dislocation of the Lens.
A dislocation downwards and inwards of a cataractous lens in a girl aged 17 (Inst. Ophthal.).

pupil and a tremulous iris with a deep anterior chamber presents itself, and on ophthalmoscopic examination the lens may be seen either as a clear globule with a dark margin or as an opaque cataractous body, lying usually in the lower part of the vitreous or resting upon the ciliary body (Fig. 329); Hildreth (1934) found that its recognition was easier using fluorescent light, an expedient profitably used by others (Duverger and Brégeat, 1948). At first it is usually movable (*lens natans*), but eventually organized membranes tend to anchor it (*lens fixata*). Provided the capsule has not been ruptured the eye may tolerate the lens in this position without apparent ill-effects for some years (30 years, Suker, 1904, and Rollet and Genet, 1913; 20 years, Cross, 1914, and Hegner, 1915; 14 years, Chandler, 1964; 11 years, Maxwell, 1951; 9 years, Jarrett, 1967) but, as after the operation of couching, degenerative changes such as choroidal sclerosis, atrophy and pigmentation may eventually destroy the vision (Werncke, 1903; Sievert, 1903; Elliot, 1919; Guillaumat and Lemaître, 1948; Rodman, 1963). Moreover, if the capsule becomes permeable or is ruptured so that the lens proteins escape, a phacotoxic uveitis with a secondary glaucoma may result, or if mechanical irritation of the ciliary body becomes evident, an iridocyclitis with raised tension is common but sympathetic ophthalmitis is exceptional (Dor and Paufique, 1932).

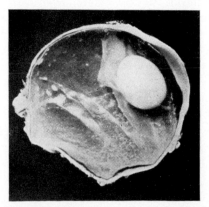

FIG. 328.—TRAUMATIC DISLOCATION OF THE LENS.

A large morgagnian cataract lies embedded in inflammatory exudate; in the exudate are many white inflammatory foci (R. H. Elliot).

FIGS. 329 and 330.—POSTERIOR DISLOCATION OF THE LENS AFTER CONTUSIONS.

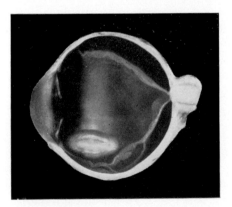
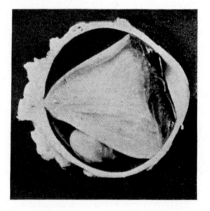

FIG. 329.—The lens lies at the bottom of the vitreous chamber; the anterior chamber is very deep (Museum, Inst. Ophthal.).

FIG. 330.—The morgagnian cataract lies beneath the retina (R. H. Elliot).

A less common location is a *subretinal luxation* when the lens slips through a retinal tear and lies in the subretinal space (Elliot, 1919; Ringelhan and Elschnig, 1931; Fralick, 1937) (Fig. 330), or inserts itself between the sclera and ciliary body (*subscleral luxation*) (Nettleship, 1881; Lawford, 1887) or occupies the cleft of a cyclodialysis.

A WANDERING LENS is an interesting phenomenon whereby the lens passes from one locality to another. The most common migration is forwards and backwards through the pupil, between the anterior vitreous and the anterior chamber. This possibility has been effective in coaxing a lens in the vitreous to traverse the pupil as an aid to its extraction by changing the patient from the prone to the supine position (Legrand, 1938; Wolfe and Mayer, 1945); but when the manœuvre occurs spontaneously an acute attack of glaucoma may result from pupillary blockage (Hilding, 1957). In other cases the patient may induce this migration with impunity by throwing his head forwards and backwards (Favory, 1952); Mitter's (1956) patient preferred his lenses in the anterior chamber, and finding them usually in the vitreous after a night's sleep, he induced them to travel through the pupil as he bent his head to wash in the morning; Gupta and Basu's (1955) patient, on the other hand, preferred to keep her lenses in the vitreous since they gave rise to a feeling of irritation in the anterior chamber.

Fralick's (1937) case was unique. A lens in the subretinal space was induced to travel through a large retinal tear and through the pupil to appear in the anterior chamber after the patient had been face-downwards for 24 hours, whence it was successfully extracted; unfortunately a subsequent operation for re-attachment of the retina proved unsuccessful.

The fate of the lens in such cases varies. We have seen that it may remain transparent for many years, and in cases of subluxation indefinitely. Degenerative changes in dislocated lenses, however, are the rule[1]; disintegration of the epithelium occurs with cleft-formation in the cortex and the gradual development of a cataract which often undergoes morgagnian changes. Calcareous impregnation and shrinkage may then follow (Halben, 1897) (Fig. 326); but partial or total absorption is a rare event (in the anterior chamber, Pagani, 1926; Maw, 1952, leaving only a wisp of capsule; in the vitreous, Snell, 1882; Augstein and Ginsberg, 1896; Harms, 1905; Maggiore, 1924).

The *complications* associated with displacement of the lens are unfortunately frequent and often serious; indeed, in all such cases they should be expected. The most common are uveitis, secondary glaucoma and retinal detachment; we have already noted the keratitis with the development of an opaque cornea which may follow dislocation into the anterior chamber.

The *uveitis* may be of two types. The lens resting on the ciliary body may cause the development of an irritative iridocyclitis, often temporary but of considerable severity, while if hypermaturity develops, a phacoanaphylactic uveitis[2] may result; both of these conditions may lead to a secondary glaucoma, in the first case acute and in the second intractable.

[1] Davey (1882), Lawford (1887), Ritter (1898), Wagenhäuser (1912), Burk (1912), Ask (1913), and others.
[2] Vol. IX, p. 501.

Secondary glaucoma is a very common sequel, which may be due to six causes, the most common of which is *pupillary blockage* by the lens or vitreous. A prolonged attack or repeated episodes may lead to the development of permanent *peripheral anterior synechiæ* and the obstruction of the drainage angle. Less commonly a *phacolytic glaucoma* may result or the rise of tension may be due to rubeosis secondary to a detachment of the retina or chorioretinal scarring. In posterior dislocations a phacolytic glaucoma is a relatively rare occurrence and it may develop several years after the displacement of the lens (8 years, Verdaguer, 1958). In post-traumatic cases, in addition to these factors a frequent cause of secondary glaucoma is the *post-concussion deformity* characterized by degeneration and sclerosis of the ciliary body and trabeculæ, often preceded by lacerations in the ciliary muscle and accompanied by the formation of a deep anterior chamber with recession of the root of the iris. The glaucoma which develops from this sequence is insidious in type and is essentially a post-concussive event, not depending primarily on the dislocation of the lens.[1] To these must be added the acute glaucoma resulting from a dislocation of the lens into the anterior chamber and the secondary glaucoma due to iridocyclitis. These developments will be discussed subsequently in the section on secondary glaucoma where the urgent problem of the treatment of the glaucoma will be considered.[2]

A *retinal detachment* is one of the worst complications which may follow a subluxation or dislocation of the lens, and treatment is frequently rendered difficult since the dislocated lens often makes it impossible to detect the areas of degeneration or the tears responsible for the condition; moreover, prior attempts to remove the lens, which may be associated with loss of the vitreous, tend to accentuate the retinal lesion. Unfortunately, this complication is by no means uncommon; thus in a series of 166 cases of subluxation and dislocation, Jarrett (1967) found 38 retinal detachments which, particularly in cases of Marfan's syndrome, may be bilateral.

The treatment of a displaced lens poses difficult questions, for its removal is no easy procedure, too frequently followed by the loss of vision or even of the eye. The dilemma whether the lens ought to be left or removed raises anxious problems varying with every patient, and no particular procedure can be advised to suit every case. In general, it may be said that if the vision is good in the other eye or reasonably good in bilateral cases and if no complications seem likely to occur, things are best left as they are; surgery should not be attempted as a routine merely because the condition is present. If surgical removal of the lens is attempted, full precautions should be undertaken to minimize a loss of vitreous by complete akinesia, the use of pre-placed sutures and of Flieringa's ring if indicated, the lowering of the intraocular pressure by carbonic anhydrase inhibitors or osmotic agents if it is

[1] p. 707.   [2] p. 659.

raised or by a peripheral iridectomy in cases of pupillary blockage, and the operation should be followed by the subsequent reconstitution of the anterior chamber with air.

In cases of subluxation without complications an attempt should be made to attain reasonable vision by optical correction of the phakic or aphakic area; owing to the irregularity of the astigmatism in the phakic area, optical correction of the latter usually affords the best results. If the aphakic area is small, the pupil can be continuously dilated by the use of weak mydriatics if the angle of the anterior chamber is open, or its area may be increased by an iridectomy (Fig. 331) or photocoagulation of the sphincter region of the iris (Straatsma *et al.*, 1966).

An alternative in young patients is a discission, but this is not usually an easy procedure since such lenses are difficult to cut and unless a wide

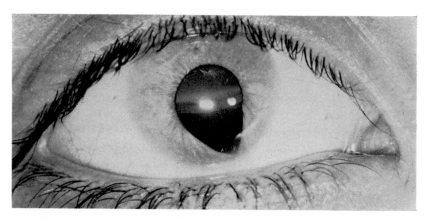

FIG. 331.—OPTICAL IRIDECTOMY FOR A DISLOCATED LENS (M. Whiting).

opening is made in the relaxed capsule this structure tends to heal and absorption of the lens ceases. The use of two needles is usually necessary, one to steady the loose lens (A. Knapp, 1941; Zeeman, 1942; Wolfe *et al.*, 1952), and the technique introduced by Sattler (1897) and extensively employed by Chandler (1951) is usually most effective. In this procedure, with the pupil widely dilated the lens is fixated by a needle passed into it from the side to which the lens is luxated and a second knife-needle opens the capsule and stirs up the cortex at the opposite free edge of the lens. Several repetitions may be necessary to obtain a sufficiently large aphakic area in the pupil; but the technique is safe and may be practised up to the age of 30 (Chandler, 1964).

Removal of a subluxated lens is much more difficult and dangerous and should not be attempted unless complications arise. The use of a vectis or a spoon is usually necessary but some loss of vitreous is very common owing to its adhesion to the lens in the young eyes in which subluxation is usually seen. It is true that many successful cases have been reported, but in almost as many the results have not been impressive and too often disappointing.

A lens dislocated into the anterior chamber is potentially in a much more dangerous position owing to the frequency of the development of corneal degeneration or of glaucoma from blockage of the pupil or closure of the drainage angle. Many cases have been reported of successful removal since the earliest extractions by Saint Yves in 1707 and J. L. Petit in 1708,[1] but there have been almost as many reports of disastrous results; in one of Axenfeld's (1914) cases, both eyes were thus lost. Discission is a safer procedure, but even in cases wherein attacks of raised tension have occurred, many surgeons have preferred to coax the lens into the posterior chamber by the methods already indicated and then to perform a peripheral iridectomy to avoid its return into the anterior chamber by preventing the occurrence of pupillary blockage, since the relative safety of a posterior dislocation may be better than the hazards of surgery (Chandler, 1964). If extraction is undertaken, the pupil should be contracted by a strong miotic such as one of the organic phosphates or by the introduction of acetylcholine into the anterior chamber lest the lens slip back into the vitreous when the anterior chamber is opened, and it may be removed by forceps after transfixation with a needle or by Lacarrère's double-pronged diathermy needle or by cryopexy. When the tension is raised, Douglas (1968) advocated its reduction during surgery by intravenous mannitol.[2]

A note should be made regarding patients with homocystinuria. In such cases major thrombo-embolic complications may follow surgical intervention (Komrower and Wilson, 1963; Carson *et al.*, 1965; Duthie, 1965); an attempt should therefore be made to replace an anteriorly dislocated lens, retaining it behind the pupil by the use of miotics (Henkind and Ashton, 1965; Spaeth and Barber, 1965). If surgical intervention is inevitable, anticoagulant therapy is indicated in order to reduce the incidence of this serious and sometimes fatal complication (Johnston, 1968).

A lens dislocated posteriorly is usually best left alone unless complications ensue; this is particularly the case if it sinks into the bottom of the vitreous and becomes adherent. By placing the patient in the prone position the earlier surgeons made many attempts to induce the lens to come forward to the anterior part of the vitreous or even through a fully dilated pupil into the anterior chamber whence it could be extracted (Higgens, 1896); but this manœuvre was rarely successful. Verhoeff (1942) adopted the original expedient of floating the lens upwards by irrigating the vitreous when it was fluid with a stream of saline, a technique occasionally successfully practised (Lindner, 1949; Hruby, 1949). The most common method, however, is to bring the lens forward into the anterior chamber with a loop (vectis) (Critchett, 1896); for this purpose Vail (1955) used a Smith's spatula. To grope blindly about the vitreous, however, is usually futile and only

[1] p. 251.   [2] p. 610.

leads to retinal damage; the removal of the lens should therefore always be attempted after a preliminary total iridectomy and direct observation with the ophthalmoscope or a binocular loupe (Eggert, 1947; Escariz, 1960), or the lens may be localized with a transilluminator held against the sclera (Rumbaur, 1957; Léopold, 1967). Other technical expedients have been adopted in place of the loop to extract such a lens, the most favoured being the double-pronged electrocoagulation needle of Lacarrère (Gardilcic, 1946; Vaz, 1947; Duverger and Brégeat, 1948; Heinsius, 1966), an erisophake (Iliff, 1957; V. Smith, 1958) or a cryopexy probe (Moreau, 1965; Ayres, 1965; Mickiewicz and Leontjewa, 1967). If the lens is obstructing the pupillary aperture in an aged and frail patient with a restricted expectation of life who cannot reasonably be subjected to a major surgical procedure, a couching operation to displace the lens to the bottom of the vitreous may be justifiable.

A very satisfactory method, however, is to fixate the lens before its removal and to guide it to the pupillary region whence it can be removed through a corneal incision by forceps, an erisophake or a cryopexy probe.

FIGS. 332 and 333.—DOUBLE-PRONGED NEEDLES.

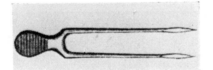

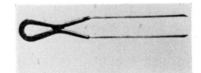

FIG. 332.—Agnew's bident.   FIG. 333.—Calhoun and Hagler's cutting-edge double needle.

The first manœuvre is usually done with the patient in the prone position; for the second, after the lens is fixed he is turned over to the supine position. The pioneer in this technique was Dixon (1853) who introduced two needles immediately behind the ciliary body to fixate the lens, and it was subsequently improved by Agnew (1885) who introduced a double-pronged needle (a " bident ") through the pars plana (Fig. 332). At first the method excited little interest (Webster, 1885; Pomeroy, 1888) and some writers objected to the trauma involved (Bull, 1890; H. Knapp, 1890), but recently with modern instruments it has been improved and is now commonly adopted[1] (Fig. 333). Dryden and his colleagues (1961) used a single needle introduced trans-sclerally for the same purpose, and Stambaugh and Nelson (1967) a triple needle with the central prong somewhat behind the other two in order to achieve more secure support of the lens. When these measures fail and the lens lies deeply in the vitreous, if removal is decided on, Stallard (1946–65) and Epstein (1963) suggested its extraction through a scleral incision after its accurate localization.

---

[1] Barraquer (1958), Calhoun and Hagler (1959), Merz *et al.* (1962), Zubero and Callahan (1962), Hollwich (1962), Krol (1966), Adler (1967).

The *prognosis* for the surgical removal of such a lens used to be so problematical that most surgeons practised it only as an alternative to excision of the globe in cases of uncontrollable glaucoma or an intractable phaco-anaphylactic reaction, but the results of these more recent techniques have made the prospects of surgery more hopeful. It should be remembered, however, that if the vision is reasonably good and complications are absent, the best prognosis results from inaction when the lens is subluxated or posteriorly dislocated; surgical extraction is followed more usually by no change or a deterioration in vision than by its improvement and may induce a retinal detachment. In general, the prognosis is somewhat better in congenital cases (as in Marfan's syndrome) than after trauma.

Adler. *Brit. J. Ophthal.*, **51**, 73 (1967).

Agnew. *Trans. Amer. ophthal. Soc.*, **4**, 69 (1885).

Ask. *Studien ü. path. Anat. d. erworbenen Linsensubluxation*, Wiesbaden (1913).

Augstein and Ginsberg. *Zbl. prakt. Augenheilk.*, **20**, 356 (1896).

Axenfeld. *Klin. Mbl. Augenheilk.*, **52**, 195 (1914).

Ayberk. *Turk. oftal. Gaz.*, **3**, 21 (1939).

Ayres. *Rev. bras. Oftal.*, **24**, 297 (1965).

Barraquer. *Arch. Soc. amer. Oftal. Optom.*, **1**, 30 (1958).

Batra, Paul and Malhotra. *Orient. Arch. Ophthal.*, **4**, 127 (1966).

Bull. *Trans. Amer. ophthal. Soc.*, **5**, 598 (1890).

Burk. *v. Graefes Arch. Ophthal.*, **83**, 114 (1912).

Busacca. *Zbl. ges. Ophthal.*, **18**, 433 (1927).

Calhoun and Hagler. *Trans. Amer. ophthal. Soc.*, **57**, 221 (1959).

Carson, Dent, Field and Gaull. *J. Pediat.*, **66**, 565 (1965).

Chandler. *Arch. Ophthal.*, **45**, 125 (1951); **71**, 765 (1964).

Critchett. *Trans. ophthal. Soc. U.K.*, **16**, 62 (1896).

Cross, A. G., and Choyce. *Brit. J. Ophthal.*, **37**, 314 (1953).

Cross, F. R. *Trans. ophthal. Soc. U.K.*, **34**, 167 (1914).

Davey. *Brit. med. J.*, **2**, 369 (1882).

Dixon. *Lancet*, **2**, 313 (1853).

Dor and Paufique. *Bull. Soc. Ophtal. Paris*, 434 (1932).

Dorsch. *Ueber angeborene u. erworben Linsenluxation u. ihre Behandlung* (Diss.), Marburg (1900).

Douglas. *Amer. J. Ophthal.*, **65**, 926 (1968).

Dryden, Perraut and Seward. *Amer. J. Ophthal.*, **52**, 468 (1961).

Duthie. *Trans. ophthal. Soc. U.K.*, **85**, 37 (1965).

Duverger and Brégeat. *Arch. Ophtal.*, **8**, 360 (1948).

Eggert. *Klin. Mbl. Augenheilk.*, **111**, 223 (1947).

Elliot. *Brit. J. Ophthal.*, **3**, 49 (1919).

Epstein. *S. Afr. med. J.*, **37**, 879 (1963).

Escariz. *Arch. Oftal. B. Aires*, **35**, 202 (1960).

Falls and Cotterman. *Arch. Ophthal.*, **30**, 610 (1943).

Favory. *Bull. Soc. Ophtal. Fr.*, 583 (1952).

Fralick. *Amer. J. Ophthal.*, **20**, 795 (1937).

Gardilcic. *Ophthalmologica*, **112**, 255 (1946).

Goondorova. *Vestn. oftal.*, No. 5, 39 (1956).

Grob. *Ueber Lageveränderung d. Linse in ætiologischer u. therapeutischer Beziehung* (Diss.), Zürich (1901).

Guillaumat and Lemaître. *Bull. Soc. Ophtal. Paris*, 90 (1948).

Gupta and Basu. *Brit. J. Ophthal.*, **39**, 566 (1955).

Halben. *Ein Beitrag zur Kenntnis d. path. Anat. d. Linsenluxation* (Diss.), Jena (1897).

Harms. *Klin. Mbl. Augenheilk.*, **43** (1), 147 (1905).

Harshman. *Amer. J. Ophthal.*, **31**, 833 (1948).

Hegner. *Beitr. Augenheilk.*, **9** (90), 707 (1915).

Heinsius. *Klin. Mbl. Augenheilk.*, **149**, 708 (1966).

Henkind and Ashton. *Trans. ophthal. Soc. U.K.*, **85**, 21 (1965).

Higgens. *Lancet*, **2**, 1812 (1896).

Hilding. *Arch. Ophthal.*, **57**, 33 (1957).

Hildreth. *Amer. J. Ophthal.*, **17**, 414 (1934).

von Hippel. *v. Graefes Arch. Ophthal.*, **20** (1), 195 (1874); **44** (3), 539 (1897).

Hirschberg. *v. Graefes Arch. Ophthal.*, **22** (1), 65 (1876).

Hollwich. *Öst. ophthal. Ges.*, **6**, 74 (1962).

Holtermann and Schmidt. *Klin. Mbl. Augenheilk.*, **143**, 832 (1963).

Hruby. *Wien. klin. Wschr.*, **61**, 605 (1949).

Iliff. *Amer. J. Ophthal.*, **43**, 126 (1957).

Jarrett. *Arch. Ophthal.*, **78**, 289 (1967).

Jess. *Klin. Mbl. Augenheilk.*, **76**, 465 (1926).

Johnston. *Brit. J. Ophthal.*, **52**, 251 (1968).

Knapp, A. *Trans. Amer. ophthal. Soc.*, **39**, 83 (1941).
    Arch. Ophthal., **27**, 158 (1942).

Knapp, H. *Arch. Ophthal.*, **19**, 53 (1890).

Knobloch. *Oftal. sborn.*, **6**, 176 (1931).

Komrower and Wilson. *Proc. roy. Soc. Med.*, **56**, 996 (1963).

Krol. *Vestn. oftal.*, **79**, 10 (1966).

Lawford. *Roy. Lond. ophthal. Hosp. Rep.*, **11**, 327 (1887).

Legrand. *Arch. Ophtal.*, **2**, 924 (1938).

Léopold. *Arch. Ophtal.*, **27**, 273 (1967).

Lindner. *Wien. klin. Wschr.*, **61**, 270 (1949).

McDonald and Purnell. *J. Amer. med. Ass.*, **145**, 220 (1951).

Maggiore. *Ann. Ottal.*, **52**, 817 (1924).

Maw. *Trans. ophthal. Soc. U.K.*, **72**, 631 (1952).

Maxwell. *Trans. ophthal. Soc. U.K.*, **71**, 780 (1951).

Meesmann. *Arch. Augenheilk.*, **91**, 261 (1922).

Merz, Zeiger and Puntenney. *Illinois med. J.*, **121**, 31 (1962).

von Michel. *Pathologisch-anatomische Befunde bei spontan oder traumatisch erworbenen Linsenverschiebungen, Gedenkschrift f. v. Leuthold*, **2**, 617 (1906).

Mickiewicz and Leontjewa. *Klin. oczna*, **37**, 499 (1967).

Mitter. *Brit. J. Ophthal.*, **40**, 253 (1956).

Mooren. *Die operative Behandlung d. naturlich u. kunstlich Gerieften Starformen*, Wiesbaden (1894).

Moreau. *Bull. Soc. Ophtal. Fr.*, **65**, 672 (1965).

Nettleship. *Trans. ophthal. Soc. U.K.*, **1**, 24 (1881).

Nirankari and Chaddah. *Amer. J. Ophthal.*, **63**, 1719 (1967).

d'Ombrain. *Brit. J. Ophthal.*, **20**, 22 (1936).

Pagani. *Boll. Oculist.*, **5**, 529 (1926).

Panas. *Traité des maladies des yeux*, Paris (1894).

Pomeroy. *Trans. Amer. ophthal. Soc.*, **5**, 168 (1888).

Rampoldi. *Ann. Univ. Med. Chir. Milano*, **261**, 49 (1882).
 Ann. Ottal., **15**, 179 (1886).

Richards and Ellis. *Arch. Ophthal.*, **60**, 472 (1958).

Ringelhan and Elschnig. *Arch. Augenheilk.*, **104**, 325 (1931).

Ritter. *Arch. Augenheilk.*, **37**, 348 (1898).

Rodman. *Arch. Ophthal.*, **69**, 445 (1963).

Rollet and Genet. *Rev. gén. Ophtal.*, **32**, 572 (1913).

Rumbaur. *Klin. Mbl. Augenheilk.*, **130**, 12 (1957).

Sattler. *Ber. dtsch. ophthal. Ges.*, **26**, 233 (1897).

Saunders. *Brit. med. J.*, **1**, 470 (1889).

Schmid. *Ophthalmologica*, **111**, 365 (1946).

Sievert. *Ueber degenerative Veränderungen d. Choroidea u. Retina bei Luxation d. Linse in d. Glaskörper* (Diss.), Freiburg (1903).

Slezak. *v. Graefes Arch. Ophthal.*, **166**, 112 (1963).

Smith, V. L. *Amer. J. Ophthal.*, **45**, 909 (1958).

Snell. *Ophthal. Rev.*, **1**, 400 (1882).

Spaeth and Barber. *Trans. Amer. Acad. Ophthal.*, **69**, 912 (1965).

Stallard. *Eye Surgery*, 1st ed. (1946); 4th ed., Bristol, 626 (1965).

Stambaugh and Nelson. *Trans. Amer. Acad. Ophthal.*, **71**, 355 (1967).

Stein. *Klin. Mbl. Augenheilk.*, **76**, 75 (1926).

Stocwer. *Z. Augenheilk.*, **5**, 181 (1901).

Straatsma, Allen, Pettit and Hall. *Amer. J. Ophthal.*, **61**, 1312 (1966).

Suker. *Ophthal. Rec.*, **11**, 412 (1904).

Vail. *Amer. J. Ophthal.*, **39** (2), 109 (1955).

Vaz. *Bol. Soc. port. Oftal.*, **5**, 209 (1947).

Veasey. *Ophthal. Rec.*, **10**, 8, 42 (1901).

Verdaguer. *Arch. chil. Oftal.*, **15**, 37 (1958).

Verhoeff. *Amer. J. Ophthal.*, **25**, 725 (1942).

Vogt. *Z. Augenheilk.*, **14**, 153 (1905).

Wagenhäuser. *Anatomische Untersuch. bei acht Fällen v. Linsenluxation* (Diss.), Tübingen (1912).

Wagenmann. *v. Graefes Arch. Ophthal.*, **35** (1), 172 (1889).

Wallmann and Ammann. *J. Génét. hum.*, **13**, 215 (1964).

Webster. *Trans. Amer. ophthal. Soc.*, **4**, 76 (1885).

Werncke. *Klin. Mbl. Augenheilk.*, **41**, Beil., 283 (1903).

Whiting. *Brit. J. Ophthal.*, **47**, 54 (1963).

Wolfe, O. R., and Mayer. *Amer. J. Ophthal.*, **28**, 193 (1945).

Wolfe, O. R. and R. M., and Spaeth. *J. int. Coll. Surg.*, **17**, 201 (1952).

Zeeman. *Acta ophthal.* (Kbh.), **20**, 1 (1942).

Zubero and Callahan. *Amer. J. Ophthal.*, **54**, 196 (1962).

SECTION II

DISEASES OF THE VITREOUS BODY

BY

SIR STEWART DUKE-ELDER

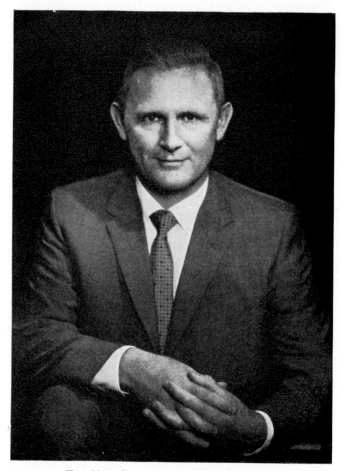

Fig. 334.—Paul Anton Cibis [1911–1965].

CHAPTER V

DISEASES OF THE VITREOUS BODY

MOST of the classical workers on the vitreous body have already been figured in this *System*; we shall therefore pay a tribute to a member of our own generation who contributed richly to modern techniques in its study and in the treatment of its disorders. PAUL ANTON CIBIS [1911–1965] (Fig. 334) was born in Silesia, at that time within Germany, and received his medical education at Breslau, Munich, Berlin and Heidelberg where he worked at the University Eye Clinic for 11 years (1938–49); in 1949 he went to the U.S.A. as a research ophthalmologist to the American Air Force in Texas and thereafter to the Washington University, St. Louis, where he remained, ultimately becoming associate professor, until his early death at the age of 53 from a massive coronary infarct. His greatest interest lay in the surgical treatment of detachment of the retina, a branch of surgery which introduced him to a concentrated study of the vitreous, gross derangements of which so often render the treatment of this condition fruitless. A fanatical worker, an able clinical observer and a surgeon of rare skill, ingenuity and daring, he did more than any person of his time to elucidate the changes which occur in the vitreous in degenerative conditions and may be said to have introduced effective intravitreal surgery into ophthalmology; this was summarized in his book, *Vitreoretinal Pathology and Surgery in Retinal Detachment*, published in the year of his death, a contribution to the advance of our specialty which was recognized throughout the world.

For the comparative anatomy of the vitreous body, the reader is referred to Vol. I of this *System* (selachians, p. 287; teleosteans, p. 304; placentals, p. 476); for the human anatomy to Vol. II, p. 294; for the embryology to Vol. III, p. 141, and for congenital anomalies, p. 761. Its physiology will be found in Vol. IV. The clinical examination of the vitreous body has also been described. Ophthalmoscopically gross changes are evident but few details can be distinguished. These can be adequately examined only with the slit-lamp assisted by a Hruby lens for the posterior region and a Goldmann's 3-mirror gonio-lens for the anterior peripheral areas.[1]

It will be noted that many pathological changes in the vitreous body have already been discussed in this *System*, particularly those associated with uveitis in Vol. IX, and the degenerative changes, especially in such conditions as the vitreo-retinal dystrophies and retinal detachments, in the previous Volume. To these the reader is referred.

GENERAL CONSIDERATIONS

As an introduction to this Section a short note on the nature of the vitreous body may be apposite. Although the normal vitreous gives the appearance of an inert transparent gel and consists of almost 99% water, it has some structural arrangement. Of the three macro-molecular constituents—collagen, soluble proteins (largely acid glycoproteins and serum proteins) and hyaluronic acid—the first represents the main structural basis

[1] Vol. VII, p. 265.

of the network of the fibrillæ which forms its essential framework, the latter two are found mainly in the peripheral layers, the third forming coil-like chains within the meshes of the collagenous framework, presumably acting as a diffusion-membrane between the body of the vitreous and the retina, and probably helping to protect the gel from cellular invasion. At the extreme periphery the collagen fibres also condense so that a concentrated surface layer is formed (the hyaloid " membrane "), which in the normal eye is intimately related to the internal limiting membrane of the retina but in the pathological eye is liable to separate from it to allow the formation of a vitreo-retinal space. Also mainly concentrated in the cortical layers are the

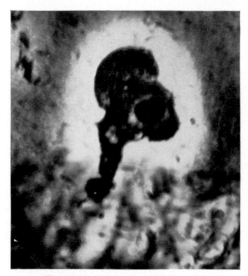

Fig. 335.—Retinal Microglia.
A retinal phagocyte migrating through a small pore in the internal limiting membrane (unstained) into the vitreous gel (× 1,000) (J. R. Wolter).

vitreous cells,[1] mainly histiocytic in origin and nature (Fig. 335); in the normal eye they seem to play an important role in the synthesis of acid mucopolysaccharides and perhaps of vitreous fibrils, while in pathological conditions they act as phagocytes (Figs. 350–51). They may proliferate into nodular aggregations and participate in the formation of preretinal fibrous tissue and the fibro-cellular membranes which may cover the inner surface of the retina and the outer face of the vitreous when it is retracted.

From the clinical point of view the normal vitreous is ophthalmo-scopically transparent and the only visible alteration which can be observed is the presence of opacities sufficiently dense to obstruct transmitted light. With the slit-lamp, however, to which the entire vitreous is readily accessible with the aid of a Hruby lens or a contact glass, the arrangement of the

[1] Vol. II, p. 305.

micellæ which make up its protein basis endows it with a complicated optical structure of pseudo-fibres and pseudo-membranes of an extremely poly-morphous nature; these appear to hang like delicate gossamer curtains of moiré silk full of folds and pleats moving slightly and characteristically in a pendulum-like motion with the movements of the eye (Fig. 336). We have already discussed the physical basis of this optical effect[1] and have seen that while a fibrillar or a membranous structure was accepted by the older ana-tomists (a deduction from the artefacts of histological coagulation), these complex appearances merely represent the optical effect in the beam of light produced by a varying arrangement of the countless colloidal micellæ which make up the basis of the gel. Where these fibrillæ are arranged indis-criminately the vitreous appears optically empty; but if they are arranged in coils or in parallel sheets they reflect the light sufficiently to give the appearance of a fibre or a membrane, a summation-effect seen most clearly in

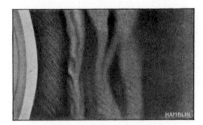

FIG. 336.—THE NORMAL VITREOUS.
Seen with the slit-lamp. The posterior surface of the lens is to the left. Dense membrane-like masses of gel are evident.

places where they are particularly condensed such as the interfaces within the vitreous body, on its outer surface and, pre-eminently, in that very condensed portion which forms the " fibres " of the zonule.

The vitreous body may thus be regarded as an extracellular substance with a complicated topography, forming a structure normally isolated to a considerable extent from the retina and aqueous humour by the chemical structure of its cortical layers. Its main function is passive for it serves as a medium to maintain the path of light between the lens and the retina free from diffusing and absorbing elements. It is essentially acellular with a metabolism so low that it cannot be measured; only in the cortex is there evidence of cellular activity. It follows that in its pathological reactions it is entirely passive, so that the old terms such as " hyalitis " connoting pathological activity should be avoided except, perhaps, when the cells in the cortical layer proliferate and participate in the development of fibrosis (Gärtner, 1962). Moreover, when lost from the adult eye it is not renewed to any extent but is replaced by intra-ocular fluid. Its reactions are therefore merely degenerative, involving changes such as liquefaction, opacification

[1] Vol. II, p. 294.

and shrinkage; but in these circumstances the very delicate balance of its colloidal structure is so readily disturbed by a great variety of changes such as an alteration in the reaction, in the carbon dioxide tension, in the salt content and by the infiltration of toxins, that these changes occur in a large number of diseases of the inner eye (Clement, 1966; Brini *et al.*, 1968).

It is to be remembered that although it is inert and takes no active part in inflammatory reactions, the vitreous body forms an excellent culture-medium so that any infective process reaching it tends to run on apace. This lack of resistance to organismal growth has been stressed by many investigators who have found that bacteria readily multiply in it and excite a severe inflammatory reaction in the surrounding tissues which rapidly proceeds to the formation of an abscess, a generalization which applies even to organisms of so low a degree of pathogenicity that elsewhere in the eye they would remain saprophytic. The pathology of these cases has already been discussed in dealing with inflammations of the uveal tract[1]; the passiveness of the vitreous body in the process is the feature of present interest.

Brini, Bronner, Gerhard and Nordmann. *Biologie et chirurgie du corps vitré*, Paris (1968).
Clement. *Fisiologia y Patologia del Vitreo*, Madrid (1966).
Gärtner. *v. Graefes Arch. Ophthal.*, **164,** 473 (1962).

GENERAL DEGENERATIONS

Fluidity of the Vitreous: Synchisis

A liquefaction of the vitreous body (SYNCHISIS; σύν, together; χέω, to pour; SYNERESIS; σύν, αἱρεῖν, to take together) is the most common degenerative change, occurring in senile and myopic conditions and after contusions as well as in most degenerative and inflammatory states of the eye. It is due to a conversion of the colloid gel into a sol and is usually associated with the development of ophthalmoscopically visible opacities formed by the colloidal micellæ which aggregate together in dust-like particles, strands or membranes. In a sense it is a dehydration rather than a hydration in so far as it represents the loss by the micellæ of their water of adsorption; this results in a destruction of the architecture of the vitreous with a collapse of the collagenous framework into shrunken lamellar condensations while the released water, containing fragmented structural elements and mucopolysaccharides, accumulates in one or more lacunæ. Once the gel has thus been disrupted there is no evidence that its normal composition and architecture can be restored. Such a breakdown may be due to purely physico-chemical factors but may also be conditioned by enzymic digestion of the protein basis of the gel.

In simple cases the only clinical symptom is the appearance of floating spots before the eyes, which instead of having a localized excursion as occurs when the elastic structure of the gel is maintained, become freer and untrammelled moving right across the field of vision. Ophthalmoscopically the

[1] Vol. IX, p. 97.

actual liquefaction produces no obvious alteration, and the vitreous may appear normal but for the fact that the opacities, if they are visible, are possessed of abnormally free and unrestrained movement. With the slit-lamp, however, the change in consistency is always obvious (Fig. 337). In uncomplicated cases when the entire gel is liquefied an absence of the usual

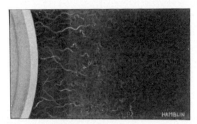

FIG. 337.—LIQUEFACTION OF THE VITREOUS.
Seen with the slit-lamp. A senile case. The gel is fluid and shows a homogeneous fibrillar degeneration.

curtain-like membranes is evident, and the whole body of the vitreous tends to become homogeneous, the primary and secondary elements being mixed so that no relatively clear retrolental space (occupied normally by the primary vitreous) exists, for the mass of vitreous comes forward immediately behind the lens. This mass, instead of showing membranous formations and folds

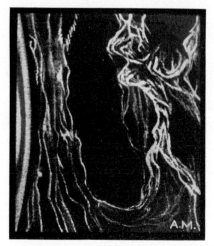

FIG. 338.—LACUNAR DEGENERATION OF THE VITREOUS (H. Goldmann).

undulating with a restricted excursion in an optically clear gel, tends to be interspersed with opacities of relatively uniform distribution, floating about with much greater freedom.

At other times a *partial liquefaction* occurs, lacunæ appearing usually in the central area, or the posterior region turning fluid (Fig. 338). In the first case the patient complains of a speck or " fly " which appears suddenly in front of his eye and floats about with a limited excursion. In the second case which is a relatively common occurrence owing to the delicacy of the vitreous framework posteriorly, the whole of the protein basis of the gel tends to be drawn anteriorly where it becomes condensed into membranous formations of considerable density and the fluid collects in the posterior region. Lacunæ filled with fluid may occupy the entire posterior segment of the globe, but in

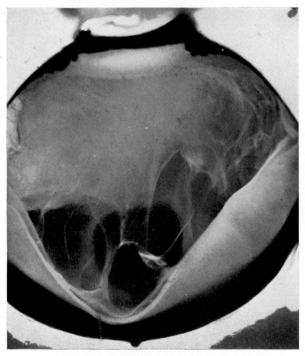

Fig. 339.—Partial Liquefaction of the Vitreous.

A gross specimen showing partial liquefaction in the posterior region, the sucker feet remaining attached to the posterior retina (S. R. Irvine).

other cases the condensed vitreous structure may constitute a dense super-ficial layer (Pischel, 1945–53; Teng, 1960) which itself may form firm adhesions to the retina at the margins of the lacunar spaces like sucker-feet (Fig. 339). These may be of considerable significance for it will be remembered that the fixation of these to the retina and the traction which they exert as they tug with movements of the eye may be causal factors in determining tears in this tissue which lead to its detachment.

The more common causes of syneresis of the vitreous may be summarized thus :

1. *Mechanical trauma* whereby the structural framework of the gel is disrupted by a concussion or the direct trauma of an intra-ocular foreign body, or ultrasonic waves (Zeiss, 1938; Kawamoto, 1947; Grün *et al.*, 1950; Lavine *et al.*, 1952).

2. *Chemical trauma*, caused particularly by the presence of two metallic cations, iron and copper. Both of these tend to depolymerize hyaluronic acid so that the effect of this substance in maintaining the stability of the gel is much reduced and the collagenous framework collapses. Similar changes may follow a hæmorrhage into the vitreous or the intravitreal injection of autogenous blood owing to the liberation of ferric ions from the hæmoglobin (Cibis and Yamashita, 1959).

3. *Thermal trauma* similarly condenses and contracts the collagenous framework resulting in areas of liquefaction, a frequent unwanted sequel to the treatment of retinal detachments by diathermic or light-coagulation. Both of these may result in a condensation of the vitreous between the fluid lacunæ and its adherence to the coagulated area of the retina with the potential danger of tearing this tissue and the development of a post-operative retinal detachment.

4. *Cold* has apparently relatively little effect on the macro- or micro-structure of the vitreous. Thus at temperatures of $-50°$ C, Oksala and Lehtinen (1958) found few significant changes in the bovine vitreous, but Dische and Zelmanes (1955) noted that the soluble glycoproteins became insoluble at $-15°$ C and were precipitated with the collagenous fibrils. Fortunately in cryosurgery the vitreous itself is not affected.[1]

5. *Radiational injuries*, particularly x- and γ-rays (1,000 to 2,000 r) and to some extent ultra-violet light, depolymerize the mucopolysaccharides in the vitreous and cause partial liquefaction of the gel (Howe, 1954; Balazs *et al.*, 1959). This effect should be remembered when radiation is applied to the posterior segment of the globe as a therapeutic measure.

6. *Immunological reactions* of the Arthus type[2] have been found to produce syneresis of the vitreous gel probably by a depolymerization of the mucopolysaccharides (Bullington *et al.*, 1960). A similar reaction follows exposure to extracellular metabolites liberated in infective processes (hyaluronidase, proteinase, streptodornase, etc.).

7. *Degenerative conditions* such as senility or high myopia and *inflammatory states* frequently involve an almost complete liquefaction of the gel. These will be discussed subsequently. Syneresis is a common association of a subluxated or dislocated lens.

Fluidity of the vitreous calls for no treatment; its clinical significance lies in the demonstration of degenerative or destructive changes in the eye, and in the possibility of the development of a detachment of the retina or the occurrence of serious complications after intra-ocular operations, for in these eyes the zonule also is usually weak, and a dislocation of the lens and prolapse of the vitreous may occur.

Balazs, Laurent, Howe and Varga. *Radiat. Res.*, **11**, 149 (1959).

Bullington, Toth and Howe. *Importance of the Vitreous Body in Retina Surgery* (ed. Schepens), St. Louis, 54 (1960).

Cibis and Yamashita. *Amer. J. Ophthal.*, **48** (2), 465 (1959).

Dische and Zelmanes. *Arch. Ophthal.*, **54**, 528 (1955).

Grün, Funder and Wyt. *Klin. Mbl. Augenheilk.*, **116**, 358 (1950).

Howe. *Acta XVII int. Cong. Ophthal.*, Montreal-N.Y., **2**, 1033 (1954).

Kawamoto. *Nip. Gank. Zas.*, **51**, 12 (1947).

Lavine, Langenstrass, Bowyer *et al.* *Arch. Ophthal.*, **47**, 204 (1952).

Oksala and Lehtinen. *Acta ophthal.* (Kbh.), **36**, 929 (1958).

Pischel. *Trans. Amer. Acad. Ophthal.*, **49**, 155 (1945).

Amer. J. Ophthal., **36**, 1497 (1953).

Teng. *Importance of the Vitreous Body in Retina Surgery* (ed. Schepens), St. Louis, 76 (1960).

Zeiss. *v. Graefes Arch. Ophthal.*, **139**, 301 (1938).

[1] Vol. X, p. 829.   [2] Vol. VII, p. 225.

Vitreous Opacities

From the clinical point of view opacities in the vitreous body are essentially secondary in origin due to a degenerative or inflammatory lesion elsewhere in the eye, usually in the uvea or retina. Ophthalmoscopically they always appear dark since they become visible by obstructing the reflected light; if they are very small they may be invisible by this method of examination although they are best seen in the unconcentrated beam of a plane mirror with a high plus lens; if they are numerous and dust-like they may obscure a view of the retina which may be seen vaguely as if through a haze; if they are many and gross the retina and, indeed, the red reflex may be totally obscured. Subjectively they are seen entoptically as MUSCÆ VOLI-TANTES, the " flies " that, if they are situated near the line of vision and an attempt is made to fixate them, dart away without ever being overtaken. They are most easily seen on looking at a bright surface or the sky and usually have a certain degree of freedom of movement with the eye, with a quick phase lasting a little over a second in the direction of movement followed by a slow phase of return to their original position lasting from 5 to 12 seconds; when the vitreous is liquefied their movement is more extensive. The optics governing their appearance and apparent movement has already been described[1] (see Contino, 1964). If they are situated in front of the centre of rotation their initial movement is with the eye and therefore appears entoptically to be in the opposite direction; if behind, they move in the opposite sense and thus appear to move in the same direction as the eye; the latter type being near the retina are more clearly observed.

The appearance of these muscæ volitantes, whether in the form of dots or lines or cobwebs, especially if they develop suddenly, may cause much anxiety to the nervous patient who not uncommonly thinks that a visual catastrophe is imminent. The phenomenon, of course, by itself is usually of little moment but is of some significance denoting a degenerative change in the vitreous gel; but occasionally, as when a small cloud appears in a specific locality in the periphery, they may indicate the sudden development of a retinal tear with a small amount of hæmorrhage.

Ætiologically vitreous opacities may be divided into three classes:

1. Congenital remnants of the hyaloid vascular system; these have already been discussed.[2]

2. Endogenous opacities:

    (*a*) coagula of the colloid basis of the gel;
    (*b*) crystalline deposits (i) asteroid bodies,
                            (ii) synchisis scintillans.

3. Exogenous opacities:

    (*a*) protein coagula—the plasmoid vitreous;
    (*b*) exudative cells;

---

[1] Vol. VII, p. 447.   [2] Vol. III, p. 769.

(c) blood;

(d) tissue cells : epithelial, histiocytic, glial;

(e) tumour cells;

(f) pigment : melanotic and hæmatogenous.

ENDOGENOUS OPACITIES

COAGULA

The endogenous opacities derived from the colloid basis of the gel with which mucopolysaccharides and proteins may be associated may be extremely small and dust-like—so small, indeed, as to be almost if not quite invisible with the ophthalmoscope—while at other times they take the form of considerable clumps or fibre-like strands and membranes (Figs. 337, 382). The fibres are arranged in irregular bundles like tangled skeins of wool which move about with optically empty spaces between them. The smaller particles probably represent the disintegration of the micellæ of the gel into granular coagula, and the fibres their agglutination into strands, for whereas in the normal condition their state of turgescence demands their massing together before they become optically visible, their higher refractive index in the coagulated form allows them to become more readily seen. The membranes, on the other hand, are typically associated with a general liquefaction of the gel posteriorly in which case the colloid basis is drawn forwards in lamellæ which fuse with the dense base of the vitreous near its ciliary attachment to form thick wavy membranous sheets which glide to and fro behind the lens. Sometimes the coagulated masses after being tossed about in the fluid vitreous for some time assume a spherical shape being agglutinated in clumps and blobs of considerable size; and many of them eventually attract cells which become adherent to them. At other times the surface condensation of the gel, which forms a limiting membrane in detachments of the vitreous, may form opacities of a definite nature.[1]

CRYSTALLINE DEPOSITS

Crystalline deposits in the vitreous were known even in pre-ophthalmoscopic days, for in pronounced cases the brilliant corpuscles were seen by focal light floating about in the pupil (*Spintheropia*, *Spintheromma*, Sichel, 1846–51; *scintillatis pupillæ*, Backer, 1851). Originally little discrimination was made between the types of crystalline deposits, and the earlier writers referred to them all as *synchisis scintillans*,[2] until Benson (1894) differentiated white spherical bodies as *asteroid hyalitis*, distinguishing them from the golden crystals typical of synchisis scintillans. The former, which are the more common, are seen in a substantially normal vitreous and appear to be deposits of calcium soaps; the latter occur in a fluid vitreous and are probably cholesterol crystals.

---

[1] p. 349.

[2] Desmarres (1845–50), Sichel (1846), Robert (1847), Hirschberg (1876), Poncet (1876), Adams (1881), and others.

ASTEROID BODIES: SCINTILLATIO ALBESCENS OR NIVEA

Although noted by such writers as Webster (1883), Cross (1886), D'Oench (1889) and Valk (1889), the occurrence of spherical or disc-shaped white bodies was first differentiated from synchisis scintillans by Benson (1894) as ASTEROID HYALITIS (*Benson's disease*); the name is an apt one to describe the appearance of " hundreds and thousands of small spheres of a light cream colour . . . like the stars in a clear night," although in the absence of inflammatory changes, the term " hyalitis " is unsuitable. Argyll Robertson (1894) described them as SNOWBALL OPACITIES, a name adopted by Holloway (1917), while Wiegmann (1918) suggested the term SCINTILLATIO ALBESCENS or NIVEA, and Rutherford (1933) aptly likened them to droplets of white paint suspended in water (Plate IV).

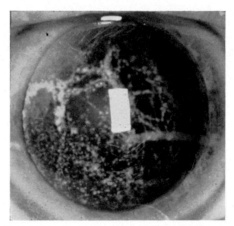

FIG. 340.—ASTEROID BODIES (Inst. Ophthal.).

The condition is not common; thus Holloway (1917–22) saw 9 cases, Feingold (1922) 8, Westpfahl (1915) recorded 40 cases from the literature, and Rutherford (1933), in reporting 18 cases seen in the Iowa Hospital in 7 years, collected reports of 58. It is essentially a senile phenomenon, for the literature shows that the age of the affected patients averages 60 years, and varies from 30 to 84; it is commonest in the 7th and 8th decades of life. So far as sex is concerned, it appears to be three times as common in males as in females; and it is much more frequently unilateral than bilateral; indeed, in only some 25% of the cases are both eyes affected.

The asteroid bodies are small discrete bodies, disc-shaped or spherical, sometimes marshalled in strands and columns, sometimes in bunches, but more usually showing no orderly arrangement (Fig. 340). With the ophthalmoscope they are seen by reflected light as creamy or white and shiny, looking like snowballs or stars in the night sky (Fig. 341); by transmitted light they are dark (Fig. 342); and in the intense focal beam of the slit-lamp

PLATE IV
Asteroid Bodies
In a man aged 72 (Inst. Ophthal.)

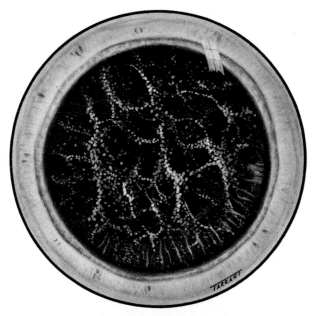

Fig. 1.—The Right Eye seen with the Ophthalmoscope.

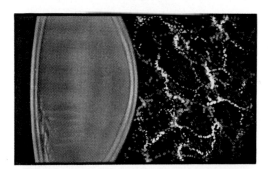

Fig. 2.—The Right Eye seen with the Slit-lamp.

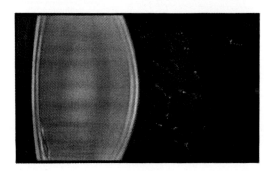

Fig. 3.—The Left Eye seen with the Slit-lamp.

[Facing p. 324

they usually appear dead-white and are round and gleam brilliantly (Erggelet, 1914; Vogt, 1921; and many others) (Plate IV). Sometimes they are bespattered with pigment granules (Pau, 1965). They may be found scattered throughout the whole vitreous or accumulated in any part of it, and they have been noted lying on a detached retina (D'Oench, 1889); sometimes there are only two or three of them to be seen, and at other times they appear to be innumerable. The vitreous itself, while usually showing some degenerative changes, retains its solidity, so that when the eye is moved the bodies move with a lazy wave-like excursion and return to their original location; they do not show an unrestrained course nor do they settle to the bottom of the vitreous chamber. They have been noted in the anterior chamber in cases of vitreous prolapse with dislocation of the

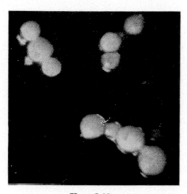   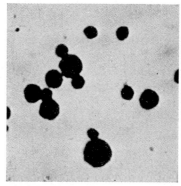

FIG. 341.   FIG. 342.

FIGS. 341 and 342.—ASTEROID BODIES.

Snowball opacities seen with reflected light in Fig. 341, by transmitted light in Fig. 342 (T. B. Holloway and W. E. Fry).

lens where they lie bound up in the jelly-like mass of vitreous (Gallenga, 1931; J. and S. Gupta, 1966). Sometimes they are associated with cellular elements which Janson (1925) considered to be derived from the retinal epithelum. The problem has been admirably summarized by Wickser (1968).

Chemical and histological examinations have been undertaken by several workers (Verhoeff, 1921; Bachstez, 1921–24; Holloway and Fry, 1929; Clapp, 1929; Gallenga, 1931; Hanssen, 1932; Rodman *et al.*, 1961), all of whom agree that these bodies are most probably *calcium soaps*, palmitate and stearate being mentioned; sodium and calcium phosphates and chlorides have been described, as well as fatty or lipid substances in various grades of stability. Tests for cholesterol, tyrosine and albumen have been negative. By polarized light they are seen to contain crystalline particles (Rodman *et al.*, 1961; Pau, 1965). The origin of these calcium-containing lipids is unknown; Krause (1935) suggested that they were derived from the lipids of degenerating leucocytes, Pau (1957–65) from pigmentary epithelial cells, and Rodman and his colleagues (1961) from the vitreous fibrils themselves. The most common association has been with diabetes, a relationship suggested by Vogt (1921); later authors have found that among such patients diabetes was present in 27% (Hatfield *et al.*, 1962; Bard, 1964) or 30% (Agarwal *et al.*, 1963), while an abnormal glucose-tolerance test was found by Smith (1958–65) in approximately 70%. Other associated ocular or general diseases seem on the whole to be coincidental, for although arterio-sclerosis (Black, 1909; Holloway, 1917–22; Verhoeff, 1921), nephritis (Stark, 1917) and other systemic diseases have been noted from time to time, and local conditions have coincided such as old choroiditis (Pollack, 1898; Holloway, 1917; Bachstez, 1924; Mathewson, 1927), cyclitis (Stark, 1924; Clapp, 1929), retinal hæmorrhages (Wiegmann, 1909; Holloway, 1917; Bailey, 1926) or venous thrombosis (Tenner, 1922), as frequently the patients have had no other discoverable lesion or disease. With insufficient evidence Stark (1917) associated them with syphilis and Bailey (1926) with tuber-culosis. The deposition may be due to changes in the composition of the blood, although the frequent unilaterality of the changes would indicate that the process must be aided by local causes in the vitreous; it may resemble the deposition of gall-stones but it may be significant that, although the phosphorus and cholesterol levels of the blood-serum have been found to be normal, a significant increase has been observed in the calcium content of the serum (Jervey and Anderson, 1965). Asteroid bodies have also been observed in primary hypercholesterolæmia (Rosen, 1952). It is interesting that calcium deposits (probably of the oxalate) are common in the retina after naphthalene poisoning in rabbits (Adams, 1930), an animal in which similar depositions can be formed by rendering the vitreous alkaline (Jess, 1922).

There is no evidence that the presence of such bodies has given rise to symptoms or has been responsible for a reduction of vision; nor that they have been modified in any way by treatment.

SYNCHISIS SCINTILLANS

SYNCHISIS SCINTILLANS is probably a rarer occurrence than asteroid bodies; moreover, it occurs in younger patients frequently under 35 years of age, and is more usually bilateral. Macnamara (1868) gave a vivid and lively description of the condition of " sparkling synchisis " wherein in-numerable particles of cholesterol floated in the vitreous like a multitude of grains of gold-leaf whisking about in all directions. In contrast to the white spheres of the asteroid bodies, these crystalline deposits have a flat, angular, crystalline appearance. Occurring in a degenerated and fluid vitreous, they may lie hidden at the bottom of the vitreous chamber while the eye remains still, and then when the globe is moved, they leap up into sight, flash about with such rapidity that exact observation of their shape is difficult, and finally settle down like a shower of glittering golden sovereigns or silvery

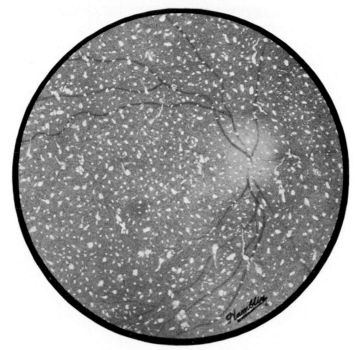

FIG. 343.—SYNCHISIS SCINTILLANS.

The shower of particles in the vitreous just after it has been disturbed.

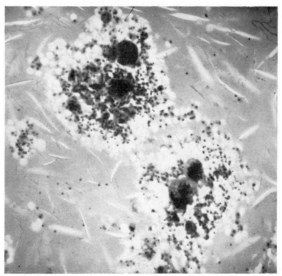

FIG. 344.—CRYSTALLINE DEPOSITS.

Showing vitreous exudate containing large numbers of cholesterol crystals associated with foreign-body giant cells. Eight years previously there had been a perforating corneal wound (H. & E.; × 120) (N. Ashton).

tinsel-like particles to the bottom of the vitreous chamber where they remain until they are disturbed again. Both with the ophthalmoscope and the slit-lamp they present a beautiful and quite characteristic picture as they flash by with a gleam as of burnished gold (Fig. 343).

It is interesting that their movements have been recorded by stereo-photography by Lijo-Pavia (1934).

Sometimes the fluid vitreous fills the anterior chamber, in which case they may form a pseudo-hypopyon gleaming with metallic reflexes (Koby, 1932), or the entire anterior chamber may be filled with the crystals (Hughes, 1937).

Microscopical and chemical examinations have shown that the crystals of this type are usually composed of *cholesterol*[1] (Fig. 344).

It is to be remembered that in contrast to asteroid bodies which appear in relatively healthy but aged eyes, this condition is secondary in that it occurs in degenerative ocular conditions; but of itself it gives rise to no symptoms and demands no treatment.

Adams, D. R. *Brit. J. Ophthal.*, **14**, 49, 545 (1930).

Adams, J. E. *Trans. ophthal. Soc. U.K.*, **1**, 135 (1881).

Agarwal, Mohan, Khosla and Gupta. *Orient. Arch. Ophthal.*, **1**, 167 (1963).

Bachstez. *Wien. med. Wschr.*, **71**, 1044 (1921). *Z. Augenheilk.*, **54**, 26 (1924).

Backer. Schmidt's *Jb. In- u. Ausl. ges. Med.*, Leipzig, **70**, 105 (1851).

Bailey. *Amer. J. Ophthal.*, **9**, 760 (1926).

Bard. *Amer. J. Ophthal.*, **58**, 239 (1964).

Benson. *Trans. ophthal. Soc. U.K.*, **14**, 101 (1894).

Berlin. *Z. vergl. Augenheilk.*, **2**, 110 (1883).

Black. *Ophthal. Rec.*, **18**, 201 (1909).

Clapp. *Arch. Ophthal.*, **2**, 635 (1929).

Contino. *G. ital. Oftal.*, **17**, 63, 129 (1964).

Cross. *Trans. ophthal. Soc. U.K.*, **6**, 376 (1886).

Desmarres. *Ann. Oculist.* (Paris), **14**, 220 (1845); **24**, 195 (1850).

D'Oench. *N.Y. med. Rec.*, **35**, 268 (1889).

Erggelet. *Klin. Mbl. Augenheilk.*, **53**, 449 (1914).

Feingold. *Amer. J. Ophthal.*, **5**, 840 (1922).

Gallenga. *Arch. Ottal.*, **38**, 398 (1931).

Gupta, J. and S. *Amer. J. Ophthal.*, **62**, 1207 (1966).

Hanssen. *Z. Augenheilk.*, **76**, 77 (1932).

Hatfield, Gastineau and Rucker. *Proc. Mayo Clin.*, **37**, 513 (1962).

Hirschberg. *Dtsch. Z. prakt. Med.*, **3**, 39 (1876).

Holloway. *Trans. Amer. ophthal. Soc.*, **15**, 153 (1917). *Arch. Ophthal.*, **47**, 50 (1918). *Amer. J. Ophthal.*, **5**, 100 (1922).

Holloway and Fry. *Arch. Ophthal.*, **2**, 521 (1929).

Hughes. *Arch. Ophthal.*, **18**, 477 (1937).

Janson. *Klin. Mbl. Augenheilk.*, **75**, 681 (1925).

Jervey and Anderson. *Sth. med. J.* (Bgham. Ala.), **58**, 191 (1965).

Jess. *Ber. dtsch. ophthal. Ges.*, **43**, 11 (1922).

Koby. *Biomicroscopie du corps vitré*, Paris, 100 (1932).

Krause. *Arch. Ophthal.*, **13**, 1022 (1935).

Lijo-Pavia. *Bull. Soc. Ophtal. Paris*, 35 (1934).

Macnamara. *Diseases of the Eye*, London, 437 (1868).

Mathewson. *Amer. J. Ophthal.*, **10**, 53 (1927).

Pau. *Klin. Mbl. Augenheilk.*, **131**, 610 (1957). *v. Graefes Arch. Ophthal.*, **161**, 64 (1959). *Ophthalmologica*, **150**, 167 (1965).

Pollack. *Beitr. Augenheilk.*, **3** (24), 375 (1898).

Poncet. *Ann. Oculist.* (Paris), **75**, 235 (1876).

Robert. *Ann. Oculist.* (Paris), **18**, 79 (1847).

Robertson, Argyll. *Trans. ophthal. Soc. U.K.*, **14**, 102 (1894).

Rodman, Johnson and Zimmerman. *Arch. Ophthal.*, **66**, 552 (1961).

Rosen. *Amer. J. Ophthal.*, **35**, 573 (1952).

Rutherford. *Arch. Ophthal.*, **9**, 106 (1933).

Sgrosso. *Rev. gén. Ophtal.*, **11**, 481 (1892).

Sichel. *Ann. Oculist.* (Paris), **15**, 167 (1846); **24**, 49 (1850); **25**, 9; **26**, 3 (1851).

Smith, J. L. *J. Amer. med. Ass.*, **168**, 891 (1958). *Trans. Amer. Acad. Ophthal.*, **69**, 269 (1965).

Stark. *Arch. Ophthal.*, **46**, 38 (1917). *Trans. Amer. ophthal. Soc.*, **22**, 315 (1924).

Stout. *Gaz. méd. Paris*, **2**, 72 (1847).

Tenner. *Arch. Ophthal.*, **51**, 507 (1922).

Valentin. *Hoppe-Seyl. Z. physiol. Chem.*, **105**, 33 (1919).

[1] Stout (1847), Poncet (1876), Berlin (1883), Sgrosso (1892), Westpfahl (1915), Valentin (1919), Koby (1932), Hughes (1937), and others.

Valk. *N.Y. med. Rec.*, **35**, 569 (1889).
Verhoeff. *Amer. J. Ophthal.*, **4**, 155 (1921).
Vogt. *Atlas d. Spaltlampenmikroskopie d. lebenden Auges*, Berlin (1921).
Webster. *Arch. Ophthal.*, **12**, 179 (1883).

Westpfahl. *Arch. Augenheilk.*, **78**, 1 (1915).
Wickser. *Docum. ophthal.*, **24**, 3 (1968).
Wiegmann. *Wschr. Therap. Hyg. Auges*, **12**, 353 (1909).
　　Klin. Mbl. Augenheilk., **61**, 82 (1918).

EXOGENOUS OPACITIES

Exogenous opacities are of various kinds.

(1) PROTEIN forming a diffuse dust-cloud or aggregating into clumps is a common accompaniment of all conditions in which the capillaries of the ciliary body are dilated. Such a *plasmoid vitreous* corresponds in every way to a plasmoid aqueous and is associated particularly with cyclitis, chorioretinitis, choroidal tumours or contusions. A powdery exudative opacity of

FIGS. 345 and 346.—AMYLOID INFILTRATION (D. Paton and J. R. Duke).

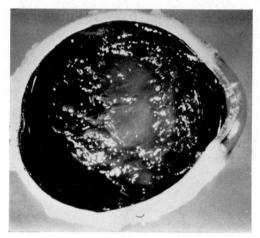

FIG. 345.—A case of primary familial amyloidosis. Opacities in the vitreous of the right eye at the time of gross examination. Lens removed during examination.

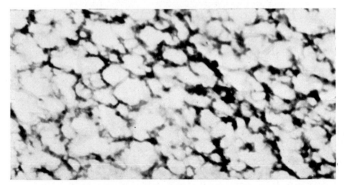

FIG. 346.—The fibrillar pattern of amyloid deposition in the vitreous of the right eye (crystal violet; × 100).

this type is frequently difficult to analyse ophthalmoscopically, for the fundus merely appears hazy with its details obscured, and the disc may seem indistinct and muzzy as if an optic neuritis were present. Subjectively a cloudiness and lowering of the visual acuity are usually remarked.

(2) AMYLOID DEPOSITS are a rarity in the vitreous. This substance, composed of closely related glycoproteins, is not usually deposited in the gel although other structures of the eye may be grossly affected.[1] In primary familial amyloidosis, however, one of the most prominent features is the appearance of vitreous opacities (Kantarjian and DeJong, 1953; Falls *et al.*, 1955; Kaufman, 1958; Paton and Duke, 1966; Wong and McFarlin, 1967; Andersson and Kassman, 1968). These may be gross and dense, globular and cell-like in the anterior vitreous and dense and wave-like resembling glass wool posteriorly where a greyish gelatinous mass may be formed in the absence of any signs of inflammation; in severe cases they may be responsible for causing virtual blindness. Histologically the deposit is seen to consist of a meshwork of coarse branching fibrils and nodules staining characteristically for amyloid (Paton and Duke, 1966) (Figs. 345–6). Attempts to replace the vitreous by cadaver vitreous (Kaufman, 1958) or liquid silicone (Paton and Duke, 1966) have not proved successful. The heroic surgical procedure of cutting a tunnel with forceps and scissors through the vitreous to the posterior pole of the eye after the cornea had been widely reflected and the lens removed was adopted with reasonably satisfactory results by Kasner and his colleagues (1968); thereafter the eye was filled with Ringer's solution.

(3) CELLULAR ELEMENTS

The cells which may invade the vitreous body from the surrounding tissues include inflammatory exudative cells, phagocytic mesodermal cells or mononuclear cells, epithelial cells, glial cells, neoplasic cells and blood cells, while formed pieces of the retina or rosettes may be found within the gel.

(*a*) EXUDATIVE CELLS, particularly lymphocytes, leucocytes and plasma cells, invade the vitreous in inflammatory conditions of the ciliary body and retina. We have already seen[2] that in cases of retinitis it is a commonplace for great quantities of such cells to break through the internal limiting membrane of the retina and become aggregated on the surface of the gel in heaps (Fig. 347) or spread into large sheets, sometimes appearing ophthalmoscopically as if they were exudative masses in the retina itself (Fig. 348). Thence the gel may become diffusely infiltrated but pathological specimens show that these cells accumulate preferentially on the walls of cavities of liquefaction or cling to the membranous septa seen in histological specimens[3] (Fig. 349). Such an infiltration may be present to any degree,

[1] Vol. IX, p. 738.　　　　　　　　　　　[2] Vol. X, p. 199.
[3] Dhai (1910), Straub (1912), Brückner (1919), Fuchs (1920). Rados (1920), Kafka (1923), Samuels (1930).

varying from a general bespattering of the vitreous so that the retina is seen
hazily, to the conversion of the entire vitreous cavity into an abscess as occurs
in panophthalmitis.   These inflammatory cells may remain unchanged for an
indefinite time; alternatively, degenerative changes ensue when they become
crenated, star-shaped and vacuolated (physaliphores), or suffer fatty changes;
and finally, when inflammatory exudation has been intense, organization and
fibrosis develop with the formation of cyclitic membranes or a pseudo-glioma.[1]
In this event giant cells, fatty globules and pigmentary deposits may appear
and vascularization, calcification, cartilage formation and eventually ossification may develop, and the contraction of the mass may lead to retinal
detachment and shrinkage of the globe.

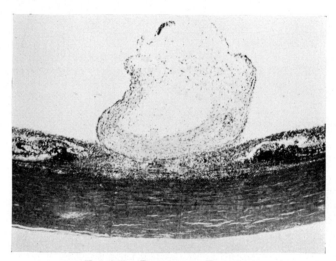

FIG. 347.—PRERETINAL EXUDATE.

An unusual case of connatal toxoplasmosis.   The retina is heavily infected with
many encysted colonies of *Toxoplasma* and there is a wad extending into the vitreous
over the active focus of chorioretinal necrotic inflammation (W. A. Manschot).

(*b*) PHAGOCYTIC CELLS (the " hyalocytes " of Balazs, 1958) are most
commonly mesodermal *microglia* from the retina (Fig. 335).   These are normally scattered uniformly around the periphery of the vitreous with a
tendency to concentrate in the neighbourhood of the retinal vessels.   In
several pathological conditions of the retina they may proliferate and are
increased in number (Gärtner, 1962) and occasionally they become enor-
mously swollen and loaded with lipids to form glitter cells (Wolter, 1960)
(Figs. 350–1).   Lipid-laden histiocytes may percolate into the vitreous in
the histiocytoses[2] (the " lipidosis bulbi " of Heath, 1933) (Fig. 352).

MONONUCLEAR CELLS, apart from their presence in inflammatory conditions, frequently invade the vitreous as phagocytes; they engulf the red

[1] Vol. IX, p. 102.   [2] Vol. VII, p. 151.

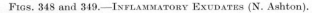

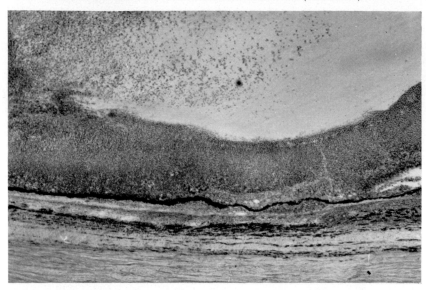

FIG. 348.—The retina is destroyed by purulent exudate and pus is present in considerable quantity in both the choroid and the vitreous (H. & E.; × 48).

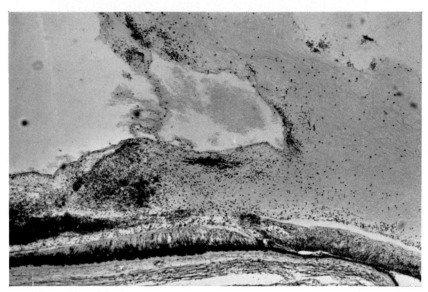

FIG. 349.—Heavy purulent exudates in the vitreous in the region of the ora serrata (H. & E.; × 48).

FIGS. 350 and 351.—VITREOUS MICROGLIA (J. R. Wolter).

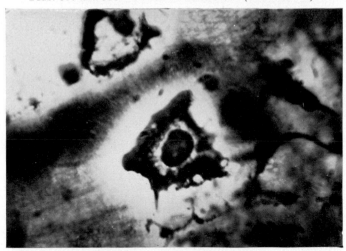

FIG. 350.—In the processes of phagocytosis, showing some vacuoles in the protoplasm.

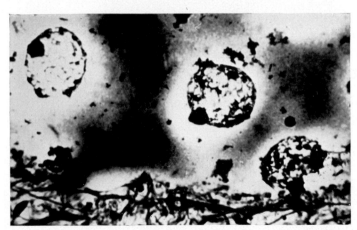

FIG. 351.—The cell has much phagocytosed substance within it and has become a glitter cell. The retina is visible in the lower part of the picture (frozen section; Hortega stain).

cells in vitreous hæmorrhages, the pigmentary granules liberated from the epithelium in the presence of choroidal tumours, as well as the debris of inflammations and are particularly common in phacolytic reactions.[1]

(c) EPITHELIAL CELLS from the ciliary body may be found in the vitreous, sometimes intact but more usually broken up, the walls being ruptured so that their small black pigment granules are set free to be engulfed by macrophages. The frequent occurrence of proliferations of the cells of the

[1] Vol. IX, p. 501.

ciliary epithelium and their migration into the vitreous gel to form floaters was first stressed by Teng and Katzin (1951) and has already been described.[1] Similarly, cells from the retinal pigmentary epithelium may migrate into the peripheral portions of the gel (Samuels, 1930).

(*d*) GLIAL CELLS may occasionally proliferate from the retina into the vitreous, usually assuming a circular shape, sometimes still attached to the retina by a pedicle and sometimes floating in the gel.

(*e*) After hæmorrhages into the vitreous at the stage of retinitis proliferans with the formation of new vessels, we have already seen that solid cords of ENDOTHELIAL CELLS and UNDIFFERENTIATED MESENCHYMAL CELLS associated with microglial phagocytes may invade the vitreous in considerable numbers as they take part in the formation of fibrous connective tissue.[2]

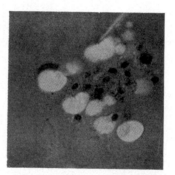

FIG. 352.—LIPID-LADEN HISTIOCYTES.
Clumps of fatty and pigmented cells in the vitreous (P. Heath).

(*f*) TUMOUR CELLS are rare visitors to the vitreous, but they may occur and may even set up metastatic deposits. Such seedings are exceptional from melanomatous and epitheliomatous neoplasms, but are much more common from retinoblastomata, being, indeed, frequent in endophytic tumours of this type.[3]

(*g*) FORMED PIECES OF THE RETINA may be seen ophthalmoscopically and with the slit-lamp and gonio-lens to be floating freely in the vitreous representing torn pieces of this tissue loosened by the traction of vitreous adhesions; these may be composed of the inner layers of the retina leaving the lamellar holes typical of cystoid degeneration, or of the entire thickness of this tissue when the operculum of a retinal tear becomes similarly detached. The detached portion of the retina may be suddenly seen entoptically as a dark floater and may cause considerable annoyance to the patient ; its appearance may be preceded by bright photopsiæ, while it may be associated with a transient dust-like haze indicating a small hæmorrhage (Simpson, 1951).

[1] Vol. X, p. 559.   [2] Vol. X, p. 150.   [3] Vol. X, p. 686.

The importance of the phenomenon lies in the possibility of the subsequent development of a retinal detachment.

A further appearance in the vitreous is ROSETTES derived from the retina, usually from its extreme periphery at the site of the ciliary ridges between the oval bays. These may become pedunculated and protrude into the vitreous and eventually may become detached to appear as discrete floating bodies (Fig. 353).

We have also seen that the inner layer of a retinoschisis may float in the vitreous resembling a semi-transparent veil.[1]

Other organized cellular elements are occasionally found, such as free wandering tubercles (Sená, 1936) or organized inflammatory tissue adhering to a detached vitreous.

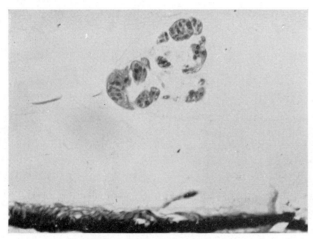

FIG. 353.—AN ORGANIZED OPACITY.
A free floater of epithelial cells in the vitreous (C. C. Teng and H. M. Katzin).

(*h*) BLOOD in the vitreous may obliterate any view of the fundus and abolish the red reflex if the hæmorrhage is massive; when it is not so profuse the blood always appears black ophthalmoscopically in the initial stages in contrast to the whitish or grey appearance of degenerative, inflammatory or neoplasic opacities, although it may gradually change to a greyish appearance after some weeks. As a rule, however, the red cells are distinguishable with the slit-lamp; these cells are remarkable for the state of preservation which they show, maintaining their shape and red colour for many months before they are finally absorbed (Samuels, 1930). The origin, appearance and behaviour of such hæmorrhages will be discussed at a later stage.[2]

(4) PIGMENT GRANULES

MELANOTIC PIGMENT GRANULES, both retinal and uveal, are found sometimes in large quantities with age, in glaucoma, after trauma and

[1] Vol. X, p. 559.   [2] p. 363.

inflammations, in retinal detachments, and with melanotic tumours. The pigmentation may be slight, comprised of a few minute and scarcely visible individual granules, or may be abundant and arranged in large clumps; the granules, which are usually of a brownish colour, frequently attach themselves to the supporting fibrils, and may produce beautiful effects as they reflect the incident light of the slit-lamp at various angles; moreover, they may be deposited extensively on the posterior capsule of the lens.

BLOOD PIGMENT may also persist for a very considerable time after hæmorrhages, sometimes in small amounts, and sometimes in sufficient quantity to change the colour of the gel and obscure the architecture of its framework.

CYSTS IN THE VITREOUS may be noted in this connection. These are usually congenital or developmental anomalies and have been previously discussed.[1] It is probable that some of those floating in the posterior part of the vitreous have been derived from the hyaloid artery or its glial sheath while others may be of pathological origin.

FIGS. 354 and 355.—THE DIAGNOSIS OF A VITREOUS HÆMORRHAGE BY ULTRASOUND (A. Oksala).

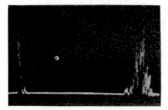
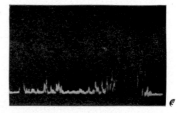

FIG. 354.—The echogram of a normal eye. On the extreme left is the echo from the posterior surface of the lens; no echoes are emitted by the vitreous space; on the right is the echo from the posterior coat of the eye.

FIG. 355.—In a recent vitreous hæmorrhage after several previous hæmorrhages. There are some low echoes from the vitreous.

These various opacities are indistinguishable separately by the ophthalmoscope, appearing merely as dust-like opacities when not sufficiently numerous to obliterate the reflex of the fundus. If they are present in great quantities, the whitish-green reflection of a purulent exudate or the dark-red glow of a hæmorrhage may be evident by focal illumination. With the slit-lamp the cells may be characterized: erythrocytes are obviously red in colour while exudative or other cells appear as brilliant white points without special form, diffusing or diffracting the light rather than reflecting it, and tending to cling to the condensed fibrillæ of the gel.

A further analysis of vitreous opacities can be made by the diagnostic use of ultrasound which may be useful when the entire vitreous body is opacified or if the cornea or lens is opaque (Baum and Greenwood, 1958; Oksala and Lehtinen, 1959; Oksala, 1960–63; Ricci and Itin, 1966).[2] The

[1] Vol. III, p. 763.   [2] Vol. VII, p. 325.

echograms indicate the site of the opacity and may provide suggestions regarding its nature. A number of low reflections is characteristic of inflammatory exudative opacities and a hæmorrhage gives a series of more accentuated waves, higher when the bleeding is fresh (Figs. 354–5). Moreover, a clear indication can be given whether the retina is in place or is detached.

The *treatment* of vitreous opacities is difficult and usually disappointing. No matter what treatment is adopted, cellular elements if not too abundant tend to disappear, and it is probable that fine dust and strands derived from the stroma may also disappear in time. Grosser opacities, however, and connective-tissue strands and membranes as well as crystalline deposits always persist. To aid the disappearance of such elements which can be dissolved, various expedients are usually suggested, but since they tend to disappear slowly of their own accord, the efficacy of any treatment is often difficult to assess. It is, however, obvious that any underlying disease of the eye should be adequately treated, and any general condition which determines the local degeneration, whether infective, toxic or sclerotic, should receive such attention as is possible. The most important treatment is ætiological—the prevention of the development of further trouble by eliminating the cause—if this can be done.

The local expedients that have been employed included heat, radiotherapy, subconjunctival injections, dionine, short-wave diathermy, ultrasonic stimulation, and other measures designed to quicken metabolic interchange and promote absorption; while as to general treatment, rest with the administration of mercury and iodine used to be the standard classical expedient, and more lately the induction of artificial fever. If there is no general contra-indication for these measures, even although their therapeutic value is based on hope rather than on proved results, they at least do the local condition no harm even if they do no good.

Operative measures have also been advocated, such as trephining with a view to accelerating tissue-interchange (G. E. and G. H. Henton, 1937; and others), or superficial diathermic coagulation of an area in the lower half of the eye followed by 10 days' immobility in the hope that the vascular reaction and increased fluidity of the gel would allow the opacities to settle over and adhere to the cauterized area (Weve, 1939; Blumenthal, 1958; Forgacs, 1962).

When the opacities are sufficiently massive to abolish vision, and all reasonable hope of spontaneous absorption has been given up, the more heroic procedure of VITREOUS REPLACEMENT may be attempted. Replacement by the vitreous of another species of animal always leads to shrinkage of the eye (Dor, 1912; and others), but the simple withdrawal of a small quantity of opacified vitreous which is made good by a transudate from the choroid has occasionally led to good results (zur Nedden, 1920–22; O'Malley,

1951–54).   Its replacement is usually more satisfactory and has been effected by physiological salt solution (Elschnig, 1911–12; Löwenstein and Samuels, 1912), serum (Sattler, 1909) or cerebro-spinal fluid (Hegner, 1928; Hu, 1951; Scuderi, 1954), solutions or emulsions of hyaluronic acid (Widder, 1960), " reconstituted vitreous " consisting of a collagen gel reinforced by hyaluronic acid (Balazs and Sweeney, 1966), cadaver vitreous which may be preserved (Cutler, 1946; Fritz, 1950; Landegger, 1950; Shafer, 1957; McKinney, 1964), or lyophilized vitreous (Paufique *et al.*, 1953–63; Stobbe and Keeney, 1960), while artificial non-absorbable fluids have been employed such as liquid silicone (Cibis *et al.*, 1962; Dufour, 1964; Moreau, 1964; and others) or polygeline (Oosterhuis *et al.*, 1966; van Haeringen *et al.*, 1966). Liquid silicone is retained permanently in the globe and until more is known of the possible complications of its long-term retention in the eye it is probably safest not to use it in supplementation procedures unless its subsequent removal is contemplated.   In rabbits, Daniele and his colleagues (1968) successfully implanted dehydrated glyceryl methacrylate hydrogel which swells to 32 times its volume after implantation.

The technique of vitreous replacement has already been described in a previous Volume[1]; the needle is introduced through the pars plana (6 mm. behind the limbus) and pushed backwards into the posterior part of the globe and the desired quantity of vitreous removed.   In this region the gel is frequently detached or liquefied and if this part of the globe is filled with foreign material the anterior part of the vitreous acts as a buffer zone between the injected material and the lens and the anterior chamber; a complicated cataract is thus avoided and some obstruction is offered to the entrance of the injected mass into the posterior and anterior chambers, particularly in aphakic eyes.   When the cloudy vitreous is withdrawn for replacement, this should always be in stages, less than one-third of the volume of the vitreous being removed each time lest a retinal detachment ensue, but it is to be remembered that phthisis of the globe is a possible sequel.   None of these methods of treatment, however, can be said to be particularly satisfactory or encouraging, and they should not be employed unless hope is abandoned that the opacities will clear and the alternative to somewhat heroic and risky surgery is virtual blindness.

Andersson and Kassman. *Acta ophthal.* (Kbh.), **46**, 441 (1968).

Balazs.   *Acta XVIII int. Cong. Ophthal.*, Brussels, **2**, 1296 (1958).

Balazs and Sweeney.   *Mod. Probl. Ophthal.*, **4**, 230 (1966).

Baum and Greenwood.   *Arch. Ophthal.*, **60**, 263 (1958).

Blumenthal.   *S. Afr. med. J.*, **32**, 296 (1958).

Brückner.   *v. Graefes Arch. Ophthal.*, **100**, 179 (1919).

Cibis, Becker, Okun and Canaan.   *Arch. Ophthal.*, **68**, 590 (1962).

Cutler.   *Arch. Ophthal.*, **35**, 615 (1946).

Daniele, Refojo, Schepens and Freeman.   *Arch. Ophthal.*, **80**, 120 (1968).

Dhai.   *Over glasoochtstof* (Thesis), Amsterdam (1910).   See *Ophthalmology*, **7**, 708 (1911).

Dor.   *Clin. Ophtal.*, **14**, 119 (1912).

Dufour.   *Ophthalmologica*, **147**, 160 (1964).

Elschnig.   *Ber. dtsch. ophthal. Ges.*, **37**, 11 (1911).

v. *Graefes Arch. Ophthal.*, **80**, 514 (1912).

Falls, Jackson, Carey *et al.*   *Arch. Ophthal.*, **54**, 660 (1955).

Forgacs.   *Ann. Oculist.* (Paris), **195**, 743 (1962).

Fritz.   *Amer. J. Ophthal.*, **32**, 45 (1950).

Fuchs.   *v. Graefes Arch. Ophthal.*, **103**, 228 (1920).

Gärtner.   *v. Graefes Arch. Ophthal.*, **164**, 473 (1962).

van Haeringen, Oosterhuis, Glasius and Jeltes.   *Exp. Eye Res.*, **5**, 235 (1966).

Henton, G. E. and G. H.   *Arch. Ophthal.*, **18**, 103 (1937).

[1] Vol. X, p. 845.

Heath. *Arch. Ophthal,*, **10**, 342 (1933).
Hegner. *Ber. dtsch. ophthal. Ges.*, **47**, 391 (1928).
Hu. *Chin. J. Ophthal.*, **1**, 117 (1951).
Kafka. *Zbl. ges. Ophthal.*, **10**, 65 (1923).
Kantarjian and DeJong. *Neurology* (Minneap.), **3**, 399 (1953).
Kasner, Miller, Taylor *et al.* *Trans. Amer. Acad. Ophthal.*, **72**, 410 (1968).
Kaufman. *Arch. Ophthal.*, **60**, 1036 (1958).
Landegger. *Amer. J. Ophthal.*, **33**, 915 (1950).
Löwenstein and Samuels. *v. Graefes Arch. Ophthal.*, **80**, 500 (1912).
McKinney. *Amer. J. Ophthal.*, **57**, 790 (1964).
Moreau. *Trans. ophthal. Soc. U.K.*, **84**, 167 (1964).
zur Nedden. *v. Graefes Arch. Ophthal.*, **101**, 145 (1920).
  Klin. Mbl. Augenheilk., **64**, 593, 846 (1920); **66**, 759 (1921); **69**, 514 (1922).
Oksala. *Amer. J. Ophthal.*, **49**, 1301 (1960).
  Klin. Mbl. Augenheilk., **137**, 72 (1960).
  Brit. J. Ophthal., **47**, 65 (1963).
Oksala and Lehtinen. *Acta ophthal.* (Kbh.), **37**, 17 (1959).
O'Malley. *Trans. ophthal. Soc. U.K.*, **71**, 773 (1951); **74**, 599 (1954).
Oosterhuis. *Arch. Ophthal.*, **76**, 374 (1966).
Oosterhuis, van Haeringen, Jeltes and Glasius. *Arch. Ophthal.*, **76**, 258 (1966).
Paton and Duke. *Amer. J. Ophthal.*, **61**, 736 (1966).

Paufique, Charleux, Manuel *et al.* *Ann. Oculist.* (Paris), **196**, 1 (1963).
Paufique, Fayet and Ravault. *Ann. Oculist.* (Paris), **192**, 241 (1959).
Paufique and Moreau. *Ann. Oculist.* (Paris), **186**, 873 (1953).
Rados. *v. Graefes Arch. Ophthal.*, **103**, 331 (1920).
Ricci and Itin. *Bull. Soc. franç. Ophtal.*, **79**, 446 (1966).
Samuels. *Arch. Ophthal.*, **4**, 838 (1930).
Sattler. *Arch. Augenheilk.*, **64**, 390 (1909).
Scuderi. *Ann. Ottal.*, **80**, 213 (1954).
Sená. *Rev. Asoc. méd. argent.*, **50**, 145 (1936).
Shafer. *Trans. Amer. Acad. Ophthal.*, **61**, 194 (1957).
Simpson. *Trans. Amer. ophthal. Soc.*, **49**, 75 (1951).
Stobbe and Keeney. *Arch. Ophthal.*, **64**, 571 (1960).
Straub. *Trans. ophthal. Soc. U.K.*, **32**, 60 (1912).
Szirmai and Balazs. *Arch. Ophthal.*, **59**, 34 (1958).
Teng and Katzin. *Amer. J. Ophthal.*, **34**, 1237 (1951).
Weve. *Trans. ophthal. Soc. U.K.*, **59**, 43 (1939).
Widder. *v. Graefes Arch. Ophthal.*, **162**, 416 (1960).
Wolter. *Amer. J. Ophthal.*, **49**, 1185 (1960).
Wong and McFarlin. *Arch. Ophthal.*, **78**, 208 (1967).

Detachments of the Vitreous Body

DETACHMENT IN THE PRESENCE OF MAJOR OCULAR DISEASE

From the earliest days of ophthalmic pathology it has been known that a gross detachment of the vitreous owing to the shrinkage of organized tissue which has proliferated into it from the uveal tract or the retina occurs as an end-result of intra-ocular disease (Müller, 1856; Iwanoff, 1869; de Wecker, 1876; and many others).   Such a gross detachment may be of four types:

(1) A relatively small *cul-de-sac detachment* occurring at any point in the circumference.

(2) An *infundibular detachment* (Milles, 1886) or funnel-shaped detachment wherein the vitreous assumes a tent-like shape, the apex being at the disc and the base round the ora (Fig. 356).   At other times the apex is situated at the site of a patch of chorioretinitis or of a perforating wound.

(3) A *posterior detachment* (Milles, 1886) wherein the attachment at the posterior pole gives way to a varying degree so that eventually the entire mass of the vitreous becomes bunched up as a hemispherical mass behind the lens (Fig. 357).

(4) An *anterior detachment* is very rare, but this portion of the vitreous may be stripped from the lens and zonule and fall back considerably; such a condition may be associated with a posterior detachment as well, in which

case the vitreous assumes the form of a broad band at the level of the ora serrata. A tearing away of the base of the vitreous from its attachment at this point is a still greater rarity and is usually due either to trauma or to the presence and presumably the contraction of pseudo-membranes in a degenerating vitreous after trauma or iridocyclitis.[1]

In these cases the vitreous is always degenerated and shrunken, and is pulled forwards by shrinking exudates and organizing fibrous tissue. Its outer surface is frequently covered by a fibro-cellular membrane similar in appearance and origin to the membranes which in similar circumstances cover the retina.[2] Occasionally in areas where organization is marked, this adventitious tissue may be of considerable thickness, and if it tears away with

FIGS. 356 and 357.—DETACHMENT OF THE VITREOUS (Museum, Inst. Ophthal.).

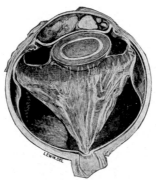 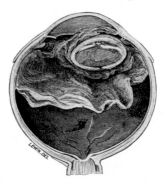

FIG. 356.—Antero-lateral and infundibular detachments of the vitreous in an eye injured 5 weeks previously.

FIG. 357.—Globular detachment of the vitreous. There is a traumatic dislocation of the lens and vitreous has passed into the anterior chamber.

the detached vitreous a dense round vitreous opacity results (Parsons, 1905; Samuels, 1930). The space between the vitreous and the retina is usually filled with a protein-rich fluid. In these cases, of course, the detachment of the vitreous is merely a pathological incident in a lesion the seriousness of which lies elsewhere.

DETACHMENT IN THE ABSENCE OF MAJOR OCULAR DISEASE

A type of detachment occurring with less obvious cause *in a vitreous not grossly degenerated* has given rise to more controversy. Most of the older pathologists, following Müller (1856) and Iwanoff (1869), considered that a detachment of this nature complicated such conditions as high myopia and staphylomata and that it was essentially a detachment *e vacuo* (Iwanoff, 1869); others again considered the pathological picture to be due to an artefact of fixation (Greeff, 1902; Elschnig, 1904). More recent histological research, however, using fixatives which involve no shrinkage (Sallmann, 1936), have

---

[1] Comberg (1924), Samuels (1930), Koby (1932), Fodor (1935), Vogt (1935), Bassin (1936), Cavka (1937).
[2] Vol. X, p. 780.

demonstrated that it does occur. It is true that an artificial posterior detachment due to post-mortem fixation does occur, but the ante-mortem variety can be differentiated histologically by the presence of albumen in the fluid between the vitreous and the retina and the occasional presence of cells.

Clinically a similar controversy arose referring particularly to myopic eyes. Early writers such as Brière (1875) and Galezowski (1877) described a grey circular opacity seen in front of the disc in myopic eyes as a detachment of the vitreous, a view strongly supported by Weiss (1885–97) who described the appearance of a reflex marking the posterior limit of the vitreous some distance in front of the retina when the posterior pole of the eye had elongated in myopia. Since his observations the circular opacity in the posterior face of the vitreous is frequently called *Weiss's ring*. A similar view was adopted by Dimmer (1882) and Dor (1898), while Masuda (1913) explained a faint opacity in this region in an emmetropic eye as probably a congenital malformation. Thereafter, however, more modern methods of optical examination by the stereoscopic ophthalmoscope and then by the slit-lamp aided by a contact glass, and eventually by the Hruby lens and the gonio-lens, opened up the vitreous to more minute inspection, and it has been definitely established that detachments of this type are relatively common, occurring not only in myopes but also in emmetropes and hypermetropes in degenerative and inflammatory conditions. The pioneer in these observations was Kraupa (1914–25) and his findings have been amply confirmed by many others.[1]

Such detachments may be of three kinds.

(1) *Anterior vitreous detachment (anterior hyaloideo-capsular separation).* It will be remembered[2] that normally the anterior face of the vitreous is separated from the posterior capsule of the lens by a potential space (of Berger) and is attached to it by a circular ring of relatively frail adherence (the hyaloideo-capsular ligament of Wieger). In certain pathological conditions this adhesion is ruptured and the potential space between the lens and the vitreous becomes a real interspace; the separation may be partial or complete (Figs. 358–9).

Such a separation is relatively rare. Weber (1942–44) found it in 0·2% of eyes, but in cases of retinal detachment it is seen more frequently (8·5%, Cibis, 1965) and also in association with a posterior vitreous detachment (Cavka, 1937) in which case the vitreous assumes the form of a broad band at the level of the ora serrata. In pathological conditions the space may contain blood or inflammatory cells (Koby, 1932) and in pigmentary glaucoma, granules of pigment may collect within it.

(2) An *antero-lateral vitreous detachment (anterior hyaloideo-retinal separation;* detachment of the base of the vitreous) (Fig. 358) is an extremely rare condition which is difficult to diagnose except with the gonio-lens. Usually occurring in a localized form it may be associated with subluxation

---

[1] Lister (1922), Pillat (1922–36), Comberg (1924), Vogt (1924–35), Isakowitz (1926–32), Amsler (1930), Koby (1932), Anderson (1933), von Rötth (1933–34), Sallmann and Rieger (1934), Fodor (1935), Baenziger (1935), Sallmann (1936), Bassin (1936), Lindner (1936–37), Cavka (1937), Churgina (1937), Kleefeld (1937), Fronimopoulos (1939), Hruby (1950–60), Pischel (1953), Schepens (1954), Favre (1955), Favre and Goldmann (1956), Busacca *et al.* (1957), Wadsworth (1957), Goldmann (1961), Rosen (1962).

[2] Vol. II, p. 295.

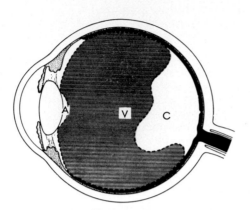

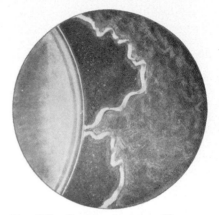

Fig. 358.—Vitreous Detachment.

A, anterior vitreous detachment; V, formed vitreous; C, posterior vitreous detachment (after P. Cibis).

Fig. 359.—Partial Anterior Vitreous Detachment.

The detachment occurred after the explosion of a bomb; seen with the slit-lamp (A. S. Philps).

or luxation of the lens or a dialysis at the ora, or may follow trauma or cataract extraction. The more common lesion in this situation, however, is a retinal detachment in the area of the ora and the pars plana.

(3) A *posterior vitreous detachment* (*posterior hyaloideo-retinal separation*) is much the most common and clinically important type, occurring frequently in myopic and almost constantly in senile eyes. It usually starts

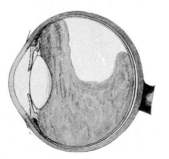

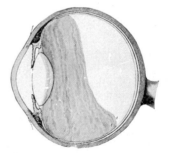

Fig. 360.—Superior detachment of the vitreous (after H. Rieger).

Fig. 361.—Posterior detachment of the vitreous (after H. Rieger).

as a *partial* detachment either at the posterior pole or often in the upper segment whence it frequently extends around the posterior pole (Figs. 360–1) and eventually may become *complete* when the hyaloid layer is separated from the retina up to the ora and the entire vitreous structure collapses, stretching as a relatively thin condensed band running across the eye behind the lens but still attached at the ora. As a rarity the attachment of

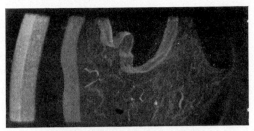

FIG. 362.—A superior detachment in an aphakic eye seen with the slit-lamp (A. Pillat).

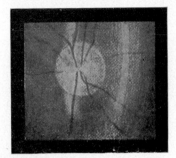

FIG. 363.—Posterior detachment seen with the ophthalmoscope (after H. Rieger).

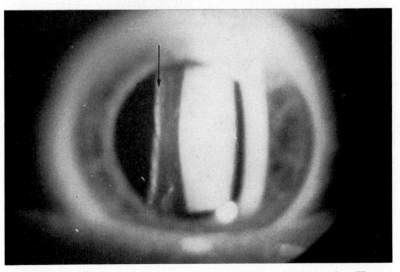

FIG. 364.—Posterior detachment: oscillation slit-lamp photograph. The arrow points to the posterior hyaloid layer (P. Cibis, *Mod. Probl. in Ophthal.*, **5**, 1967, S. Karger, Basel).

the vitreous to the optic disc may persist so that a funnel-shaped infundibular detachment may result.

The primary cause of such a retraction of the vitreous and its detachment is usually a degeneration of the gel with syneresis and the formation of cavities in its structure filled with fluid. Goldmann (1961) has described how these lacunæ gradually enlarge, occupying a considerable proportion of the vitreous until they eventually burst posteriorly emptying themselves into the hyaloideo-retinal space; meantime the gel itself retracts and its marginal hyaloid layer becomes much thickened so that its contour may be discernible by focal illumination (Figs. 362–4). At other times it collapses completely into a shrunken tangle of fibrillæ (Figs. 365–6); such an

FIGS. 365 and 366.—VITREOUS DETACHMENT WITH COLLAPSE (H. Goldmann).

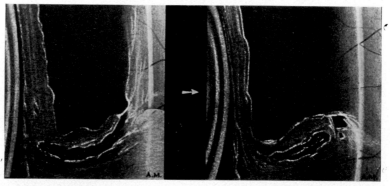

FIG. 365.   FIG. 366.

FIG. 365.—A large lacuna is seen to develop in the posterior part of the gel.
FIG. 366.—The lacuna communicates with the retro-vitreal space and the gel collapses to become concentrated behind the lens.

event usually occurs suddenly, sometimes in a matter of minutes. Sometimes the separation of the vitreous from its bed is complete; but in other cases adhesions remain where the shrunken gel still adheres to the retina (Fig. 367), particularly in the region where the superior oblique muscle is attached or where adhesions already exist in areas of cystoid or lattice degeneration of the retina or at old foci of chorioretinitis. Traction on these adhesions with movements of the globe may lead to the formation of horseshoe retinal tears, the importance of which in the causation of a detachment of the retina can easily be appreciated (Fig. 368); if in the process a blood vessel is torn a hæmorrhage will result, a relatively common event which will be discussed elsewhere.[1]

A second but less frequent complication is the development of retinal œdema at the posterior pole which possibly occurs if separation from the optic disc or macula has been difficult (Jaffe and Light, 1967; Jaffe, 1967); after

[1] p. 363.

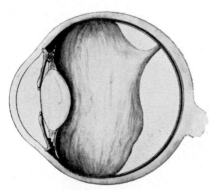 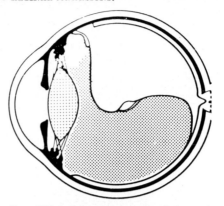

FIG. 367.—An adhesion occurring after vitreous retraction (after K. Hruby).

FIG. 368.—A horseshoe tear of the retina caused by the retinal flap adhering to the surface of a detached vitreous (H. Goldmann).

the vitreous has become detached the œdema usually subsides but if it has persisted for some time, cystoid degeneration of the macula may ensue. Indeed, there is some evidence that syneresis and shrinkage of the posterior part of the vitreous with adherence of its cortical layer to the retina at the macula so that traction exists may be a factor in the pathogenesis of serous

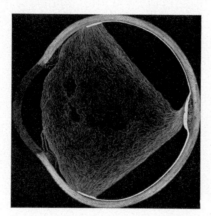

FIG. 369.—SEROUS DISCIFORM DETACHMENT OF THE MACULA.

There are vitreo-retinal adhesions over the macula in aphakia; the straight surface of the posterior vitreous indicates considerable tension (F. I. Tolentino et al.).

or hæmorrhagic central retinopathy and a cause of its frequent tendency to recur (Tolentino et al., 1967) (Fig. 369) and perhaps also in the formation of a retinal hole near the posterior pole (Jaffe, 1967).

Such detachments of the vitreous are usually associated with a thickening and opacification of its limiting hyaloid layer, which may be blurred, indefinite and shaggy, or clearly defined and even thrown into delicate folds.

Frequently holes appear in this layer (HYALOID HOLES), sometimes a single hole and sometimes an area showing a mosaic. Not uncommonly a membranous opacity is seen floating freely in the vitreous representing a torn area of this limiting layer; these may be thickened to form discrete masses which may originate from glial tissue from the optic disc or from fibro-cellular membranes situated elsewhere in the fundus, particularly from areas of

FIGS. 370 to 373.—CONDENSATION OF THE HYALOID LAYER.

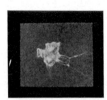

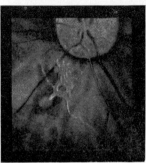

FIG. 370.—Vitreous detachment with opacity.

FIG. 371.—Vitreous detachment with condensation opacity (H. Rieger).

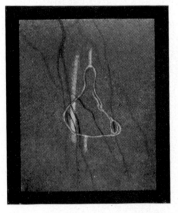

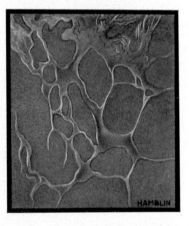

FIG. 372.—Vitreous detachment with hole (H. Rieger).

FIG. 373.—Vitreous detachment with trellis-work opacity.

inactive choroiditis (Figs. 370–3). Thus in posterior detachments the vitreous separates from its frail anchorage at the margin of the disc tearing away at the wide funnel-shaped expansion of Cloquet's canal. Such a ring-shaped aperture is commonly present in myopic and senile eyes and is best seen ophthalmoscopically with the plane mirror or with the slit-lamp used with a Hruby lens. The ring hovers at a variable distance in front of the optic disc, its edges forming an opacity which when seen from the side may appear oval and distorted, and with the passage of time it may alter in density, shape and position. Vogt (1924), who called the appearance the *senile ring*, considered it as characteristic of age as circumpapillary choroidal atrophy and lenticular opacities; he thought that the opacity was rendered dense by the adherence of glial tissue detached from the optic disc. Similarly, in optic neuritis a ring-shaped opacity of this type may be formed (Cavka, 1937), as well as in association with localized foci of chorioretinal disease or degeneration situated at the macula or in the periphery.[1]

We have seen that a vitreous detachment is an almost invariable accompaniment of a *detachment of the retina* and it has been found to occur in 41 out of 58 patients with adult retinoschisis (Shea *et al.*, 1960) and in 20% of 200 patients with all types, juvenile and adult, of this condition (Cibis, 1965). An unfortunate sequence may occur in long-standing retinal detachments wherein an extensive syneresis of the posterior vitreous occurs leaving its cortical layer adherent to the retina as a membrane while the main mass of the vitreous is condensed anteriorly behind the lens; in such a massive preretinal detachment of the vitreous, subsequent degeneration and contraction of the cortical layer which remains adherent to the retina always provides difficult problems for remedial surgery (Tolentino *et al.*, 1967). A vitreous detachment may also occur, although less frequently, in widespread retinal degenerations such as pigmentary dystrophy (Elschnig, 1904; Rieger, 1936–43; Bonavolontà, 1951).

In *aphakic eyes* a posterior detachment of some degree is always found (Hauer and Barkay, 1964; Tolentino and Schepens, 1965; Jaffe and Light, 1966). This complication usually occurs without incident but an œdema of the macular area or retinal hæmorrhages may occasionally occur (Fig. 369).

It is, of course, possible for a detachment to occur owing to the pushing forward of the vitreous by fluid collecting between it and the retina—as by a chorioretinal exudate, a subhyaloid hæmorrhage or a pooling of aqueous at the posterior pole.

The only *clinical symptom* associated with such detachments is the appearance of vitreous floaters and the occurrence of photopsiæ at the time of their development due to adherence of the internal limiting membrane of the retina to the face of the collapsed vitreous—the " subjective lightning streaks " of Foster Moore (1935), usually most obvious in the temporal field. Sometimes the detachment is accompanied by the development of a haze of vitreous opacities or a retinal hæmorrhage; and occasionally the ring-like formation of a posterior detachment or more irregular opacities are seen entoptically. *Treatment* is not indicated.

The main clinical interest, however, of such conditions is their *relation to*

[1] Kraupa (1914–25), Purtscher (1919), Lister (1922), Goldstein (1923), Bedell (1925), Isakowitz (1926), Anderson (1933), Rieger (1936), Goldmann (1961), and others.

retinal detachments, for an adhesion of the limiting membrane of a retracted vitreous to the retina whether at an area of degeneration or old inflammation is one of the frequent causes of the formation of horse-shoe tears in this tissue with their dangerous potentialities (see Linder, 1966).

Amsler. *Bull. Soc. franç. Ophtal.,* **43,** 315 (1930).
Anderson. *Brit. J. Ophthal.,* **17,** 460 (1933).
Baenziger. *v. Graefes Arch. Ophthal.,* **134,** 23 (1935).
Bassin. *Klin. Mbl. Augenheilk.,* **97,** 599 (1936).
Bedell. *Trans. ophthal. Soc. U.K.,* **45,** 646 (1925).
Bonavolontà. *Ann. Ottal.,* **77,** 15 (1951).
Brière. *Ann. Oculist.* (Paris), **74,** 138 (1875).
Busacca, Goldmann and Schiff-Wertheimer. *Biomicroscopie du corps vitré et du fond de l'œil,* Paris (1957).
Cavka. *v. Graefes Arch. Ophthal.,* **137,** 472 (1937).
Churgina. *Vestn. oftal.,* **11,** 13 (1937).
Cibis. *Vitreoretinal Pathology and Surgery in Retinal Detachment,* St. Louis (1965).
Comberg. *Klin. Mbl. Augenheilk.,* **72,** 692 (1924).
Dimmer. *Klin. Mbl. Augenheilk.,* **20,** 259 (1882).
Dor. *Ber. dtsch. ophthal. Ges.,* **27,** 321 (1898).
Elschnig. *Klin. Mbl. Augenheilk.,* **42** (2), 529 (1904).
Favre. *Ophthalmologica,* **129,** 291 (1955).
Favre and Goldmann. *Ophthalmologica,* **132,** 87 (1956).
Fodor. *Klin. Mbl. Augenheilk.,* **94,** 651 (1935).
Fronimopoulos. *v. Graefes Arch. Ophthal.,* **140,** 482 (1939).
Galezowski. *Gaz. méd. Paris,* **6,** 167 (1877).
Goldmann. *Brit. J. Ophthal.,* **45,** 449 (1961).
Goldstein. *Arch. Ophthal.,* **52,** 271 (1923).
Greeff. *Anleitung z. mikr. Untersuch. d. Auges,* 2nd ed., Berlin (1902).
Hauer and Barkay. *Brit. J. Ophthal.,* **48,** 341 (1964).
Hruby. *v. Graefes Arch. Ophthal.,* **143,** 224 (1941); **154,** 283 (1953).
Spaltlampen-Mikroscopie d. hinteren Augenabschnittes, Vienna (1950).
Importance of the Vitreous Body in Retina Surgery (ed. Schepens), St. Louis, 94 (1960).
Isakowitz. *Klin. Mbl. Augenheilk.,* **77,** 121 (1926); **88,** 369 (1932).
Iwanoff. *v. Graefes Arch. Ophthal.,* **15** (2), 1, 31 (1869).
Jaffe. *Trans. Amer. Acad. Ophthal.,* **71,** 642 (1967).
Jaffe and Light. *Arch. Ophthal.,* **76,** 541 (1966).
Kleefeld. *Bull. Soc. belge Ophtal.,* No. 74, 21; No. 75, 116 (1937).
Koby. *Microscopie du corps vitré,* Paris (1932).

Kraupa. *Z. Augenheilk.,* **31,** 149 (1914); **88,** 224 (1936).
Klin. Mbl. Augenheilk., **70,** 716 (1923); **72,** 476 (1924); **75,** 708 (1925).
Linder. *Acta ophthal.* (Kbh.), **44,** Suppl. 87 (1966).
Lindner. *v. Graefes Arch. Ophthal.,* **135,** 332, 462 (1936); **137,** 157 (1937).
Lister. *Int. Cong. Ophthal.,* Washington, 50 (1922).
Masuda. *Klin. Mbl. Augenheilk.,* **51** (1), 452 (1913).
Milles. *Roy. Lond. ophthal. Hosp. Rep.,* **11,** 26 (1886).
Moore. *Brit. J. Ophthal.,* **19,** 545 (1935).
Müller. *S.-B. phys.-med. Ges. Würzburg* (1856). See *v. Graefes Arch. Ophthal.,* **15** (2), 3 (1869).
Parsons. *Trans. ophthal. Soc. U.K.,* **25,** 99 (1905).
Pillat. *Klin. Mbl. Augenheilk.,* **69,** 429 (1922); **96,** 396; **97,** 60 (1936).
Z. Augenheilk., **57,** 347 (1925); **58,** 443 (1926); **61,** 105 (1927); **84,** 259 (1934); **89,** 244 (1936).
Pischel. *Amer. J. Ophthal.,* **36,** 1497 (1953).
Purtscher. *Z. Augenheilk.,* **42,** 256 (1919).
Rieger. *v. Graefes Arch. Ophthal.,* **131,** 410 (1934); **136,** 119 (1936); **146,** 305 (1943).
Z. Augenheilk., **89,** 245 (1936).
Klin. Mbl. Augenheilk., **96,** 396, 695 (1936).
Rosen. *Amer. J. Ophthal.,* **54,** 837 (1962).
von Rötth. *Klin. Mbl. Augenheilk.,* **91,** 682 (1933); **93,** 47 (1934).
Sallmann. *v. Graefes Arch. Ophthal.,* **135,** 593 (1936).
Sallmann and Rieger. *v. Graefes Arch. Ophthal.,* **133,** 75 (1934).
Samuels. *Arch. Ophthal.,* **4,** 838 (1930).
Schepens. *Amer. J. Ophthal.,* **38,** 8, 37 (1954).
Shea, Schepens and von Pirquet. *Arch. Ophthal.,* **63,** 1 (1960).
Tolentino, Freeman and Schepens. *Arch. Ophthal.,* **78,** 23 (1967).
Tolentino and Schepens. *Arch. Ophthal.,* **74,** 781 (1965).
Tolentino, Schepens and Freeman. *Arch. Ophthal.,* **78,** 16 (1967).
Vogt. *Klin. Mbl. Augenheilk.,* **72,** 212 (1924); **75,** 463 (1925); **95,** 94 (1935); **102,** 516 (1939).
v. Graefes Arch. Ophthal., **134,** 1 (1935).
Z. Augenheilk., **88,** 1 (1935).
Wadsworth. *Arch. Ophthal.,* **58,** 725 (1957).
Weber. *Klin. Mbl. Augenheilk.,* **108,** 710 (1942).

Weber. *Ophthalmologica*, **107,** 108 (1944).

de Wecker. *Graefe-Saemisch Hb. d. ges. Augenheilk.*, 1st ed., Leipzig, **4,** 715 (1876).

Weiss. *v. Graefes Arch. Ophthal.*, **31** (3), 239 (1885).
Ueber d. Vorkommen v. scharfbegrenzten Ektasien im Augengrunde . . . . bei hochgradiger Myopie, Wiesbaden (1897).

Organized Membranes

In the previous Volume on diseases of the retina we have already encountered several conditions wherein organized membranes, sometimes vascularized from the retina, surround the vitreous, both when the gel remains adherent to the retina and when it is detached. The membranes usually run along the surface for, as we have seen,[1] the cortical layer of the gel with its high content of glycoproteins and hyaluronic acid offers a considerable resistance to cellular invasion unless it is torn. The membrane may run over the internal limiting membrane of the retina, between it and the gel, line both surfaces when the vitreous is detached as if converting the retrovitreal space into a cell-lined cavity, or occasionally line the inner surface of a shrunken and detached vitreous (Figs. 374–6).

The development of such membranes has long been known, not only at the vitreo-retinal interface but on the surface of a detached vitreous (Theodore Carl, 1879), and their nature has excited much discussion. Iwanoff (1865) considered that they were composed of endothelial cells probably derived from the endothelium of the retinal vessels, a view supported by several writers (Nordenson, 1887; Tepljaschin, 1894; Krückmann, 1896; Parsons, 1905; and others). Leber (1882), on the other hand, as we have seen,[2] concluded that they were of inflammatory origin (a " pre-retinitis "), their cells being derived from the epithelium of the pars ciliaris, augmented by the proliferation of the vitreous cells. It is now generally agreed that the cells partaking in such membranes may have a variegated origin—from the pigmented or unpigmented cells of the ciliary epithelium or the pigmentary retinal epithelium, from mesodermal elements of the retinal vascular system, from fibrous or fibro-glial tissue derived from the retina, and from cellular elements of the vitreous or inflammatory cells which have migrated into it.[3]

Such membranes may be found in several inflammatory or degenerative conditions.

In *chorioretinitis* the stage of healing may be accompanied by the proliferation of mesodermal tissues associated with the retinal vessels, and sometimes also those of the choroid when Bruch's membrane has been destroyed and these two tissues are fused into a single scar. The resultant fibro-glial scar may proliferate to form a delicate avascular membrane running along the interface between the retina and the vitreous or lying in the vitreous itself (Knapp, 1937) and sometimes, particularly when the

[1] p. 316. [2] Vol. X, p. 779.
[3] von Hippel (1900–8), Gonin (1904–34), Leber (1916), Samuels (1938), Wadsworth (1952), Klien (1955), Hagedoorn and Sieger (1956), Smith (1960).

FIGS. 374 and 375.—VITREOUS MEMBRANES.

(P. A. Cibis, *Vitreoretinal Pathology and Surgery in Retinal Detachment*, C. V. Mosby & Co., St. Louis.)

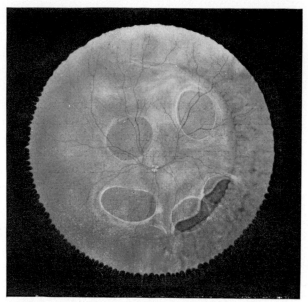

FIG. 374.—An epiretinal and preretinal membrane of fibroplasic tissue in a 12-year-old patient with 13–15 trisomy.

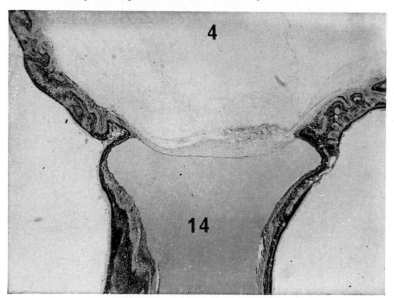

FIG. 375.—Histological section of a case of a completely detached retina, showing the fibroplasic membrane lining the posterior surface of the retracted vitreous, forming a concentric post-equatorial ring and fusing with the epiretinal membrane. 4, retracted vitreous; 14, hyaloideo-retinal space.

inflammation has involved the region around the optic disc where mesodermal tissue is abundant, the inflammatory tissue may proliferate into the substance of the vitreous to form the picture of retinitis proliferans.[1]

In a *proliferative retinopathy*, particularly in diabetes, a similar new formation may result (Figs. 377–9). The new vessels first proliferate along the surface of the retina and as this occurs adhesions tend to form with the hyaloid surface of the vitreous (Davis, 1965; Tolentino *et al.*, 1966). It is essentially when the vitreous shrinks and becomes detached that these new

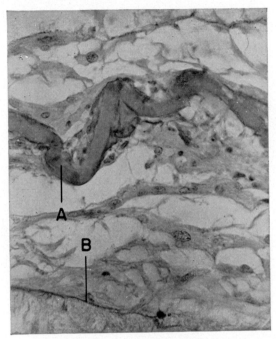

FIG. 376.—VITREOUS MEMBRANE.

In a case of retinal detachment. A condensed glassy membrane of the vitreous, A, is seen with cells on either side attached to the internal limiting membrane of the retina, B (T. R. Smith, Schepens's *Importance of the Vitreous Body in Retina Surgery*, C. V. Mosby & Co., St. Louis).

vessels are torn and hæmorrhages result; and if the cortical layer of the vitreous is ruptured the bleeding percolates into the substance of the gel. Similar membranes may develop in other proliferative lesions, such as retrolental fibroplasia. In proliferative diabetic retinopathy in the absence of hæmorrhages, opaque avascular bands may be formed (Duke-Elder and Dobree, 1968); some of these are scimitar-shaped adherent to the retina at both ends by broad expansions (Fig. 377), others evolve as amorphous star-shaped masses separated from the retina by clear fluid, some of their exten-

[1] Vol. X, p. 150.

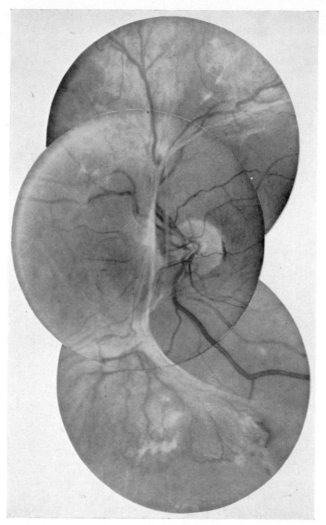

Fig. 377.—Avascular Connective-tissue Bands in the Vitreous

A large scimitar-shaped band running through the vitreous from the upper to the lower temporal quadrant of the retina, in a case of proliferative diabetic retinopathy (S. Duke-Elder and J. H. Dobree).

sions being anchored to this tissue (Figs. 378–9). The hyaloid face of the vitreous may be responsible for some of the tissue in the former; but the latter appear to be constituted entirely of condensations of the posterior face of the vitreous and their importance lies in revealing the presence of a posterior vitreous detachment.

Extensive *vitreous hæmorrhages* may result in the formation of such membranes, as have been produced experimentally in rabbits by creating

FIGS. 378 and 379.—AVASCULAR CONNECTIVE-TISSUE BANDS IN THE VITREOUS.
(S. Duke-Elder and J. H. Dobree.)

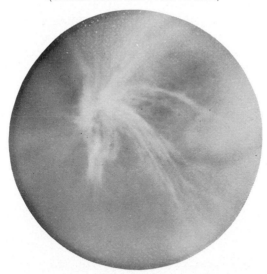

FIG. 378.—Photograph in the plane of the mid-vitreous, showing avascular strands forming on the posterior surface of a detached vitreous, in a case of proliferative diabetic retinopathy.

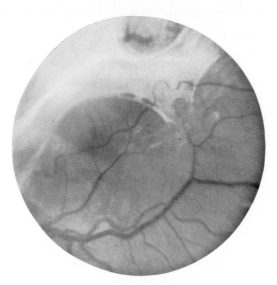

FIG. 379.—The same case, showing the anchorage of some of the upper bands into the retina itself.

bleeding artificially or injecting autogenous blood into the eyes of rabbits (Freeman *et al.*, 1967).

In *degenerative conditions* the formation of membranes is a commonplace; and in these the cellular population varies. In the condition of epithelial proliferation from the pars plana of the ciliary body, these cells may spread over the surface of the peripheral retina throughout areas of considerable size leading to adhesions between the retina and vitreous which by their traction may lead to the development of retinal holes (Teng and Katzin, 1951). A similar membrane in which glial elements are common has been seen in the dominant type of *vitreo-retinal dystrophy* (of Wagner) (Franceschetti *et al.*, 1963) (Fig. 380). Membranes composed of cells resembling endothelium may grow over the retina in *pigmentary dystrophy* (Gonin, 1902–3; Cogan, 1949; Wolter, 1957–58) and in cases of *chronic*

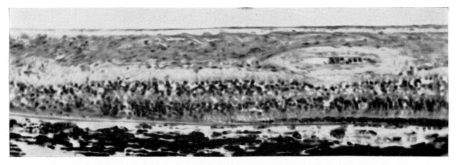

FIG. 380.—THE HYALOIDEO-RETINAL DYSTROPHY OF WAGNER.

Section of the retina to show a thick cellular preretinal membrane, thickening of the outer layer of the vitreous and atrophy of the retina (H. R. Bohringer *et al.*).

glaucoma (Smith, 1960). In cases of *detached retina* the extent of such membranes may be very striking.

The presence of such membranes in the causation and prognosis of a detachment of the retina is important. The development of adhesions between this tissue and the vitreous, particularly when it becomes detached, is a frequent cause of retinal tears and subsequent detachment, while the fixed retinal folds resulting from their contraction render the prospect of a successful reposition of the retina much more slender. If these are extensive and cannot be overcome by a buckling operation, the only hope of successful surgery may lie in the heroic procedure of detaching the membrane from the retina and filling the interspace between the two structures with an injection such as silicone (Cibis, 1965), or alternatively, cutting such membranes directly with scissors with miniature blades on a long handle introduced through the pars plana under the control of binocular indirect ophthalmoscopy (Freeman *et al.*, 1967). The importance of this complication and the surgical possibilities of overcoming it have already been discussed in the previous Volume.

Carl, Theodore. *v. Graefes Arch. Ophthal.*, **25**, 111 (1879).

Cibis. *Vitreoretinal Pathology and Surgery in Retinal Detachment*, St. Louis, 199 (1965).

Cogan. *Trans. Amer. Acad. Ophthal.*, **54**, 629 (1949).

Davis. *Arch. Ophthal.*, **74**, 741 (1965).

Duke-Elder and Dobree. *Bibl. ophthal.*, No. 76, 133 (1968).

Franceschetti, François and Babel. *Les hérédo-dégénérescences chorio-rétiniennes*, Paris, **2**, 861 (1963).

Freeman, Anastopoulou, Schepens and Morales. *Arch. Ophthal.*, **77**, 677 (1967).

Freeman, Schepens and Anastopoulou. *Arch. Ophthal.*, **77**, 681 (1967).

Gonin. *Ann. Oculist.* (Paris), **128**, 90 (1902); **129**, 24 (1903); **132**, 30 (1904).
    Le décollement de la rétine, Lausanne (1934).

Hagedoorn and Sieger. *Amer. J. Ophthal.*, **41**, 660 (1956).

von Hippel. *v. Graefes Arch. Ophthal.*, **51**, 132 (1900); **68**, 38 (1908).

Iwanoff. *v. Graefes Arch. Ophthal.*, **11**, 135 (1865).

Klien. *Amer. J. Ophthal.*, **40**, 515 (1955).

Knapp. *Arch. Ophthal.*, **18**, 558 (1937).

Krückmann. *v. Graefes Arch. Ophthal.*, **42**, 293 (1896).

Leber. *Int. med. Cong.*, London, **3**, 75 (1882). *Graefe-Saemisch Hb. d. ges. Augenheilk.*, 2nd ed., Leipzig, **7A** (2), 1374 (1916).

Nordenson. *Die Netzhautablösung*, Wiesbaden (1887).

Parsons. *The Pathology of the Eye*, London, **2**, 542 (1905).

Samuels. *Arch. Ophthal.*, **21**, 273 (1938).

Smith, T. R. *Importance of the Vitreous Body in Retina Surgery* (ed. Schepens), St. Louis, 61 (1960).

Teng and Katzin. *Amer. J. Ophthal.*, **34**, 1237 (1951).

Tepljaschin. *Arch. Augenheilk.*, **28**, 354 (1894).

Tolentino, Lee and Schepens. *Arch. Ophthal.*, **75**, 238 (1966).

Wadsworth. *Trans. Amer. Acad. Ophthal.*, **56**, 370 (1952).

Wolter. *Arch. Ophthal.*, **57**, 539 (1957). *Acta XVIII int. Cong. Ophthal.*, Brussels, **1**, 435 (1958).

SPECIFIC DEGENERATIONS

SENILE DEGENERATIONS

In old age some degree of vitreous degeneration is universal. The essential changes are a liquefaction (syneresis) of the gel with the development of cavitation, a thickening of the boundary layer and its separation from the retina, usually giving rise to a posterior detachment and sometimes an anterior detachment with a condensation of the collagenous framework into membranes or clumps; these changes are represented diagramatically in Fig. 381.

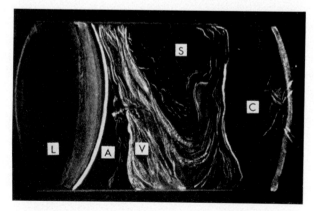

FIG. 381.—SENILE CHANGES IN THE VITREOUS.

L, lens; A, anterior vitreous detachment; V, the formed condensed vitreous; S, a cavitation of liquefied vitreous to form a lacunar space; C, posterior vitreous detachment (after P. A. Cibis).

The formation of lacunæ which grow in size and increase in number in the second half of adult life is so common as to be considered physiological (Samuels, 1930; Baurmann, 1935; Pau, 1951; Sanna and Nervi, 1965; Andersen and Edmund, 1966); the logical sequel to this change, a posterior detachment with a collapse of the gel, has been found to be present, usually bilaterally, in over 50% of eyes with no evident ocular disease over the age of 50 years (Z'Brun, 1921; Colyear, 1965), in 50 to 70% of those from 50 to 70 years of age (Hauer and Barkay, 1964; Linder, 1966) and in most otherwise normal eyes of people over 75 years (Goldmann, 1961–62); while condensation of the framework of the gel to form entoptically visible floaters is constant in the aged (Fig. 382). It is interesting that these senile changes have been found to occur prematurely in cases of acromegaly (Gärtner and Löpping, 1967).

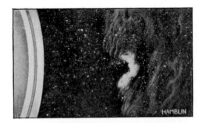

FIG. 382.—THE SENILE VITREOUS.
Irregular fibrillar appearance with condensations appearing ophthalmoscopically as opacities. Seen with the slit-lamp.

The thickening and degeneration of the marginal layer of the vitreous in senile eyes is of importance especially in the anterior region where the retina itself so frequently shows degenerative changes. Macroscopic examination shows that there is usually a considerable amount of degeneration and liquefaction of the gel so that only a ring-shaped layer of the peripheral vitreous remains attached to retina forming senile peripheral vitreous adhesions (Teng and Chi, 1957; Wadsworth, 1957). Histologically this is seen to contain a dense network of fibrillæ, and Wolter (1959) found that these adhesions were cemented by the extension of some of the fibres into the substance of the retina (Figs. 383–4). On electron-microscopic examination Gärtner (1965) confirmed these senile changes in the surface layer of the gel, and it is evident that in the presence of degenerative lesions in the retina the pull of the anchored vitreous strands could well precipitate the formation of a retinal tear and the development of a detachment.

Clinically, with the ophthalmoscope the slighter degrees of degeneration may be invisible, but with the slit-lamp and the Hruby lens a filamentous structure is usually very obvious, the fibres being long and wavy and running in all directions (Fig. 337). Sometimes they are aggregated into clumps which may be visible ophthalmoscopically while their relatively free mobility betrays the liquefaction of the gel (Koeppe, 1918; Vogt, 1924; Comberg, 1924) (Fig. 337); at other times minute white irregularities are seen on the strands as if they had been sprinkled with sugar—the *senile peppering* of Koby (1932). In rare cases, snowball-like asteroid bodies are present.[1]

Symptoms are absent except for the entoptic appearance of vitreous floaters which, although they cause no visual disability and show little tendency to progress, sometimes give rise to anxiety; they are, however, constantly present in aged eyes if visual conditions are favourable for entoptic

FIGS. 383 and 384.—THE MERGENCE OF THE VITREOUS WITH THE PERIPHERAL RETINA
(J. R. Wolter.)

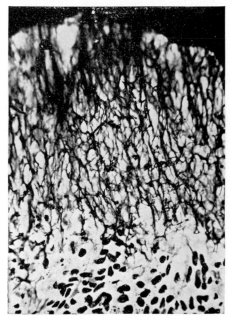 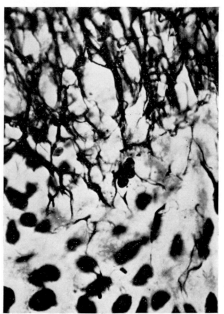

FIG. 383.—Lower-power view of the fibrillar structures of the dense vitreous within the peripheral retina.

FIG. 384.—High-power view of Fig. 383, showing the branching and root-like anchoring of the vitreous fibrillæ within the retina (Hortega stain).

vision. Their first appearance is usually sudden and unless the gel is widely liquefied they usually remain relatively stationary with movements of the eye; the suddenness of their appearance may be due to the local dissolution of the gel by a minimal trauma or a sharp rotation of the globe so that a part of its colloidal framework gives way. A posterior detachment of the vitreous may give rise to the *senile annular opacity* (of Vogt, 1925)—a small annular opacity situated near the disc which probably represents the result of a detachment of the gel from the nerve-head, a subject which has already been discussed.[2]

[1] p. 324.   [2] p. 346.

The *diagnosis* of senile changes in the vitreous from inflammatory opacities can be accomplished only with the slit-lamp, whereby their fibrillar constitution can be observed as well as the absence of inflammatory cells. It has been claimed, however, that the diagnosis can be verified by the presence of a number of small spikes in the echogram (Gärtner and Löpping, 1967). No *treatment* is of any value, nor is any required.

MYOPIC DEGENERATION

The highly myopic eye suffers a degeneration of the vitreous very similar to the senescent eye, for in both cases the changes are due to disintegration of the gel and the opacities are endogenous. Liquefaction is the rule, a process seen first and most extensively at the posterior pole, and the tendency is for the colloid basis of the gel, condensed into membranous formations, to accumulate anteriorly, causing a posterior vitreous detachment.[1] This is found in direct proportion to the degree of myopia and the age of the patient; Rieger (1936), out of a total of 321 eyes, found it present in 189

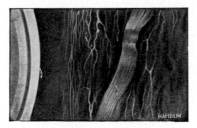

FIG. 385.—Micro-fibrillar degeneration of the vitreous in myopia; seen with the slit-lamp.

and probably present in 24, the average age of its onset being 70 years in cases of −5D or less, 38 years in those of −10D, 28 years in those of −20D, and 23 years in those of −30D.

Immediately behind the lens the slit-lamp usually reveals numerous and irregular filaments showing nodes and thickenings running typically in a vertical direction, behind which more or less well-developed and extensive diaphanous membranes are almost constantly seen, sometimes showing an irregular fibrillation (*micro-fibrillar degeneration*) (Fig. 385) (Koeppe, 1918; Streiff, 1924; Comberg, 1924; Vogt, 1924; Koby, 1932; and others). Pathologically such a vitreous body, while showing punctate and fibrillar coagula and a few incidental cellular elements, reveals nothing characteristic (von Graefe, 1854; Greeff, 1902–6; Terrien, 1906; Cattaneo, 1931; and others); the lesions are not histological but physico-chemical.

Apart from the degenerative processes associated with high myopia, mechanical factors enter into the ætiology of these changes in the vitreous.

[1] Sallmann and Rieger (1934), Lindner (1936–37), Fronimopoulos (1939), Hruby (1950–53), Favre and Goldmann (1956), Busacca *et al.* (1957), Goldmann (1961), and others.

If the tensile strength of the fibrillar framework is not sufficient to keep pace with the lengthening of the globe, the architecture of the vitreous collapses and lacunæ of syneresis form, but gross pathological alterations do not occur until the hyaloideo-retinal adherence is disrupted and a posterior vitreous detachment results; thereupon irreversible degenerative changes develop with fibrillar condensations and, if adhesions between the gel and the retina persist in the periphery in areas of degeneration or old inflammation, their traction leads to retinal tears and subsequent detachment of this tissue (Baurmann, 1935).

The subjective *symptoms* of such a condition may cause the patient much annoyance, and the appearance of spots and streamers in front of the eyes may not only become a nuisance but also give rise to some anxiety, while in the more severe forms the vision may be considerably affected. Nor is the anxiety completely without foundation, for it may be that while a solid or completely fluid vitreous is relatively safe, the membranes and strands of a semi-fluid vitreous, if adherent to the retina, may have serious consequences.   No *treatment* is applicable.

RETINAL DETACHMENT

Although the vitreous may occasionally be relatively normal in an eye with a recent retinal detachment, in the majority of cases, particularly in myopic and senile eyes and eventually in all cases, definite signs of degenera-

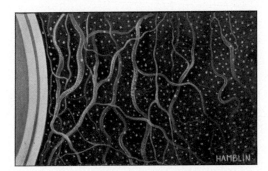

FIG. 386.—THE VITREOUS IN RETINAL DETACHMENT.

tion are seen.   Frequently evidences of vitreous degeneration including syneresis and posterior detachment, often with hyaloideo-retinal adhesions, precede the detachment; and when this has existed for any length of time these degenerative changes are present invariably and in increasing degree as the lesion advances with age (Leber, 1882–1916).   In addition to the usual evidences of liquefaction with the formation of endogenous opacities, Koby (1932) described as an almost constant phenomenon the development of tube-like anastomosing strands looking as if they represented rolled-up membranes (Fig. 386); in addition, punctate opacities are always evident, some of them white and round and many of them pigmented and stellate, probably representing depositions of pigment from the retinal epithelium on the fibrillar framework.

INFLAMMATORY CONDITIONS

In any intra-ocular inflammation of some standing and severity the vitreous shows changes due to the appearance of exogenous opacities; in more severe cases when liquefaction of the gel occurs, endogenous opacities

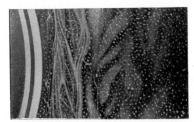

FIG. 387.—THE VITREOUS IN ACUTE ANTERIOR UVEITIS.
Showing punctate and membranous opacities.

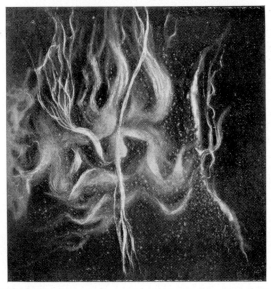

FIG. 388.—THE VITREOUS IN CHRONIC CYCLITIS (A. J. Bedell).

are added to these. It used to be said that syphilis—particularly syphilitic chorioretinitis—was the most common cause of such opacities but, while they are numerous and pronounced in this disease, it by no means holds a monopoly.

In the early stages of an iridocyclitis, a chorioretinitis or a papillitis the entire vitreous may assume an opalescent appearance due to its being flooded with a protein-rich fluid from the dilated capillaries, while it is permeated by minute opacities appearing in the beam of the slit-lamp as small, brilliantly white dots, rounded or stellate, lying free in the gel or encrusting its fibrillar structure (Fig. 387). Histological examination shows these to be leucocytes, mainly polymorphonuclear cells in the earlier stages of the disease and lymphocytes and plasma cells in the later (Fig. 389). As time goes on they become yellowish and brownish, and if the inflammation dies down they may slowly disappear. During this time the structure of the vitreous may be relatively normal, but if the inflammation is prolonged the gel eventually

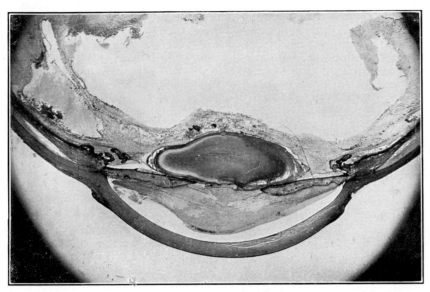

FIG. 389.—INFLAMMATORY EXUDATES.

In the more chronic stage of a post-traumatic condition showing the exudation in the anterior chamber and the shrinkage of the vitreous which contains a cavity to the right, the wall of which is lined by leucocytes (M. Straub).

breaks down and liquefies throwing down filamentous and membranous opacities, until eventually the combination of the two types may produce an intense opacification. Occasionally the exudative opacities are confined almost exclusively to Cloquet's canal (Butler, 1928; Koby, 1932). So long as these inflammatory opacities remain fine and dust-like, the choroidal inflammation is usually superficial with a good prognosis; if they are coarse they indicate the presence of an acute and severe lesion; and such opacities may be the first sign and for a period the only sign of a chronic cyclitis.

In advanced cases the combination of the two types of opacity may produce a dense and muddy haze with disastrous effects upon vision. With the slit-lamp the picture may be complicated (Fig. 388); an abundance of minute white specks, spangles and threads are mingled with large agglutinations like tangled skeins of wool, broad sinuous bands, wavy membranes, and extremely dense floating clouds, the whole oscillating slightly and swaying across the pupil with movements of the eyes.

The observation of the early opacities may sometimes be of great clinical importance. They may, for example, form a very early symptom of *sympathetic ophthalmitis*, in which disease, in conjunction with corneal precipitates and similar cells circulating in the aqueous, a multitude of minute opacities in the anterior vitreous and deposited on the posterior capsule of the lens may form a diagnostic sign of great value (Vogt, 1921); these vitreous opacities may be the first sign to appear and, indeed, cases have been reported in which they have formed the only evidence of sympathetic disturbance (Motolese, 1924; Alajmo, 1929). *Heterochromic cyclitis* is peculiar in that although the exudative opacities may be numerous and particularly dense over many years, the structure of the gel may remain indefinitely intact.

A third clinical appearance of considerable interest is the sudden occurrence of opacities of the exogenous type, sometimes in great quantity, *without apparent cause*. Such a happening is of common and general occurrence. It is presumably due to peripheral foci of anterior choroiditis, so minute as to have escaped notice or so far forward as not to have been ophthalmoscopically detected, of which the disturbance of the vitreous forms the only clinical evidence. The importance of the syndrome is that it may well form the prelude to a series of similar attacks each involving the disability of further vitreous opacities or to more serious and widespread uveal inflammation of a recalcitrant and chronic nature unless the ætiology is discovered and combatted—in many cases a task of no small difficulty.

TUMOURS

Intra-ocular tumours affecting the posterior segment of the eye always cause some disorganization of the vitreous, somewhat resembling senile degeneration. In addition, however, in melanotic tumours a fine yellowish dust of pigment may be seen; but with an endophytic retinoblastoma the cloud of opacities may be so dense as to obscure the details of the fundus.[1] So thickly, indeed, may these accumulate that a vitreous abscess may be simulated (Lemoine, 1947). The individual opacities are white or yellowish-white in colour and generally represent neoplasic cells or even formed nodules (Scheel, 1925; Reese, 1963). Since a severe chorioretinitis is rare in young children, such an appearance should always give rise to the suspicion of retinoblastoma (Chandler, 1951).

Alajmo. *Boll. Oculist.*, **8**, 358, 400 (1929).
Andersen and Edmund. *Acta ophthal.* (Kbh.), Suppl. 84, 25 (1966).
Baurmann. *Klin. Mbl. Augenheilk.*, **95**, 259 (1935).
  v. Graefes Arch. Ophthal., **134**, 201 (1935).
Busacca, Goldmann and Schiff-Wertheimer. *Biomicroscopie du corps vitré et du fond de l'œil*, Paris (1957).
Butler. *Trans. ophthal. Soc. U.K.*, **48**, 409 (1928).
Cattaneo. *Boll. Oculist.*, **10**, 265 (1931).
Chandler. *Trans. Amer. ophthal. Soc.*, **49**, 351 (1951).

Colyear. *Controversial Aspects of the Management of Retinal Detachment* (ed. Schepens and Regan), Boston, 45 (1965).
Comberg. *Klin. Mbl. Augenheilk.*, **72**, 692 (1924).
Favre and Goldmann. *Ophthalmologica*, **132**, 87 (1956).
Fronimopoulos. *v. Graefes Arch. Ophthal.*, **140**, 482 (1939).
Gärtner. *v. Graefes Arch. Ophthal.*, **168**, 529 (1965).
Gärtner and Löpping. *v. Graefes Arch. Ophthal.*, **172**, 254; **173**, 282 (1967).
Goldmann. *Brit. J. Ophthal.*, **45**, 449 (1961).

[1] Vol. X, p. 686.

Goldmann. *Ophthalmologica*, **143**, 253 (1962).
von Graefe. *v. Graefes Arch. Ophthal.*, **1** (1), 390 (1854).
Greeff. *Die pathologische Anatomie d. Auges*, Berlin (1902–6).
Hauer and Barkay. *Brit. J. Ophthal.*, **48**, 341 (1964).
Hruby. *Spaltlampen-Mikroscopie d. hinteren Augenabschnittes*, Vienna (1950).
v. Graefes Arch. Ophthal., **154**, 283 (1953).
Koby. *Biomicroscopie du corps vitré*, Paris (1932).
Koeppe. *v. Graefes Arch. Ophthal.*, **96**, 232 (1918).
Leber. *Int. Med. Cong.*, London, **3**, 75 (1882).
Graefe-Saemisch Hb. d. ges. Augenheilk., 2nd ed., Leipzig, **7A** (2), 1374 (1916).
Lemoine. *Amer. J. Ophthal.*, **30**, 52 (1947).
Linder. *Acta ophthal.* (Kbh.), **44**, Suppl. 87 (1966).
Lindner. *v. Graefes Arch. Ophthal.*, **135**, 332, 462 (1936); **137**, 157 (1937).
Motolese. *Boll. Oculist.*, **3**, 1029 (1924).
Pau. *v. Graefes Arch. Ophthal.*, **152**, 201 (1951).

Reese. *Tumors of the Eye*, 2nd ed., N.Y. (1963).
Rieger. *v. Graefes Arch. Ophthal.*, **136**, 119 (1936).
Sallmann and Rieger. *v. Graefes Arch.Ophthal.*, **133**, 75 (1934).
Samuels. *Arch. Ophthal.*, **4**, 838 (1930).
Sanna and Nervi. *Ann. Ottal.*, **91**, 1031 (1965).
Scheel. *Klin. Mbl. Augenheilk.*, **75**, 670 (1925).
Streiff. *Klin. Mbl. Augenheilk.*, **73**, 703 (1924).
Teng and Chi. *Amer. J. Ophthal.*, **44**, 335 (1957).
Terrien. *Arch. Ophtal.*, **26**, 737 (1906).
Vogt. *Atlas d. Spaltlampenmikroskopie d. lebenden Auges*, Berlin (1921).
Klin. Mbl. Augenheilk., **72**, 212 (1924); **75**, 463 (1925).
Wadsworth. *Arch. Ophthal.*, **58**, 725 (1957).
Wolter. *Amer. J. Ophthal.*, **47**, 153 (1959).
Z'Brun. *v. Graefes Arch. Ophthal.*, **107**, 61 (1921).

VITREOUS HÆMORRHAGES

Whether it is small or large a vitreous hæmorrhage occurs suddenly and unexpectedly, a mode of onset which distinguishes it clinically from most other vitreous opacities. If the hæmorrhage is minute a cloud of opacities may suddenly appear; if it is larger strands of blood may be ophthalmoscopically visible which tremble on movements of the globe if the gel remains solid but swirl about with marked changes in their shape if it is fluid; and when the bleeding is massive the red reflex is partly or completely abolished behind the clear lens. Whether the hæmorrhage is initially directly into the vitreous itself or is subhyaloid in location and bursts into the gel some time after it is formed, the end-result is the same. If localized to the periphery of the vitreous the red cells may take up a lamellar arrangement (Lindner, 1934–36), and the canal of Cloquet may be preferentially distended with them (Hoffmann, 1926; Barkan, 1928). The deposition of blood cells as a thin layer on the posterior surface of the lens is also the rule, and there they may remain unchanged for a long time, sometimes for years; the blood may be scattered over the posterior capsule indiscriminately at first, but in time there is a tendency for it to settle down into a crescentic band near the periphery at the line where the vitreous normally comes into contact with the capsule (Egger's line). Any large hæmorrhage liquefies the gel, and even when absorption has proceeded so far as to allow the return of normal vision, some opacities, usually coloured with blood pigment, always remain as a permanent legacy.

After a few days or weeks a vitreous hæmorrhage shows signs of absorbing.[1] Ophthalmoscopically, a profuse hæmorrhage may change from a jet-

[1] See also p. 335.

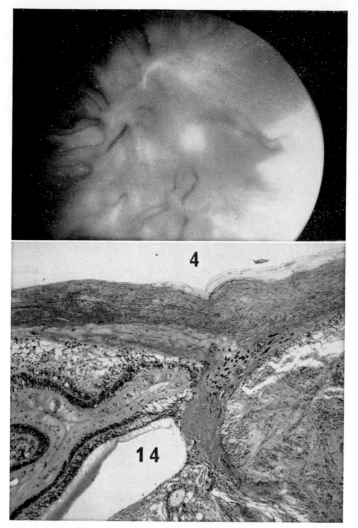

Fig. 390.—Epiretinal Membrane.

The upper figure shows fibroplasic membranes in an eye operated on for retinal detachment forming deep folds in the retina. The lower figure is from a similar eye wherein the epiretinal membrane shows layers of various densities of fibrous tissue. 4, vitreous; 14, hyaloideo-retinal interspace (P. A. Cibis, *Vitreo-retinal Pathology and Surgery in Retinal Detachment*, C. V. Mosby & Co., St. Louis).

black to a whitish colour, and if the bleeding is sparse it tends to break up into smaller particles which may be difficult to distinguish from degenerative endogenous opacities. There is a tendency for the blood to sink into the lower half of the vitreous chamber where it may be disturbed on movements of the eye; for this reason the vision is often best on waking in the morning and again becomes misty when the patient moves about. Absorption is slow, depending on the fluidity of the gel, for diffusion within it—even of hæmo-globin—is sluggish (Fischer, 1932; von Sallmann, 1948–50). If the bleeding has been massive, although occasionally the absorption of a hæmorrhage may be surprisingly rapid, several years may elapse before sufficient clarity results to allow a return of useful vision and sometimes, especially if repeated hæmorrhages have occurred, this may never be regained.

While a vitreous hæmorrhage may gradually absorb without compli-cations, in this process two mischances may occur. The first is a *fibroblastic reaction* leading to the formation of organized tissue. This may remain avascular when strands of fibrous tissue may develop on the surface of the retina confined to the hyaloideo-retinal space where a dense epiretinal membrane may be formed, the contraction of which may deform the retina into stellate or contraction folds[1] (Fig. 390), or a similar reaction may occur whereby fibroblasts are stimulated to invade the gel and may lead to the formation of intravitreal strands the contraction of which may detach the retina. The final picture, occurring particularly in the presence of irritative factors such as infection, is that of retinitis proliferans when blood vessels proliferate from the retina, usually from the optic disc, being held together by delicate sheets of connective tissue, as has already been described.[2]

The second complication which may develop after a considerable time is the reaction of *hæmosiderosis*, essentially similar in pathology to the siderosis which follows the presence of a particle of iron within the eye (von Hippel, 1894; Richter, 1957; Cibis *et al.*, 1959). This is caused by blood cells which tend to find their way to the angle of the anterior chamber where the resul-tant reaction may lead to sclerosis of the trabeculæ and obliteration of the drainage channels and the development of *hæmolytic glaucoma*. A retinal degeneration may also occur (Brégeat *et al.*, 1966).

The *causes* of hæmorrhages into the vitreous always lie outside the gel itself and depend essentially on degenerative, inflammatory or neoplasic diseases of the retina or choroid. These have all already been noted so that only a brief summary is required here.

(1) A *tearing of the retina*, with or without its detachment, due to a contraction and detachment of the vitreous is the commonest cause; when the hæmorrhage occurs, therefore, the tear is already formed. We have already seen that adhesions between the hyaloid layer of the gel and the retina are particularly strong at the site of the retinal vessels where, indeed, they may be reinforced by the prolongation of vitreous fibrillæ into the retina itself (Wolter, 1964) (Fig. 391).[3] When the vitreous detaches the vessels may be dragged bodily out of the retina (Davanger, 1961; Dobree, 1964), but more usually a sudden separation of the two structures at these points may result in the development of a hæmorrhage. These are usually small and disappear in a few days, but the gravitation of the erythrocytes

[1] Vol. X, p. 802.   [2] Vol. X, p. 150.   [3] Vol. X, p. 779.

in the subhyaloid space may stimulate the entoptic appearance of a rising cloud or a shower of sparks (Cibis, 1965). Similarly, when an anchored vitreous strand tears the retina and forms a horse-shoe-shaped hole, the hæmorrhage is usually sparse for the peripheral vessels are small and in the area of adhesion they share in the degenerated state of the retina. Only occasionally is the bleeding profuse with the formation of an intra- or extra-hyaloid hæmorrhage (Vogt, 1939). In the absence of other retinal disease, it follows that when such a hæmorrhage occurs a most careful search should be made for such a tear and, if necessary, the patient should ideally be immobilized until a clear view of the fundus can be obtained in the hope that a relatively simple prophylactic operation may prevent the occurrence of a

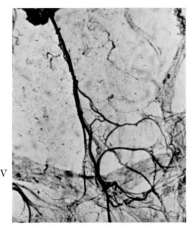

FIG. 391.—A VITREOUS STRAND.

Extending through an (unstained) limiting membrane to form a meshwork around the blood vessels of the retina, V (trypsin digestion; silver staining) (J. R. Wolter).

retinal detachment or, if it has occurred, it may be treated at the stage when it is still limited.

(2) *Vascular diseases of the retina* are a frequent cause of vitreous hæmorrhages, most commonly diabetic or hypertensive retinopathy, retinal perivasculitis (including Eales's disease), occlusion of the central retinal vein, and the erosion of a vessel in an acute chorioretinitis or, more rarely, the rupture of a vessel in a necrotic neoplasm. In most of these cases the retinal disease is bilateral and if the fundus is obscured by the hæmorrhage the diagnosis can be made with a considerable amount of certainty by examination of the other eye. These conditions have all been described in the previous Volume, and the hæmorrhage forms an incident which of itself requires no special treatment, although its presence may delay the recovery of useful vision.

(3) The *hæmopoietic diseases* may give rise to a retinal hæmorrhage

which percolates into the vitreous—the anæmias, the leucæmias, the purpuras, sickle-cell Hb-C disease, and polycythæmia.[1]

(4) In cases of *subarachnoid hæmorrhage* the rupture of a subhyaloid hæmorrhage may result in a considerable infiltration of the vitreous. This condition has already been noted[2] and will be discussed fully in a subsequent Volume.[3]

(5) The frail *new vessels* of vascular proliferations into the vitreous of whatever cause may give way, sometimes leading to massive hæmorrhages.

(6) A *choroidal hæmorrhage*, if sufficiently profuse, may rupture through the pigmentary epithelium and the retina and percolate into the vitreous body.

(7) Vitreous hæmorrhages have been reported occurring before, or vicariously in place of *menstruation* (Rusinowa and Gustowski, 1965).

(8) *Trauma*, either a concussion or a perforating injury, may cause such an accident.[4]

The *treatment* of a vitreous hæmorrhage, apart from dealing with its cause, particularly if it is recurrent, is difficult. In severe cases when the prognosis seems to be unfavourable, a removal of some of the gel or its replacement may be indicated.[5] Ricci (1960) suggested injections of oxygen into the vitreous, Drozdowska (1964) practised the disintegration of the hæmorrhage by ultrasound, while Falkowska and her colleagues (1967–68) advocated photocoagulation, preferentially using the laser.

An interesting case was reported by Michaelson (1960). A woman aged 50 years had a massive vitreous hæmorrhage and after a cataract extraction and four vitreous aspirations without replacement, a dense membrane remained within the vitreous obscuring the fundus; this was successfully divided under observation with the slit-lamp by a needle inserted through the pars plana.

Barkan. *Arch. Ophthal.*, **57**, 502 (1928).
Brégeat, Regnault and Perdriel. *Bull. Soc. franç. Ophtal.*, **79**, 437 (1966).
Cibis. *Vitreoretinal Pathology and Surgery in Retinal Detachment*, St. Louis (1965).
Cibis, Yamashita and Rodriguez. *Arch. Ophthal.*, **62**, 180 (1959).
Davanger. *Acta ophthal.* (Kbh.), **39**, 1 (1961).
Dobree. *Brit. J. Ophthal.*, **48**, 367 (1964).
Drozdowska. *Klin. oczna*, **34**, 33 (1964).
Falkowska and Kecik. *Klin. oczna*, **37**, 39 (1967).
Falkowska, Kecik, Malinowska and Szretter. *Brit. J. Ophthal.*, **52**, 450 (1968).
Fischer. *Arch. Augenheilk.*, **105**, 431 (1932).
von Hippel. *v. Graefes Arch. Ophthal.*, **40** (1), 123 (1894).

Hoffmann. *Klin. Mbl. Augenheilk.*, **77**, 641 (1926).
Lindner. *Ber. dtsch. ophthal. Ges.*, **50**, 86 (1934).
— *v. Graefes Arch. Ophthal.*, **135**, 332 (1936).
Michaelson. *Brit. J. Ophthal.*, **44**, 634 (1960).
Ricci. *Minerva Oftal.*, **2**, 133 (1960).
Richter. *J. exp. Med.*, **106**, 203 (1957).
Rusinowa and Gustowski. *Klin. oczna*, **35**, 467 (1965).
von Sallmann. *Amer. J. Ophthal.*, **31**, 90 (1948).
— *Arch. Ophthal.*, **42**, 583 (1949); **43**, 638 (1950).
Vogt. *Klin. Mbl. Augenheilk.*, **102**, 516 (1939).
Wolter. *Acta ophthal.* (Kbh.), **42**, 971 (1964).

[1] Vol X, p. 373. [2] Vol X, p. 145.
[3] Vol. XII. [4] Vol. XIV.
[5] p. 337.

PROLAPSE OF THE VITREOUS BODY (VITREOUS HERNIA)

An INTERNAL PROLAPSE or HERNIA, wherein the gel comes forward into the anterior chamber, occurs commonly in three conditions:

(1) Most commonly following an intracapsular extraction of cataract (Fig. 392).
(2) Following a complete discission of the lens or a capsulotomy (Fig. 393).
(3) In cases of dislocation or subluxation of the lens[1] (Figs. 318, 398).

It may be said always to occur in some degree after extraction of the lens when the posterior capsule is opened or removed, and is always a post-traumatic or post-operative condition. The prolapse may assume three

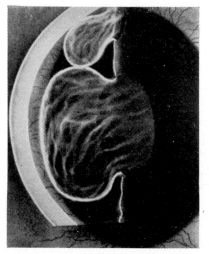

FIG. 392.—A DIFFUSE HERNIATION OF THE VITREOUS.
Through the pupil and the peripheral iridectomy (above) after an intracapsular extraction of a cataract; the gel is maintained within the elastic hyaloid layer (N. S. Jaffe and D. S. Light).

forms; a general bulging, a sacculated form, and an unrestrained pouring of the gel into the anterior chamber.

A GENERAL HERNIATION OF THE VITREOUS is the more common type, wherein after an uncomplicated intracapsular extraction the anterior face of the vitreous loses its support and while previously concave becomes convex in configuration.[2] A considerable hernia bulging into the anterior chamber occurs as a rule after both an intracapsular extraction (Fig. 392) or a discission operation (Fig. 393), and after some days may recede so that eventually the anterior face of the vitreous returns to the plane of the pupil;

[1] p. 295.
[2] Kubik (1929), Vannas (1932), Reese (1949), Leahey (1951), deRoetth (1958), Paufique and Royer (1960), Otradovec and Zicha (1960), Werner (1961), Jaffe and Light (1966), and others.

there it may remain or the hernia may reappear later and persist (Kubik, 1929; Vannas, 1932). In the same way after a capsulotomy the retrolental space, which was abolished immediately after the operation, tends to be re-formed so that there is a clear space between any capsular remnants and the anterior surface of the vitreous. Sallmann (1936) associated the original large protrusion after extraction and its subsequent recession with the development and disappearance of a post-operative choroidal detachment,[1] and it is always accompanied by a posterior detachment of the vitreous body (Jaffe and Light, 1966). It was reported by Walser (1959) that such a prolapse occurs more frequently after the use of chymotrypsin (65%) than without the use of this enzyme (12%) in the operation. Gentle massage of the globe will push out a prolapse further into the anterior chamber, and a

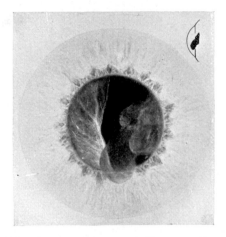

Fig. 393.—After-cataract and Vitreous Prolapse.
After discission of a congenital cataract (A. J. Bedell).

sudden trauma, a physical exertion, or even a maximal dilatation of the pupil may be sufficient to increase it or induce a prolapse when formerly none existed.

The extent and density of the prolapse may vary considerably. It may be so delicate as to escape observation unless specially sought. It may seem to have a single membranous covering representing the normal hyaloid layer, or it may be grossly laminated, as if composed of a series of pseudo-membranes of some thickness, each showing a glassy contour and each bestrewn by fine pigmentary remnants. The surface may be smooth or may have a round attenuated area corresponding to the anterior portion of Cloquet's canal in which folds or plicæ may be visible. Such a herniation may not only bulge through the pupil but also through a peripheral iridectomy (Fig. 392). The protrusion of the gel may form a continuous bulge or

[1] Vol. IX, p. 951.

it may be constricted by thickened bands resulting from the organization of post-operative inflammatory exudates (Jaffe and Light, 1966). After some time the visual acuity may be further diminished by consolidation and the development of opacities in the face of the vitreous (Reese, 1949; deRoetth, 1958).

A factor which may increase the prolapse of the vitreous particularly when a condition of pupillary blockage has occurred, is the pooling of aqueous in the hyaloideo-retinal space when the posterior vitreous is liquefied and detached; in such a case the aqueous from the ciliary body cannot reach the anterior chamber and drain away, and the pressure thus exerted in the posterior chamber of the eye may be a contributory cause in the development of the secondary glaucoma which may result (Christensen and Irvine, 1966; Sugar, 1966).

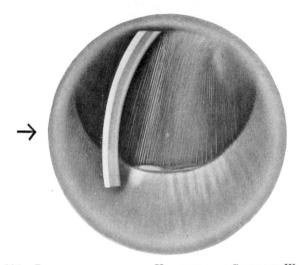

FIG. 394.—INCORPORATION OF THE VITREOUS IN A CATARACT WOUND.
Vertical lines of tension are seen in the vitreous running towards a detached retina (after C. D. Shapland).

A not uncommon event at any time after the operation for cataract is the prolapse of the vitreous enclosed in the hyaloid layer into the inner surface of the surgical wound, the posterior lips of which have remained open. This may be an insidious development and may be accompanied by an incorporation of the iris into the wound or a retroversion of this tissue, and may be followed by some cloudiness of the upper part of the cornea (Fig. 394). A secondary glaucoma may be the result of this complication owing to blockage of the drainage angle, and may require surgical treatment.

Complications may arise from these events. Particularly if the anterior chamber is shallow but sometimes when it is of normal depth the herniated vitreous may lie in apposition to the cornea, a gross type of prolapse the development of which is aided by a dilated pupil. In this event a progressive corneal œdema tends to develop, sometimes culminating in a *disc-shaped opacity* appearing 24 to 48 hours after the operation associated with wrinkling of Descemet's membrane forming a type of striate keratopathy[1]; this may be limited to the central part of the cornea or may be more extensive. The sequence is often accompanied by lacrimation, photophobia and signs of a mild iridocyclitis. Such an opacity may show no amelioration with the passage of time and may become permanent and disabling and may ultimately be associated with a bullous keratopathy if the adherence of the hyaloid membrane to the cornea is not relieved (Reese, 1949; Leahey, 1951); but it develops only if the hyaloid layer is intact and not from the presence of free vitreous in the anterior chamber, and has been found to occur most readily if the corneal endothelium is dystrophic as in Fuchs's combined dystrophy[2] or cornea guttata.[3] In rare instances a similar herniation may occur some years after an intracapsular extraction, sometimes after a history of trauma (Werner, 1961) and sometimes for no apparent reason (Reese, 1949).

The treatment of such a complication is difficult after it has persisted for some time, but prophylactic measures at the time of surgery should include the induction of full miosis and filling the anterior chamber with air immediately after the wound has been closed. If the condition has recently developed a strong miotic frequently reduces the hernia, particularly if the patient is confined to bed in the supine position. If it is not thus resolved Reese (1949) advised a dilatation of the pupil with 10% phenylephrine followed by DFP (di-isopropyl-phosphorofluoridate), a manœuvre which may be aided by the injection of air into the anterior chamber. In well-established cases it may be necessary to open the eye and free the vitreous from the cornea with a spatula or even to excise the prolapsed vitreous, either procedure being followed by the injection of air (Paufique and Royer, 1960). In all cases resolution of the prolapse may be furthered by osmotically reducing the volume of the vitreous by the intravenous injection of such substances as mannitol or urea (Kornblueth and Gombos, 1962) or the oral administration of glycerol (Jaffe and Light, 1966).

A second complication is the development of a *pupillary block* associated with an iris bombé (Bowman, 1865; Knapp, 1895). This is due to an obstruction of the pupil owing to the hernia through its aperture, a consequent over-distension of the posterior chamber with a bulging forward of the iris, and the subsequent formation of peripheral synechiæ of the iris to the cornea obliterating the angle (Hudson, 1911) (Fig. 395). The treatment of the resulting secondary glaucoma is discussed elsewhere.[4]

A SACCULATED or " BEAD " PROLAPSE, on the other hand, is more rare (Fig. 396).[5] In this type one or more distinct sac-like pouches are formed

---

[1] Vol. VIII, p. 705.   [2] Vol. VIII, p. 957.
[3] Vol. VIII, p. 952.   [4] p. 718.
[5] Siegfried (1898), Haab (1900), Hesse (1919), Cowan (1932), Butler (1933), Paula-Santos (1936), Irvine (1953), Kirsch and Steinman (1954), Jaffe and Light (1966), and others.

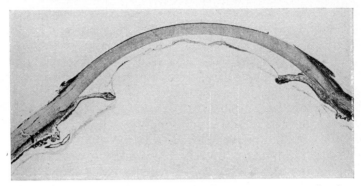

FIG. 395.—VITREOUS PROLAPSE AFTER DISLOCATION OF THE LENS.

After a couching operation. Note the marked condition of iris bombé with the prolapse of the vitreous, and the secondary formation of peripheral synechiæ (A. C. Hudson).

which protrude into or hang down in the anterior chamber and may contain some hæmorrhage (Fig. 397). In these cases the anterior limiting layer of the vitreous has ruptured but its indiscriminate protrusion forward has been prevented by the rapid formation of a weaker superficial condensation of sufficient tensile strength to retain the gel within it (Cowan, 1932). The apparently distinct surface membrane is probably a mechanical effect

FIGS. 396 and 397.—SACCULATED PROLAPSE.

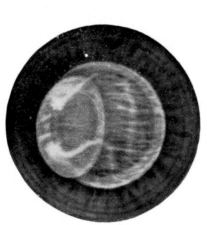

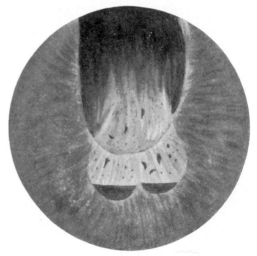

FIG. 396.—After an intracapsular extraction of a cataract. There is a herniation of the contents of the anterior part of Cloquet's canal through the hole in the anterior hyaloid layer, the herniation being retained by a new limiting border (N. S. Jaffe and D. S. Light).

FIG. 397.—A biloculate pouch of vitreous prolapsing into the anterior chamber containing blood after a cataract extraction (T. Harrison Butler).

of the tension and stress created by the hernia on the micellar structure of the gel causing a rearrangement or re-orientation and a condensation of its fibrillar elements; these ruptures were found by Jaffe and Light (1966) to occur in 33% of cases of intracapsular extractions usually within the first 6 weeks after surgery. Such a hernia may remain localized and be retained behind a stout newly formed hyaloid layer (Irvine, 1957). At other times the anterior surface is frayed and broken showing teased-out cotton-like fibres which may wave freely in the anterior chamber or become adherent

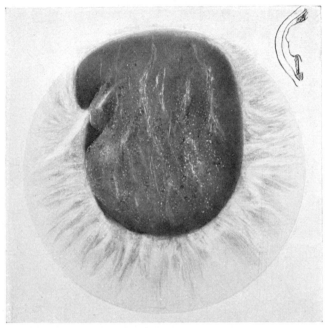

FIG. 398.—VITREOUS PROLAPSE.

After dislocation of the lens and an iridectomy for secondary glaucoma. The vitreous face, powdered with blood-cells, almost touched the cornea (A. J. Bedell).

to the capsule or the iris. Again, vitreous debris may appear on the posterior surface of the cornea as a frayed white dust. Occasionally this surface condensation ruptures and through it the semi-fluid vitreous pours freely into the anterior chamber (Samuels, 1930; Bassin, 1936; Kirsch and Steinman, 1954). The rupture may be small and symptomless, but if it occurs suddenly and fluid vitreous spills into the anterior chamber, a considerable amount of pain and evidences of iridocyclitis may result, particularly if the vitreous prolapses into the surgical wound, sometimes persisting with remissions and exacerbations over a period varying from months to years and occasionally resulting in macular œdema and degeneration (Irvine, 1953).

Finally, in a COMPLETE PROLAPSE the entire anterior chamber may be filled with a formless gelatinous mass. In all cases there tend to be some cellular elements and a considerable amount of pigment both of uveal and hæmorrhagic origin in the herniated gel (Fig. 398).

The *rise of tension* following an extraction of cataract or a capsulotomy or associated with a prolapse of the vitreous is dealt with elsewhere (Chapter IX).

An EXTERNAL PROLAPSE of the vitreous body out of the globe may occur into a perforating wound when the gel may bulge through the opening in the selera ; this condition will be discussed more fully in the Volume on injuries to the eye.[1]

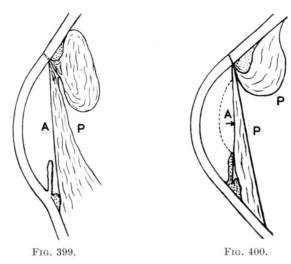

FIG. 399.   FIG. 400.

FIGS. 399 and 400.—INCARCERATION OF THE VITREOUS.

Diagrammatic representation of incarceration of the vitreous in the scar after an operation for cataract. In Fig. 399 the anterior surface membrane of the vitreous (A) is incarcerated and the posterior (P) is not ; this is a relatively (but not invariably) safe condition. In Fig. 400 the posterior membrane is also incarcerated, a circumstance liable to lead to detachment of the retina (H. Goldmann).

In this connection a prolapse of the vitreous through the wound during an operation for the extraction of cataract should be noted when a dense band of the gel may run to the scar where it remains adherent. As a rule such an incorporation leads to the development of lines of stress in the hyaloid layer which may cause a retinal detachment. In adults this sequel usually occurs only where, after a previous posterior vitreous detachment, the posterior hyaloid membrane becomes caught in the wound (Goldmann, 1961 ; Iliff, 1966) (Figs. 399–400) ; it is essentially the tautness of this membrane and its adherence to the retina that cause retinal tears and detachment which are by no means easy to treat.

[1] Vol. XIV.

Bassin. *Klin. Mbl. Augenheilk.*, **97**, 599 (1936).

Bedell. *Trans. ophthal. Soc. U.K.*, **45**, 646 (1925).

Bowman. *Roy. Lond. ophthal. Hosp. Rep.*, **4**, 332 (1865).

Butler. *Brit. J. Ophthal.*, **17**, 343 (1933).

Cheney. *Ophthalmology*, **5**, 28 (1909).

Christensen and Irvine. *Arch. Ophthal.*, **75**, 490 (1966).

Cowan. *Amer. J. Ophthal.*, **15**, 125 (1932).

deRoetth. *Amer. J. Ophthal.*, **45**, 59 (1958).

Goldmann. *Brit. J. Ophthal.*, **45**, 449 (1961).

von Graefe. *v. Graefes Arch. Ophthal.*, **15** (3), 108 (1869).

Haab. *Z. Augenheilk.*, **3**, 113 (1900).

Hesse. *Z. Augenheilk.*, **42**, 191 (1919).

Hudson. *Roy. Lond. ophthal. Hosp. Rep.*, **18**, 203 (1911).

Iliff. *Amer. J. Ophthal.*, **62**, 856 (1966).

Irvine. *Amer. J. Ophthal.*, **36**, 599 (1953).

Symposium on Diseases and Surgery of the Lens (ed. Haik), St. Louis (1957).

Jaffe and Light. *Arch. Ophthal.*, **75**, 370; **76**, 541 (1966).

Kirsch and Steinman. *Amer. J. Ophthal.*, **37**, 657 (1954).

Knapp, H. *Arch. Augenheilk.*, **30**, 1 (1895).

Kornblueth and Gombos. *Amer. J. Ophthal.*, **54**, 753 (1962).

Kubik. *Klin. Mbl. Augenheilk.*, **82**, 592 (1929).

Leahey. *Arch. Ophthal.*, **46**, 22 (1951).

Otradovec and Zicha. *Csl. Ofthal.*, **16**, 352 (1960).

Paufique and Royer. *Ann. Oculist.* (Paris), **193**, 545 (1960).

Paula-Santos. *Arch. Ophtal.*, **53**, 876 (1936).

Reese. *Amer. J. Ophthal.*, **32**, 933 (1949).

Sallmann. *v. Graefes Arch. Ophthal.*, **135**, 602 (1936).

Samuels. *Arch. Ophthal.*, **4**, 838 (1930).

Siegfried. *Beitr. Augenheilk.*, **3** (22), 45 (1898).

Sugar. *Amer. J. Ophthal.*, **61**, 435 (1966).

Vannas. *Klin. Mbl. Augenheilk.*, **89**, 318 (1932).

Walser. *Klin. Mbl. Augenheilk.*, **134**, 524 (1959).

Werner. *Trans. ophthal. Soc. U.K.*, **81**, 85 (1961).

SECTION III

GLAUCOMA AND HYPOTONY

BY

SIR STEWART DUKE-ELDER

AND

BARRIE JAY

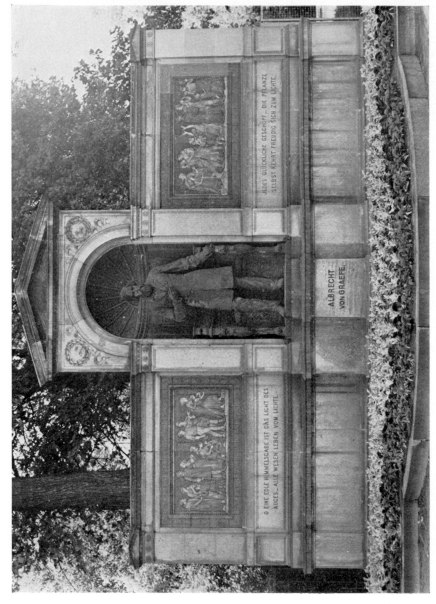

FIG. 401.—The monument to Albrecht von Graefe in the garden of the Charité Hospital in Berlin (by courtesy of Prof. K. Velhagen).

CHAPTER VI

INTRODUCTION

Few readers would question the suggestion of the frontispiece that in the history of glaucoma the greatest name is Albrecht von Graefe. He created a revolution in ophthalmology the most dramatic aspect of which was the transformation of the acute form of the disease from a painful and tragic condition into one for which there was a hope of cure. He died at the early age of 42, but his memory is immortal, and to perpetuate it the monument seen in Fig. 401 was unveiled in 1882 in the garden of the Charité Hospital in Berlin which fortunately survived the destruction of the second World War with only little harm. In his right hand he holds the ophthalmoscope of von Helmholtz, while his left hand rests on the arm of an antique chair. In the panels on either side vision is described as a gift from heaven, for all nature yearns for light : on his right are depicted the blind seeking his help ; on the left the cured rejoicing

The term GLAUCOMA does not connote a disease-entity but *embraces a composite congeries of pathological conditions which have the common feature that their clinical manifestations are to a greater or less extent dominated by the height of the intra-ocular pressure and its consequences.*[1] The degree of raised pressure which assumes a pathological significance is impossible to define since it varies within wide limits from one eye to another : it may be taken as *that pressure which the tissues of the particular eye in question are unable to withstand without damage to their structure or impairment of their function.*

It is to be remembered that an intra-ocular pressure that is generally accepted as being within the normal range may produce the typically pathological effects at the optic disc and in the visual fields when the nerve-head is unduly vulnerable as may occur, for example, in myopic eyes ; these cases properly come under the definition of glaucoma. On the other hand, the intra-ocular pressure may be higher than that generally considered to be within the normal range without any evidence of pathological signs or symptoms and without any variation in the diurnal rhythm greater than 5 mm. Hg or any rise on provocative tests and with a normal facility of aqueous outflow ; by this definition these should be considered not as glaucomatous but as *hypertensive eyes.* Moreover, cases exist wherein the typical changes at the optic disc and defects in the visual fields occur while the level of the ocular tension is normal or even subnormal and is never elevated spontaneously as in its diurnal variations nor can be raised by provocative tests when account is taken of ocular rigidity. These have been termed *low-tension glaucoma* or *pseudo-glaucoma,* as was suggested by

---

[1] In view of this composite nature, some writers such as Sugar (1951) prefer to use the term " the glaucomas ", a somewhat unnecessary expedient unless such terms as " pain " and " diarrhœa " are to be used in the plural since their ætiology and clinical manifestations are equally composite.

de Wecker (1896); this is an unfortunate contradiction in terms which is best avoided. Such cases are usually seen bilaterally in later adult life and are due to affections of the optic nerve from various causes; they are generally due to vascular insufficiency and will be discussed in the subsequent Volume as *ischæmic optic neuropathy*.[1]

HISTORY

When discussing the history of cataract[2] we have already seen that the Classical and Alexandrian Greeks did not recognize the specific disease which we now know as glaucoma. In the Hippocratic Aphorisms[3] the term glaucoma (γλαύκωμα) was used to describe blindness coming on in advancing years associated with a glazed appearance of the pupil—" If the pupil becomes sea-coloured sight is destroyed and blindness of the other eye often follows." The word has usually been interpreted as implying a greenish or bluish hue, but it is more probable that to the Greeks it indicated no specific colour but the dull sheen or " glaze " of blindness. The term, however, was used without any specific pathological connotation and represented no morbid entity, but probably included absolute glaucoma among other conditions ; glaucoma as we know it today was vaguely classified as amblyopia, amaurosis, or gutta serena. Originally, indeed, it was undifferentiated from cataract; both diseases were located in the lens, then considered the essential organ of vision, and both depended on a disturbance of the visual spirits. Only at a later date was it recognized by Celsus [25 B.C.– A.D. 50] and Rufos of Ephesus [*c.* A.D. 95–117] and later by Galen [A.D. 131– 210] and other writers of the early Christian centuries that the morbid conditions situated behind the pupil which gave rise to blindness could be differentiated into two groups, " suffusions " (ὑποχύμα) or cataracts which were amenable to operative treatment, and the glaucomas which were not. The first was due to the presence of an evil humor in front of the lens, the second to a drying up of the visually important lens itself; in the first the pupil became white, in the second bluish-green ; in the first the patient could perceive light, but in the second he could not and the blindness was incurable. The most hazy ideas were prevalent about the pathology of the condition, but the classical dogma was transmitted into early European thought by Benevenutus Grassus (Grapheus) of Jerusalem [*c.* 12th to 14th century], the Salernian scholar who transcribed much of Greek and Arabic learning in his *Practica oculorum* which became the standard textbook in the Christian West for centuries. In Europe it was thus generally accepted that this type of amaurosis was associated with the lens, a view maintained by the great French oculist, Antoine Maître-Jan, in his classical textbook as late as 1707. To Michael Brisseau (1709) of Paris[4] must go the credit for first showing that cataract was an opacification of the lens and disproving any

---

[1] Vol. XII.   [2] p. 65.
[3] *Aphorismi*, Sect. iii, 31.   [4] p. 66.

lenticular abnormality in glaucoma by the anatomical examination of the eyes of Bourdelot, the blind physician of Louis XIV. Even the astute Boerhaave (1748) described glaucoma as a type of cataract which began with pain and ended with blindness without any mention of hardness of the eye.

The first suggestion of a disease associated with a rise in intra-ocular pressure and thus corresponding to what is now known as glaucoma seems to occur in the Arabian writings of At-Tabari [10th century] who wrote in the " Book of Hippocratic treatment " of a chronic inflammatory condition of the eye with raised tension, and of Sams-ad-Din [?–1348] of Cairo who, among the 153 diseases of the eye and its adnexa, described with the oph- thalmias a " migraine of the eye " or " headache of the pupil ", an illness associated with pain in the eye, hemicrania and dullness of the humours, and followed by dilatation of the pupil and cataract; if it became chronic, tenseness of the eye and blindness supervened. The first original and clear recognition of such a condition in European writings, however, is due to Richard Banister (1622) (Fig. 402), an itinerant English oculist and author of the first book on ophthalmology in English to contain original teaching[1]; he clearly differentiated between curable cataract (gutta obscura) and gutta serena wherein " the humour settled in the hollow nerves, be growne to any solid or hard substance, it is not possible to be cured ", and gave a tetrad of features—tension (" if one feele the Eye by rubbing upon the Eie-lids, that the Eye be growne more solid and hard than naturally it should be "), as well as the long duration of the disease, the absence of perception of light and the presence of a fixed pupil. This very excellent description, however, passed unnoticed although the same four points were plagiarized from Banister's *Breviary* by the unoriginal and illiterate quack, Sir William Read (1706), who became the oculist to Queen Anne and held that glaucoma " proceeds from the viciated crystalline humour "; not without boasting, he extolled the good results obtained on a patient, Jeremiah Puttiford, in 1705, by the administration of vegetable decoctions, depletion and couching.

All through the 18th century the term " glaucoma " was merely a label applied to an inflamed eye wherein the pupil appeared greenish-blue and the visual prognosis was bad, but the tension of the eye was not stressed. Thus in his textbook, Charles Saint-Yves (1722) described glaucoma as an acute inflammation wherein the pupil was sea-coloured and the vision became foggy, a condition followed by a defect in the visual field wherein objects could be seen only partially " du coin de l'œil " and the pain was severe. It is true that hardness of the eye was noted by Johann Zacharias Platner

---

[1] This book contained four parts—Banister's original " Breviary of the Eyes ", a (partially acknowledged) translation of Jacques Guillemeau's *Traité des maladies de l'oeil* (1585), the third an (unacknowledged) reprint of Walter Bailey's *Briefe Treatise concerning the Preseruation of the Eie-Sight,* and several other reprints and translations. The description of gutta serena is in Banister's own work.

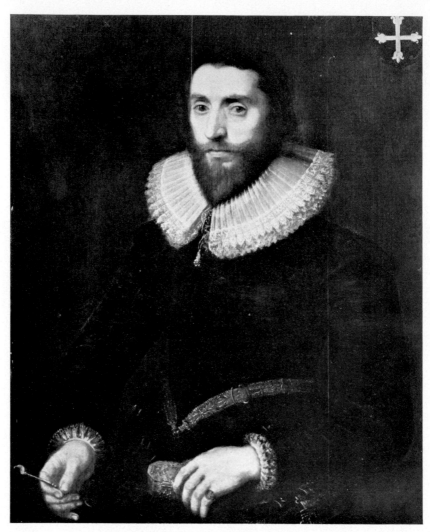

FIG. 402.—RICHARD BANISTER
[?–1626].
(From the Royal College of Surgeons of England.)

(1738) of Leipzig, who distinguished two types of the disease, one due to swelling of the lens wherein the eye became hard, and the other to swelling of the vitreous wherein the eye became soft. Arrachart (1786), a member of the Royal Academy of Surgery of Paris, also described the clinical picture of acute glaucoma wherein the eye became painful and inflamed, the iris lost its colour, the pupil was dilated and assumed a greenish hue, and a progressive visual deterioration led to blindness. The best clinical description of this disease given during this century, however, was due to Josef Beer of Vienna (1792)[1] who accurately wrote of a form of acute " iritis " with the distinctive symptoms of acute glaucoma evolving into the absolute stage, but he made no mention of the ocular tension and with his belief in diatheses he attributed it to a gouty origin.

It was not until the beginning of the 19th century that the first excellent description of glaucoma with a raised ocular tension was given by Antoine-Pierre Demours (1818) in a treatise which incorporated the teaching of his father, Pierre Demours, and himself; the credit for this probably largely belongs to the father, but it must be equally shared. The clinical picture was fully detailed; he noted that " *le globe devient dur au toucher* ", and described for the first time the appearance of the colours of a rainbow (" *l'arc-en-ciel* ") around lights.

Because of this first complete clinical description we are inserting the portrait of PIERRE DEMOURS [1702–1795] (Fig. 403), who was born in Marseilles, educated in Paris and Avignon, and practised ophthalmology for 50 years in Paris. He earned his great reputation for his work on ocular anatomy, describing the posterior membrane of the cornea at about the same time as Descemet; he became physician to the King and a fellow of the Academy of Sciences. His equally celebrated son, ANTOINE-PIERRE DEMOURS [1762–1836], was not an investigator as was his father but became a better surgeon and among his many writings the most famous is his *Traité des maladies de yeux* (1818) in 4 volumes which contained hundreds of carefully annotated cases studied during the 50 years of his father's and the 20 years of his own practice. The many beautiful plates in these volumes were the best that had hitherto appeared in our literature.

Thereafter the central concept of a rise in the intra-ocular pressure became fully established. In Germany Karl Heinrich Weller (1826) of Dresden wrote of the hardness of the eye not only in the established but also in the developing condition, combining the descriptions of Beer and Demours and describing two entities, arthritic ophthalmia without a greenish pupil and glaucoma wherein this was present. But the most important interpretations of the disease came from Britain. In London, G. J. Guthrie (1823) recognized hardness of the eye as characteristic of a disease which he called GLAUCOMA, while Sir William Lawrence (1826–30), like Weller, described an acute inflammatory syndrome affecting the vitreous and choroid as arthritic ophthalmia and a chronic form of the same condition corresponding to the picture now called absolute glaucoma. For the former he

[1] Vol. IX, Fig. 1.

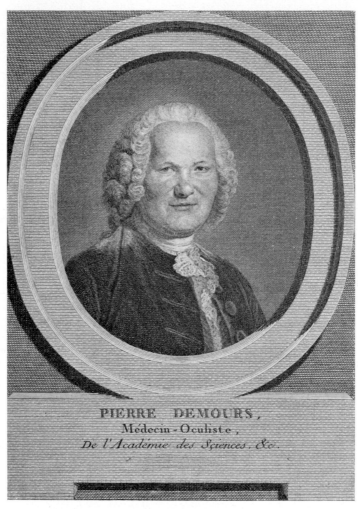

PIERRE DEMOURS,
Médecin-Oculiste,
De l'Académie des Sciences, &c.

FIG. 403.—PIERRE DEMOURS
[1702–1795].

PLATE V

The Optic Disc in Glaucoma

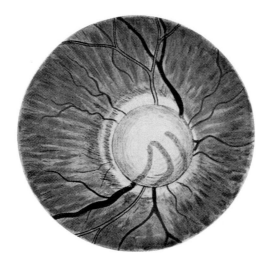

A reproduction of Fig. 34 from Eduard Jaeger's *Ueber Staar und Staaroperationen*, Wien (1854), showing 'amaurosis arthritica (glaucomatosa)'. Note that the (cupped) optic disc is pictured as swollen.

introduced the term *acute glaucoma* and for the first time the two were recognized as belonging to the same clinical entity; it was not until 30 years had passed that Donders recognized that the non-congestive (simple) type of the disease was a member of the same family. Finally, the essential feature of raised tension was fully established by William Mackenzie (1835) who, in the second edition of his classical and widely read textbook, ascribed the raised tension in both chronic (congestive) and acute glaucoma as defined by Lawrence to an increase in the watery contents of the globe owing to a serous choroiditis, and employed puncture of the vitreous for its relief. To this great Scottish clinician must be given the credit for the final and generally accepted establishment of the diagnosis between cataract and glaucomatous amaurosis, the propounding of a presumptive pathology of the latter condition, and a reasoned suggestion for its relief.

Of these early British observers, historical credit belongs to RICHARD BANISTER [?–1626] whose portrait appears in Fig. 400. Since pictures of Lawrence[1] and Mackenzie[2] have already appeared in this *System*, we are also including here a photograph of GEORGE JAMES GUTHRIE [1785–1856] (Fig. 404) who, in his deservedly famous book, *Lectures on the Operative Surgery of the Eye* (London, 1823), described " glaucoma "—a disease consisting essentially in an alteration of the component parts of the vitreous humour— as characterized thus: " If the eye is examined by the touch, it will be found rather firmer or harder than natural ". Guthrie had an extraordinary career. He qualified as a Member of the Royal College of Surgeons of England at the age of 16, of which he was later to become President on three occasions (1833, 1840, 1854); after qualification he joined the army where he remained for 15 years serving with distinction in both the American and Penninsular Wars; he then returned to London and in 1816 founded " The Royal Westminster Infirmary for the Cure of Diseases of the Eye ", where at first he was the only surgeon on the staff, and his old General, the Duke of Wellington, acted as President. This institution now forms part of Moorfields Eye Hospital.

The next epoch in the history of glaucoma followed the introduction of the ophthalmoscope, when clinical observations on the glaucomatous cup began to accumulate (Jacobson, 1853; Jaeger, 1854; von Graefe, 1854–57; Weber, 1855; and others), observations which were confirmed by the pathological researches of Heinrich Müller (1856) on the phenomenon of cupping of the optic disc. It is interesting that both Jaeger (1854) and von Graefe (1854) originally described the appearance as a swelling of the disc (Plate V), a mistake corrected by Weber (1855) and by von Graefe himself in the same year. When this had been established, the fact that hypertension was the essential cause of glaucoma was universally admitted. It must be remembered, however, that up to this time the disease was confined to clinical pictures dominated by signs of inflammation and congestion; these von Graefe (1857) divided into three categories—acute, chronic and secondary, and the anomaly that the ophthalmoscope had lately revealed in eyes with no signs of congestion, he described as " amaurosis with excavation of the

[1] Vol. VIII, Fig. 664.　　　　[2] Vol. IX, Fig. 400.

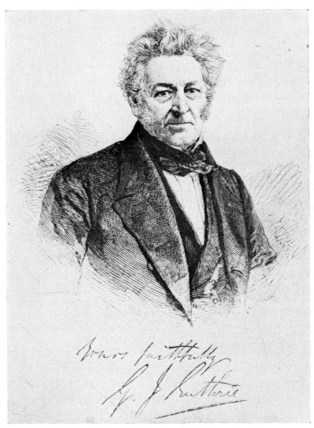

FIG. 404.—GEORGE JAMES GUTHRIE
[1785–1856].

optic nerve". The final important clinical observation in this epoch was the unifying concept of Donders (1862) (Fig. 405), who recognized the last condition wherein an incapacitating increased tension occurred without any inflammatory symptoms as *simple glaucoma*.

Thereafter the ætiology of the disease attracted much attention. A great variety of suggestions followed that of Beer's (1792) gouty iritis, and Mackenzie's (1835) serous choroiditis—irritation of the secretory nerves of the eye (Donders, 1862; de Weckcr, 1863), thickening of the sclera (Coccius, 1863; Adamük, 1867), a disease of the vitreous (Wardrop, 1818; Guthrie, 1823; Lawrence, 1826–30; Middlemore, 1835; Stilling, 1868), and so on—all of which stimulated an immense amount of research on the nature of the intra-ocular fluid, a subject which is only now being clarified. The first clue initially noted by Heinrich Müller (1858) and based on proved pathological facts was announced by Max Knies (1876) of Freiburg and Adolf Weber (1877) (Fig. 511) of Darmstadt, working independently, who discovered the frequency of obstruction of the angle of the anterior chamber in glaucoma; Knies thought that the adhesion of the iris to the cornea at the angle was a primary change due to pre-existing inflammation, while Weber interpreted it as a secondary change induced by an abnormally swollen ciliary body. This second clue was taken up and elaborated by Priestley Smith (1879–91) of Birmingham (Fig. 597). The classical researches of this author, who dcvoted much of his lifetime to the subject and stressed faulty drainage rather than the theory of the overproduction of fluid generally accepted since the time of Mackenzie, sought the immediate cause of glaucoma in abnormalities at the angle of the anterior chamber. In secondary glaucoma these were usually obvious; in the primary type he placed great importance upon the combination of a small globe and a large lens leading to a shallow anterior chamber and obstruction at its angle.

For some decades thereafter the general concept prevailed that primary glaucoma of all types was due to an obstruction to the drainage of the aqueous humour, most commonly to the formation of peripheral anterior synechiæ as taught by Knies and Weber. A new thought, however, suggested by Erich Seidel (1920) in Heidelberg, was elaborated by E. J. Curran (1920) of Kansas who introduced the idea of blockage of the pupil, and J. G. Raeder (1923) of Kristiania. Reasoning from the position occupied by the lens, Raeder divided primary glaucoma into two types, one with a shallow anterior chamber due to increased pressure behind the lens, and the other with a deep anterior chamber wherein the obstruction to the drainage of the aqueous occurred in the anterior chamber so that pressure was built up in front of the lens. In the meantime, with the aid of early types of gonioscope, Salzmann (1914–15), Troncoso (1925–35), Thorburn (1927) and particularly Sigurd Werner (1932) of Helsingfors pointed out that in some glaucomatous eyes the angle of the anterior chamber was closed while in others it was open. Finally, Otto Barkan (1938) (Fig. 543) of San Francisco, with an improved type of gonioscope used with a contact lens, exploited this concept further and divided the condition into glaucoma with, on the one hand, a deep anterior chamber and an open angle and, on the other hand, a shallow anterior chamber the drainage angle of which became closed to produce a rise of tension; he further suggested that in the second type closure of the angle was due to obstruction of the flow of aqueous through the pupil ("increased physiological seclusion of the pupil"), and advised a peripheral iridectomy to re-establish communication between the posterior and anterior chambers as a means of surgical cure, an operation which had been previously advocated by Curran (1920). From these revolutionary ideas grew the contemporary classification of primary glaucoma into the simple and closed-angle types and the realization of the importance of pupillary blockage in the latter. Thereafter, during the last two decades our knowledge of the defects arising in the drainage channels at the angle of the anterior chamber has been increased both by the investigation of the minute structure of this important region by such techniques as micro-injection and electron microscopy, and the fuller investigation of the dynamics of the aqueous humour, a complex and fascinating subject discussed in a previous Volume.[1]

The history of the treatment of glaucoma will be discussed in a subsequent Section.

CLASSIFICATION

An attempt to classify the different clinical manifestations of glaucoma was first made by von Graefe (1857) who divided them into three types, acute, chronic (or absolute) and secondary, all of which were characterized by congestion of the eye which, following Mackenzie, he thought was caused by a serous choroiditis; the condition now known as simple glaucoma he called "excavation of the optic nerve" and it was not considered as a manifestation of glaucoma until the classical paper by Donders (1862). Thereafter it became generally accepted that two main types of the disease existed, *primary glaucoma* occurring without other obvious disease of the eye, *secondary glaucoma* occurring as the result of other ocular disease, as well as *congenital glaucoma*. For many years the standard classification of primary glaucoma embraced two categories—*chronic simple* and *congestive*—the latter being divided into two phases, acute and chronic; the ultimate stage of both was known as *absolute glaucoma*. Other terminological variations were proposed to designate the two main types, such as *lymphostatic* and *hæmostatic* by Heerfordt (1911), terms which, being ætiologically wrong, never received wide acceptance, or *compensated* and *incompensated* by Elschnig (1928) which for a time were commonly used. Thus matters remained until the concept of acute glaucoma established by Barkan (1938) as being anatomically determined by pupillary blockage and closure of the drainage

[1] Vol. IV.

angle introduced a more satisfactory terminology based on the ætiology. Barkan suggested the terms *wide-angle* and *narrow-angle*, or subsequently, *open-angle* and *closed-angle* glaucoma.

The value of this classification soon became widely recognized owing to the popularization of gonioscopy, but differences arose regarding the terminology. Barkan's phraseology has the value of dramatic contrast, but it can be criticized. A narrow angle by itself need not be pathological or even potentially pathological and simple glaucoma can occur in such an eye; indeed, this disease bears no relation to the configuration of the angle of the anterior chamber and the term " any-angle " would be appropriate. Moreover, the term " simple glaucoma " is hallowed by age and can appropriately be retained until its ætiology is more fully elucidated. Certainly the term " congestive " should be eliminated since it describes a phase which may occur in either type of primary glaucoma. The closed-angle type may well be divided into four stages: (1) *pre-glaucoma* (Gradle, 1924–46), wherein the narrowness of the angle, although allowing adequate drainage, potentially leads to attacks of raised tension or intermittent attacks; (2) *intermittent*, with periodic transient attacks of raised tension which cause no organic or functional damage; (3) *acute*, during an acute phase of raised tension; and (4) *chronic*, closed-angle glaucoma wherein the drainage is permanently blocked by peripheral anterior synechiæ.

We shall therefore base our classification on the terminology adopted by the International Symposium on Glaucoma in 1954 (Duke-Elder, 1955) as follows:

I. PRIMARY GLAUCOMA—not due to obvious disease in the eye.
    (*a*) Simple glaucoma.
    (*b*) Closed-angle glaucoma, which may include four phases—
        (1) pre-glaucoma, (2) intermittent, (3) acute, and (4) chronic.

II. SECONDARY GLAUCOMA due to pre-existing ocular disease; it may be either of the open- or closed-angle type.

III. CONGENITAL GLAUCOMA (BUPHTHALMOS) due to obstruction of drainage by congenital anomalies.

Buphthalmos has already been described in a previous Volume[1]; the others will be discussed here.

An adequate understanding of glaucoma demands a knowledge of the anatomy of the drainage channels from the eye and the physiology of the formation, circulation and drainage of the aqueous humour; all these subjects have been discussed in previous Volumes of this *System* so that repetition is unnecessary. The detailed anatomy of the drainage channels, the angle of the anterior chamber, the trabeculæ, the canal of Schlemm and

[1] Vol. III, p. 548.

its exit channels through the intrascleral venous plexus and the aqueous veins will be found in Vol. II, p. 186 ff. The dynamics of the aqueous humour and the circumstances determining its outflow, largely at the angle of the anterior chamber and partially through the uveo-scleral channels of exit (a small fraction of the drainage which varies little with the intra-ocular pressure) are described in Vol. IV. The theory of the methods of measuring the intra-ocular pressure will also be found in Vol. IV, where stress is placed on the accuracy of applanation tonometry compared with impression tonometry owing to the elimination of the complicating factor of ocular rigidity; as also are the site, variations and measurement of the facility of aqueous outflow by the somewhat unreliable technique of tonography. The practical clinical application of tonometry is described in Vol. VII, p. 336.

The physiology of the intra-ocular pressure is also discussed in Vol. IV, its normal maintenance as a balance between the formation of aqueous and the ease of its drainage, a factor determined largely by the resistance offered by the drainage channels and to a minor extent by the pressure in the episcleral veins, the physiological changes it undergoes including the rhythmic changes depending on the diurnal variation (and to a less extent on the menstrual rhythm), as well as the physiological and experimental factors which cause alterations in its level.

It will be remembered that in man the normal intra-ocular pressure is generally accepted as being in the region of 15 to 16 mm. Hg, its limiting values being usually taken as 10 and 21 mm. Hg; a level of over 21 mm. Hg may be regarded as suspicious and of 24 mm. Hg or over as tested by applanation tonometry is usually considered as abnormal. We have also seen that a difference of more than 3 mm. Hg is rarely seen in health between the two eyes, that sex exerts little effect, and that after the first 6 weeks of life (when the tension may reach 30 mm. Hg or more) there is little difference with age; a rise of 1 mm. Hg may be expected to occur in men and of 2 mm. Hg in women between the ages of 40 and 75 years.

Adamük. *Ann. Oculist.* (Paris), **58**, 5 (1867).

von Ammon. *Klinische Darstellungen d. Krankheiten u. Bildungsfehler d. mensch. Auges*, Berlin (1838).

Arrachart. *Cours et traité générale historique et pratique des maladies des yeux*, Paris (1786).

Banister. *A Treatise of One Hundred and Thirteen Diseases of the Eyes and Eyeliddes*, London (1622).

Barkan. *Amer. J. Ophthal.*, **19**, 951 (1936); **21**, 1099 (1938); **36**, 445 (1953).

Beer. *Die Lehre v. d. Augenkrankheiten*, Wien (1792).

Boerhaave. *Prælectiones publicæ de morbis oculorum*, Paris, 107, 112, 139 (1748).

Brisseau. *Traité de la cataracte et du glaucome*, Paris (1709).

Coccius. *v. Graefes Arch. Ophthal.*, **9** (1), 1 (1863).

Curran. *Arch. Ophthal.*, **49**, 131 (1920).

Demours. *Traité des maladies des yeux*, Paris, **1**, 470 (1818).

Donders. *See* Hoffmanns. *v. Graefes Arch. Ophthal.*, **8** (2), 124 (1862).

Duke-Elder. *Glaucoma: a Symposium*, Oxon., 315 (1955).

Elschnig. *v. Graefes Arch. Ophthal.*, **120**, 94 (1928).

Gradle. *Amer. J. Ophthal.*, **7**, 603 (1924); **29**, 520 (1946).

von Graefe. *v. Graefes Arch. Ophthal.*, **1** (1), 371; (2), 299 (1854); **2** (1), 248 (1855); **3** (2), 456 (1857).

Guthrie. *Lectures on the Operative Surgery of the Eye*, London, 214 (1823).

Heerfordt. *v. Graefes Arch. Ophthal.*, **78**, 413 (1911).

Jacobson. *De glaucomate* (Diss.), Königsberg (1853).

Jaeger. *Ueber Staar u. Staaroperationen*, Wien (1854).

Knies. *v. Graefes Arch. Ophthal.*, **22** (3), 163 (1876).

Lawrence. *Lancet*, **10**, 262, 483 (1826); **2**, 711 (1829–30).
A Treatise on Diseases of the Eye, London (1833).

Mackenzie. *A Practical Treatise on the Diseases of the Eye*, 2nd ed., London, 826 (1835).

Maître-Jan. *Traité des maladies de l'œil*, Troyes (1707).

Middlemore. *A Treatise on the Diseases of the Eye*, London, **2**, 12 (1835).

Müller, H. *S.B. physiol.-med. Ges. Würzburg* (1856). See *Gesammelte u. hinterlassene Schriften z. Anatomie u. Physiologie d. Auges*, Leipzig, **1**, 340 (1872).
v. Graefes Arch. Ophthal., **4** (1), 366; (2), 22 (1858).

Platner. *De motu ligamenti ciliaris in oculo*, Leipzig (1738).

Raeder. *v. Graefes Arch. Ophthal.*, **112**, 29 (1923).

Read. *A Treatise of the Eyes*, London (1706).

Saint-Yves. *Nouveau traité des maladies des yeux*, Paris, 266 (1722).

Salzmann. *Z. Augenheilk.*, **31**, 1 (1914); **34**, 26, 160 (1915).

Seidel. *v. Graefes Arch. Ophthal.*, **102**, 415 (1920).

Smith, Priestley. *Glaucoma, its Causes, Symptoms, Pathology and Treatment*, London (1879).
The Pathology and Treatment of Glaucoma, London (1891).

Stilling. *v. Graefes Arch. Ophthal.*, **14** (3), 259 (1868).

Sugar. *The Glaucomas*, N.Y. (1951).

Thorburn. *Svenska läk. Handl.*, **53**, 252, 273 (1927).

Troncoso. *Amer. J. Ophthal.*, **8**, 433 (1925); **18**, 103 (1935).

Tyrrell. *A Practical Work on the Diseases of the Eye*, London (1840).

Wardrop. *Essays on the Morbid Anatomy of the Human Eye*, London, **2** (1818).

Weber. *v. Graefes Arch. Ophthal.*, **2** (1), 133 (1855); **23** (1), 1 (1877).

de Wecker. *Traité théoretique et pratique des maladies des yeux*, Paris (1863–7).
Ann. Oculist. (Paris), **116**, 249 (1896).

Weller. *Die Krankheiten d. mensch. Auges*, 3rd ed., Berlin, 295, 474 (1826).

Wenzel. *Manuel de l'oculiste*, Paris (1808).

Werner. *Acta ophthal.* (Kbh.), **10**, 427 (1932).

CHAPTER VII

SIMPLE GLAUCOMA

WE are introducing this Chapter on simple glaucoma with a photograph of FRANS CORNELIS DONDERS [1818–1889] (Fig. 405), who occupied the Chair of Ophthalmology at Utrecht and was one of the greatest ophthalmologists in history; together with his contemporaries and friends, Albrecht von Graefe and Sir William Bowman, he was one of the masters who guided ophthalmology at the stage when it was emerging as a science into the maturity of an established branch of medicine. We have seen that to von Graefe and his predecessors glaucoma was essentially associated with congestion of the globe—acute, absolute or secondary—while the condition of a chronically raised tension in a quiet eye was termed " amaurosis with excavation of the optic disc ". To Donders belongs the credit of recognizing this condition wherein an incapacitating raised tension occurred without inflammatory signs as belonging to the same family and calling it *simple chronic glaucoma*.

We have already taken especial note of the conspicuous part he played together with Listing in elucidating the mechanism of the movements of the eye and, more particularly, in introducing to our profession the importance of the assessment of refractive errors and their correction by spectacles. In the latter connection his classical photograph appears elsewhere in this *System*[1]; the photograph reproduced here, however, is unique, taken by Bramine Hubrecht whom he subsequently married.

By SIMPLE GLAUCOMA we mean a chronic condition wherein the ocular tension is raised above a level compatible with the continued health and function of the eye, associated with a gonioscopically open angle and a reduced facility of aqueous outflow, and not due to any obvious disease of the eye. If present over a sufficient period it causes characteristic pathological changes at the optic disc and in the visual fields and can be expected ultimately to end in absolute glaucoma and blindness.

Incidence

Glaucoma is a common disease in most countries of the world and an extensive literature on its incidence has been built up over the past half-century. Much of this literature is impossible to assess critically; some of it, unfortunately, is worthless, because the criteria accepted for the diagnosis of glaucoma vary considerably from one author to another, because many of the series investigated consist of selected subjects, and in some instances because the incidence of diseases of the eye other than glaucoma influences the statistics. A universal agreement on criteria for the diagnosis of glaucoma is urgently needed and it is hoped that one will be forthcoming in the foreseeable future.

Bearing in mind these reservations, the most informative and useful

---

[1] Vol. V.

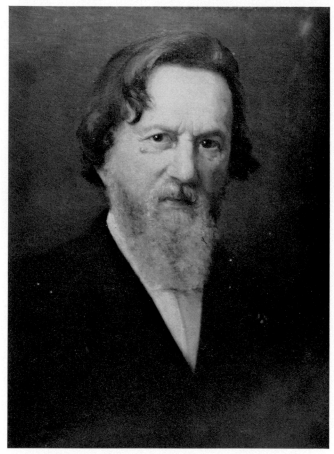

FIG. 405.—FRANS CORNELIS DONDERS
[1818–1889].
(Photographed by Bramine Hubrecht whom he later married; by courtesy of
Prof. H. J. M. Weve.)

statistics are those resulting from the surveys of large numbers of un-selected subjects which have been carried out over the past 20 years in Europe and in North America. The variations in incidence appear to depend to a large extent on the criteria for the diagnosis of glaucoma and also on the average age of the sample surveyed. The following figures are representative:

	Size of Sample	Incidence of Glaucoma	Comments
Brav and Kirber (1951) . . .	10,000	1·53%	40–65 years of age
Wolpaw and Sherman (1954) . .	12,000	2%	Over 45 years
Kostenoja (1955)	600	4·6%	Over 64 years
Vaughan et al. (1955) . . .	1,000	1·9%	Inmates of mental hospital
Bendor-Samuel and Reed (1956) . .	1,000	3·5%	Out-patients over 40 years
Richter and Sautier (1956) . . .	1,981	1·26%	Out-patients not known to have glaucoma
Foote (1957)	30,741	2·32%	
Kornzweig et al. (1957) . . .	1,068	5·3%	Old people
Smillie et al. (1957) . . .	1,054	0·8%	Over 40 years
Vaughan et al. (1957) . . .	7,943	2·01%	Over 40 years
Porter (1958)	2,000	2·6%	Over 40 years
Packer et al. (1959) . . .	13,155	2·06%	Non-ophthalmic patients
Eggink (1959)	1,000	2·3%	Over 40 years
Leydhecker (1959) . . .	10,000	1·47%	All ages
	5,561	2·31%	Over 40 years
Bendor-Samuel et al. (1960) . .	5,000	1·7%	
Gray (1960)	21,197	1·8%	Over 40 years
Havener et al. (1960) . . .	8,535	1·6%	Over 40 years
Garner and Dressler (1961) . .	1,440	2·3%	
Kishida and Nakajima (1961) .	2,295	1·31%	Factory workers
Lukić (1961)	3,386	1·33%	All ages
Leikovsky (1961) . . .	1,357	1·4%	
Perlis (1961)	3,196	3·2%	Post Office workers
Eggink (1962)	9,995	2·25%	62 of 224 eyes had field loss
Satz (1963)	43,323	1·13%	General population
Blumenthal and Kornblueth (1965) .	2,200	1·73%	Over 40 years
McDonald and Johnsos (1965) .	10,090	2·4%	Over 40 years
Kasparov (1965) . . .	90,644	1·3%	Over 40 years
Frydman et al. (1966) . . .	67,193	1·4%	
Hollows and Graham (1966) . .	4,231	0·84%	40–75 years old (0·43% simple glau-coma)
Luntz et al. (1966) . . .	2,308	0·9%	All ages
Segal and Skwierczyńska (1967) .	15,695	0·95%	Over 30 years
Bankes et al. (1968) . . .	5,941	0·93%	Over 40 years (0·71% simple glau-coma)

It appears from these surveys that between 1% and 2% of the popu-lation over the age of 40 have glaucoma and that the incidence of the disease increases with age. In most of the surveys, however, the diagnosis of glaucoma was made merely by measuring the ocular tension and it is possible that cases of ocular hypertension have inflated these figures. It is also true that in most of the surveys the type of glaucoma is not specified, and although most cases will be of simple glaucoma, cases of chronic closed-angle and of secondary glaucoma will have been included; where this has been analysed the incidence of simple glaucoma in a population over 40 years of age is somewhat less than 1%.

The statistics of Bankes and his colleagues (1968) were very adequately controlled, the sample of 5,941 persons over 40 years of age being derived from the ordinary population of an English town although with some degree of selection. The criteria adopted for the diagnosis of simple glaucoma were conservative—a tension by applanation tonometry over 21 mm. Hg or a difference of more than 5 mm. Hg between the two eyes, suspicious or cupped optic discs, a defect in the visual field typical of glaucoma and an open angle of the anterior chamber. In this series of individuals, mostly

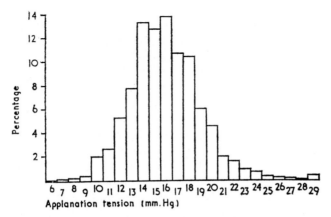

Fig. 406.—The Applanation Ocular Tension in a Population.

The frequency-distribution of the ocular tension among the subjects of a glaucoma survey. The curve has a skew to the right in favour of high readings (J. L. K. Bankes *et al.*).

without ocular symptoms, both types of primary glaucoma were diagnosed in 0·93%; 0·71% had simple glaucoma, 0·17% closed-angle glaucoma and the remainder had "low-tension glaucoma" (Fig. 406). Of the patients of similar age and completely unselected from village populations in Wales analysed by Hollows and Graham (1966) using similar criteria, 0·84% had glaucoma of all types, 0·43% being diagnosed as affected by simple glaucoma and 0·10% as closed-angle glaucoma. In Central Europe, recent figures perhaps not so strictly controlled have been higher. Thus in Germany Frühauf and his colleagues (1967) concluded that 1·5 to 2% of people over the age of 40 have unsuspected glaucoma, while in Poland Dziuba and Rudobielski (1967) diagnosed incipient glaucoma in 1·7% of 6,796 ophthalmic out-patients and in 0·87% of 2,295 industrial workers.

Race

The racial incidence is even more difficult to assess from the extensive literature, although Fuchs (1962) and Mann (1966) have attempted this formidable task. It is possible, however, in the present state of our knowledge, to draw certain broad conclusions. Simple glaucoma is rare in Australoids and Pacific Islanders (Mann and Loschdorfer, 1955; Ward, 1955; Holmes, 1956–61; Elliott, 1959; Mann, 1960–66) and in Mongoloids including American Indians (Holmes, 1960–61; Fuchs, 1962; Mann, 1966), while it is common in Negroids (Rodger, 1958; Fuchs, 1962; Mann, 1966; Turner, 1967) and in Caucasoids. In this last racial group simple glaucoma appears to be particularly common in Iceland (Skulason, 1933; Björnsson, 1955–67; Sveinsson, 1956–59), Norway (Fuchs, 1962) and certain parts of Russia (Fuchs, 1962). Further surveys to determine the incidence of simple glaucoma in the general population, not in a selected population such as one which attends hospital, are still needed from many parts of the world before a more accurate picture can be drawn of the relationship between this disease and race.

Sex

In the incidence of simple glaucoma there is no marked sex-difference, but in most reported series of cases there appears to be a slight preponderance of males. Thus Priestley Smith (1879) found in non-congestive glaucoma 253 males and 223 females. Similarly Carvill (1932) found 54% of the non-congestive cases were in men. In more recent series Holst (1947) found 62·3% male, Sveinsson (1959) about twice as many males as females, Leydhecker (1959) 58% male, and Perkins and Jay (1960) 56·5% male. Most of the reports show a similar distribution, although Nelander (1933) and Kurland and Taub (1957) found twice as many females as males in their series, while several authors have reported an approximately equal distribution between the sexes (Lehrfeld and Reber, 1937; Posner and Schlossman, 1948; Suda, 1963). The preponderance of males is more marked in patients under 50 years of age (under 50, 68·2% male, over 50, 53·5% male—Perkins and Jay, 1960).

Age

Simple glaucoma is a disease of late middle life occurring most commonly in the seventh decade. Although its overall incidence increases rapidly from the age of 40 to 70 and thereafter becomes less common, its frequency increases gradually over the age of 40 until it involves a considerable percentage of the population over the age of 70 and becomes a common disease in the 80's.

Thus Lehrfeld and Reber (1937) found 12·2% of cases in the fifth, 23·6% in the sixth, 37·4% in the seventh, 23·6% in the eighth, and 3·2% in the ninth decades. The percentages of affected individuals in each decade vary in the different surveys, but all show the same trend. The following are representative : Leydhecker (1959)—0·35% in the third, 0·65% in the fourth, 1·45% in the fifth, 2·84% in the sixth, and 4·48% in the seventh decades; Leikovsky (1961)—0·65% in the fifth, 0·9% in the sixth, 2·6% in the seventh decades, and 4% in those over 70; Wright (1966)—0·22% in the fifth, 0·10% in the sixth, 0·57% in the seventh, 2·81% in the eighth decades, and 14·29% in those over 80; Bankes and his associates (1968)—0·02% in the fifth, 0·31% in the sixth, 0·9% in the seventh, 2·82% in the eighth decade and 10·0% in those over 80 years of age. Harrison and Wolf (1964) also found a high incidence of simple glaucoma in the very old—13% in those between 74 and 92 years. Other authors have commented upon the increasing frequency of simple glaucoma with age (Ascher, 1962; Strömberg, 1962; Björnsson, 1964; and others).

The occurrence of the disease in young people is referred to as JUVENILE GLAUCOMA, an unsatisfactory term partly because different writers put varying age-limits to this category with its onset anywhere between 20 and 40 years, and partly because the term has been used in the literature to embrace all types of primary and secondary glaucoma. Glaucoma occurring in young people is not common, but many cases have been reported since von Graefe's (1862) observation in a girl aged 10 years. Opinions have varied regarding its nature; thus Posner and Schlossman (1948) considered it to be related to adult, not infantile glaucoma, while Ellis (1948) found a developmental abnormality of the angle of the anterior chamber in his cases and therefore classified the condition as a delayed form of buphthalmos. Since the advent of routine gonioscopy, however, juvenile glaucoma has usually been accepted as *a simple glaucoma of early onset or a congenital glaucoma of late onset* (François, 1954; Boles Carenini, 1965).

Despite the unsatisfactory nature of the terminology, juvenile glaucoma tends to occur in a characteristic type of eye. Many cases are myopic, this type of refraction being either as common as hypermetropia[1] or more so,[2] while a marked degree of pigmentation in the trabecular meshwork has been noted by a number of authors (Krouwels, 1951; François, 1954; and others). Some of the earlier observers found that other congenital ocular deformities frequently occurred (Löhlein, 1913; Haag, 1915) but in the majority of recent cases this is not so. Heredity appears to exert an influence on its occurrence (Löhlein, 1913; Ellis, 1948); in most families the disease is transmitted as an autosomal dominant and only rarely as an autosomal recessive trait.

It appears, therefore, that juvenile glaucoma denotes little more than the age of onset of the raised ocular tension, that some cases are delayed forms of congenital glaucoma, others should be regarded as examples of simple or primary closed-angle glaucoma of early onset, while others represent various forms of the secondary type. There remains, however, a characteristic group which typically presents with a myopic eye and

---

[1] Löhlein (1913), Keerl (1920), Carvill (1932).
[2] Nettleship (1888), Haag (1915), Wurdemann (1935), Cappetta and Motolese (1936), Lehrfeld and Reber (1937), Ellis (1948), Crombie and Cullen (1964).

a heavily pigmented trabecular meshwork, a clinical picture not unlike that of pigmentary glaucoma. a condition which will be discussed at a later stage.[1]

Bilaterality

The earlier reports in the literature suggested that simple glaucoma sometimes affected one eye; thus in a series of 1,023 cases Lehrfeld and Reber (1937) found that on their first appearance at hospital 50·7% of patients showed unilateral and 49·3% bilateral involvement. Since more accurate methods of diagnosing early glaucoma have come into use, however, such an assessment can no longer be accepted as valid and when long periods of observation have been available, for one eye can be affected some considerable time before its fellow, it must be concluded that simple glaucoma is essentially a bilateral disease. Adequate series of cases to explore this question are sadly lacking. In 575 patients diagnosed as simple glaucoma Rohrschneider and Bauermann (1957) found 40 apparently unilateral of which 22 were available for follow-up; of these, 8 were post-concussive, but from their observations it would seem to follow that simple glaucoma can remain unilateral for a period up to 15 years. Such cases, however, are exceptional and their apparent occurrence should arouse the suspicion that they are secondary rather than primary in type. On the other hand, Drance and his colleagues (1968) concluded that in some of these cases the causal factor determining the onset of the disease in one eye was vascular disease which produced the changes characteristic of simple glaucoma with little or no elevation of the intra-ocular pressure.

Heredity

Although the familial occurrence of various forms of glaucoma has been recognised for almost a century, albeit as an uncommon event, it is only recently that the role of heredity in simple glaucoma has become well established (Becker *et al.*, 1960; Miller and Paterson, 1962; François and Heintz-de Bree, 1966); indeed, the incidence of familial glaucoma is probably about 20% of cases (François, 1966). The numerous reports in the literature of familial glaucoma which appeared prior to the advent of routine gonioscopy or were published in more recent years lacking gonioscopic examination cannot be critically assessed although many are probable examples of simple glaucoma.[2] On the other hand, Becker and his colleagues (1960) diagnosed glaucoma tonographically in 5·5% of the relatives of patients with the disease. Miller and Paterson (1962) diagnosed it in 8% of siblings of such

---

[1] p. 486.
[2] Kummer (1871), Pflüger (1875), Jacobson (1886), Nettleship (1888–1906), Story (1893), Priestley Smith (1894), Nolte (1896), Rogman (1899), Lawford (1907), Calhoun (1914), Plocher (1918), Bartels (1922), Holland (1924), James (1927), Dérer (1930), Courtney and Hill (1931), Berg (1932), Zorab (1932), Allmaras (1938), Strehler (1938), Biró (1939), Briggs (1939), Korte (1939), Casini (1940), Stokes (1940), Glees and Ried (1941), Posner and Schlossman (1949), Penzani (1955) and many others.

patients and in 2·7% of their descendants, and Leighton (1968) in 5·3% of siblings and 4% of their offspring. In a few instances an autosomal recessive inheritance has been postulated[1] (Fig. 408), but in the majority of cases transmission occurred through two or more generations, signifying an autosomal dominant transmission (Fig. 407). Examples of gonioscopically verified simple glaucoma transmitted in this way have now been reported on a number of occasions.[2] X-linked recessive transmission is exceptional

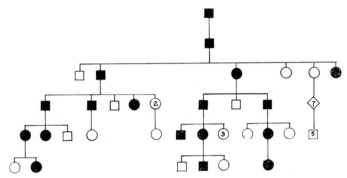

Fig. 407.—SIMPLE GLAUCOMA.
Dominant inheritance (after L. Hambresin and C. Schepens, 1946).

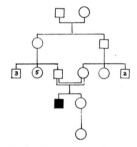

Fig. 408.—PRESENILE GLAUCOMA.
Recessive inheritance with consanguinity (after P. J. Waardenburg, 1949).

(Sveinsson, 1959). A few of the published pedigrees purported to show anticipation, as was first noted by von Graefe (1869), wherein the mean age of onset of the disease among children was earlier than in the parent. It is now generally accepted, however, that anticipation is the result of a bias of ascertainment and has no biological basis (McKusick, 1966).

[1] Pimentel (1941), Waardenburg (1950), Goldschmidt (1951), Biró (1951), Huber (1952), Weekers et al. (1955), François (1958), Becker et al. (1960), Bessière and Le Goff (1963), Beiguelman and Prado (1963).
[2] François et al. (1950–66), Havener (1955), Weekers et al. (1955), Miller and Paterson (1962), Stanković and Dergenc (1967).

At this point it is relevant to discuss the ocular hypertension induced by the topical application of steroids, a subject which permeates much of the recent literature on the heredity of simple glaucoma. The clinical occurrence, features and treatment of this type of glaucoma will be discussed presently,[1] but in the meantime it may be stated that in clinically normal subjects with no family history of glaucoma, applications of topical dexamethasone or betamethasone result in three magnitudes of rise in ocular tension: 5 mm. Hg or less (low responders), 6–15 mm. (intermediate responders), 16 mm. or more (high responders). Armaly (1965) found that the percentages of normal subjects in each group were 66%, 29% and 5% respectively, an assessment confirmed by Becker (1965). On the other hand, François and his co-workers (1966), studying a similar group of subjects, found that only 17·9% showed a rise in ocular tension of over 5 mm. Hg. Armaly (1965) proposed that the magnitude of the dexamethasone-induced rise in the ocular tension is determined by a pair of allelic genes, P^L and P^H, where P^L determines the low pressure response and P^H the high; the corresponding genotypes will therefore be $P^L P^L$ for low responders, $P^L P^H$ for

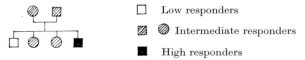

FIG. 409.—THE RESPONSES IN A FAMILY TO DEXAMETHASONE.
After 4 weeks of the topical application of dexamethasone 0·1% t.i.d. (M. F. Armaly).

intermediate and $P^H P^H$ for high responders. The validity of this genetic foundation for the steroid-induced rise in ocular tension was established by a study of the response of parents and offspring to topical dexamethasone (Armaly, 1966) (Fig. 409). Indeed, the clinically normal offspring of patients with simple glaucoma frequently respond to dexamethasone or betamethasone with a magnitude of hypertension similar to their glaucomatous parents (Armaly, 1963; Becker and Hahn, 1964). It may not be, however, that the hypertensive response to these corticosteroids is entirely governed by genetic factors; this was suggested by Spaeth (1967) who found such a response to be relatively frequent after traumatic recession of the angle of the anterior chamber.

Becker and Mills (1963) postulated that simple glaucoma is a heritable trait and represents the homozygous recessive state (*gg*) with a frequency of 4%. The heterozygous state (*ng*) will then have a frequency of 32%, and the homozygous dominant (*nn*) a frequency of 64%. They proposed that this genetic composition could be separated into two groups identifiable by the steroid effect on the ocular tension: a group with a less magnitude of response corresponding to the genotype (*nn*), and a group with a greater

[1] p. 701.

magnitude of response corresponding to the genotypes (ng) and (gg). In support of this hypothesis was the finding that the distribution of the rise of tension in normal eyes suggested a bimodal pattern with an anti-mode at approximately 6 mm. Hg. It was also found that the frequency of the greater magnitude of response in normal subjects was 30%, corresponding to the genotype (ng). Becker (1965) studied the response to betamethasone of the offspring of patients with simple glaucoma and found they consisted of two populations: 81% had an ocular tension of less than 31 mm. Hg, while in 19% the tension rose to 31 mm. or higher. These two populations were believed to correspond to the genotypes (ng) and (gg). Becker and Ballin (1965) found that the second group, which exhibited the high response to betamethasone, demonstrated remarkable similarities to patients with simple glaucoma not only in the degree of the elevation of the ocular tension following the instillation of steroids, but also when subjected to testing for the ability to taste phenylthiocarbamide and also to water-provocative tonography. François and his colleagues (1966) found that 31·2% of apparently normal subjects from families with simple glaucoma showed a rise of ocular tension of over 5 mm. Hg when subjected to topical steroids, while Paterson (1965) studied the response to dexamethasone of siblings and children of patients with simple glaucoma. She used Armaly's (1965) classification and found that in the siblings 33·3% were low responders, 44·5% were intermediate responders, and 22·2% were high responders. In the children the percentages in the three groups were respectively 33·3, 58·3, and 8·3.

The question of the identity of P^H and (g) thus arises. Armaly and Becker (1965) studied the dexamethasone-induced rise of ocular tension in patients with simple glaucoma and found three magnitudes of response, but the frequencies of their occurrence differed markedly from those observed in subjects with clinically normal eyes. They suggested that the heritable trait was not the disease, simple glaucoma itself, but only the steroid-induced rise of ocular tension. The relationship of the genotypes $P^L P^L$, $P^L P^H$, and $P^H P^H$ to simple glaucoma will therefore be indirect, albeit intimate. Simple glaucoma can occur in the presence of any of the three genotypes, but the chances of its occurrence are considerably reduced if the individual has the genotype $P^L P^L$, and considerably greater if his genotype is $P^H P^H$ (Armaly, 1965; Miller, 1966).

It appears probable, therefore, that the genetically determined steroid-induced ocular hypertension bears some relationship to simple glaucoma, although this is indirect. It also appears possible that the conflicting reports on this relationship and also on the transmission of the disease are indications of the genetic heterogeneity of simple glaucoma and also of its possible multifactorial inheritance. The situation is further complicated by the observations that the cup-disc ratio of the optic nerve is probably genetically determined in a multifactorial manner (Armaly, 1967) and that the intra-ocular pressure and the facility of aqueous outflow in normal eyes are similarly transmitted (Armaly, 1967–68).

Be that as it may, it is now established that simple glaucoma is genetically determined and that the appreciable familial incidence of this condition behoves us to examine with particular care the relatives of affected individuals, so that if the disease develops it is treated at as early a stage as possible.

It is interesting that Podos and his associates (1966) found a similar abnormal hypertensive response to topical steroids in high myopia as in families with glaucoma, a suggestive finding that raises possibilities of a relationship between these two conditions.

Allmaras. *Z. Augenheilk.*, **95**, 276 (1938).
Armaly. *Arch. Ophthal.*, **70**, 482, 492 (1963); **75**, 32 (1966); **78**, 35, 187, 193 (1967); **80**, 354 (1968).
Invest. Ophthal., **4**, 187 (1965).
Armaly and Becker. *Fed. Proc.*, **24**, 1274 (1965).
Ascher. *Klin. Mbl. Augenheilk.*, **140**, 516 (1962).
Bankes, Perkins, Tsolakis and Wright. *Brit. med. J.*, **1**, 791 (1968).
Bartels. *Z. Augenheilk.*, **48**, 298 (1922).
Becker. *Invest. Ophthal.*, **4**, 198 (1965).
Becker and Ballin. *Arch. Ophthal.*, **74**, 621 (1965).
Becker and Hahn. *Amer. J. Ophthal.*, **57**, 543 (1964).
Becker, Kolker and Roth. *Amer. J. Ophthal.*, **50**, 557 (1960).
Becker and Mills. *J. Amer. med. Ass.*, **185**, 884 (1963).
Beiguelman and Prado. *J. Génét. hum.*, **12**, 53 (1963).
Bendor-Samuel, May and Reed. *Brit. med. J.*, **1**, 853 (1960).
Bendor-Samuel and Reed. *Winnipeg Clin. Quart.*, **9**, 144 (1956).
Berg. *Acta ophthal.* (Kbh.), **10**, 568 (1932).
Bessière and Le Goff. *Bull. Soc. Ophtal. Fr.*, **63**, 789 (1963).
Biró. *Ophthalmologica*, **98**, 43 (1939); **122**, 228 (1951).
Björnsson. *Amer. J. Ophthal.*, **39**, 202 (1955). *Lœknabladid*, **48**, 97 (1964). *Acta ophthal.* (Kbh.), Suppl. 91 (1967).
Blumenthal and Kornblueth. *Amer. J. Ophthal.*, **60**, 87 (1965).
Boles Carenini. *Ann. Ottal.*, **91**, 140 (1965).
Brav and Kirber. *J. Amer. med. Ass.*, **147**, 1127 (1951).
Briggs. *Brit. J. Ophthal.*, **23**, 649 (1939).
Calhoun. *J. Amer. med. Ass.*, **63**, 290 (1914).
Cappetta and Motolese. *Boll. Oculist.*, **15**, 911 (1936).
Carvill. *Trans. Amer. ophthal. Soc.*, **30**, 71 (1932).
Casini. *Arch. Ottal.*, **47**, 1 (1940).
Courtney and Hill. *J. Amer. med. Ass.*, **97**, 1602 (1931).
Crombie and Cullen. *Brit. J. Ophthal.*, **48**, 143 (1964).

Dérer. *Ophthal. Sborn.*, **5**, 112 (1930).
Drance, Wheeler and Pattullo. *Amer. J. Ophthal.*, **65**, 891 (1968).
Dziuba and Rudobielski. *Klin. oczna*, **37**, 665 (1967).
Eggink. *Ophthalmologica*, **138**, 225 (1959); **143**, 113 (1962).
Elliott. *Trans. ophthal. Soc. N.Z.*, **12**, 87 (1959).
Ellis. *Amer. J. Ophthal.*, **31**, 1589 (1948).
Foote (1957). *Quoted in* Leydhecker, *Glaukom*, Berlin, 32 (1960).
François. *Acta XVII int. Cong. Ophthal.*, Montreal-N.Y., **2**, 1145 (1954).
François. *L'hérédité en ophtalmologie*, Paris (1958).
Amer. J. Ophthal., **61**, 652 (1966).
François, Deweer and van den Berghe. *Bull. Soc. belge Ophtal.*, No. 96, 665 (1950).
François and Heintz-de Bree. *Amer. J. Ophthal.*, **62**, 1067 (1966).
François, Heintz-de Bree and Tripathi. *Amer. J. Ophthal.*, **62**, 844 (1966).
Frühauf, Groeschel and Müller. *Klin. Mbl. Augenheilk.*, **151**, 403 (1967).
Frydman, Clower, Fulghum and Hester. *J. Amer. med. Ass.*, **198**, 1237 (1966).
Fuchs. *Geography of Eye Diseases*, Vienna (1962).
Garner and Dressler. *Sight-sav. Rev.*, **31**, 41 (1961).
Glees and Ried. *v. Graefes Arch. Ophthal.*, **142**, 495 (1941).
Goldschmidt. *J. Hered.*, **42**, 271 (1951).
von Graefe. *v. Graefes Arch. Ophthal.*, **8** (2), 242 (1862); **15** (3), 108 (1869).
Gray. *Penn. med. J.*, **63**, 205 (1960).
Haag. *Klin. Mbl. Augenheilk.*, **54**, 133 (1915).
Harrison and Wolf. *Amer. J. Ophthal.*, **57**, 235 (1964).
Havener. *Amer. J. Ophthal.*, **40**, 828 (1955).
Havener, Johnson and Keller. *Ohio St. med. J.*, **56**, 497 (1960).
Holland. *Indian med. Gaz.*, **59**, 408 (1924).
Hollows and Graham. *Glaucoma: Epidemiology, Early Diagnosis and some Aspects of Treatment* (ed. Hunt), Edinb., 24 (1966).

Holmes. *Amer. J. Ophthal.*, **42**, 393 (1956); **51**, 253 (1961).
VI Cong. Pan-Amer. Ophthal., Caracas, Reports, 129 (1960).
Holst. *Nord. Med.*, **34**, 847 (1947).
Huber. *Ophthalmologica*, **123**, 198 (1952).
Jacobson. *v. Graefes Arch. Ophthal.*, **32** (3), 96 (1886).
James. *Brit. J. Ophthal.*, **11**, 438 (1927).
Kasparov. *Vestn. Oftal.*, **78**, 45 (1965).
Keerl. *Das Glaukom der Jugendlichen* (Diss.), Leipzig (1920).
Kishida and Nakajima. *Acta Soc. ophthal. jap.*, **65**, 1682 (1961).
Kornzweig, Feldstein and Schneider. *Amer. J. Ophthal.*, **44**, 29 (1957).
Korte. *Klin. Mbl. Augenheilk.*, **102**, 664 (1939).
Kostenoja. *Acta ophthal.* (Kbh.), **33**, 650 (1955).
Krouwels. *Ned. T. Geneesk.*, **95**, 1745 (1951).
Kummer. *Korresp.-Bl. schweiz. Aerzte*, 280 (1871).
Kurland and Taub. *Amer. J. Ophthal.*, **43**, 539 (1957).
Lawford. *Roy. Lond. ophthal. Hosp. Rep.*, **17**, 57 (1907).
Lehrfeld and Reber. *Arch. Ophthal.*, **18**, 712 (1937).
Leighton. *Proc. roy. Soc. Med.*, **61**, 542 (1968).
Leikovsky. *Vestn. Oftal.*, **74** (4), 4 (1961).
Leydhecker. *Docum. ophthal.*, **13**, 357 (1959).
Löhlein. *v. Graefes Arch. Ophthal.*, **85**, 393 (1913).
Lukić. *Rev. oftal. venez.*, **5**, 22 (1961).
Luntz, Sevel and Lloyd. *Glaucoma: Epidemiology, Early Diagnosis and some Aspects of Treatment* (ed. Hunt), Edinb., 18 (1966).
McDonald and Johnsos. *Amer. J. Ophthal.*, **59**, 875 (1965).
McKusick. *Heritable Disorders of Connective Tissue*, 3rd ed., St. Louis, 6 (1966).
Mann. *Report on a Survey of the Cocos Keeling Islands*, Canberra (1960).
Culture, Race, Climate and Eye Disease, Springfield (1966).
Mann and Loschdorfer. *Ophthalmic Surveys of the Territories of Papua and New Guinea*, Port Moresby (1955).
Miller. *Trans. ophthal. Soc. U.K.*, **86**, 425 (1966).
Miller and Paterson. *Brit. J. Ophthal.*, **46**, 513 (1962).
Nelander. *Acta ophthal.* (Kbh.), **11**, 370 (1933).
Nettleship. *Roy. Lond. ophthal. Hosp. Rep.*, **12**, 215 (1888).
Ophthalmoscope, **4**, 549 (1906).
Nolte. *Beitr. z. Lehre v. d. Erblichkeit d. Augenkrankungen* (Diss.), Marburg (1896).
Packer, Deutsch, Lewis et al. *J. Amer. med. Ass.*, **171**, 1090 (1959).
Paterson. *Trans. ophthal. Soc. U.K.*, **85**, 295 (1965).

Penzani. *G. ital. Oftal.*, **8**, 53 (1955).
Perkins and Jay. *Trans. ophthal. Soc. U.K.*, **80**, 153 (1960).
Perlis. *Vestn. Oftal.*, **74** (6), 12 (1961).
Pflüger. *Klin. Mbl. Augenheilk.*, **13**, 111 (1875).
Pimentel. *Ophtalmos*, **2**, 329 (1941). See *Amer. J. Ophthal.*, **25**, 904 (1942).
Plocher. *Klin. Mbl. Augenheilk.*, **60**, 592 (1918).
Podos, Becker and Morton. *Amer. J. Ophthal.*, **62**, 1039 (1966).
Porter. *Trans. Amer. Acad. Ophthal.*, **62**, 54 (1958).
Posner and Schlossman. *Amer. J. Ophthal.*, **31**, 915 (1948).
Arch. Ophthal., **41**, 125 (1949).
Richter and Sautier. *Klin. Mbl. Augenheilk.*, **129**, 218 (1956).
Rodger. *Amer. J. Ophthal.*, **45**, 343 (1958).
Rogman. *Clin. Ophtal.*, **5**, 73 (1899).
Rohrschneider and Bauermann. *Klin. Mbl. Augenheilk.*, **130**, 189 (1957).
Satz. *Vestn. Oftal.*, **76**, 31 (1963).
Segal and Skwierczyńska. *Ophthalmologica*, **153**, 336 (1967).
Skulason. *Um Glaukenblinde*, Reykjavik (1933).
Smillie, Roth, Blum and Gates. *Amer. J. Ophthal.*, **44**, 20 (1957).
Smith, Priestley. *Glaucoma*, London (1879). *VIII int. Cong. Ophthal.*, Edinb., 33 (1894).
Spaeth. *Arch. Ophthal.*, **78**, 714 (1967).
Stanković and Dergenc. *Acta ophthal. iugosl.*, **5**, 71 (1967).
Stokes. *Arch. Ophthal.*, **24**, 885 (1940).
Story. *Ophthal. Rev.*, **12**, 69 (1893).
Strehler. *Zwei Stammbäume von Glaucoma simplex* (Diss.), Zürich (1938).
Strömberg. *Acta ophthal.* (Kbh.), Suppl. 69 (1962).
Suda. *Kumamoto med. J.*, **16**, 145 (1963).
Sveinsson. *Lœknabladid*, **40**, 1 (1956). *Acta ophthal.* (Kbh.), **37**, 191 (1959).
Turner. *Amer. J. Optom.*, **44**, 56 (1967).
Vaughan, Asbury, Hoyt et al. *Trans. Pac. Cst. oto-ophthal. Soc.*, **36**, 99 (1955).
Vaughan, Shaffer, Asbury et al. *Sight-sav. Rev.*, **27**, 145 (1957).
Waardenburg. *Genetica*, **15**, 79 (1950).
Ward. *Ophthalmic Survey of Fiji* (Colonial Office Rep.), London (1955).
Weekers, Gouguard-Rion and Gouguard. *Bull. Soc. belge Ophtal.*, No. 110, 255 (1955).
Wolpaw and Sherman. *Sight-sav. Rev.*, **24**, 139 (1954).
Wright. *Glaucoma: Epidemiology, Early Diagnosis and some Aspects of Treatment* (ed. Hunt), Edinb., 12 (1966).
Wurdemann. *Amer. J. Ophthal.*, **18**, 1173 (1935).
Zorab. *Trans. ophthal. Soc. U.K.*, **52**, 446 (1932).

Predisposing Factors

Several factors have been said to predispose to the development of simple glaucoma, particularly the refractive state, especially the presence of myopia, the chemical properties of the blood, the state of the capillaries, the presence of systemic diseases such as arteriosclerosis, and the influence of the sympathetic and endocrine systems. We shall see that there is little conclusive evidence yet available that any of these bears a specific relation to the ætiology of the disease; it is a field wherein idiosyncrasy has weighed more heavily than critical assessment.

1. THE REFRACTION

Although the influence of refractive errors in the ætiology of simple glaucoma is not as marked as it is in primary closed-angle glaucoma wherein hypermetropia is the predominant error and myopia is distinctly uncommon, there appears to be some evidence either that the myopic eye is particularly sensitive to the effects of raised ocular tension or that myopia and simple glaucoma are related in some direct or indirect manner. The early literature on the incidence of myopia in simple glaucoma is difficult to assess because before the advent of routine gonioscopy it was impossible to determine the type of glaucoma with any degree of accuracy, and also because the diagnosis of the disease was often missed until it had reached a late stage. Several reasons contributed to this. The low ocular rigidity, particularly in high degrees of myopia,[1] resulted in misleadingly low estimations of ocular tension by Schiøtz tonometry; the appearance of the optic disc was often misinterpreted as being due to the atrophy accompanying myopic changes; and the areas of myopic degeneration in the fundus are mirrored in the visual field thus tending to confuse the search for glaucomatous field defects, while the optical aberrations of the corrected or uncorrected eye may give rise to bizarre field defects (Jayle and Ourgaud, 1953; Jayle and Bérard, 1955).

In the earlier literature the incidence of myopia in simple glaucoma has varied widely in different series. Gala (1930) found the incidence of myopia in primary glaucoma to be as low as 1·6%, while Lehrfeld and Reber (1937) found 14% of patients with simple glaucoma to be myopic. Some authors believed that the myopic patient was just as liable to glaucoma as one with emmetropia or hypermetropia (Löhlein, 1913), while others have recorded impressive percentages of myopia in simple glaucoma—Lange (1896) 43% myopes in patients with simple glaucoma, Goldschmidt (1923) 57% of 60 cases, while Knapp (1925) reported a series of 25 cases, and a considerable number has been noted wherein the degree of myopia was high (Ischreyt, 1910; Gilbert, 1912; Rolandi, 1913; Lacroix, 1922; and many others). We have already seen that many patients with juvenile

[1] Vol. IV, p. 272.

glaucoma are myopic (Nettleship, 1888, almost 66% of his young patients; Wurdemann, 1935, 5 out of 6 patients under 30 years of age; Cappetta and Motolese, 1936, 47% of 17 patients with juvenile glaucoma).

More recently, Sugar (1957) stated that the incidence of myopia in simple glaucoma is the same as that in the general population, while Schepens and Marden (1966) found that it varied between 5% and 18% in different series. Davenport (1959) reported that over 10% of patients with simple glaucoma had at least —3 D of myopia, while Perkins and Jay (1960) found that 22% of 205 patients with simple glaucoma over the age of 50 were myopic; under the age of 50 the incidence of myopia was 37·8% (40% in males, 31·4% in females). There have also been recent reports of the high incidence of simple glaucoma in myopic subjects (15% of 52 eyes with myopia of over —5 D, Weekers et al., 1958; 27·8% of 144 eyes with myopia of over —10 D, Diaz-Dominguez, 1961). Diaz-Dominguez (1966) noted a particularly high incidence of glaucoma in eyes with myopia of more than —20 D and suggested that malignant myopia may be a specific form of congenital glaucoma.

Podos and his co-workers (1966) have recently reported a high incidence of positive responders to topical corticosteroids[1] in patients with more than —5 D of myopia without evidence or family history of glaucoma, the distribution of the response being similar to that of close relatives of patients with simple glaucoma and significantly different from that of normal volunteers.

There appears little doubt, therefore, that simple glaucoma is at least as common in myopic patients as it is in the rest of the population, and is probably more common in patients with high degrees of myopia, and that myopia is more common in the younger group than in older patients with simple glaucoma. There also appears to be a relationship between myopia and the response of the ocular tension to topical corticosteroids. It may well become evident on further investigation that the relationship between myopia and simple glaucoma is more intimate than has hitherto been believed.

2. THE PROPERTIES OF THE BLOOD

A great deal of work has been done on the physico-chemical properties of the blood in glaucoma with a view to determining ætiological factors, but it must be said at once that an analysis of the literature yields extremely meagre and incomplete results, frequently confusing and contradictory, from which no definite conclusions can be drawn.

With regard to the *cellular constitution of the blood* reports are few. Passow (1930) reported an increase in erythrocytes, and Massoud (1937) of mononuclears, findings which are probably of no significance.

[1] p. 400.

With regard to the *chemistry of the blood*, it would appear that there is probably no abnormality in the proteins (Schumacher, 1967), sugar, sodium and phosphorus (Cohen *et al.*, 1932); Vanýsek and Moster (1964), however, found that glaucomatous patients had an increase in the serum proteins with a preponderance of globulins over albumins, and Ascher (1922) claimed that the chlorides were slightly diminished, while Passow (1930), Giannantoni (1932) and Popov (1951) found them increased. There have been several investigations into the cholesterol content and the reports have not been unanimous; Cogan and Freed (1961), for example, found a raised blood cholesterol in 45 out of 60 patients with simple glaucoma, but this has not been the usual finding; indeed, it would seem that the conclusion is legitimate that a hypercholesterolæmia is not usually present.[1] Moreover, treatment with an antilipæmic drug such as Atromid-S (clofibrate), despite some favourable reports (Orbán *et al.*, 1966, in acute glaucoma; Cullen, 1967), has not been generally successful (Gloster *et al.*, 1968). More interest has attached to the calcium and potassium, partly because a lowering of the potassium-calcium quotient inclines towards alkalinity, while a decrease of calcium increases the excitability of the sympathetic nervous system and the permeability of the capillaries. A diminution of the calcium and an increase of the potassium have been reported by Biffis (1933), Trematore (1934), Trovati (1935), and others; more indeterminate results were recorded by Rossi (1932), Cohen and his colleagues (1932), and Tron and Odnasheva (1937), while the opposite relation was claimed by Fradkin and his associates (1930). More recently, Dienstbier and Balík (1951) and Vanýsek and Moster (1964) have reported a normal potassium-calcium quotient in patients with glaucoma, although the latter workers found a low potassium-magnesium quotient and a high magnesium-calcium quotient in these patients. It would appear, therefore, that these variations, if they occur at all, are by no means constant and, at most, not sufficiently great to alter seriously the alkaline reserve or raise the sympathetic tonus.

With reference to the *physical properties of the blood* most attention has been devoted to the reaction. Some authors have claimed to have found an increased alkalinity[2] while others have obtained indeterminate results.[3] The osmotic pressure was thought to be slightly below the normal level in glaucomatous patients by Hertel and Citron (1921) and Pletneva (1923); but in all these cases sufficiently consistent material is lacking to lead to any pragmatic conclusion or to justify the opinion that the blood of the glaucomatous subject differs from the normal to any significant degree.

3. THE CAPILLARY SYSTEM

A considerable literature has been amassed over the years suggesting a possible disturbance of the capillary system in glaucomatous subjects. Scheerer (1924–25), for example, came to the conclusion that every case of glaucoma showed some pathological change in structure or in function of the capillaries of the skin where there was constriction of the arterial part and dilatation of the venous part of the capillary loops, tending especially towards stasis, dilatation and increased permeability. Scheerer also concluded that there was a lack of regular pulsation in the perimacular capillaries when they were viewed entoptoscopically. This claim was supported by capillaroscopic and oscillometric observations by several workers who noted other general signs of a disturbance of the vascular

---

[1] Salvati (1928), Petersen and Levinson (1930), Muselevic (1930), Passow (1930), Trovati 1935), Vannas and Tarkkanen (1960).

[2] Meesmann (1926), Trovati (1935), and others.

[3] Seidel (1927), Jasiński (1927), Schmerl (1928), Wegner and Endres (1928) and others.

system[1]; while Dieter (1928), using a subjective method of measurement, found the capillary pressure in the eye always raised in glaucoma. In more recent years Magitot (1947–54), Cristini (1947–59) and many others have supported the concept of capillary dysfunction in simple glaucoma, but the evidence does not bear critical examination, and Keeney and Leopold (1952) among others concluded that capillary fragility and morphology are normal in this disease.

4. SYSTEMIC DISEASES

The influence of systemic diseases on the development of simple glaucoma is difficult to evaluate. It must be remembered that although statistics can be quoted showing a high percentage of arteriosclerosis, hypertension, nephritis, diabetes and other conditions in glaucomatous subjects, the figures given are rarely higher than would be expected in any sample group of the population of the same age. In the past, *focal sepsis* was frequently associated with the ætiology of simple glaucoma,[2] but any part which this plays in the ætiology is highly questionable. With regard to the *vascular and metabolic diseases* the position may be somewhat different, and many authorities maintain, although with decreasing insistence, that simple glaucoma is essentially a local symptom of a systemic disease of this type.

A *high blood-pressure* has from time to time been considered to be ætiologically associated with simple glaucoma, largely because of the close physiological relationship between it and the intra-ocular pressure. In non-glaucomatous cases, however, it is found that a raised systemic pressure is not associated with a high intra-ocular pressure (Foster Moore, 1915). In glaucomatous subjects reports vary. The first investigators to examine the problem found, as most of their successors have done, that many cases are not associated with a high blood-pressure, and concluded that there was no causal relationship between the two (Terson and Campos, 1898). Their immediate followers differed somewhat, some finding the blood-pressure to be high,[3] while others such as Krämer (1910), Craggs and Taylor (1913) and MacRae (1915) found little difference from controls. Subsequent statistical evidence has shown that although a high blood-pressure and a high intra-ocular pressure are frequently associated, the relationship between them is accidental rather than essential.[4] It may be taken, therefore, that the systemic blood-pressure is not a primary or even an important factor in the ætiology of glaucoma.

It certainly appears true, however, that simple glaucoma is frequently

[1] Pletneva (1926), Horniker (1928), Schmidt (1929), Wegner (1930), Petersen and Levinson (1930), Goldenburg (1931), de Saint-Martin and Mériel (1932), Ferrari (1932), Mészáros and Tóth (1933), Towbin and Wilenski (1933).

[2] Kerry (1925), Geiger and Roth (1928), Levy (1930), Rossi (1932), Bhatt (1951), and many others.

[3] Joseph (1904), Frenkel and Garipuy (1906), Kümmell (1911), Gilbert (1912).

[4] Elschnig (1917), Wessely (1918), Jackson (1918), Viguri (1923), Kahler and Sallmann (1923), Vele (1933), Weinstein (1935), and many others.

associated with *arteriosclerosis*, usually of a widespread nature. Charlin (1923), indeed, from an extensive clinical study, concluded that 90% of such patients showed well-marked degenerative and diseased conditions in the vascular system, while Calhoun (1929) put the incidence at 95%. More recently, although several authors[1] have confirmed this association of arteriosclerosis with simple glaucoma, others have denied it (Sunde, 1951; Luntz *et al.*, 1965). In the earlier literature there are also reports of the association of simple glaucoma with *nephritis* (Calhoun, 1929) and with *syphilis*,[2] but these associations are almost certainly fortuitous. Although it is unquestionably the case that many patients with simple glaucoma are also the victims of vascular sclerosis, this is not surprising because of their usual age; the evidence for a direct association between these two conditions is therefore far from strong.

5. THE NEURO-VEGETATIVE SYSTEM

Ever since Adamük's experiments (1866–67) indicating a preliminary rise in the intra-ocular pressure on stimulation of the sympathetic nerve, an abnormality of the sympathetic system has been stressed as a characteristic of glaucomatous patients. Particular emphasis was thrown upon this by Félix Lagrange (1922), who went so far as to say that " at the basis and at the beginning of every glaucoma there is an intervention of the sympathetic nerve "; this view has been advocated by many writers, both in the earlier literature,[3] and in more recent times.[4] Although it has so far been impossible either to prove or disprove this hypothesis, we have already seen[5] that the influence of the sympathetic nervous system on the pressure in the normal human eye is probably small so long as the angle of the anterior chamber is not narrow and, this being the case, it is difficult to accept that a disturbance of the neuro-vegetative system is the underlying cause of simple glaucoma, or that it even plays any significant part in its ætiology.

6. THE ENDOCRINE GLANDS

Closely related to the hypothetical imbalance of the neuro-vegetative system and its effects on vasomotor control is a lack of stability in the endocrine system, and a host of authors has called attention to this factor

[1] Dienstbier *et al.* (1950), Sugar (1950), Gasparri (1952), Cristini (1953), Brand (1954), Mackie (1958), Weinstein (1963), Manuelli and Paganoni (1964), Faraldi (1965), and others.

[2] Pflüger (1885), Elschnig (1913), Hirschberg (1919), Charlin (1923), Carlotti (1923), Arnoux (1924), Espildora Luque (1929), Calhoun (1929), Mazal (1931).

[3] Pichler (1917), Abadie (1923), de Andrade (1924), Hamburger (1924–25), H. Lagrange (1925), Scalinci (1926), Thiel (1926), Bistis (1930), H. G. Smith and Barkan (1930), and many others.

[4] Hess (1947), Magitot (1947), Marquez (1947), Zondek and Wolfsohn (1947), Filbry (1948–49), Moreu (1948), Posner and Schlossman (1948), Schmerl and Steinberg (1948), Courtis and Nuñez (1950), Niedermeier (1950), Popov (1952), Thiel (1952), Lowenstein (1955), Duke-Elder (1957), Agarwal (1958), Cristini (1959), Dienstbier (1964), and many others.

[5] Vol IV, p. 295.

in glaucomatous subjects[1]; Passow (1930), for example, claimed to have demonstrated an excess of iodine in the blood in 83% of glaucomatous cases indicating the presence of thyrotoxicosis. In the more recent literature there are several reports of the association of simple glaucoma and thyroid dysfunction.[2] Some of these reports are difficult to assess because the criteria for diagnosing disturbances of the thyroid are either not stated or not critical. Becker and his co-workers (1966), however, have shown a remarkable prevalence of low values of the protein-bound iodine in patients with simple glaucoma and Pohjanpelto (1968) concluded that hypothyroidism is sometimes associated with an increased intra-ocular pressure, although Cheng and Perkins (1967) found only two patients with simple glaucoma in 155 with various forms of thyroid disease. Dollfus and Séguy (1936) found an abnormal quantity of folliculin in the urine, although Radnót and Csillag (1949) could discover no abnormality in the circulating gonadotropic hormone and œstrin in glaucomatous patients, a negative finding paralleled by Boros and Valkó (1959) on the estimation of the urinary 17-ketosteroids. Some authors[3] have claimed that the incidence of simple glaucoma in diabetics is the same as in non-diabetics, while others have found an increased incidence in these patients,[4] and Traisman and his colleagues (1967) noted a significantly higher intra-ocular pressure in juvenile cases. There have also been a few reports of a high incidence of simple glaucoma in patients with acromegaly, with pituitary tumours or Cushing's syndrome,[5] but this is by no means invariable (Lutsker et al., 1968), and in this connection a note should be made of the hypertensive effect of certain steroids.[6] The possible influence of endocrine disorders in determining the incidence of simple glaucoma is difficult to evaluate, and until further research has clarified the position it is pointless to speculate on the significance of some of these observations.

There are, in the recent literature, several references to the association of glaucoma and AUDITORY DISTURBANCES, particularly hypo-acousia.[7] There have also been occasional reports of glaucoma, usually of the closed-angle variety, and Ménière's disease occurring in the same patient (Godtfredsen, 1949–50; Fontana and Cristiani, 1950). It is impossible to assess the significance of these observations although it is possible that many of the associations are fortuitous.

[1] Hertel (1918), Imre (1921–24), Paltracca (1921), F. Lagrange (1922), v. Csapody (1923), Müller (1924), Scalinci (1924), Brana (1925), H. Lagrange (1925), Lamb (1926), Salvati (1928), Passow (1930), Mossa (1934), and many others.
[2] Haselmann (1949), Gördüren (1962), Rogova (1964), McLenachan and Davies (1965), Vasilieva (1965), Becker et al. (1966).
[3] Waite and Beetham (1935), Palomar (1956), Armaly and Baloglou (1967), Bankes (1967), Lieb et al. (1967).
[4] Armstrong et al. (1960), Safir et al. (1964), Sugar (1964), Cristiansson (1965), Kordic (1966), Pur (1966).
[5] Arén and Skanse (1955), Pagliarani and Fiorini (1960), van Bijsterveld and Richards (1964), Howard and English (1965), Kovalev and Shpakov (1966), Bayer and Neuner (1967).
[6] p. 400.
[7] G. and W. Cristini (1950), Ferraris de Gaspare and Maffei (1951), ten Doesschate and Lansberg (1954), Beretta and Cerabolini (1957), Zolog et al. (1961), Lampé et al. (1963), Gärtner (1964), Krejci et al. (1964), Wójcik-Mazurowska and Knapik-Fialkowska (1966).

In summary, therefore, while it must be admitted that many of these observations are scanty and somewhat perfunctory, it may be said in general terms that *simple glaucoma is a genetically determined condition tending to occur in persons over middle age,* and that its incidence increases with age. There is some inconclusive evidence that it occurs more commonly in highly myopic eyes and that it may have a vague association with certain endocrine abnormalities.

Abadie. *Clin. Ophtal.*, **12**, 303 (1923).

Adamük. *Zbl. med. Wiss.*, **4**, 561 (1866); **5**, 433 (1867).

Agarwal. *Acta 1st Afro-Asian Cong. Ophthal.* (Cairo), 159 (1958).

de Andrade. *Ann. Oculist.* (Paris), **161**, 771 (1924).

Arén and Skanse. *Acta ophthal.* (Kbh.), **33**, 295 (1955).

Armaly and Baloglou. *Arch. Ophthal.*, **77**, 493 (1967).

Armstrong, Daily, Dobson and Girard. *Amer. J. Ophthal.*, **50**, 55 (1960).

Arnoux. *Clin. Ophtal.*, **13**, 440 (1924).

Ascher. *v. Graefes Arch. Ophthal.*, **107**, 247 (1922).

Bankes. *Brit. J. Ophthal.*, **51**, 557 (1967).

Bayer and Neuner. *Dtsch. med. Wschr.*, **92**, 1791 (1967).

Becker, Kolker and Ballin. *Amer. J. Ophthal.*, **61**, 997 (1966).

Beretta and Cerabolini. *Riv. oto-neuro-oftal.*, **32**, 662 (1957).

Bhatt. *Proc. All-India ophthal. Soc.*, **12**, 135 (1951).

Biffis. *Ann. Ottal.*, **61**, 109, 284 (1933).

van Bijsterveld and Richards. *Amer. J. Ophthal.*, **57**, 267 (1964).

Bistis. *Arch. Ophtal.*, **47**, 96 (1930).

Boros and Valkó. *Szemészet*, **96**, 51 (1959).

Brana. *Z. Augenheilk.*, **56**, 68 (1925).

Brand. *Ophthalmologica*, **128**, 281 (1954).

Calhoun. *Amer. J. Ophthal.*, **12**, 265 (1929).

Cappetta and Motolese. *Boll. Oculist.*, **15**, 911 (1936).

Carlotti. *Clin. Ophtal.*, **12**, 428 (1923).

Charlin. *Klin. Mbl. Augenheilk.*, **70**, 123 (1923).

Cheng and Perkins. *Brit. J. Ophthal.*, **51**, 547 (1967).

Cogan and Freed. *Helmholtz ophthal. Inst., Sci. Notes* (Moscow), **6**, 89 (1961).

Cohen, Killian and Halpern. *Arch. Ophthal.*, **8**, 39 (1932).

Courtis and Nuñez. *Acta XVI int. Cong. Ophthal.*, London, **2**, 854 (1950).

Craggs and Taylor. *Ophthalmoscope*, **11**, 350 (1913).

Cristiansson. *Acta ophthal.* (Kbh.), **43**, 224 (1965).

Cristini, G. *Ann. Oculist.* (Paris), **180**, 530 (1947).
Acta XVI int. Cong. Ophthal., London, **2**, 865 (1950).

Cristini. *Rev. oto-neuro-oftal.*, **28**, 1 (1953); **34**, 3 (1959).

Cristini, G. and W. *Riv. oto-neuro-oftal.*, **25**, 421 (1950).

von Csapody. *Klin. Mbl. Augenheilk.*, **70**, 111 (1923).

Cullen. *Lancet*, **2**, 892 (1967).

Davenport. *Trans. ophthal. Soc. U.K.*, **79**, 3 (1959).

Diaz-Dominguez. *Ann. Oculist.* (Paris), **194**, 597 (1961).
Arch. port. Oftal., **18**, 13 (1966).

Dienstbier. *Cs. Oftal.*, **20**, 403 (1964).

Dienstbier and Balík. *Cs. Oftal.*, **7**, 395 (1951).

Dienstbier, Balík and Fischer. *Cs. Oftal.*, **16**, 289 (1960).

Dienstbier, Balík and Kafka. *Brit. J. Ophthal.*, **34**, 47 (1950).

Dieter. *Arch. Augenheilk.*, **99**, 678 (1928).

ten Doesschate and Lansberg. *Bull. Soc. belge Ophtal.*, No. 107, 205 (1954).

Dollfus and Séguy. *Bull. Soc. Ophtal. Paris*, 299 (1936).

Duke-Elder. *Trans. ophthal. Soc. U.K.*, **77**, 205 (1957).

Elschnig. *Prag. med. Wschr.*, **38**, 377 (1913).
v. Graefes Arch. Ophthal., **92**, 101, 237 (1917).

Espildora Luque. *Arch. Oftal. hisp-amer.*, **30**, 545 (1929).

Faraldi. *Rass. ital. Ottal.*, **32**, 209 (1965).

Ferrari. *Arch. Ottal.*, **39**, 147 (1932).

Ferraris de Gaspare and Maffei. *Riv. oto-neuro-oftal.*, **26**, 294 (1951).

Filbry. *Klin. Wschr.*, **60**, 30 (1948).
Klin. Mbl. Augenheilk., **115**, 506 (1949).

Fontana and Cristiani. *Riv. oto-neuro-oftal.*, **25**, 341 (1950).

Fradkin, Krasnov and Cheifez. *Russ. Arch. Oftal.*, **7**, 786 (1930).

Frenkel and Garipuy. *Arch. Ophtal.*, **26**, 615 (1906).

Gärtner. *Ophthalmologica*, **147**, 393 (1964).

Gala. *Oftal. sborn.*, **5**, 119 (1930).

Gasparri. *Boll. Oculist.*, **31**, 175 (1952).

Geiger and Roth. *Illinois med. J.*, **53**, 110 (1928).

Giannantoni. *Lettura Oftal.*, **9**, 319 (1932).

Gilbert. *v. Graefes Arch. Ophthal.*, **82**, 389 (1912).

Gloster, Hartley and Perkins. *Brit. J. Ophthal.*, **52**, 793 (1968).

Godtfredsen.   *Acta oto-laryngol.*, **37**, 533 (1949).
Bull. Soc. franç. Ophtal., **63**, 295 (1950).
Gördüren.   *Brit. J. Ophthal.*, **46**, 491 (1962).
Goldenburg.   *Amer. J. Ophthal.*, **14**, 944 (1931).
Goldschmidt.   *Der Refraktionszustand beim Glaukom* (Diss.), Halle (1923).
Hamburger.   *Med. Klin.*, **20**, 274 (1924). *Dtsch. med. Wschr.*, **51**, 186 (1925).
Haselmann.   *Klin. Mbl. Augenheilk.*, **115**, 527 (1949).
Hertel.   *Ber. dtsch. ophthal. Ges.*, **41**, 57 (1918).
Hertel and Citron.   *v. Graefes Arch. Ophthal.*, **104**, 149 (1921).
Hess.   *Arch. Ophthal.*, **37**, 324 (1947).
Hirschberg.   *Zbl. prakt. Augenheilk.*, **43**, 129 (1919).
Horniker.   *v. Graefes Arch. Ophthal.*, **119**, 488; **121**, 347 (1928).
Howard and English.   *Arch. Ophthal.*, **73**, 765 (1965).
Imre.   *Arch. Augenheilk.*, **88**, 155 (1921). *Klin. Mbl. Augenheilk.*, **71**, 777 (1923); **73**, 206 (1924). *Arch. Ophthal.*, **53**, 205 (1924).
Ischreyt.   *v. Graefes Arch. Ophthal.*, **73**, 566 (1910).
Jackson.   *Amer. J. Ophthal.*, **1**, 373 (1918).
Jasiński.   *Klin. oczna*, **5**, 97, 110 (1927).
Jayle and Bérard.   *Ann. Oculist.* (Paris), **188**, 431 (1955).
Jayle and Ourgaud.   *Bull. Soc. Ophtal. Fr.*, 513 (1953).
Joseph.   *Recherches cliniques sur le glaucome primitif dans ses rapports avec l'artériosclerose et l'imperméabilité rénale* (Thèse), Paris (1904).
Kahler and Sallmann.   *Wien. klin. Wschr.*, **36**, 883 (1923).
Keeney and Leopold.   *Arch. Ophthal.*, **47**, 720 (1952).
Kerry.   *Trans. ophthal. Soc. U.K.*, **45**, 355 (1925).
Knapp, A.   *Trans. Amer. ophthal. Soc.*, **23**, 61 (1925).
Kordic.   *Arch. chil. Oftal.*, **23**, 12 (1966).
Kovalev and Shpakov.   *Vestn. Oftal.*, **79**, 51 (1966).
Krämer.   *v. Graefes Arch. Ophthal.*, **73**, 349 (1910).
Krejcí, Siroký, Krejcová and Novák.   *Cs. Oftal.*, **20**, 268 (1964).
Kümmell.   *v. Graefes Arch. Ophthal.*, **79**, 183 (1911).
Lacroix.   *Ann. Oculist.* (Paris), **159**, 730 (1922).
Lagrange, F.   *Du glaucome et de l'hypotonie*, Paris (1922).
Lagrange, H.   *Brit. J. Ophthal.*, **9**, 398 (1925).
Lamb.   *Trans. Amer. ophthal. Soc.*, **24**, 105 (1926).
Lampé, Tomits and Csüllög.   *Szemészet*, **100**, 145 (1963).

Lange.   *Vossius's Samml. zwangl. Abhandl. Geb. Augenheilk.*, **1** (6) (1896).
Lehrfeld and Reber.   *Arch. Ophthal.*, **18**, 712 (1937).
Levy.   *Amer. J. Ophthal.*, **13**, 991 (1930).
Lieb, Stärk, Jelinek and Malzi.   *Acta ophthal.* (Kbh.), Suppl. 94 (1967).
Löhlein.   *v. Graefes Arch. Ophthal.*, **85**, 393 (1913).
Lowenstein.   *Ann. Oculist.*, **188**, 981 (1955).
Luntz, Sevel and Lloyd.   *Brit. J. Ophthal.*, **49**, 128 (1965).
Lutsker, Merkova and Klimenko.   *Vestn. Oftal.*, **81**, 33 (1968).
Mackie.   *Brit. J. Ophthal.*, **42**, 1 (1958).
McLenachan and Davies.   *Brit. J. Ophthal.*, **49**, 441 (1965).
MacRae.   *Ophthalmoscope*, **13**, 168 (1915).
Magitot.   *Ann. Oculist.* (Paris), **180**, 1 (1947); **186**, 385 (1953); **187**, 1 (1954).
Manuelli and Paganoni.   *Ann. Ottal.*, **90**, 710 (1964).
Marquez.   *Ophthal. ibero Amer.*, **9**, 123 (1947).
Massoud.   *Brit. J. Ophthal.*, **21**, 559 (1937).
Mazal.   *Brat. lek. listy*, **11**, 82 (1931).
Meesmann.   *Arch. Augenheilk.*, **97**, 1 (1926).
Mészáros and Tóth.   *Klin. Mbl. Augenheilk.*, **90**, 67 (1933).
Moore, Foster.   *Roy. Lond. ophthal. Hosp. Rep.*, **20**, 108 (1915).
Moreu.   *Arch. Soc. oftal. hisp-amer.*, **8**, 64 (1948).
Mossa.   *Rass. ital. Ottal.*, **3**, 28 (1934).
Müller, L.   *Wien. klin. Wschr.*, **37**, 1270 (1924).
Muselevic.   *Russ. Arch. oftal.*, **7**, 529 (1930).
Nettleship.   *Roy. Lond. ophthal. Hosp. Rep.*, **12**, 215 (1888).
Niedermeier.   *Ber. dtsch. ophthal. Ges.*, **56**, 134 (1950).
Orbán, Hanisch and Vereb.   *Klin. Mbl. Augenheilk.*, **149**, 847 (1966).
Pagliarani and Fiorini.   *Rev. oto-neuro-oftal.*, **35**, 140 (1960).
Palomar.   *Arch. Soc. oftal. hisp.-amer.*, **16**, 827 (1956).
Paltracca.   *Arch. Ottal.*, **28**, 129 (1921).
Passow.   *Arch. Augenheilk.*, **103**, 111 (1930).
Perkins and Jay.   *Trans. ophthal. Soc. U.K.*, **80**, 153 (1960).
Petersen and Levinson.   *Arch. Path.*, **9**, 282, 395 (1930).
Pflüger.   *Ber. dtsch. ophthal. Ges.*, **17**, 91 (1885).
Pichler.   *Arch. Augenheilk.*, **82**, 194 (1917).
Pletneva.   *Russ. oftal. J.*, **2**, 7 (1923). *Festschr. für Prof. Awerbach*, Moscow, 5 (1926).
Podos, Becker and Morton.   *Amer. J. Ophthal.*, **62**, 1039 (1966).
Pohjanpelto.   *The Thyroid Gland and Intraocular Pressure*, Helsinki (1968).
Popov.   *Vestn. oftal.*, **30** (2), 13 (1951); **31** (4), 10 (1952).
Posner and Schlossman.   *Amer. J. Ophthal.*, **31**, 915 (1948).

Pur. *Cs. Oftal.*, **22**, 427 (1966).
Radnót and Csillag. *Ophthalmologica*, **118**, 998 (1949).
Rogova. *Vestn. oftal.*, **77**, 38 (1964).
Rolandi. *Ann. Ottal.*, **42**, 303 (1913).
Rossi. *Arch. Ottal.*, **39**, 1, 51 (1932).
Safir, Paulsen and Klayman. *Diabetes*, **13**, 161 (1964).
de Saint-Martin and Mériel. *Arch. Ophtal.*, **49**, 705 (1932).
Salvati. *G. Ocul.*, **9**, 54 (1928).
Scalinci. *G. Ocul.*, **5**, 33 (1924).
   Ann. Ottal., **54**, 235 (1926).
Scheerer. *Klin. Mbl. Augenheilk.*, **73**, 67 (1924); **74**, 688 (1925).
Schepens and Marden. *Amer. J. Ophthal.*, **61**, 213 (1966).
Schmerl. *Arch. Augenheilk.*, **98**, 565 (1928).
Schmerl and Steinberg. *Amer. J. Ophthal.*, **31**, 155 (1948).
Schmidt. *Arch. Augenheilk.*, **100–1**, 190 (1929).
Schumacher. *Ophthalmologica*, **154**, 51 (1967).
Seidel. *v. Graefes Arch. Ophthal.*, **119**, 15 (1927).
   Klin. Mbl. Augenheilk., **78**, 77 (1927).
Smith, H. G., and Barkan. *Amer. J. Ophthal.*, **13**, 1076 (1930).
Sugar. *Acta XVI int. Cong. Ophthal.*, London, **2**, 846 (1950).
   The Glaucomas, 2nd ed., London, 103 (1957).
   Sorsby's *Modern Ophthalmology*, London, **4**, 554 (1964).
Sunde. *Acta ophthal.* (Kbh.), **29**, 213 (1951).
Terson and Campos. *Arch. Ophtal.*, **18**, 209 (1898).

Thiel. *Klin. Mbl. Augenheilk.*, **77**, 753 (1926).
   Ophthalmologica, **123**, 195 (1952).
Towbin and Wilenski. *Z. Augenheilk.*, **80**, 141 (1933).
Traisman, Alfano, Andrews and Gatti. *Amer. J. Ophthal.*, **64**, 1149 (1967).
Trematore. *Lettura oftal.*, **11**, 161 (1934).
Tron and Odnasheva. *Vestn. oftal.*, **11**, 3 (1937).
Trovati. *Ann. Ottal.*, **63**, 641 (1935).
Vannas and Tarkkanen. *Acta ophthal.* (Kbh.), **38**, 452 (1960).
Vanýsek and Moster. *Cs. Oftal.*, **20**, 280 (1964).
Vasilieva. *Vestn. oftal.*, **78**, 70 (1965).
Vele. *Ann. Ottal.*, **61**, 511 (1933).
Viguri. *An. Soc. mex. Oftal.*, **4**, 114 (1923).
Waite and Beetham. *New Engl. J. Med.*, **212**, 367, 429 (1935).
Weekers, Lavergne and Prijot. *Ann. Oculist.* (Paris), **191**, 26 (1958).
Wegner. *Arch. Augenheilk.*, **103**, 511 (1930).
Wegner and Endres. *Z. Augenheilk.*, **64**, 43 (1928).
Weinstein. *Arch. Ophthal.*, **13**, 181 (1935).
   Docum. ophthal., **17**, 303 (1963).
Wessely. *Arch. Augenheilk.*, **83**, 99 (1918).
   Ber. dtsch. ophthal. Ges., **41**, 80 (1918).
Wójcik-Mazurowska and Knapik-Fialkowska. *Pol. Tyg. lek.*, **21**, 1719 (1966).
Wurdemann. *Amer. J. Ophthal.*, **18**, 1173 (1935).
Zolog, Salomon and Atanasescu. *Oftalmologia* (Buc.), **5**, 11 (1961).
Zondek and Wolfsohn. *Amer. J. Ophthal.*, **30**, 596 (1947).

Pathology

The study of the pathology of simple glaucoma has been rendered difficult by the fact that until recently almost all the histological material was derived from eyes which had been excised in the absolute stage of the disease, long after the presence of a high tension had produced extensive and widespread degenerative changes. As we shall see, it has been demonstrated by various techniques that the site of obstruction to the outflow of the aqueous in simple glaucoma must lie between the anterior chamber and the episcleral venous plexus, and during the past few years several authors have described histological changes in the angle of the anterior chamber and in the outflow channels to account for this. These will be reviewed first, and then a résumé will be given of the pathological changes which result from the continued action of an increased intra-ocular pressure from any cause.

In the earlier literature the angle of the anterior chamber excited a great deal of interest since the importance of its occlusion in the ætiology of glaucoma was suggested by Knies (1876) and Weber (1877), and a vast amount of investigation was devoted to it (Brailey, 1880; Priestley Smith,

1880–91; Birnbacher and Czermak, 1886; and many others). The
formation of extensive peripheral anterior synechiæ was known to occur
most constantly and rapidly in the type of the disease now known as primary
closed-angle glaucoma and to be rarer in the simple type where peripheral
synechiæ may occur only at a late stage (Barkan, 1938–54; Reese, 1944;
Sugar, 1951; François, 1955) (Fig. 410), are more commonly partial so that
much of the angle remains free, or are altogether absent. This absence has
been verified anatomically (Priestley Smith, 1879) and gonioscopically. In
all cases of long-standing glaucoma, degenerative changes in the trabecular
meshwork are the rule. They include a sclerosis and thickening of the
trabeculæ (Henderson, 1910; Rønne, 1913; Verhoeff, 1915; Maggiore,

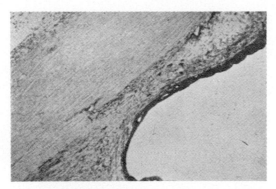

FIG. 410.—OBLITERATION OF THE ANGLE IN ABSOLUTE GLAUCOMA.

In a man aged 75 with simple glaucoma. The angle is obliterated by anterior
synechiæ; there is extreme narrowing of the vessels, the scleral fibres are sclerosed
and hypertrophied and pigment outlines the external collector channels which are
now rendered useless (G. Dvorak-Theobald and H. Q. Kirk).

1917) and a deposition of pigment, sometimes in considerable quantity, in
its meshes (Levinsohn, 1909–22; Rønne, 1913; Schieck, 1918; and others)
(Fig. 411).

More recently, changes of a more intimate type have been investigated.
Teng and his co-workers (1955–57) described a primary degeneration in the
angle of the anterior chamber, which increased with age and was present in
12 to 13% of eyes over the age of 50. They believed that this started in the
collagen of the external trabecular region and then spread to the canal of
Schlemm, to the collector channels and to the intrascleral plexus. The
changes consisted of granularity followed by fragmentation of the collagen,
proliferation of the endothelial cells of the trabeculæ, and the formation of
adhesions between the walls of the canal of Schlemm. Following this report
several authors have described various changes in the angle of the anterior
chamber affecting the trabeculæ, including a general thickening and sclerosis

of the tissues,[1] endothelial proliferation,[2] degenerative changes in the endothelial cells with vacuolization and swelling of the cytoplasm and thickening of the glass membrane[3] (Figs. 412–13); all these changes are associated with narrowing of the intertrabecular spaces. These changes in the trabeculæ were described by Speakman (1961–62) and Speakman and Leeson (1962) as a progressive nodular dystrophy of the collagen somewhat resembling the

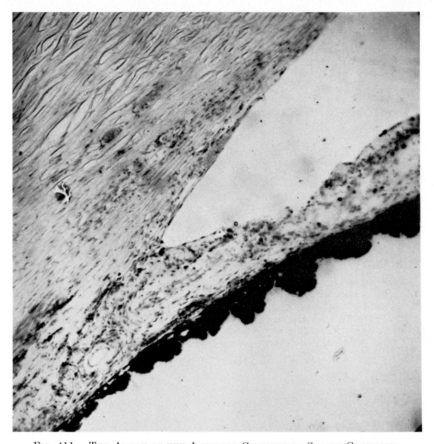

FIG. 411.—THE ANGLE OF THE ANTERIOR CHAMBER IN SIMPLE GLAUCOMA.

The trabeculæ are sclerosed, the canal of Schlemm and its efferent channels are compressed. The iris shows a considerable amount of atrophy (N. Ashton).

formation of the Hassall-Henle bodies of the corneal endothelium, with fragmentation and coiling of the fibre-bundles, while Wolter (1963) suggested that they might be due to a contraction or compression of the trabecular

[1] Dvorak-Theobald and Kirk (1956), Kornzweig et al. (1957–58), Flocks (1958), Becker (1959), Wolter (1959–60), Speakman (1961), Speakman and Leeson (1962), Wolter et al. (1963).
[2] Rohen and Unger (1958), Wolter (1959), Unger and Rohen (1960).
[3] Ashton (1959–60), Becker (1959), Garron (1959), Unger and Rohen (1960), Rohen and Straub (1967).

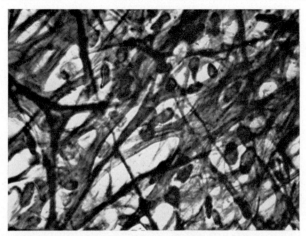

Fig. 412.—The deeper parts of the uveal meshwork in a patient aged 40, showing an extensive proliferation of the trabecular endothelium and some sclerosis of the trabeculæ (J. R. Wolter).

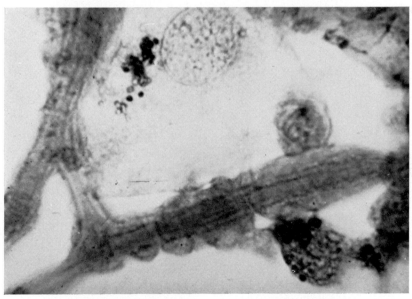

Fig. 413.—There are marked swellings and irregularities of the fibres of the uveal trabeculæ largely due to changes in the hyaline membrane (N. Ashton).

fibres as a result of the collapse of the filtering meshwork. A number of authors also described narrowing and partial obstruction of the canal of Schlemm (Dvorak-Theobald and Kirk, 1956; Kornzweig, 1957; Flocks, 1958), but the most dramatic changes tend to be localized in the inner wall of this canal. Indeed, in cases of absolute glaucoma Unger and Rohen (1960)

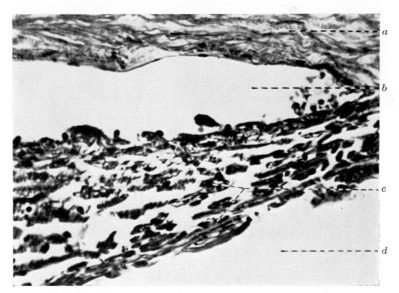

FIG. 414.—THE NORMAL TRABECULÆ.

In a woman aged 47 years. *a*, sclera; *b*, canal of Schlemm; *c*, trabeculæ;
d, anterior chamber (J. Rohen and H. H. Unger).

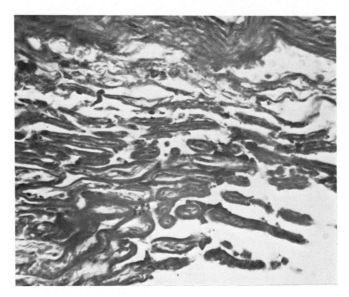

FIG. 415.—THE TRABECULÆ IN SIMPLE GLAUCOMA.

The trabeculæ in a patient aged 74 suffering from absolute glaucoma. Note
the extreme thickening of the trabecular lamellæ (J. Rohen and H. H. Unger).

found the degenerative changes to be so marked that the entire meshwork was replaced by amorphous tissue (Figs. 414–8). Pathological changes in the nerve fibres of the trabecular meshwork have been described by Wolter (1959–60) and Wolter and his associates (1963): the normally regular nerves were found to be distorted with irregular thickenings and degenerative end-

FIGS. 416 and 417.—THE TRABECULÆ IN SIMPLE GLAUCOMA (J. Rohen and H. H. Unger).

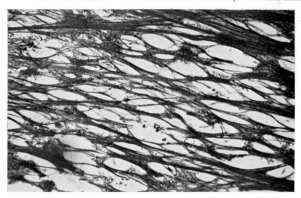

FIG. 416.—Flat section of the trabeculæ in a normal woman aged 49 years.

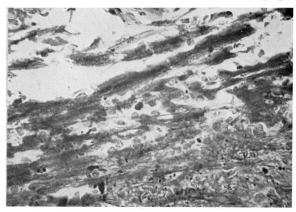

FIG. 417.—Flat section of the trabeculæ in a patient aged 62 with simple glaucoma.

bulbs were present as well as peculiar large terminal swellings at the ends of the interrupted trabecular nerves (Fig. 419). Ashton (1959–60) found that in early simple glaucoma the trabecular meshwork may appear histologically normal and he suggested that some of the changes described by previous workers may have been the result of post-mortem changes or of fixation arte-facts. Although this criticism may be valid for some of the earlier reports, more recent workers have taken care to obtain adequate fixation of trephine buttons and excised eyes wherein similar pathological changes have

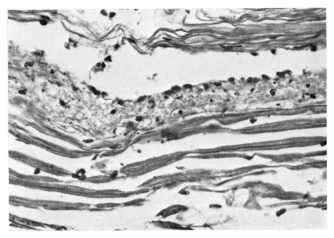

FIG. 418.—THE TRABECULÆ IN SIMPLE GLAUCOMA.

The trabecular spaces are in good condition but there is swelling of the hyaline
membrane and a striking thickness and foamy appearance of the trabecular wall of
Schlemm's canal (H. H. Unger and J. Rohen).

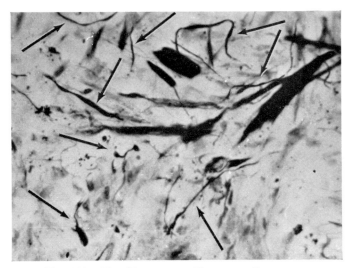

FIG. 419.—THE TRABECULAR NERVES IN GLAUCOMA.

The many abnormal nerve fibres (arrowed) with an abnormal course and calibre
at the base of the trabeculæ (tangential section; Hortega stain) (J. R. Wolter *et al*).

been found. It appears, therefore, that in established simple glaucoma the
intertrabecular spaces are narrowed as a result of thickening of the
trabeculæ, and Becker (1959) has shown that there is a positive correlation
between trabecular pathology and a reduction in the outflow of the aqueous,
a result confirmed by Bárány and Rohen (1963) in vervet monkeys with
secondary glaucoma.

Electron-microscopic studies have confirmed these changes, particularly in the inner wall of Schlemm's canal[1] (Figs. 420–4). These changes include a thickening of the basement membrane of the endothelium, a relative reduction in the endothelial cells, a corresponding increase in the extra-cellular elements, particularly a gross accumulation of amorphous hyalin-like material beneath the endothelium containing collagen-like fibrils ("curly collagen"), and a deficiency of pinocytotic vesicles in the endothelial cells. Electron-microscopic studies have confirmed the presence of these vesicles first remarked by Speakman (1960) in the endothelium of the inner wall of the canal in normal eyes[2] and they have been shown by Fine (1964) to transport ferritin molecules (and presumably aqueous) across the endothelial cytoplasm and, by rupture, to discharge them into the canal (Figs. 420–2). In advanced simple glaucoma these vacuoles have been found to be few or absent (Tripathi, 1968) (Figs. 423–4). This layer of relative impermeability in the trabecular wall of the canal and the absence of endothelial vesicles in this region would appear to be of some significance.

While these changes have been found in cases of advanced simple glaucoma, in the early stages of the disease they may be too subtle to be demonstrated by current techniques, and Kayes (1967), in an electron-microscopic study of the trabecular meshwork of a patient who gave a positive response to topical steroids, found no abnormality in the outflow channels. A further observation of considerable interest is the demonstration of the presence of gamma globulin and of plasma cells in the trabecular meshwork of eyes with simple glaucoma (Becker, 1959; Becker et al., 1963). These observations raise the possibility of an immunological component in the pathogenesis of this disease.

In addition to these various observations on the pathology of the trabecular meshwork, narrowing and obliteration of the intrascleral vessels, originally described by a number of earlier workers,[3] have been subsequently confirmed. The constriction of the venous outlets draining from Schlemm's canal was dramatically shown by subsequent observers, particularly Dvorak-Theobald and Kirk (1956). They found that the collector channels were initially narrowed and eventually obliterated, to be represented only by a line of nuclei, while the episcleral vessels became constricted; these changes were often found in addition to sclerosis of the trabeculæ but were sometimes markedly present when the trabecular changes were minimal. Since these intrascleral veins are merely slits in the sclera lined with a single layer of endothelium which may be preserved on their obliteration, they concluded that their constriction must be due to changes in the surrounding

[1] Bárány and Rohen (1963), Fine (1964), Yamashita and Rosen (1965), Boles Carenini and Orzalesi (1967), Rohen and Straub (1967), Tripathi (1968).
[2] Missotten (1964), Holmberg (1965), Yamashita and Rosen (1965), Kayes (1967), and others.
[3] Birnbacher and Czermak (1886), Elschnig (1896), Heerfordt (1911–12), Hussels (1912), Hanssen (1918), and others.

FIGS. 420 to 422.—SCHLEMM'S CANAL AND THE TRABECULÆ IN THE NORMAL EYE
(R. C. Tripathi.)

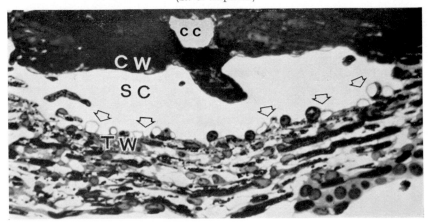

FIG. 420.—In an 80-year-old human eye. CC, collector channels in the corneo-sclera; CW, corneo-scleral wall of Schlemm's canal; SC, lumen of Schlemm's canal; TW, trabecular wall of Schlemm's canal; the arrows point to vacuolated cells lining the wall (× 560).

FIGS. 421 and 422.—Vacuolated cells lining the trabecular wall of Schlemm's canal. Normotensive eye, Rhesus monkey (electronmicrographs, × 18,000).

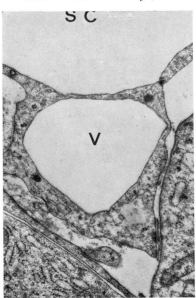

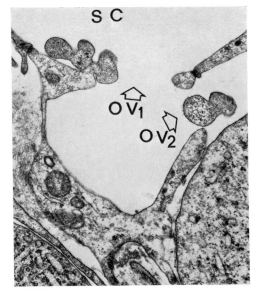

FIG. 421.—SC, lumen of Schlemm's canal; V, a vacuole.

FIG. 422.—OV$_1$, open communication of the vacuole with lumen of Schlemm's canal; OV$_2$, open communication of the vacuole with an open space in the endothelial meshwork.

FIGS. 423 and 424.—SCHLEMM'S CANAL AND THE TRABECULAR MESHWORK
IN A LATE STAGE OF SIMPLE GLAUCOMA (R. C. Tripathi).

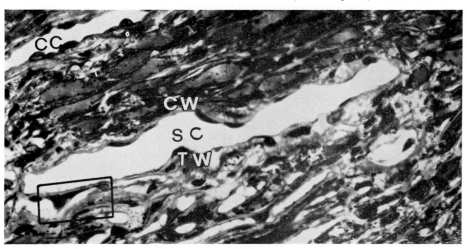

FIG. 423.—In an 82-year-old human eye with simple glaucoma. CC, collector
channels in the corneo-sclera; CW, corneal wall of Schlemm's canal; SC, lumen of
Schlemm's canal; TW, trabecular wall of Schlemm's canal. Note the absence of
vacuoles compared with Fig. 420 (× 560).

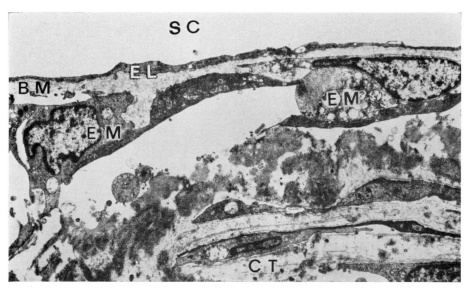

FIG. 424.—Electronmicrograph of the enclosed area in Fig. 423. BM, basement
membrane; CT, corneo-scleral trabeculæ; EL, endothelial cells lining Schlemm's
canal; EM, endothelial meshwork; SC, lumen of Schlemm's canal (× 6,000).

Figs. 425 and 426.—Schlemm's Canal and its Efferent Channels.
Shown by the injection of Indian ink (N. Ashton).

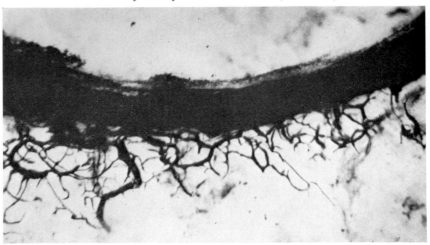

Fig. 425.—The normal eye.

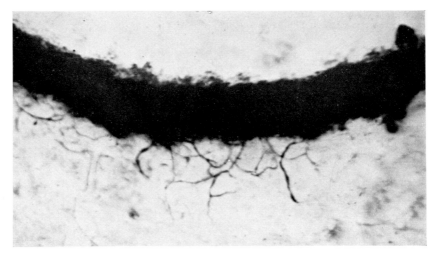

Fig. 426.—An advanced case of simple glaucoma.

tissue, probably resulting from sclerosis and thickening of the scleral collagen such as is seen normally in advanced age. Vannas and Teir (1960), on the other hand, demonstrated mucopolysaccharides in the vicinity of the exit veins and suggested that this substance may have compressed these channels. Whatever the cause—most probably the first—the obliteration of these exit channels was well demonstrated by Ashton (1955–60) in his injection experiments in normal and glaucomatous eyes (Figs. 425–6).

It would seem, therefore, with the somewhat scanty evidence yet available in the study of established cases of the disease that the most likely site of the blockage of drainage is either in the region of the inner (trabecular) wall of the canal of Schlemm or in the exit channels or both. Nevertheless, although there appears to be little doubt that pathological changes of one sort or another can be demonstrated in the outflow channels of eyes in which the disease has become established, it has not yet been determined with certainty that those changes are the cause of the raised tension rather than the result of it.

THE PATHOLOGICAL RESULTS OF INCREASED PRESSURE

In the CORNEA the epithelium almost invariably becomes œdematous in conditions of unrelieved high tension, as in absolute glaucoma, and an

FIGS. 427 and 428.—EPITHELIAL ŒDEMA IN GLAUCOMA (J. H. Parsons).

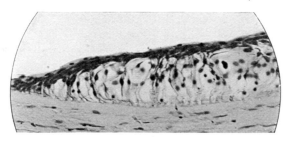

FIG. 427.—The basal cells are elongated, vacuolated, and separated by droplets of fluid. To the left they have completely disappeared, only the flattened superficial cells remaining ($\times$ 200).

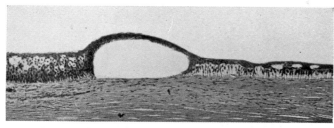

FIG. 428.—Advanced vesicular keratopathy. On the left the middle epithelial cells are elongated and vacuolated. The lamellæ are separated by fluid and Bowman's membrane has disappeared except towards the extreme right which is near the centre of the cornea ($\times$ 66).

intractable bullous keratopathy develops with its ultimate sequel of degenerative glaucomatous pannus (Figs. 427–33). In pigmentary glaucoma the rise of ocular tension may be sufficient to produce an epithelial œdema similar to that seen in primary closed-angle glaucoma. The corneal œdema which may accompany any form of glaucoma is probably the result of endothelial damage (Redslob, 1936; Cogan, 1940–41). Earlier writers had assumed

Figs. 429 to 432.—The Corneal Epithelium in Congenital Glaucoma.
In the rabbit (L. B. Sheppard and W. M. Shanklin).

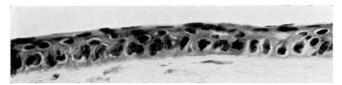

Fig. 429.—The epithelium in the normal rabbit.

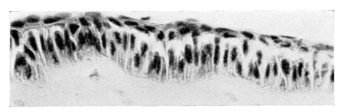

Fig. 430.—Early glaucomatous œdema showing cleavage of the superficial
from the basal cellular layer.

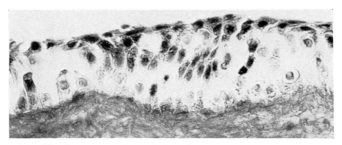

Fig. 431.—Further separation of the cellular layers and increase in the
thickness of the epithelium.

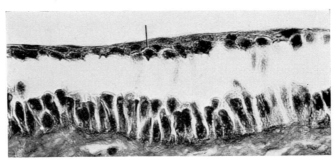

Fig. 432.—Complete detachment of the superficial from the basal cellular
layer. The arrow points to a wing-shaped polygonal cell.

that the phenomenon was due to the mechanical forcing of aqueous into the cornea through the trabeculæ and its traversing Bowman's membrane by way of the nerve-canals (Sgrosso and Antonelli, 1890; Newolina, 1908), or alternatively, was trophic in nature due to the anæsthesia of the corneal nerves (Birnbacher and Czermak, 1886).

Hydration of the cornea becomes abnormal if the endothelium is damaged although the intimate mechanism is unknown since the details of the interaction between the intra-ocular pressure, swelling pressure and the active dehydrating mechanism of the cornea are at present not fully elucidated. It can be readily appreciated, however, that a raised intra-ocular pressure could well outbalance the opposing forces and thus tend to drive more water than usual into the tissues of the cornea.[1]

The process was studied histologically first by von Graefe (1853), Leber (1878), and Fuchs (1881–1902). The œdema appears first as droplets between the basal epithelial cells and then between the polygonal cells, forcing them apart with the formation of vesicles until large bullæ are formed when the entire layer of cells may be elevated from Bowman's membrane and eventually exfoliated. At the same time, degenerative changes in the cells—turgescence, shrinkage, necrosis and vacuolation— are manifold. The corneal stroma itself becomes vacuolated and the interstitial cells degenerate (Courtis, 1933); while the endothelium becomes rarefied and eventually proliferates in places, especially near the angle. On its inner surface there are frequently found cells and pigment from the degenerated iris.

The histology of these progressive œdematous changes in the corneal epithelium has been studied in glaucoma in animals by Rochon-Duvigneaud (1921), Beckh (1935) and Sheppard and Shanklin (1968) (Figs. 429–32). Initially the œdema separates the basal cells from each other and then from the superficial layers of cells which become completely detached, while the basal cells themselves become percolated with fluid, until finally all the epithelium is cast off.

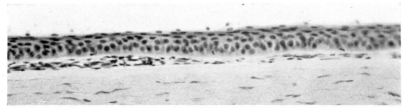

FIG. 433.—GLAUCOMATOUS PANNUS (J. A. C. Wadsworth).

In long-standing cases degenerative changes of a more permanent character appear which are termed *glaucomatous* (or degenerative) *pannus*[2] (Fig. 433). The corneal surface becomes rough and uneven and is frequently

[1] Anseth and Dohlman (1957), Harris (1962), Maurice (1962), Ytteborg and Dohlman (1965).

[2] Baas (1900), Bietti (1908), Gilbert (1909), Fuchs (1916), and others.

broken by the bursting of vesicles. Histologically the essential change is the appearance of connective tissue at first between Bowman's membrane and the degenerated epithelium; this invades the epithelium to form bullæ and encloses islands of epithelial cells in its meshes; it also penetrates inwards, eroding Bowman's membrane and infiltrating the substantia propria. The terminal result may be the formation of an opaque homogeneous mass showing large areas of hyaline and amyloid degeneration.

The entire UVEAL TRACT usually shows an extensive degree of atrophy in chronic glaucoma of any type, either congenital or acquired, wherein there has been a long-standing rise in ocular tension. In clinical cases an obliteration of the choriocapillaris has been demonstrated and a diminution of blood volume has been found by biohæmophotometric techniques (Cristini, 1950;

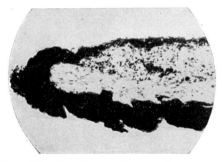

FIG. 434.—THE IRIS IN SIMPLE GLAUCOMA.

Showing general sclerosis with ectropion of the pigment layer and migration of pigment towards the anterior surface (R. Castroviejo).

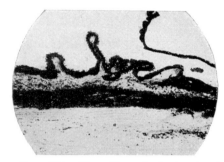

FIG. 435.—The ciliary body in simple glaucoma. Showing marked atrophy (R. Castroviejo).

Cristini *et al.*, 1962). This obliteration of the capillary circulation was demonstrated by François and Neetens (1964) using micro-angiography and was dramatically duplicated by Kalvin and his associates (1966) in their experiments[1] on producing high tension in the eyes of monkeys[1] (Figs. 562–9).

In advanced cases the changes become more pronounced. In these the iris is uniformly thinned and atrophic, vascular sclerosis is usually marked and retraction of the tissue results in ectropion of the pigment layer which may sometimes be extreme (Knies, 1876; Birnbacher and Czermak, 1886; Licskó, 1923) (Figs. 434–5); occasionally entropion results from shrinkage of connective tissue on the posterior surface of the iris (Dvorak-Theobald, 1959). The stromal melanocytes become rounded and gradually disappear, and the epithelial pigmentary cells disintegrate, liberating their pigment which is scattered over the surface of the iris, powdering the corneal endothelium and collecting in the angle of the anterior chamber. The muscular

[1] p. 628.

tissue disappears, the stroma becomes rarefied, and eventually advanced degeneration and atrophy result in the appearance of dehiscences and the formation of a tissue comprised of little more than fibroblasts. As a rule this process is widespread, but small spots of intense atrophy may occur in the stroma and defects in the pigment epithelium may show a patchy distribution, while the process may be evident only in large isolated plaques resulting in a picture resembling iridoschisis. Similarly the ciliary processes retract and shrink, the muscular tissue atrophying and being replaced by fibrous tissue so that the entire ciliary body becomes flattened. The non-pigmented epithelium atrophies and the cells of the pigmentary epithelium

FIGS. 436 to 438.—RETINAL DEGENERATION IN SIMPLE GLAUCOMA.

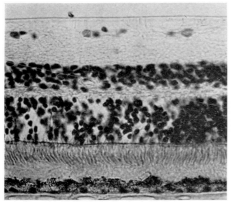

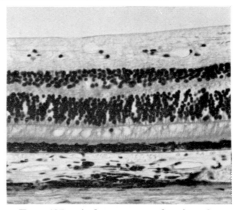

FIG. 436.—The ganglion cells are beginning to disappear. They are reduced in number and some are pyknotic (J. A. C. Wadsworth).

FIG. 437.—A later stage showing fewer ganglion cells and fewer elements in the inner nuclear layer (N. Ashton).

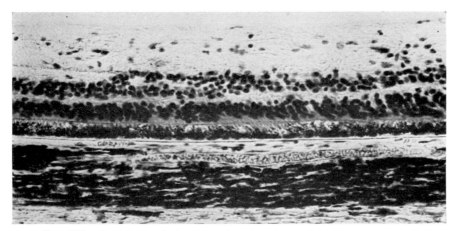

FIG. 438.—An advanced stage showing almost complete disappearance of the ganglion cells, disruption of the inner nuclear layer and diminution of the outer nuclear layer (N. Ashton).

disintegrate, scattering their melanin granules. The choroid also atrophies and may become so thin that histologically it is represented by little more than a pigmented line.

One feature of the whole uveal tract is the appearance around the capillaries and veins of concentric deposits of albuminous and fibrinous exudates which may undergo hyalinization, and of a perivascular infiltration.

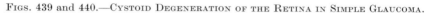

Figs. 439 and 440.—Cystoid Degeneration of the Retina in Simple Glaucoma.

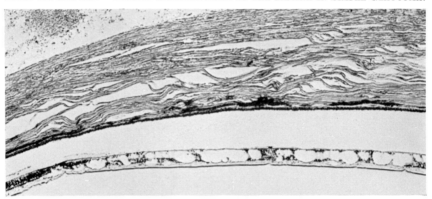

Fig. 439.—In the region of the ora serrata (J. A. C. Wadsworth).

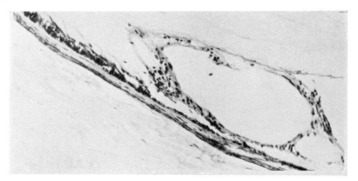

Fig. 440.—At the junction of the retina and the ciliary epithelium (F. Vrabec).

A striking feature of routine histological preparations of chronic glaucomatous eyes in the final stages of the disease is the frequent occurrence of uveal angiosclerosis and atrophy, these changes being particularly common in the posterior choroid and in the shrunken hyalinized ciliary body (Ashton, 1955).

The RETINA shows degenerative changes as soon as hypertension becomes established. The first evidences are seen in the ganglion cells, which become vacuolated, atrophic and finally disappear (Figs. 436–8); the plexiform layers then degenerate allowing the nuclear layers to fuse, a change followed by the

FIGS. 441 to 445.—GLIOSIS IN SIMPLE GLAUCOMA (J. R. Wolter).

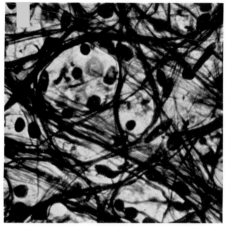

FIG. 441.—Proliferated astroglia in the ganglion cell layer.

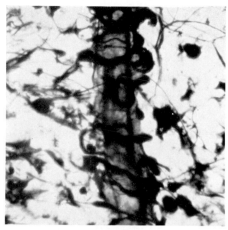

FIG. 442.—Hypertrophic perivascular glia around a retinal capillary.

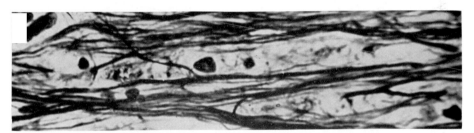

FIG. 443—Proliferated lemmocytes in the nerve-fibre layer.

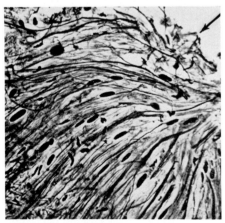

FIG. 444.—New-formed glial cells on the inner limiting membrane of the retina at the margin of the optic disc (arrowed).

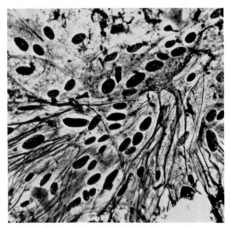

FIG. 445.—A new-formed layer of glia in the inner part of the retina.

appearance of cystoid degeneration[1] first at the macula, plentifully at the ora serrata and eventually indiscriminately[2] (Figs. 439–40). The arcuate nerve-fibre layer also shows degenerative changes at an early stage, due to a combination of the increased ocular tension and the poor blood supply so that this layer is eventually replaced by connective tissue and glial cells (Dvorak-Theobald, 1959); indeed, the hypertrophy of the glial tissue throughout the retina may become very marked (Figs. 441–5) (Wolter, 1959; Ikui et al., 1967). The rods and cones become matted together and lie flattened almost parallel to the surface (Berenstein, 1900; von Hippel, 1901), while the vessels show advanced sclerosis and hyaline degeneration

FIGS. 446 and 447.—THE RETINA IN ABSOLUTE GLAUCOMA.

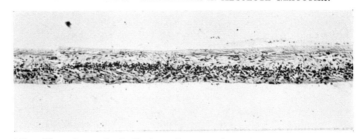

FIG. 446.—There is marked gliosis and a complete absence of ganglion cells as well as of visual elements (J. A. C. Wadsworth).

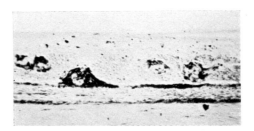

FIG. 447.—Showing complete atrophy of the neural tissues and the migration of pigment into the retina (M. L. Hepburn).

(Gilbert, 1915–19; Hanssen, 1918; and others) (Fig. 446). The pigmentary epithelium remains unchanged for a considerable time, but eventually also undergoes degenerative changes, the pigment migrating into the retina; defects appear, among which the most obvious is around the optic disc forming the *circumpapillary glaucomatous halo*, which to a certain extent resembles the circumpapillary atrophy of senile eyes (Elschnig, 1928) (Fig. 447). In the stage of absolute glaucoma micro-aneurysms are abundant in the retinal vessels (Unger and Jankovsky, 1967) (Figs. 448–50).

The retinal changes resulting from an acutely high tension were well

[1] Vol. X, p. 543.
[2] Schreiber (1906), Hanssen (1918), Verhoeff (1925), Castroviejo (1931).

FIGS. 448 to 450.—CAPILLARY ANEURYSMS IN GLAUCOMA.
(H.-H. Unger and F. Jankovsky.)

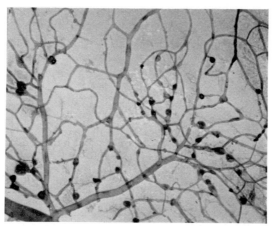

FIG. 448.

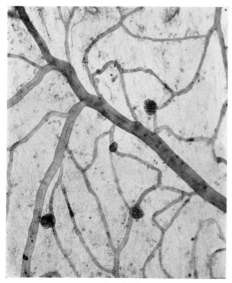

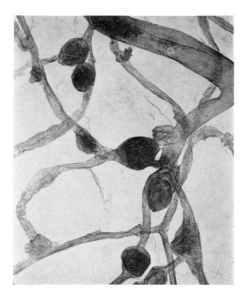

FIG. 449.   FIG. 450.

demonstrated by Kalvin and his associates (1966) in their experiments on monkeys (Fig. 564); the ganglion cells are seen to disappear at an early stage and the disintegration of the rods and cones is dramatic.

The response of the SCLERA to an increased ocular tension depends to some extent upon the age of the patient. We have already seen that in the eyes of infants the sclera readily and uniformly stretches under the influence of hypertension so that a buphthalmic globe is produced; in the fully developed eye, however, an ectasia is a late result, is only partial, and is probably largely due to ischæmic degeneration. It used to be thought that the sclera was excessively rigid in glaucomatous eyes, but as we have already seen[1] there is little convincing evidence that this is so. Investigations into the influence of age on the ocular rigidity[2] have also given conflicting results and it is probably true to say that it varies little in this respect. The *staphylomata* which may appear in the later stages of absolute glaucoma are first small and localized, but under the influence of continued pressure eventually become confluent and even annular. Two main types occur, ciliary staphylomata and intercalary staphylomata[3] (Birnbacher and

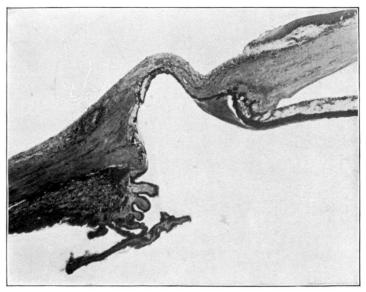

Fig. 451.—Intercalary Staphyloma in Absolute Glaucoma (J. H. Parsons).

Czermak, 1886) (Fig. 451). In the former the sclera covering the ciliary region becomes stretched, and the thinned-out ciliary body lines the inner surface of the bulge; in the latter the sclera anterior to the ciliary body suffers distension and the iris appears to become separated from the ciliary body. This is due to the fact that in the cases of long-standing glaucoma wherein it occurs, peripheral synechiæ bind the root of the iris to the part of the sclera which has become ectatic, so that the staphyloma is coated on the inside with a pigmented layer representing the atrophic remnants of the adherent iris, while the free part of the iris lies anterior to it. As extensive peripheral synechiæ are necessary for the development of an intercalary staphyloma, this condition is more commonly seen in long-standing closed-angle rather than in simple glaucoma. Equatorial staphylomata are rare,

[1] Vol. IV, p. 263.   [2] Vol. IV, p. 274.   [3] Vol. VIII, p. 999.

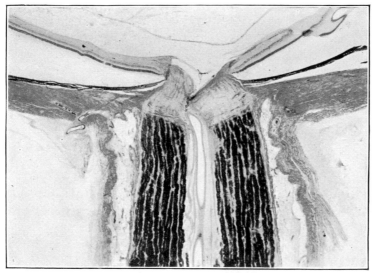

FIG. 452.—THE NORMAL OPTIC NERVE (Weigert's stain) (J. H. Parsons).

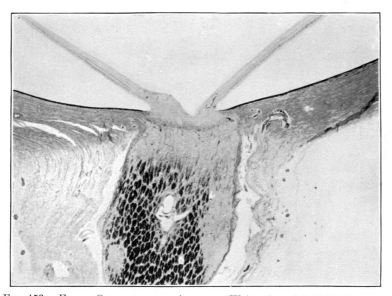

FIG. 453.—EARLY GLAUCOMATOUS ATROPHY (Weigert's stain) (J. H. Parsons).

and usually develop in the neighbourhood of a vortex vein; all of them show histologically an extremely attenuated sclera which forms a thin membrane on the inner surface of which the stretched and atrophied uvea is recognizable only as a pigmented line. A spontaneous rupture is a pathological curiosity (Stölting, 1888; Knape, 1910; Meller, 1918).

A dilatation of the anterior ciliary arteries has been described as an almost constant finding in simple glaucoma when the ocular tension was above 60 mm. (Dobree, 1954). The perforating branches of the arteries are particularly involved and, after reduction of the ocular tension, the dilatation takes at least some days to regress. The episcleral veins show little change in advanced simple glaucoma, but in absolute glaucoma they are frequently greatly distended. The arterial dilatation seems to be a compensatory change consequent upon the raised tension, while the venous dilatation probably indicates that much of the blood destined for the interior of the globe has been short-circuited into the superficial veins.

The OPTIC NERVE shows pathological changes so constantly in established simple glaucoma that the *cupped appearance of the disc* is one of the primary diagnostic features of the disease. The changes were first described

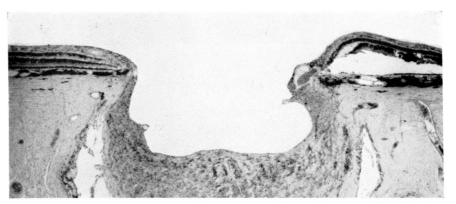

FIG. 454.—CUPPING OF THE OPTIC NERVE-HEAD IN SIMPLE GLAUCOMA (N. Ashton).

by H. Müller (1856–58) and comprise two essential features—an atrophy of the nerve fibres and an ectasia of the disc (Figs. 452–4). The atrophy of the nerve fibres commences at an early stage, is most marked at first on the temporal side, but ultimately involves the entire nerve, the neural tissue being replaced by glia (Wolter, 1957) (Fig. 455). In their experiments producing acute glaucoma in monkeys[1] Lampert and his colleagues (1968) found that the sequence was, first, a hydropic swelling and degeneration of the axons, followed after some days by a cystic transformation of the necrotic tissue causing its dissolution in focal areas, the degenerated axons and debris being removed by phagocytes some of which were hæmatogenous macrocytes. The ectasia starts with the formation of a concavity by the lamina cribrosa, so that the scleral ring forms the lateral edge of the cup and eventually constitutes a prominent overhanging lip jutting out over the excavated nerve-head. As a general rule the cup is empty and is occupied by

[1] p. 628.

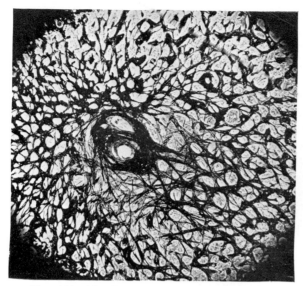

FIG. 455.—THE LAMINA CRIBROSA IN GLAUCOMA.

In a case of advanced secondary glaucoma, showing the extreme hypertrophy
of the connective tissue with atrophy of the nerve fibres (J. R. Wolter).

vitreous; but sometimes its surface is covered with proliferated neuroglial
tissue, which in exceptional cases may even fill it and project into the
vitreous cavity (Römer, 1901; Behr, 1914). An important exception to this
general configuration may be seen in myopic eyes; in these the cupping

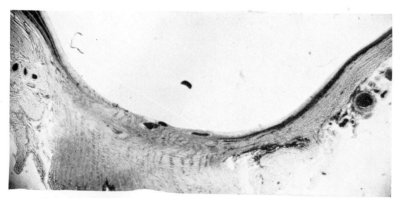

FIG. 456.—GLAUCOMATOUS CUPPING IN A HIGHLY MYOPIC EYE.
(R. K. Blach and B. Jay.)

may be gradual with sloping edges without any overhanging lip, giving the
appearance that the optic disc has partaken in the posterior staphyloma
(Blach and Jay, 1965) (Fig. 456).

Originally it was generally accepted that the ectasia of the optic disc was a *mechanical pressure-effect* by which a hernia was produced at the weakest spot in the ocular coats, while the atrophy of the nerve fibres was also regarded as a secondary result of pressure, partly due to degeneration of the ganglion cells and partly owing to a combination of the effects of pressure and stretching as the fibres pass over the rim and sides of the cup at the nerve-head.[1] That this mechanical influence undoubtedly plays a part is seen in the fact that an excavation can be produced in the dead eye by raising the intra-ocular pressure (Laker, 1886; Birnbacher and Czermak, 1886) or, conversely, by suddenly decreasing the intracranial pressure (Szymánski and Wladyczko, 1925). Fuchs (1911–16) explained the differences in the appearance and depth of various cups, particularly those in the formation of which a rise in pressure has been slight, by variations in the anatomical configuration of the supporting tissue of the nerve-head; the lamina itself may be far forward or far back, while in some eyes the supporting tissue is made up essentially of strong transversely running laminæ, and in others of frailer bundles of glial tissue running longitudinally. From histological studies he concluded that the sequence of events was first a disappearance of the delicate anterior glial fibres and then of the deeper fibres incorporated in the lamina; this was followed by the bending backward of the connective tissue lamellæ which at first became sclerosed and then thinner and atrophic and eventually broken up, sometimes with the formation of spaces, under the influence of continued pressure. While the supporting framework of the intra-ocular portion of the nerve was undergoing these changes, pressure-atrophy began to be apparent in the nerve fibres. He suggested that this may occur extensively at an early stage when only the anterior glial fibres have disappeared and the connective tissue lamina is still in a normal position, producing the clinical appearance of an increased physiological cup with atrophy. On the other hand, when the lamina is weak it may yield while the nerve fibres are still intact, producing a deep cup associated with little defect in the visual field, and in extreme cases it may yield to a normal intra-ocular pressure.

Schnabel (1892–1908), however, put forward the opposite view, claiming that *the primary process is a neuritic atrophy*, the degeneration of the nerve fibres leading to the formation of small empty spaces which finally coalesce (CAVERNOUS DEGENERATION) (Figs. 457–8); he claimed that these lacunæ appear at a very early stage before any excavation of the disc is visible. At the same time, a proliferation of the interstitial connective tissue occurs which becomes vascularized and then contracts, so that the lamina is not pushed back by the intra-ocular pressure but is pulled back by the shrinking connective tissue of the atrophic nerve. He pointed out that the cavernous degeneration is very apparent in the region of the lamina, where by the coalescence of clefts the lamina itself is exposed, and eventually a single

[1] Müller (*1856*), Birnbacher and Czermak (1886), Stock (1908–27), Fuchs (1916), Kapuściński (*1930*), and others.

large cavern results in this situation—the glaucomatous excavation. His views were to a large extent supported by many observers,[1] and the occurrence of atrophy some considerable distance in the extra-ocular portion of the nerve would seem to indicate the action of some factor other than the intra-ocular pressure. Elschnig (1928) claimed that glaucomatous atrophy differed from other forms by the reduction in the capillary circulation, an ischæmic condition seen in the lessening and eventual absence of fluorescence over the surface of the optic disc on fluorescein angiography (Figs. 473–475) and confirmed histologically by Cristini (1950–51) (Figs. 459–62)

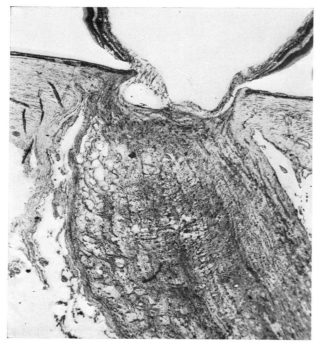

Fig. 457.—Cavernous Optic Atrophy in Simple Glaucoma (N. Ashton).

after staining with benzidine, by François and Neetens (1964–66) by microangiography, and in monkeys with experimental acute glaucoma by Kalvin and his associates (1966) (Fig. 568). Moreover, it must be remembered that cavernous changes are by no means specific for glaucoma, and when they occur in the presence of a normal ocular tension and a normal facility of aqueous outflow, it is now believed that they are generally due to sclerotic vascular disease within the optic nerve and should therefore be termed *ischæmic optic neuropathy*.[2]

[1] Elschnig (1895–1928), Hummelsheim and Leber (1901), Schnaudigel (1904), Evans (1939), Wolff (1947), and others.
[2] Vol. XII.

Lagrange and Beauvieux (1925), indeed, considered that the changes in the nerve were secondary to vascular changes which were themselves secondary to pressure. They found that the cup terminated in a deep conical projection penetrating backwards alongside the vessels, a process which caused vascular obliteration and sclerosis and resulted in neuro-retinal atrophy. The blood supply to the lamina and the anterior part of the optic nerve is derived from anastomosing branches between the central

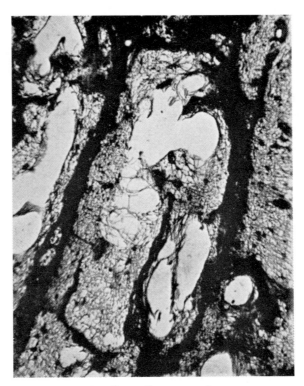

FIG. 458.—GROSS CAVERNOUS ATROPHY.
In a case of secondary glaucoma. The cavernous spaces have run together
to form large cavities (E. Wolff).

artery of the retina—or the central artery of the optic nerve if it is present —and the circle of Zinn (François and Neetens, 1954; Hayreh, 1963). It has been argued that the ocular tension can influence the blood vessels within the eye but not those behind the lamina or outside the optic nerve, so that an increased ocular tension can result in the shunting of blood away from the optic nerve-head, leading to degeneration of the glial supporting tissue and the neurons (Gafner and Goldmann, 1955; Goldmann, 1956–59; Nordmann, 1960; Becker and Shaffer, 1965). This theory is supported by the observation that in patients with systemic hypertension

FIGS. 459 to 462.—THE OPTIC NERVE IN SIMPLE GLAUCOMA (G. Cristini).

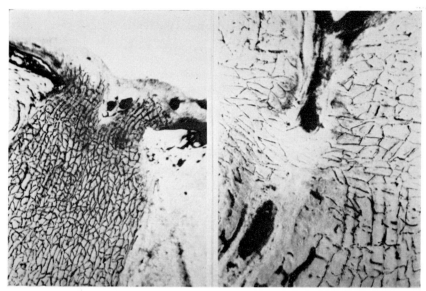

FIG. 459.   FIG. 460.

FIG. 459.—The capillary network in the normal optic nerve (benzidine method).

FIG. 460.—Magnification of the capillary network in the region of the lamina in the normal eye.

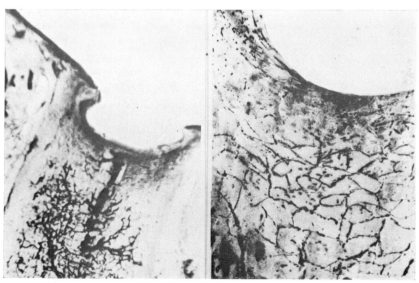

FIG. 461.   FIG. 462.

FIG. 461.—A reduction in the number of capillaries in simple glaucoma.

FIG. 462.—The fragmentary capillary network in simple glaucoma. Compare Figs. 562–9.)

and simple glaucoma, a lowering of the blood pressure can result in a rapid deterioration of the visual fields (McLean, 1957; Harrington, 1959; Lobstein *et al.*, 1960; and others). On the other hand, some investigators believe that the changes in the optic nerve-head result from vascular lesions within the nerve and that a raised ocular tension, when present, is an incidental occurrence (Magitot, 1947–53; Marquez, 1947; Cristini, 1947–50; Redslob, 1955; and others); while others, including Duke-Elder (1949–62), consider that the vascular system is the essential site of the pathology, and that changes in the nerve, and therefore in the visual field, depend on a relative vascular insufficiency which varies as the ratio between the intra-ocular pressure and the capillary pressure. We have just seen that the evidence is strong that glaucomatous atrophy is associated with an obliteration of the capillary bed in the optic nerve; but the fact that this effect is seen in experimental glaucoma as induced in monkeys by Kalvin and his associates (1966), Hamasaki and Fujino (1967) and Zimmerman and his co-workers (1967) suggests that it may follow as a result of ischæmic necrosis associated with a high pressure. One peculiar difference, however, exists between the picture seen after an occlusive infarct and that evident in acute glaucoma experimentally produced in monkeys (Zimmerman *et al.*, 1967; Lampert *et al.*, 1968): in an ischæmic infarct there is a macrophagic and glial reaction and the cavernous spaces contain no hyaluronic acid, while in acute glaucoma the microglial and astrocytic response is negligible and the cavernous spaces contain hyaluronic acid. These observers therefore suggested that cavernous degeneration seen in acute glaucoma was a special type of infarct resulting from ischæmia of the nerve into the necrotic tissues of which hyaluronic acid was forced by pressure from the vitreous. It is interesting that Teng (1964) postulated that glaucomatous cupping is mainly the result of loss of tissue due to the degenerative effect of the vitreous on the nerve fibres and collagen, but it would seem probable that the increased intra-ocular pressure and the vascular obstruction play the primary role.

These changes in the optic nerve, particularly when associated with the histological picture of cavernous atrophy, bear some resemblance to lacunar atrophy of the cerebral cortex, a disease affecting the same type of patient who suffers from simple glaucoma and due to insufficiency of the cerebral circulation. This similarity was pointed out by Morax (1916), Magitot (1929), Marchesani (1935), Redslob (1941), and particularly by Sjøgren (1946) who found similar changes in the optic nerve and cortex in the same patients, some of whom would be classed as " glaucoma without hypertension "; Cavka (1955–56) made similar confirmatory observations.

It appears, therefore, from our present knowledge, that a raised ocular tension causes or is associated with vascular changes in the optic nerve leading to a condition of localized ischæmia, and that any coincidental vascular sclerosis within the nerve intensifies this damage. Changes within the nerve-head consequent upon vascular insufficiency, without a raised ocular tension at any time and without a reduced coefficient of aqueous outflow, should not be considered as due to glaucoma but to ischæmic vascular disease.

Anseth and Dohlman. *Acta ophthal.* (Kbh.), **35**, 85 (1957).

Ashton. *Glaucoma: a Symposium* (ed. Duke-Elder), Oxon. (1955).
Glaucoma (IV Macy Fdn. Conf., ed. Newell), N.Y., 89 (1959).
Proc. roy. Soc. Med., **52**, 69 (1959).
Trans. ophthal. Soc. U.K., **80**, 397 (1960).

Baas. *Klin. Mbl. Augenheilk.*, **38**, 417 (1900).

Bárány and Rohen. *Arch. Ophthal.*, **69**, 630 (1963).

Barkan. *Amer. J. Ophthal.*, **21**, 1099 (1938); **24**, 768 (1941); **37**, 724 (1954).

Becker. *Glaucoma* (IV Macy Fdn. Conf., ed. Newell), N.Y., 223 (1959).

Becker and Shaffer. *Diagnosis and Therapy of the Glaucomas*, 2nd ed., St. Louis (1965).

Becker, Unger, Coleman and Keates. *Arch. Ophthal.*, **70**, 38 (1963).

Beckh. *Amer. J. Ophthal.*, **18**, 1144 (1935).

Behr. *Klin. Mbl. Augenheilk.*, **52**, 790 (1914).

Berenstein. *v. Graefes Arch. Ophthal.*, **51**, 186 (1900).

Bietti. *Klin. Mbl. Augenheilk.*, **46** (1), 337 (1908).

Birnbacher and Czermak. *v. Graefes Arch. Ophthal.*, **32** (2), 1; (4), 1 (1886).

Blach and Jay. *Trans. ophthal. Soc. U.K.*, **85**, 161 (1965).

Boles Carenini and Orzalesi. *Boll. Oculist.*, **46**, 653 (1967).

Brailey. *Roy. Lond. ophthal. Hosp. Rep.*, **10**, 10 (1880).

Castroviejo. *Arch. Ophthal.*, **5**, 189 (1931).

Cavka. *Ber. dtsch. ophthal. Ges.*, **59**, 112 (1955).
Ophthalmologica, **132**, 76 (1956).
Arch. Ophtal., **16**, 507 (1956).

Cogan. *Arch. Ophthal.*, **23**, 918 (1940); **25**, 552, 941 (1941).

Courtis. *Arch. Oftal. B. Aires*, **8**, 399 (1933).

Cristini. *Ann. Oculist.* (Paris), **180**, 530 (1947).
Acta XVI int. Cong. Ophthal., London, **2**, 865 (1950).
Brit. J. Ophthal., **35**, 11 (1951).

Cristini, Forlani and Scardovi. *Brit. J. Ophthal.*, **46**, 99 (1962).

Dobree. *Brit. J. Ophthal.*, **38**, 500 (1954); **40**, 1 (1956).

Duke-Elder. *Arch. Ophthal.*, **42**, 538 (1949).
Amer. J. Ophthal., **33**, 11 (1950).
Ulster med. J., **22**, 3 (1953).
Canad. med. Ass. J., **82**, 293 (1960).
Trans. ophthal. Soc. U.K., **82**, 307 (1962).

Dvorak-Theobald. *Symposium on Glaucoma* (ed. Clark), St. Louis, 26 (1959).

Dvorak-Theobald and Kirk. *Amer. J. Ophthal.*, **41**, 11 (1956).

Elschnig. *Ber. dtsch. ophthal. Ges.*, **24** 149 (1895).
Arch. Augenheilk., **33**, Erg., 187 (1896).
Henke-Lubarsch *Hb. d. spez. path. Anat. u. Histol.*, Berlin, **11** (1), 873 (1928).

Evans. *Brit. J. Ophthal.*, **23**, 745 (1939).

Fine. *Invest. Ophthal.*, **3**, 609 (1964).

Flocks. *Trans. Amer. Acad. Ophthal.*, **62**, 556 (1958).

François. *Glaucoma: a Symposium* (ed. Duke-Elder), Oxon., 169 (1955).

François and Neetens. *Brit. J. Ophthal.*, **38**, 472 (1954).
Arch. Ophthal., **71**, 219 (1964).
Increased intra-ocular pressure and optic nerve atrophy, Brussels (1966).

Fuchs. *v. Graefes Arch. Ophthal.*, **27** (3), 66 (1881); **91**, 435; **92**, 145, 197 (1916).
Trans. ophthal. Soc. U.K., **22**, 15 (1902).
Z. Augenheilk., **25**, 108 (1911).

Gafner and Goldmann. *Ophthalmologica*, **130**, 357 (1955).

Garron. *Glaucoma* (IV Macy Fdn. Conf., ed. Newell), N.Y., 11, 231 (1959).

Gilbert. *v. Graefes Arch. Ophthal.*, **69**, 1 (1909); **82**, 389 (1912); **90**, 76 (1915).
Arch. Augenheilk., **85**, 74 (1919).

Goldmann. *Triangle*, **2**, 274 (1956).
Amer. J. Ophthal., **48** (2), 213 (1959).

von Graefe. *v. Graefes Arch. Ophthal.*, **2** (1), 206 (1853).

Hamasaki and Fujino. *Arch. Ophthal.*, **78**, 369 (1967).

Hanssen. *Klin. Mbl. Augenheilk.*, **61**, 509 (1918).

Harrington. *Amer. J. Ophthal.*, **47** (2), 177 (1959).

Harris. *Invest. Ophthal.*, **1**, 151 (1962).

Hayreh. *Brit. J. Ophthal.*, **47**, 651 (1963).

Heerfordt. *v. Graefes Arch. Ophthal.*, **78**, 413 (1911); **83**, 149 (1912).

Henderson. *Glaucoma*, London (1910).

von Hippel. *v. Graefes Arch. Ophthal.*, **52**, 498 (1901); **74**, 101 (1910).

Holmberg. *Docum. ophthal.*, **19**, 339 (1965).

Hummelsheim and Leber. *v. Graefes Arch. Ophthal.*, **52**, 336 (1901).

Hussels. *Z. Augenheilk.*, **27**, 213, 354 (1912).

Ikui, Uga and Nakao. *Folia ophthal. jap.*, **18**, 898 (1967).

Kalvin, Hamasaki and Gass. *Arch. Ophthal.*, **76**, 82, 94 (1966).

Kapuściński. *Arch. Ophtal.*, **47**, 779 (1930).

Kayes. *Invest. Ophthal.*, **6**, 381 (1967).

Knape. *Finska Läk. Sällsk. Handl.*, **52** (2), 547 (1910).

Knies. *v. Graefes Arch. Ophthal.*, **22** (3), 163 (1876); **23** (2), 62 (1877).

Kornzweig. *Ophthal. ibero-amer.*, **19**, 290 (1957).

Kornzweig, Feldstein and Schneider. *Amer. J. Ophthal.*, **46**, 311 (1958).

Lagrange and Beauvieux. *Arch. Ophtal.*, **42**, 129 (1925).

Laker. *Klin. Mbl. Augenheilk.*, **24**, 187 (1886).

Lampert, Vogel and Zimmerman. *Invest. Ophthal.*, **7**, 199 (1968).

Leber. *v. Graefes Arch. Ophthal.*, **24** (1), 252 (1878).

Levinsohn. *Arch. Augenheilk.*, **62**, 131 (1909).
Z. Augenheilk., **40**, 344 (1918).
Klin. Mbl. Augenheilk., **61**, 174 (1918); **68**, 471 (1922).

Licskó. *Klin. Mbl. Augenheilk.*, **71**, 456 (1923).

Lobstein, Bronner and Nordmann. *Ophthalmologica*, **139**, 271 (1960).

McLean. *Amer. J. Ophthal.*, **44**, 323 (1957).

Maggiore. *Ann. Ottal.*, **46**, 317 (1917).

Magitot. *Ann. Oculist.* (Paris), **166**, 356, 439, 565, 609 (1929); **180**, 1, 321 (1947); **186**, 385 (1953).

Marchesani. *Klin. Mbl. Augenheilk.*, **95**, 389 (1935).

Marquez. *Ophthal. ibero-amer.*, **9**, 123 (1947).

Maurice. *Int. Ophthal. Clin.*, **2** (3), 561 (1962).

Meller. *Klin. Mbl. Augenheilk.*, **60**, 458 (1918).

Missotten. *Bull. Soc. belge Ophtal.*, No. 136 (1), 5 (1964).

Morax. *Ann. Oculist.* (Paris), **153**, 25 (1916).

Müller, H. (1856). See *Gesammelte u. hinterlassene Schriften zur Anatomie u. Physiologie d. Auges*, Leipzig, **1**, 340 (1872).
v. Graefes Arch. Ophthal., **4** (2), 1 (1858).

Newolina. *Klin. Mbl. Augenheilk.*, **46** (2), 360 (1908).

Nordmann. *Ann. Oculist.* (Paris), **193**, 17 (1960).

Redslob. *Bull. Soc. franç. Ophtal.*, **49**, 145 (1936).
Ann. Oculist. (Paris), **177**, 323 (1941); **188**, 781 (1955).

Reese. *Amer. J. Ophthal.*, **27**, 1193 (1944).

Rochon-Duvigneaud. *Ann. Oculist.* (Paris), **158**, 401 (1921).

Römer. *v. Graefes Arch. Ophthal.*, **52**, 514 (1901).

Rønne. *Klin. Mbl. Augenheilk.*, **51** (2), 505 (1913).

Rohen and Straub. *v. Graefes Arch. Ophthal.*, **173**, 21 (1967).

Rohen and Unger. *Amer. J. Ophthal.*, **46**, 802 (1958).

Schieck. *Klin. Mbl. Augenheilk.*, **61**, 332 (1918).

Schnabel. *Arch. Augenheilk.*, **24**, 273 (1892).
Z. Augenheilk., **14**, 1 (1905); **19**, 556 (1908).

Schnaudigel. *v. Graefes Arch. Ophthal.*, **59**, 344 (1904).

Schreiber. *v. Graefes Arch. Ophthal.*, **64**, 237 (1906).

Sgrosso and Antonelli. *Ann. Ottal.*, **19**, 166 (1890).

Sheppard and Shanklin. *Amer. J. Ophthal.*, **65**, 406 (1968).

Sjøgren. *Acta ophthal.* (Kbh.), **24**, 239 (1946).

Smith, Priestley. *Roy. Lond. ophthal. Hosp. Rep.*, **10**, 25 (1880).
Glaucoma, London (1879; 1891).

Speakman. *Canad. med. Ass. J.*, **84**, 1066 (1961).
Brit. J. Ophthal., **44**, 513 (1960); **46**, 31 (1962).

Speakman and Leeson. *Brit. J. Ophthal.*, **46**, 321 (1962).

Stock. *Klin. Mbl. Augenheilk.*, **46** (1), 342 (1908); **78**, Beil., 61 (1927).

Stölting. *v. Graefes Arch. Ophthal.*, **34** (2), 135 (1888).

Sugar. *The Glaucomas*, N.Y. (1951).

Szymánski and Wladyczko. *Klin. oczna*, **3**, 145 (1925).

Teng. *Amer. J. Ophthal.*, **58**, 181, 379 (1964).

Teng, Katzin and Chi. *Amer. J. Ophthal.*, **43**, 193 (1957).

Teng, Paton and Katzin. *Amer. J. Ophthal.*, **40**, 619 (1955).

Tripathi. *Exp. Eye Res.*, **7**, 335 (1968).

Unger and Jankovsky. *v. Graefes Arch. Ophthal.*, **173**, 323 (1967).

Unger and Rohen. *Amer. J. Ophthal.*, **50**, 37 (1960).

Vannas and Teir. *Amer. J. Ophthal.*, **49**, 411 (1960).

Verhoeff. *Arch. Ophthal.*, **44**, 129 (1915); **54**, 20 (1925).

Weber. *v. Graefes Arch. Ophthal.*, **23** (1), 1 (1877).

Wolff. *Trans. ophthal. Soc. U.K.*, **67**, 133 (1947).

Wolter. *Amer. J. Ophthal.*, **44** (2), 48 (1957); **48** (2), 370 (1959); **49**, 1089 (1960).
Arch. Ophthal., **62**, 99 (1959); **69**, 595 (1963).

Wolter, Pfister and Fechner. *Brit. J. Ophthal.*, **47**, 1 (1963).

Yamashita and Rosen. *Amer. J. Ophthal.*, **60**, 427 (1965).

Ytteborg and Dohlman. *Arch. Ophthal.*, **74**, 375, 477 (1965).

Zimmerman, de Venecia and Hamasaki. *Invest. Ophthal.*, **6**, 109 (1967).

Clinical Features

SIMPLE GLAUCOMA varies little in its clinical manifestations in different patients, as a rule developing slowly, quietly and insidiously, and may indeed have arrived at a far advanced stage in both eyes before anything amiss is noticed by the patient in the appearance of the eye, in subjective symptoms of pain and discomfort, or in apparent functional efficiency. Signs of congestion are completely absent and the eye is white, unless the ocular tension is very high when the anterior ciliary vessels may be dilated. The anterior chamber may be deep or shallow and its angle is almost always open, unless peripheral anterior synechiæ have formed following surgery or as a result of the development of absolute glaucoma when they are seldom extensive or unless a hæmorrhagic glaucoma supervenes. The iris is occasionally atrophic, particularly in the so-called pigmentary glaucoma.[1] Sooner or later the disc tends to become cupped and atrophic, while the ocular tension is almost always found to be above normal. Meantime, although the central vision may remain good until a late stage, a shrinkage of the peripheral field develops or paracentral scotomata become annoying. Apart, however, from a vague feeling of fullness or headache, a slight increase in presbyopia and a loss of rapid adaptation to dim illumination, the patient may be little inconvenienced.

The initial symptoms of simple glaucoma as encountered in the Glaucoma Clinic at the Institute of Ophthalmology in London are seen in Table III; unfortunately, most of them are not experienced until the disease is well established.

TABLE III

EARLY SYMPTOMS OF SIMPLE GLAUCOMA (in percentages)

Blurred vision—permanent . . .	44
Difficulty in reading	20
Scotoma	13
Eye-ache	13
No symptoms	10

As the disease progresses, the choroid may show evidences of depigmentation, particularly around the disc where a non-pigmented ring, the *circumpapillary glaucomatous halo*, forms and the excavation and atrophy of the nerve-head increase. The shrinkage of the visual field may now cause considerable embarrassment and the patient walks hesitatingly, turning his head repeatedly from side to side, fumbling for objects and stumbling over obstacles in his path. A gradual progression of all these symptoms occurs, usually exceedingly slowly over a period of many years, until eventually, and usually not without the intervention of headache and pain, the eye becomes intensely hard, all vision is lost and a state of absolute glaucoma is reached.

p. 486.

The condition of ABSOLUTE GLAUCOMA from every point of view is quite without hope. The sclera is porcelain-white and on it the anterior ciliary vessels, dilated and varicose, show up vividly by contrast in an irregular anastomotic circle; the cornea is insensitive; the anterior chamber is deep or shallow and its angle may occasionally be occluded by peripheral anterior synechiæ; the pupil is widely dilated and immobile; the iris, bounded by a dark rim of pigmented epithelium, has receded almost behind the scleral rim and has become depigmented and assumed the slate-grey appearance of advanced atrophy; the fundus has become markedly tesselated, and the dead-white disc shows a deep excavation with a prominent overhanging edge; and vision is permanently and completely lost. Unfortunately pain and headache are usually constant and severe exacerbations with the recurrence of congestive attacks are liable to occur.

Finally *degenerative changes* complete the picture. Hyalin-like opacities appear on the cornea, running in a band-shape across it or spreading irregularly over its surface; chronic œdema results in the formation of bullæ which periodically rupture; or opacification may be completed by the development of a degenerative pannus.[1] The lens becomes opaque and the iris extremely atrophic. Eventually, advancing degeneration in the sclera may result in its yielding before the sustained pressure with the formation of equatorial, ciliary or intercalary staphylomata. It is the exception for relief from the continued pain to be obtained by the bursting of the globe owing to mild trauma; more usually, if the eye is allowed to remain, further intra-ocular degenerative changes—hæmorrhages, anterior uveitis, or panophthalmitis—complicate the sufferings of the patient, or alternatively the cornea may disintegrate in a degenerative or hypopyon ulcer, in which event perforation may result. In most cases if the eye survives sufficiently long, the tension falls and it may even become soft owing partly to stretching but mainly to general degenerative changes; in other cases a persistent uveitis results in phthisis bulbi, but here again relief from pain is not always obtained owing to the shrinkage of the eye. The picture is indeed tragic and its pathos is intensified by the fact that simple glaucoma is a bilateral disease.

EXTERNAL EXAMINATION

The CONJUNCTIVA shows little change in simple glaucoma. Continued hypertension may induce a visible dilatation of the anterior ciliary arteries, uncommon when the tension is below 40 mm. Hg and almost invariable when above 60 mm. (Dobree, 1954) (Figs. 463–6). This involves particularly the perforating branches of the arteries and, after reduction of the ocular tension, the arterial dilatation takes at least some days to regress. In longstanding cases of absolute glaucoma the episcleral veins, in addition to the arteries, are greatly distended, and the constant engorgement leads to permanent dilatation and the formation of new anastomoses, the end-

---

[1] Vol. VIII, p. 681.

FIGS. 463 to 466.—THE ANTERIOR CAPILLARY CIRCULATION IN SIMPLE GLAUCOMA
(J. H. Dobree.)

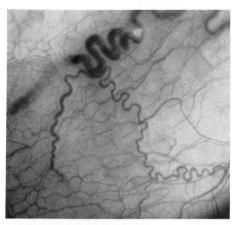

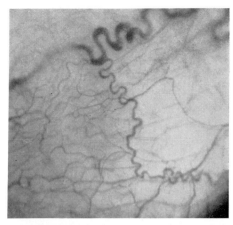

FIG. 463.—An untreated case, tension 63 mm. Hg Schiøtz.

FIG. 464.—The same case after pilocarpine therapy for two weeks, tension 22 mm. Hg Schiøtz.

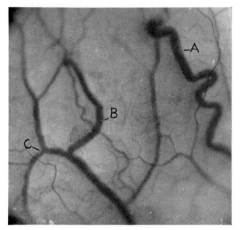

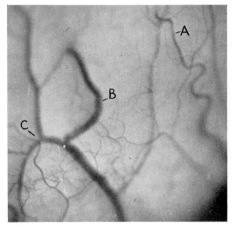

FIG. 465.—An untreated case, tension 80 mm. Hg Schiøtz.

FIG. 466.—The same case after operation, tension 25 mm. Hg Schiøtz.

A, anterior ciliary artery; B, vein from deep scleral plexus; C, vein from superficial episcleral venules.

result being the development of a prominent, tortuous and irregular circle of venous anastomoses—the *Medusa head* (Heerfordt, 1911; Köllner, 1922) (Fig. 467). At this stage the conjunctiva has become atrophied and brittle, and the sclera, owing to the progress of sclerotic and degenerative changes, assumes a delicate bluish-white appearance like porcelain. The further degeneration and consequent stretching of this tissue to form staphylomata has already been discussed.

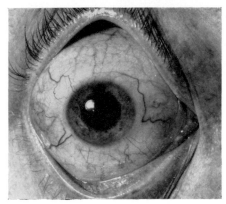

FIG. 467.—PASSIVE HYPERÆMIA IN SIMPLE GLAUCOMA (Inst. Ophthal.).

In the CORNEA two evidences of raised pressure are occasionally seen—haziness and anæsthesia—the pathology of which has already been described[1]: clinically a steaminess and irregularity of the surface lead to an appearance resembling ground glass, sometimes with the occurrence of large bullæ (Fig. 468). Although these corneal changes are usually indicative of closed-angle glaucoma, they may occur in simple glaucoma, particularly when it develops under the age of 50 when the onset of the raised tension

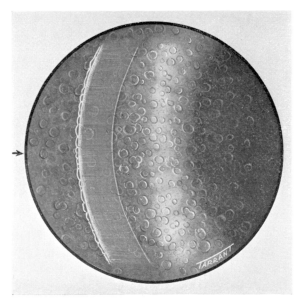

FIG. 468.—EPITHELIAL ŒDEMA IN GLAUCOMA.

Slit-lamp drawing to show the vesicles by direct focal illumination and transillumination (Inst. Ophthal.).

[1] p. 423.

appears in many cases to be more abrupt. This œdema is largely responsible for the entoptic appearance of haloes and the transient periods of misty vision that may occur in these patients, although in pigmentary glaucoma it has been suggested that the haloes may sometimes be due to the presence of the pigmented spindle on the posterior surface of the cornea (Sugar, 1966). In absolute glaucoma corneal œdema and anæsthesia are commonly present.

It has been claimed that in cases of cornea guttata the facility of outflow is decreased (Buxton *et al.*, 1967) and that simple glaucoma is an abnormally frequent occurrence in patients with this condition (10 to 15% of cases of Fuchs's dystrophy, Becker and Shaffer, 1965).

In the IRIS some degree of atrophy is frequently seen, particularly in pigmentary glaucoma and in the glaucoma associated with pseudo-exfoliation of the lens capsule. The atrophy involves the layer of pigmented epithelium and can be most readily demonstrated by transillumination; in glaucoma associated with pseudo-exfoliation the loss of pigment is near the pupil while in pigmentary glaucoma the iris transilluminates in a patchy manner in the mid-periphery. In far-advanced and absolute glaucoma of any type the degree of the atrophic changes in the iris is more marked;

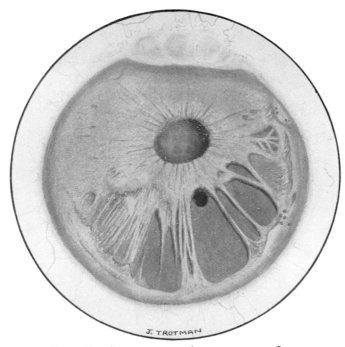

Fig. 469.—Glaucomatous Atrophy of the Iris.

Unilateral stationary iridoschisis in an eye with simple glaucoma. The bleb of a trephine operation done 16 years previously is seen above. During this time the atrophic process remained stationary (J. Winstanley).

its structure loses its delicate architecture, the crypts and the collarette disappear and eventually large patches of advanced atrophy become apparent (Fig. 469). This has already been discussed,[1] as also has the shrinkage which results in an ectropion of the uveal layer, the almost constant pigmentary disturbance causing transparent lacunæ in the iris on transillumination, and the liberal besprinkling of its anterior surface as well as the angle of the anterior chamber with pigmentary deposits (Bergler, 1925).

The ANTERIOR CHAMBER in simple glaucoma varies considerably in depth, the variation being similar to that seen in non-glaucomatous individuals of the same age,[2] although there are possibly more cases with shallow anterior chambers than in the general population (Törnquist and Brodén, 1958). As a general rule in the young the anterior chamber is normal or deep, while in the old it becomes more shallow; in emmetropes it tends to be normal, in myopes deep, and in hypermetropes shallow. In the angle of the anterior chamber the question of the formation of peripheral anterior synechiæ has already been discussed, where it was pointed out that gonioscopic examinations have made it clear that in general they are uncommon and of late formation. It is interesting that many cases show an absence of blood-filling of Schlemm's canal[3]; in such cases the presumption is that this phenomenon is due to sclerosis of the outflow channels.

The PUPIL is said to undergo subtle changes in simple glaucoma. At first it may appear normal, but close examination reveals in early cases a bilateral reduction in the later phases of pupillary constriction, while in advanced simple glaucoma all phases of constriction may be sluggish and the latent period of constriction increased (Lowenstein and Schoenberg, 1942–44); these authors concluded that this reaction was a fatigue phenomenon affecting the sympathetic pathways in the hypothalamus. In absolute glaucoma the pupil, as we have seen, becomes widely dilated and fixed.

In the LENS the most interesting feature in certain cases of simple glaucoma, particularly in those from Scandinavian countries, is the occurrence of pseudo-exfoliation of the capsule, a degenerative phenomenon which we have already discussed at length.[4] In absolute glaucoma the development of a cataract is the rule, starting at first as a general haze especially in the posterior cortex but eventually progressing to form a complicated cataract.[5]

OPHTHALMOSCOPIC EXAMINATION

In simple glaucoma several changes of considerable importance occur in the fundus. After the existence of prolonged pressure there is always

---

[1] Vol. IX, p. 680.
[2] Löhlein (1913), Haag (1915), Raeder (1923), Rosengren (1930–55), Aizawa (1960), Weekers and Grieten (1961), and others.
[3] Bangerter and Goldmann (1941), Kronfeld et al. (1942), Kronfeld (1949), Smith (1956).
[4] p. 45.　　　　[5] p. 227.

some degree of atrophy of the choroid and the pigmentary epithelium, so that eventually the larger choroidal vessels are exposed and a tesselated appearance results. This atrophy is frequently accentuated in two situations —around the disc where a *circumpapillary halo* marks a ring of extreme atrophy which allows the sclera to shine through; and at the points of exit of vortex veins where a whitish or yellow areola appears. Apart from these general changes two phenomena require special mention—the pallor and cupping of the disc and the condition of the retinal vessels.

The OPTIC DISC presents one of the most important diagnostic features in glaucoma of some standing. It undergoes two marked changes—atrophy and cupping (Figs. 470-5). We have already discussed the pathology of these changes and have concluded that a raised ocular tension damages the optic nerve initially by producing vascular changes within it. From the clinical point of view, the degree of pallor, indicating the extent of atrophy of the nerve fibres, is of great importance, particularly as a prognostic indication. The presence of optic atrophy is a most constant clinical sign of established glaucoma, but it does not occur only in the presence of a raised tension for, as we have already mentioned, pallor with excavation may be extremely marked in ischæmic optic neuropathy.[1]

The cupping of the disc is also the result of a combination of the same two factors of mechanical pressure and ischæmia acting in various cases to varying degrees. From the clinical point of view the commencement of cupping is betrayed by the presence of a kink in the vessels as they cross the edge of the disc, particularly on the temporal side and often in its upper quadrant. In its fully developed form the excavation appears as a deep cup involving the whole of the area of the disc with straight sides and usually an overhanging rim, while the floor is pale and may show the markings of the lamina or be covered with glial tissue. The course of the blood vessels is important: as a rule they are dragged over in a bundle towards the nasal side and climb over the sharp edge with an acute bend. When the cup is deep the rim obscures the sides so that the vessels disappear as they climb from the floor to the rim, to reappear again as they bend sharply over the edge. In doing so they appear to suffer an apparent discontinuity in their direction, a phenomenon best explained pictorially in Figs. 476-7.

The actual fact of cupping may be easily verified by the method of parallactic displacement using direct or indirect ophthalmoscopy,[2] and the depth of the excavation may be measured by the direct method, by focusing a vessel on the rim of the excavation and then on the floor. A difference of as much as 5 dioptres is sometimes found between the two levels, indicating a depth of 1·6 mm., while depths of 6 D (Stock, 1910; Klar, 1940) or 7 D (Kayser, 1933) are exceptional. The extent of this will be realized when it is remembered that the diameter of the disc is 1·5 mm.; in such cases the floor of the cup extends beyond the outer surface of the sclera, and in excising

---

[1] p. 437.   [2] Vol. VII, p. 316.

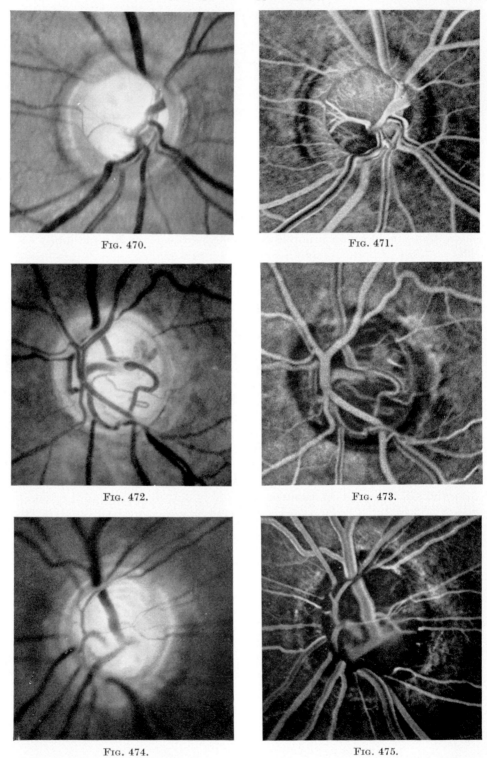

FIGS. 470 to 475.—THE OPTIC DISC IN SIMPLE GLAUCOMA (J. A. Oosterhuis).
(For legends see opposite page.)

FIG. 470.

FIG. 471.

FIG. 472.

FIG. 473.

FIG. 474.

FIG. 475.

such an eye it is not impossible to cut through a cup of this type and open the globe instead of cutting the optic nerve.

An accurate assessment of the degree of cupping is of immense importance in following the course of a case of simple glaucoma; this should be done by repeated careful drawings or, better, by serial photography. An increase in the size of the cup is of importance as well as its depth. It is generally agreed that this is static in the normal eye with age (Pickard, 1935–48; Snydacker, 1964); an increase in size as measured by serial photography using an ophthalmoscopic graticule is an abnormality indicating the presence and progress of glaucoma (Parr, 1965; Hollows and Graham, 1966) (Fig. 478).

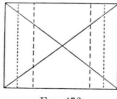
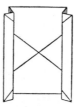

Fig. 476.   Fig. 477.

Figs. 476 and 477.—To Illustrate the Displacement of Vessels in a Glaucomatous Cup.

The sheet of paper with diagonal lines seen in Fig. 476 is folded at right angles first along the broken line and then along the dotted line. The resulting appearance (Fig. 477) shows how the apparent displacement of the diagonal lines corresponds to that of the vessels.

The RETINAL VESSELS frequently show the phenomenon of pulsation at the disc. Venous pulsation is common in normal eyes and may be absent in conditions of high tension, but it is of importance that an arterial pulse is usually more readily evoked by finger-pressure upon the globe than in the normal eye and may, indeed, be spontaneous. This phenomenon of arterial pulsation in glaucoma was first noted by von Graefe (1855) and its study was continued by Jacobi (1876), Ballantyne (1913), Krämer (1920) and

Fig. 470.—A case of early glaucoma; a man aged 48 with normal visual acuity, slight restriction of the visual field and no paracentral scotomata.

Fig. 471.—Fluorescence angiogram of the case in Fig. 470, showing fluorescence over most of the floor of the disc except the lower segment.

Fig. 472.—Fully excavated optic disc in a man aged 70, showing some new vessels. The disc flattened after an Elliot trephining four years previously. There was a small central visual field and a temporal residual field.

Fig. 473.—Fluorescence angiogram of the case in Fig. 472, showing almost complete absence of fluorescence on the floor of the disc with the exception of the retinal vessels and some fluorescence in the peripapillary glaucomatous halo.

Fig. 474.—A totally excavated optic disc with peripapillary atrophy in a woman aged 56. The visual acuity was 1/60 and the field was restricted to a small temporal remnant.

Fig. 475.—Fluorescence angiogram of the case in Fig. 474. There is complete absence of fluorescence on the floor of the disc and a considerably mottled fluorescence in the circumpapillary atrophic halo.

others. It must be remembered that a spontaneous arterial pulse is not diagnostic of glaucoma, for it may be conditioned by many factors such as a low diastolic blood pressure.[1] When the intra-ocular and diastolic pressures are normal, the amplitude of pulsation present in the central artery of the retina is too slight to be observed unless the ophthalmoscopic image is highly magnified (de Speyr, 1914); the significance of the phenomenon of easily observable pulsation is that it indicates that the intra-ocular pressure has approached or exceeded the diastolic arterial pressure. In this event the expansile pulse becomes complete at the disc, the arteries emptying at diastole and filling at systole, and the blood-column flashing out of sight across the disc to appear again as suddenly. Attempts have been made to estimate the height of the blood pressure in the ophthalmic arteries by ophthalmodynamometry, and to correlate the difference between the

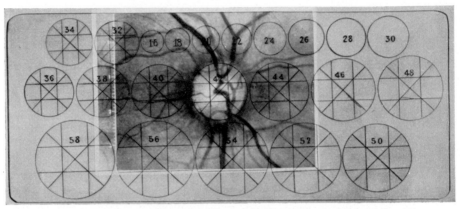

Fig. 478.—Photographic graticule measurement of the proportion of the optic disc involved in an excavation (F. C. Hollows and P. A. Graham).

pressure in the central retinal artery and the intra-ocular pressure with the progression of changes in the visual field in glaucoma.[2] If this difference in pressure is small, some authors have suggested that this indicates that the circulation in the optic nerve-head is poor and that deterioration in the visual fields may be rapid (Dupont, 1959; Lobstein et al., 1960; Belmonte González, 1962), although others could find no relationship between this difference and the visual defects (Bronner, 1959). The presence of a spontaneous or readily produced arterial pulse in the eye, however, indicates a small margin of pressure-head in the ocular circulation. Ophthalmoscopically the arteries usually show little change in calibre in simple glaucoma, but the arteries and veins are frequently engorged and congested to a degree often varying with the height of the tension when this is variable, being dilated when the tension is high and constricted when it is reduced, presumably a compensatory mechanism to maintain the circulation (Dobree,

[1] Vol. IV, p. 7.   [2] p. 471.

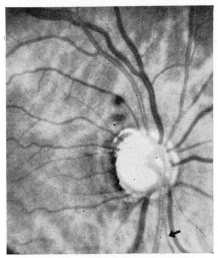

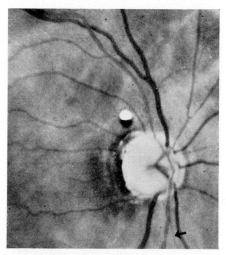

Fig. 479.—The arteries and veins are dilated; tension 73 mm. Hg Schiøtz.

Fig. 480.—Loss of dilatation in the same case; ocular tension reduced by operation to 22 mm. Hg Schiøtz. The arrow (below) indicates a very small arteriole.

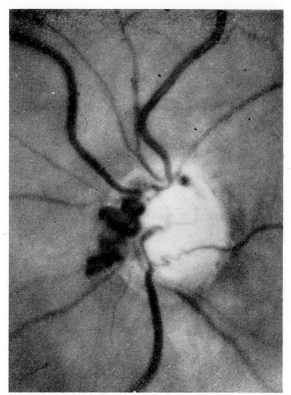

Fig. 481.—Vascularization of the Optic Disc in Simple Glaucoma.

In a case of simple glaucoma with an ocular tension of 60 mm. Hg. New coiled vessels and groups of dilated capillaries are present unassociated with any defect in the visual field (J. H. Dobree).

1956) (Figs. 479–80). In advanced cases this venous stasis may be apparent in the region of the optic disc by the appearance of large vascular loops or tortuosities or of new anastomotic channels[1] (Fig. 481). It is interesting that occlusion of the central retinal vein is a not uncommon finding in established simple glaucoma.[2]

Aizawa. *Acta Soc. ophthal. jap.*, **64**, 869 (1960).

Axenfeld. *Z. Augenheilk.*, **25**, 362 (1911).

Ballantyne. *Ophthalmoscope*, **11**, 271, 338, 460 (1913).

Bangerter and Goldmann. *Ophthalmologica*, **102**, 321 (1941).

Becker and Shaffer. *Diagnosis and Therapy of the Glaucomas*, St. Louis, 214 (1965).

Belmonte González. *Arch. Soc. oftal. hisp.-amer.*, **22**, 1072 (1962).

Bergler. *Arch. Augenheilk.*, **95**, 35 (1925).

Bloch. *Klin. Mbl. Augenheilk.*, **44** (2), 413 (1906).

Bronner. *Bull. Soc. Ophtal. Fr.*, 937 (1959).

Buxton, Preston, Riechers and Guilbault. *Arch. Ophthal.*, **77**, 602 (1967).

Dobree. *Brit. J. Ophthal.*, **38**, 500 (1954); **40**, 1 (1956).

Dupont. *Ann. Oculist.* (Paris), **192**, 651 (1959).

von Graefe. *v. Graefes Arch. Ophthal.*, **1** (1), 362 (1854); (2), 299 (1855).

Haag. *Klin. Mbl. Augenheilk.*, **54**, 133 (1915).

Heerfordt. *v. Graefes Arch. Ophthal.*, **78**, 413 (1911).

Hollows and Graham. *Brit. J. Ophthal.*, **50**, 570 (1966).

Hormuth. *Klin. Mbl. Augenheilk.*, **41**, Beil., 255 (1903).

Jacobi. *v. Graefes Arch. Ophthal.*, **22** (1), 111 (1876).

Kayser. *Klin. Mbl. Augenheilk.*, **91**, 589 (1933).

Klar. *Ber. dtsch. ophthal. Ges.*, **53**, 162 (1940).

Köllner. *Arch. Augenheilk.*, **91**, 181 (1922).

Krämer. *v. Graefes Arch. Ophthal.*, **103**, 14 (1920).

Kraupa. *Arch. Augenheilk.*, **78**, 182 (1915).

Kronfeld. *Arch. Ophthal.*, **41**, 393 (1949).

Kronfeld, McGarry and Smith. *Amer. J. Ophthal.*, **25**, 1163 (1942).

Lobstein, Bronner and Nordmann. *Ophthalmologica*, **139**, 271 (1960).

Löhlein. *v. Graefes Arch. Ophthal.*, **85**, 393 (1913).

Lowenstein and Schoenberg. *Arch. Ophthal.*, **28**, 1119 (1942); **31**, 384, 392 (1944).

Parr. *Trans. ophthal. Soc. N.Z.*, **18**, 93 (1965).

Pickard. *Trans. ophthal. Soc. U.K.*, **55**, 599 (1935).
Brit. J. Ophthal., **32**, 355 (1948).

Raeder. *v. Graefes Arch. Ophthal.*, **112**, 29 (1923).

Rosengren. *Acta ophthal.* (Kbh.), **8**, 99 (1930); **9**, 103 (1931).
Arch. Ophthal., **44**, 523 (1950).
Ber. dtsch. ophthal. Ges., **59**, 128 (1955).

Sengupta. *Brit. J. Ophthal.*, **38**, 685 (1954).

Smith, R. *Brit. J. Ophthal.*, **40**, 358 (1956).

Snydacker. *Amer. J. Ophthal.*, **58**, 958 (1964).

de Speyr. *Ann. Oculist.* (Paris), **152**, 419 (1914).

Stock. *Klin. Mbl. Augenheilk.*, **48**, Beil., 124 (1910).

Sugar. *Amer. J. Ophthal.*, **62**, 499 (1966).

Törnquist and Brodén. *Acta ophthal.* (Kbh.), **36**, 309 (1958).

Weekers and Grieten. *Bull. Soc. belge Ophtal.*, No. 129, 361 (1961).

THE OCULAR TENSION

In simple glaucoma the ocular tension may vary within wide limits, and it must be emphasized that the actual height of the tension may have little bearing on its pathological effects, either upon the structure or function of the eye. One eye may withstand a pressure of over 30 mm. Hg for some years without apparent damage, while another will progress to blindness with intermittent periods of raised tension that may never be higher than the low 20s or even the high teens. In any particular case *that tension is pathological which the tissues of the eye in question cannot withstand without damage.*

[1] von Graefe (1854), Hormuth (1903), Bloch (1906), Axenfeld (1911), Kraupa (1915) Sengupta (1954).
[2] Vol. X, p. 101.

In the clinical investigation of the ocular tension three methods of tonometry are in common use: digital, indentation and applanation. The use of the first, digital tonometry, in the routine examination of patients is to be deplored, for although the experienced examiner can frequently estimate gross departures from normal, he is unable to assess small variations within the range that may be significant. We have already discussed the theoretical basis[1] and the practical application[2] of indentation and applanation tonometry and have concluded that the latter is the more reliable.

Schiøtz tonometry has several disadvantages: there are appreciable instrumental and observer errors; the curvature and thickness of the cornea may affect the results; considerable errors may occur due to variations in the ocular rigidity; and, since the indentation of the eye expresses some aqueous, repeated readings within a short space of time are unreliable as they become increasingly lower. The greatest errors arise from variations in the ocular rigidity; if this is high the intra-ocular pressure is overestimated and the converse is true if it is low. Even the method suggested by Friedenwald (1954–57) to overcome this by *differential tonometry*, whereby successive readings are made using different weights on the plunger, while theoretically sound, introduces other errors, among which must be counted the disastrous effect of misreading the scale of the tonometer by as little as half a scale

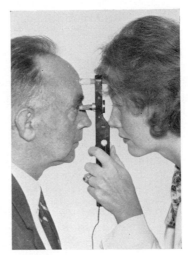

FIG. 482.—APPLANATION TONOMETRY.

A portable instrument: at the top there is a head-rest; in the middle the applanation tonometer applied to the eye, its manipulation controlled from the handle of the instrument (E. S. Perkins).

division (Gloster, 1966). A shorthand method for the estimation of ocular rigidity by this technique is provided by Friedenwald's nomogram (1957) which is illustrated and its use is described in the Appendix.[3] Factors in favour of Schiøtz tonometry are the simplicity of the technique and the cheapness and portability of the instrument.

Applanation tonometry with Goldmann's instrument is more reliable than Schiøtz tonometry although there are a few patients, particularly those with irregularities of their corneal surface and those with marked epiphora, in whom applanation tonometry is difficult or even impossible. The Goldmann tonometer, however, is expensive and not portable, difficulties being overcome by the recent introduction of portable applanation tonometers (Fig. 482) (Perkins, 1965; Draeger, 1967) which correlate well with the readings obtained with the Goldmann instrument (Wallace and

[1] Vol. IV, p. 231.   [2] Vol. VII, p. 336.   [3] p. 750.

Lovell, 1968). A romer was described by Woodhouse (1968) to construct applanation calibration curves on Friedenwald's tonographic nomogram.

We have already seen[1] that the average pressure in the healthy human eye is in the region of 15 to 16 mm. Hg, that values between 21 and 24 mm. should be regarded with suspicion, and that pressures of more than 24 mm. are abnormal. It must be remembered, however, that these figures were obtained from the examination of a large number of subjects, and that there is a small number of eyes, in particular those that have already sustained damage to their optic nerves, that will not tolerate pressures considered to be within the normal range.

Not only is the height of the intra-ocular pressure of importance; its variation is also of great significance. Thus in the healthy eye the tension should not differ materially from that of its fellow and should not vary more than 3 or 4 mm. at different times of the day. In recent studies of normal subjects, for example, Goedbloed and his colleagues (1961) found that a difference in pressure between the two eyes of more than 3·5 mm. occurred in only 3 to 4%, while Davanger (1965) observed differences of more than 4, 5 or 6 mm. in only 1·7%, 0·9% and 0·4% respectively of normal individuals, but a difference of more than 6 mm. in 10% of patients with glaucoma.

THE DIURNAL VARIATION

We have already discussed the normal diurnal variation of the intra-ocular pressure,[2] in which, as was first pointed out by Maslenikow (1904), the pressure is usually highest in the morning before getting out of bed and lowest late in the evening; each variation tends to occur in two steps, a sharp fall at first, followed by a gradual decline throughout the day, and a slow rise at night, tending to become accentuated towards morning (Fig. 483).

The mechanism controlling the diurnal variation of the intra-ocular pressure, as well as daily variations in many other physiological " constants " (circadian fluctuations), appears to be situated at some distance from the eye, possibly in the hypothalamus, and might act upon the intra-ocular pressure by producing changes in one or more of three factors determining variations in the " steady state "—the production of aqueous, the resistance to aqueous outflow, or the episcleral venous pressure—but the exact mechanism is not yet clear. It is probable that the variation is partly due to changes in the rate of production of aqueous. In the phase of raised pressure this was found to be increased by Grant (1955) using tonography, a finding confirmed by Ericson (1958) in normal subjects by using the suction-cup technique, when he showed that there was a correlation between changes in the flow of aqueous and the diurnal variation of tension, the production being lowest at midnight and 4 a.m. Moreover, in rabbits Anjou (1961) found an inverse relationship between the aqueous flare, an indication

[1] Vol. IV, p. 238. [2] Vol. IV, p. 277.

of its content of protein, and the ocular tension.   Studies on the resistance
to the outflow of aqueous have yielded inconsistent results: some authors
have found a direct relationship between this and the ocular tension
(Stepanik, 1954; Boyd, 1964; Boyd and McLeod, 1964), others concluded
that any variation with the resistance was not in phase with the diurnal

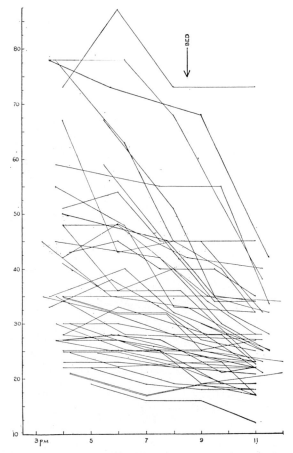

FIG. 483.—THE DIURNAL VARIATION IN TENSION IN SIMPLE GLAUCOMA.

Superimposed curves of the intra-ocular pressure of 45 glaucomatous eyes showing the decline in tension towards the late evening. They were hospital patients and
the arrow indicates when the community went to bed (D. A. Langley and H.
Swanljung).

variation in tension (Kronfeld, 1952; Newell and Krill, 1964), while others
again have found that the resistance was unchanged throughout the day
(deRoetth, 1954; Boles-Carenini, 1955; Grant, 1955).   Finally, with regard
to the pressure in the episcleral veins, although Thomassen (1947–48),
Thomassen and his associates (1950) and Bain (1954) claimed to have

observed an increase in venous pressure preceding the rising phase in the diurnal variation, others have detected little change and certainly no direct relationship between the two (Goldmann, 1951; Linnér, 1956; Leith, 1963).

It is obvious that the mechanism of the diurnal variations is not yet clear; but it is evident that small changes, as in the formation of the aqueous, will give rise to great alterations in the intra-ocular pressure when it is high and particularly if the drainage is impeded.

The magnitude of the diurnal variation in glaucomatous eyes has been extensively investigated. The earlier work on this subject, before gonioscopic examination of these eyes was performed routinely, is of no more than

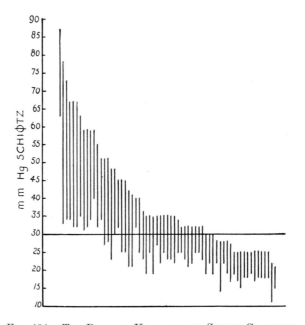

FIG. 484.—THE DIURNAL VARIATION IN SIMPLE GLAUCOMA.

The vertical lines represent the highest and lowest tension recorded in 63 unoperated eyes with simple glaucoma (D. A. Langley and H. Swanljung).

historical interest,[1] but more recent investigations have confirmed the view of these earlier workers that their magnitude is greater in cases of simple glaucoma than in normal eyes (Fig. 484). Drance (1960) found that the mean diurnal variation in normal eyes was 3·7 mm. $\pm$ 1·8 mm., while in 138 patients with untreated simple glaucoma it was 11 mm. $\pm$ 5·7 mm. In the glaucomatous patients the diurnal variation was less than 5 mm. in 6%, 5–9 mm. in 48%, 10–14 mm. in 28%, 15–19 mm. in 12%, 20–24 mm. in 5%, and 25 mm. or more in 3%. These findings have been confirmed by Kata-

[1] Pisarello (1915), Köllner (1916–18), Thiel (1922–25), Hagen (1924), Raeder (1925), Löhlein (1926), Serr (1927), Andrezen (1928), Lauber (1928), Sallmann and Deutsch (1930), and others.

Fig. 485 to 487. The Diurnal Variation in Simple Glaucoma
(D. A. Langley and H. Swanljung).

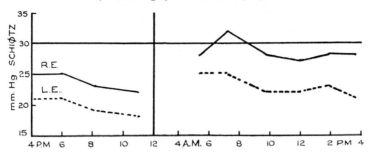

Fig. 485.—The falling type of curve.

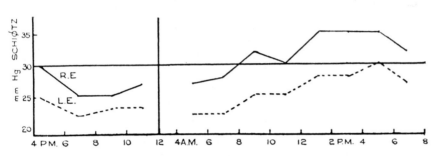

Fig. 486.—The rising type of curve.

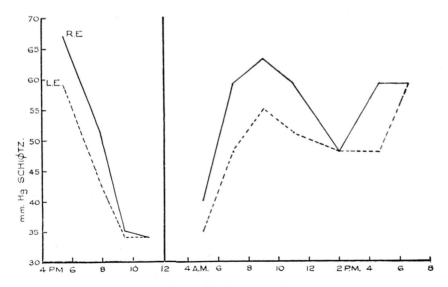

Fig. 487.—The double-variation type of curve.

visto (1964) and Étienne (1967). Huerkamp (1956) and Davanger (1964) found that the diurnal variation increased in proportion to the mean ocular tension and in certain cases it has been found to reach an excursion of 50 to 60 mm. Hg (Duke-Elder, 1952).

In addition to the increased diurnal variation commonly seen in simple glaucoma, the pattern of the variation may also become altered. Although the normal rhythm of the diurnal curve with its highest point in the morning before arising and its lowest later in the evening may be seen in some patients

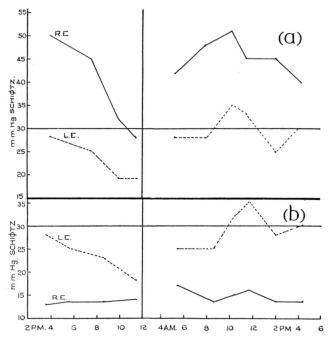

FIG. 488.—THE DIURNAL VARIATION IN BILATERAL SIMPLE GLAUCOMA.

(a) Before operation. (b) After operation on the right eye (D. A. Langley and H. Swanljung).

with simple glaucoma, it is not unusual to observe a peak at other times of the day, and various types of diurnal curve have been described. A reversal of the curve, with the highest tension in the evening, has been reported on several occasions,[1] while other authors have described a number of different patterns occurring in simple glaucoma. Langley and Swanljung (1951), for example, differentiated four types of diurnal curve (Figs. 485–7): (1) a falling type maximal at 6–8 a.m., followed by a continuous decline, (2) a rising type maximal at 4–6 p.m., (3) a double variation type with two peaks

[1] Thiel (1925), Sallmann and Deutsch (1930), Weiss (1931), Magitot (1938), Langley and Swanljung (1951), Kaneda and Kiritoshi (1953), MacDonald (1955), Huerkamp (1956), Hager (1958), Suda *et al.* (1962), Katavisto (1964), and others.

at 9–11 a.m. and 6 p.m., and (4) a flat type of curve. Similar types of curve were described by Kaneda and Kiritoshi (1953), while Suda and his colleagues (1962) and Katavisto (1964) divided their cases of simple glaucoma into those with a regularly periodic curve, the peak of tension being in the morning, during the day, or at night, and those with an irregular curve of a varying or a flat type. It appears, therefore, that the type of diurnal curve in simple glaucoma is of little practical interest; what is important is that the variation may be large and that the ocular tension may reach its maximal value at any time of the day or night.

It is interesting that the diurnal variation in tension persists even in the absolute stage of the disease when all vision has been lost, and is also seen, although muted in degree, after successful surgical intervention showing that, although the tension has been lowered, the instability persists (Fig. 488).

THE FACILITY OF AQUEOUS OUTFLOW

In so far as the theoretical basis of tonography and the perilimbal suction-cup technique has already been discussed in detail in another

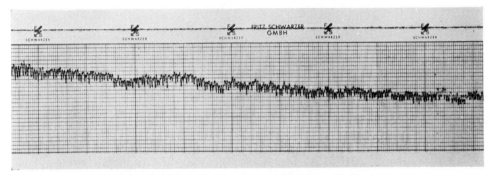

FIG. 489.—A TYPICAL TONOGRAPHIC RECORD (J. Gloster).

Volume of this *System*,[1] it only remains to discuss here the clinical importance of a reduced facility of aqueous outflow in the diagnosis and management of simple glaucoma. Although it has been known for some years that repeated applications of a Schiøtz tonometer to the eye will result in measurements indicating steadily decreasing pressures (Schiøtz, 1909), it is only since the introduction of " electronic " tonometers that satisfactory continuous records of the reduction in ocular tension have been obtained and analysed, thus allowing the facility of aqueous outflow to be calculated in the living human eye (Grant, 1950).

The technique of TONOGRAPHY as introduced by Morton Grant (1950) following the use of the electronic tonometer by Moses and Bruno (1950) is a simple means of determining the rate of flow of the aqueous.

[1] Vol. IV, p. 248.

The patient lies comfortably on a couch in the supine position, the eye is lightly anæsthetized and fixation is maintained by the other eye by observing a suitably placed light or other object. An electronic tonometer, usually bearing the 5·5 G. weight and recording a continuous tracing, is placed upon the eye and retained for a period of 4 minutes, the initial and final pressures being noted.[1] The consequent elevation of the intra-ocular pressure causes some aqueous to be expelled from the eye at a rate more rapid than normal so that the pressure progressively falls and the tonometric indentation of the cornea becomes progressively deeper, increasing the scale-reading (Fig. 489). The rate at which the pressure falls is partly determined by the resistance to aqueous outflow; this factor was expressed by Grant as its reciprocal which he termed the *facility of outflow* (C). It follows that a glaucomatous eye with a high resistance to outflow has a low value of C. The drop in the plunger during the 4 minutes, expressed as the mean of the scale-readings at the beginning and end of the recording, is used to calculate the volumetric change of the aqueous (in µl./min.) in terms of the average pressure-gradient between the anterior chamber and the episcleral veins.

The calculation is based on Poiseuille's equations which have been described in a previous Volume.[2] The fundamental expression for the normal eye is

$$F = \frac{P_0 - P_v}{R} = C(P_0 - P_v) \text{ or } C = \frac{F}{P_0 - P_v}$$

when F is the rate of flow, P_0 the pressure in the undisturbed eye, P_v the pressure in the episcleral veins, R the resistance and C the facility of outflow. During a 4-minute tonography the final equation is

$$C = \frac{(V_{c4} - V_{c0}) + \dfrac{1}{K}(\log P_{t0} - \log P_{t4})}{\left(\dfrac{P_{t0} + P_{t4}}{2} - P_0 - \triangle P_v\right)t}$$

when V_{c0} and V_{c4} represent the volume of corneal indentation at the beginning and end of tonography, K is Friedenwald's coefficient of ocular rigidity (assumed to be 0·0215), P_{t0} and P_{t4} the pressures in the undisturbed eye and after the test, $\triangle P_v$ is the average rise in the episcleral venous pressure during the test (assumed to be 1·25 mm. Hg), and t the duration of the test in minutes.

Fortunately, in clinical practice the considerable calculations required in each individual case are unnecessary, for the value of C can be obtained from the initial reading and the change in scale-reading as calculated for eyes of average ocular rigidity by reference to the tables prepared by Grant (1950).[3] It is to be noted that, apart from the time (t), each of the eight terms on the right-hand side of this equation is inaccurate, a point stressed originally by Grant himself who emphasized the importance of these errors and stated clearly that he regarded the technique as suitable for clinical research but doubted its applicability to the diagnosis and management of the disease. It is doubtful if Poiseuille's law, which defines the flow of a

[1] Vol. VII, p. 347, Fig. 280.   [2] Vol. IV, p. 192.   [3] p. 750.

simple fluid through a system of straight rigid tubes of uniform bore, is applicable to the complex drainage channels of the eye. Again, the fall of pressure may not be linear so that the arithmetic mean between the initial and final values may not give an adequate assessment. Moreover, the existence of a *uveo-scleral outflow*[1] ensures that the drainage of aqueous humour is not entirely through the trabeculæ and Schlemm's canal, while the elevation of the intra-ocular pressure expels a certain amount of blood from the uveal tract which tends to return to its original volume during the course of the test, and the same factor suppresses the formation of aqueous, an effect making the facility of outflow appear greater than it really is, which was called *pseudo-facility* by Bárány (1963).[2] Since neither of these factors is catered for, it follows that the volumetric change does not entirely reflect the drainage of aqueous. Moreover, an average assessment of the coefficient of ocular rigidity may lead to large errors in individual cases, since this factor may greatly influence the rate at which the intra-ocular pressure falls.

Finally, an inexact assessment is made of the pressure in the episcleral veins based on an average height of 10 to 12 mm. Hg and an average rise of 1·25 mm. Hg during tonography. There is, however, a considerable individual variation in the pressure in these veins which was estimated by Weigelin and Löhlein (1952) to vary between 9 and 16·8 mm. Hg; there is little consensus of opinion regarding the change during tonography (Goldmann, 1959; Leith, 1963), and small differences will have profound effects on the results. There is evidence that the application of the tonometer to the eye disturbs its normal hydrodynamics (Stocker, 1958); while the common practice of testing one eye may upset the other by a consensual reaction so that a subsequent test to the second may be misleading (Berry *et al.*, 1967; Kronfeld, 1968). It will be realized that these inaccuracies add up to a formidable list; the technique pushes the use of an instrument such as a tonometer to, if not beyond, its limits of reliability (Moses and Bruno, 1950), and the computation is a good example of the difficulty and danger of expressing biological processes in terms of mathematical equations with their deceptive aura of accuracy.

Several expedients have been suggested to obtain more reliable results. The fact that most tonographic records do not show a regular fall of pressure without irregularities has given rise to suggestions to replace the acceptance of the arithmetic mean of the initial and final pressures as an index of the fall in pressure (Merté, 1957–58; Stepanik, 1961), but the complications thereby introduced have led to no more satisfactory conclusions. For the same reason, the duration of tonography has been extended, notably by Leydhecker (1957–58) who increased the time to 7 minutes and used the results derived from the last 4 minutes largely to avoid the rapid fall which generally occurs in the first half of a 4-minute test; this, however, introduces

[1] Vol. IV, p. 127.   [2] Vol. IV, p. 255.

other sources of error and would appear to be no more accurate (Armaly, 1964). A correction for the ocular rigidity was suggested by Moses and Becker (1958) by taking the initial pressure with an applanation tonometer and using Friedenwald's nomogram for ocular rigidity by the method illustrated in the Appendix,[1] but there is considerable doubt that this method of deduction is correct (Gloster, 1966). Indeed, studies of the ocular rigidity during tonography have led to varied conclusions: that it rises (Tuovinen, 1961), falls (Ytteborg, 1960) or does not change (Stepanik, 1957). To eliminate the question of ocular rigidity Gloster (1962) introduced an *applanation outflow test* wherein the eye was compressed and applanation readings of the pressure were taken before, during and after the compression; but thereby further sources of error are introduced (Gloster, 1966). Other procedures have been suggested such as *isotonography* whereby the intra-ocular pressure is not allowed to fall during the test by progressively increasing the plunger-weight (Moses, 1958; van Beuningen, 1958) or the pressure is similarly restored at the end of the test to its original level (Prijot, 1958–59; Kessler, 1959); but again, similar errors arise. In order to avoid the effect of consensual reactions when the second eye is tested, Draeger (1959) suggested *binocular tonography* whereby two electronic tonometers, two tonographers and an unusually cooperative patient are required; a more practical alternative is to test the second eye an hour later than the first or on a subsequent visit.

It is thus evident that in tonography there are many sources of error which are virtually impossible to assess, and that the various methods of eliminating these are by no means free from other errors. It is probably best—and certainly simplest—to use the original tables of Morton Grant (1950)[2] and base clinical conclusions upon these as specific figures without ascribing to them a precise value representing the number of microlitres of aqueous expressed each minute on raising the intra-ocular pressure by 1 mm. Hg. Considered as such, recognizing that errors exist in some eyes and interpreting the results as corroborative but not conclusive evidence, we shall see that the technique is the most useful available for estimating the facility of outflow of the aqueous.

It would appear that there is a wide range in the facility of outflow in healthy human eyes. Prijot (1961), for example, found that C varied between 0·12 and 0·66 in 339 non-glaucomatous subjects; Becker and Christensen (1956) calculated that the average value was 0·31 but that 6% of normal subjects gave a value of less than 0·20 and 1% a value of less than 0·15, and similar average values have been observed by other workers (Leydhecker, 1958—0·28 ± 0·071; Prijot, 1961—0·28; Tuovinen, 1961—0·33).

Grant (1951) found that in patients with untreated simple glaucoma the facility of outflow was reduced, and this observation has been con-

---

[1] p. 748.
[2] p. 748.

firmed by numerous subsequent workers.[1] It is difficult to compare any
but the most recent measurements for it is only in the past few years that
the 1955 calibration tables for the Schiøtz tonometer have been generally
used; and because of the wide variations encountered in normal subjects,
it is difficult to place a lower limit on this measurement beyond which a
pathological obstruction can be assumed. Becker and Shaffer (1965) considered that a facility of less than 0·18 was probably pathological and one of
less than 0·13 definitely so, Gloster (1966) believed that a value of less than
0·15 was suspicious of glaucoma while one of less than 0·12 was diagnostic

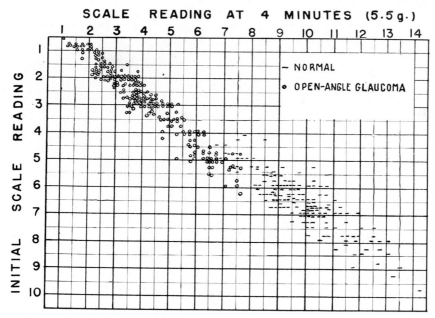

FIG. 490.—TONOMETRIC READINGS ON NORMAL AND SIMPLE GLAUCOMATOUS EYES
(W. Morton Grant).

of the disease, while Leydhecker (1966) calculated that a facility of 0·13 was
probably pathological and one of 0·09 or less was certainly so. Leydhecker's
(1958–66) results are not strictly comparable with those of the other workers
quoted as his technique for performing tonography differed from theirs in
that he performed the tonography for 7 minutes and calculated the facility of
outflow from the results of the last 4 minutes.

   As would be expected from these variable values the differentiation
between glaucomatous and healthy eyes is not definite (Prijot, 1961;

[1] Goldmann (1951), Prijot and Weekers (1951), Kronfeld (1952), deRoetth and Knighton
(1952), Becker and Friedenwald (1953), Mansheim (1953), Weekers and Prijot (1953), Horwich
and Breinin (1954), Scheie et al. (1955), Roberts (1958), Leydhecker (1958), Newell and Krill
(1964), Osterczy-Sliwińska (1965), Gloster (1966), and many others.

Stepanik, 1961); Figs. 490–1 give some of Grant's values. To achieve a better differentiation on the basis of tonometric results, Becker and Christensen (1956) and Leydhecker (1957) introduced the use of the *ratio* P_0/C. On the assumption that a glaucomatous eye will have both a high pressure and a lower facility, this empirical ratio, without expressing any specific physical property of the eye, exaggerates the difference between the pathological and the normal. According to Becker and Christensen (1956) the P_0/C ratio should be less than 100 in normal eyes; in Gloster's (1966) view a ratio of more than 125 should be regarded with suspicion while a ratio over 150 is pathological.

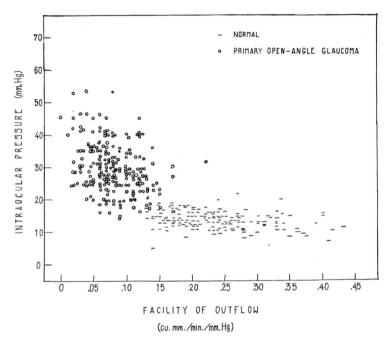

FIG. 491.—THE FACILITY OF AQUEOUS OUTFLOW IN NORMAL AND SIMPLE GLAUCOMATOUS EYES (W. Morton Grant).

With all its limitations tonography has proved to be a useful clinical technique when its results are properly interpreted. Its greatest value has been the unequivocal demonstration that the primary factor in determining a rise in the intra-ocular pressure in simple glaucoma is an increase in the resistance to the drainage of the aqueous. As we shall see presently, however, its greatest limitation is in the diagnosis of borderline cases wherein the rise of tension is marginal, the appearance of the optic disc is equivocal and visual damage has not occurred, for in these a small decrease in the facility of the outflow need not connote a glaucomatous eye. In such cases, however, a high facility indicates the absence of glaucoma; moreover, the technique is of some value in prognosis, in the need for surgical interference and the mechanical value of this when it has been done. Again, the presence of a low facility in an eye which cannot otherwise be examined (as because of cataract) is a very useful confirmation of the suspected presence of the disease.

The Perilimbal Suction-cup Technique. In a previous Volume[1] we have already discussed the theoretical basis of this technique devised by Rosengren (1956) and developed by Ericson (1958). Thereby the outflow channels are occluded by the application of a suction cup at the limbus thus raising the intra-ocular pressure, and following its removal the rate of decay of the ocular tension is measured and thus provides an estimation of the resistance to the outflow of aqueous. It has been established by this technique that there is a resistance to the outflow of aqueous in simple glaucoma[2] and the magnitude of this resistance appears similar to that derived from tonography. It seems probable, therefore, that this technique is useful in the early diagnosis of simple glaucoma, particularly in those patients in whom fixation of the eye is difficult and tonography inaccurate.

A FLUOROMETRIC METHOD of estimating the facility of outflow was adopted by Goldmann (1951) whereby 4 ml. of a 10% solution of sodium fluorescein is injected intravenously and the concentration of the dye in the anterior chamber is estimated at short intervals with a slit-lamp fluorometer while at the same time measurements are made of the free fluorescein in an ultrafiltrate of the blood. From the relation of these two concentrations Goldmann estimated the turnover rate of fluorescein in the anterior chamber which he found to average 2·2 μl. per minute in normal eyes. It follows that the resistance to outflow ($R = 1/C$) can be calculated from the formula

$$R = \frac{P_0 - P_v}{F}.$$

This is probably a more accurate method than that employed by Weekers and Delmarcelle (1953) who adapted the technique introduced by Langley and MacDonald (1952) of instilling fluorescein into the conjunctival sac, since the concentration of the dye in the cornea is unknown. The fluorometric method has the great advantage that the eye remains undisturbed, but it is too difficult a technique and requires so much complicated apparatus that it cannot be easily used as a routine clinical practice.

A further OUTFLOW PRESSURE TEST introduced by Goldmann (1951) was to measure the rise of intra-ocular pressure necessary to produce the slightest observable increase in the diameter of an aqueous vein; but again, this difficult technique has not been generally adopted in the investigation of simple glaucoma.

Andrezen. *Russ. oftal. Z.*, **7**, 303 (1928).
Anjou. *Acta ophthal.* (Kbh.), **39**, 507 (1961).
Armaly. *Invest. Ophthal.*, **3**, 77 (1964).
Bain. *Brit. J. Ophthal.*, **38**, 129 (1954).
Bárány. *Invest. Ophthal.*, **2**, 584 (1963).
Becker and Christensen. *Arch. Ophthal.*, **56**, 321 (1956).

Becker and Friedenwald. *Arch. Ophthal.* **50**, 557 (1953).
Becker and Shaffer. *Diagnosis and Therapy of the Glaucomas*, 2nd ed., St. Louis (1965).
Berry, Drance and Wiggins. *Canad. J. Ophthal.*, **2**, 411 (1967).

[1] Vol. IV, p. 195.
[2] Galin *et al.* (1961–63), Pasmanik *et al.* (1962–64), Mikuni *et al.* (1963), Fukuchi (1964), Mikuni (1964), Langham and Maumenee (1964), MacFaul (1966), Mikawa (1967), and others.

van Beuningen. *Klin. Mbl. Augenheilk.*, **133**, 723 (1958).

Boles-Carenini. *Amer. J. Ophthal.*, **39**, 793 (1955).

Boyd. *Canad. med. Ass. J.*, **90**, 467 (1964).

Boyd and McLeod. *Ann. N.Y. Acad. Sci.*, **117**, 597 (1964).

Davanger. *Acta ophthal.* (Kbh.), **42**, 764 (1964); **43**, 299 (1965).
Intraocular Pressure in Normal Eyes and in Eyes with Glaucoma Simplex, Bergen (1965).

Draeger. *Öst. ophthal. Ges.*, **4**, 23 (1959).
Invest. Ophthal., **6**, 132 (1967).

Drance. *Arch. Ophthal.*, **64**, 494 (1960); **70**, 302 (1963).

Duke-Elder. *Amer. J. Ophthal.*, **35**, 1 (1952).

Ericson. *Acta ophthal.* (Kbh.), **36**, 381; Suppl. 50 (1958).

Étienne. *Ann. Oculist.* (Paris), **200**, 977 (1967).

Friedenwald. *Decennial Report of the Com. on the Standardization of Tonometers*, *Amer. Acad. Ophthal.* (1954).
Trans. Amer. Acad. Ophthal., **61**, 108 (1957).

Fukuchi. *Acta Soc. ophthal. jap.*, **68**, 101, 170, 265 (1964).

Galin, Baras and McLean. *Trans. Amer. Acad. Ophthal.*, **66**, 230 (1962).

Galin, Baras, Nano and Cavero. *Arch. Ophthal.*, **70**, 202 (1963).

Galin, Nano and Baras. *Rev. bras. Oftal.*, **20**, 177 (1961).

Gloster. *Trans. ophthal. Soc. U.K.*, **82**, 315 (1962).
Tonometry and Tonography, London (1966).

Goedbloed, Schappert-Kimmijser, Donders *et al.* *Ophthalmologica*, **141**, 481 (1961).

Goldmann. *Ophthalmologica*, **111**, 146; **112**, 344 (1946); **119**, 65; **120**, 150 (1950); **145**, 88 (1963).
Docum. ophthal., **5–6**, 278 (1951); **13**, 236 (1959).
Amer. J. Ophthal., **48** (2), 213 (1959).

Grant. *Arch. Ophthal.*, **44**, 204 (1950); **46**, 113 (1951).
Glaucoma: a Symposium (ed. Duke-Elder), Oxon. (1955).

Hagen. *Acta ophthal.* (Kbh.), **2**, 199 (1924).

Hager. *Die Behandlung d. Glaucoms mit Miotica*, Stuttgart (1958).

Horwich and Breinin. *Arch. Ophthal.*, **51**, 687 (1954).

Huerkamp. *Klin. Mbl. Augenheilk.*, **128**, 394 (1956).

Kaneda and Kiritoshi. *Acta Soc. ophthal. jap.*, **57**, 236 (1953).

Katavisto. *Acta ophthal.* (Kbh.), Suppl. 78 (1964).

Kessler. *Amer. J. Ophthal.*, **47**, 233 (1959).

Köllner. *Arch. Augenheilk.*, **81**, 120 (1916); **83**, 135 (1918).

Kronfeld. *Arch. Ophthal.*, **48**, 393 (1952).
Invest. Ophthal., **7**, 319 (1968).

Langham and Maumenee. *Trans. Amer. Acad. Ophthal.*, **68**, 277 (1964).

Langley and MacDonald. *Brit. J. Ophthal.*, **36**, 432 (1952).

Langley and Swanljung. *Brit. J. Ophthal.*, **35**, 445 (1951).

Lauber. *Lijecn. Vjesn.*, **50**, 140 (1928). See *Zbl. ges. Ophthal.*, **20**, 246 (1929).

Leith. *Brit. J. Ophthal.*, **47**, 271 (1963).

Leydhecker. *Docum. ophthal.*, **10**, 174 (1956).
Ber. dtsch. ophthal. Ges., **61**, 327 (1957).
Klin. Mbl. Augenheilk., **132**, 77 (1958).
Trans. ophthal. Soc. U.K., **78**, 553 (1958).
Glaucoma in Ophthalmic Practice, London (1966).

Linnér. *Amer. J. Ophthal.*, **41**, 646 (1956).

Löhlein. *Klin. Mbl. Augenheilk.*, **77**, Beil., 1 (1926).

MacDonald. *Trans. canad. ophthal. Soc.*, **7**, 178 (1955).

MacFaul. *Brit. J. Ophthal.*, **50**, 12 (1966).

Magitot. *Docum. ophthal.*, **1**, 411 (1938).

Mansheim. *Arch. Ophthal.*, **50**, 580 (1953).

Maslenikow. *Vestn. Oftal.*, **21**, 237 (1904).

Merté. *Ber. dtsch. ophthal. Ges.*, **61**, 381 (1957).
Acta XVIII int. Cong. Ophthal., Brussels, **2**, 1523 (1958).

Mikawa. *Folia ophthal. jap.*, **18**, 958 (1967).

Mikuni. *Trans. Asia-Pac. Acad. Ophthal.*, **2**, 244 (1964).

Mikuni, Iwata and Fukichi. *Rinsho Ganka*, **17**, 719 (1963).

Moses. *Arch. Ophthal.*, **59**, 527 (1958).

Moses and Becker. *Amer. J. Ophthal.*, **45**, 196 (1958).

Moses and Bruno. *Amer. J. Ophthal.*, **33**, 389 (1950).

Newell and Krill. *Trans. Amer. ophthal. Soc.*, **62**, 349 (1964).

Osterczy-Sliwińska. *Klin. oczna*, **35**, 183 (1965).

Pasmanik and Galin. *Arch. chil. Oftal.*, **19**, 50 (1962).

Pasmanik, Rojas, de Camino and Miranda. *Arch. chil. Oftal.*, **21**, 12 (1964).

Pasmanik, Verdaguer and Riveros. *Arch. chil. Oftal.*, **19**, 155 (1962).

Perkins. *Brit. J. Ophthal.*, **49**, 591 (1965).

Pisarello. *Ann. Ottal.*, **44**, 544 (1915).

Prijot. *Ophthalmologica*, **136**, 266 (1958).
Arch. Ophthal., **61**, 536 (1959).
Contribution à l'étude de la tonométrie et de la tonographie en ophtalmologie, Hague (1961).

Prijot and Weekers. *Bull. Soc. belge Ophtal.*, No. 98, 353 (1951).

Raeder. *Klin. Mbl. Augenheilk.*, **74**, 424 (1925).

Roberts. *Glaucoma* (Trans. 3rd Macy Conf., ed. Newell), N.Y., 203 (1958).

deRoetth. *Arch. Ophthal.*, **51**, 740 (1954).

deRoetth and Knighton. *Arch. Ophthal.*, **48**, 148 (1952).

Rosengren. *Trans. ophthal. Soc. U.K.*, **76**, 65 (1956).

Sallmann and Deutsch. *v. Graefes Arch. Ophthal.*, **124**, 624 (1930).

Scheie, Spencer and Helmick. *Trans. Amer. ophthal. Soc.*, **53**, 265 (1955).

Schiøtz. *Arch. Augenheilk.*, **62**, 317 (1909).

Serr. *Ber. dtsch. ophthal. Ges.*, **46**, 398 (1927).

Stepanik. *Amer. J. Ophthal.*, **38**, 629 (1954).
Klin. Mbl. Augenheilk., **130**, 585 (1957).
Adv. Ophthal., **11**, 120 (1961).

Stocker. *Amer. J. Ophthal.*, **45**, 192 (1958).

Suda, Ootsuba, Sawada *et al. Rinsho Ganka*, **16**, 11 (1962).

Thiel. *Klin. Mbl. Augenheilk.*, **68**, 244 (1922); **70**, 766 (1923).
v. Graefes Arch. Ophthal., **113**, 329, 347 (1924).
Arch. Augenheilk., **96**, 331 (1925).

Thomassen. *Acta ophthal.* (Kbh.), **25**, 221 (1947).

Thomassen. *Trans. ophthal. Soc. U.K.*, **68**, 75 (1948).

Thomassen, Perkins and Dobree. *Brit. J. Ophthal.*, **34**, 221 (1950).

Tuovinen. *Acta ophthal.* (Kbh.), Suppl. 67 (1961).

Wallace and Lovell. *Brit. J. Ophthal.*, **52**, 568 (1968).

Weekers and Delmarcelle. *Ophthalmologica*, **125**, 425 (1953).

Weekers and Prijot. *Ann. Oculist.* (Paris), **186**, 596 (1953).

Weigelin and Löhlein. *v. Graefes Arch. Ophthal.*, **153**, 202 (1952).

Weinstein and Forgács. *Brit. J. Ophthal.*, **37**, 444 (1953).

Weiss. *Russ. oftal. Z.*, **14**, 93 (1931).

Woodhouse. *Brit. J. Ophthal.*, **52**, 492 (1968).

Ytteborg. *Acta ophthal.* (Kbh.), **38**, 562 (1960).

THE VISUAL FIELDS

The study of the visual fields in glaucoma, although started by von Graefe (1855–69), owes its detailed analysis to ophthalmologists in Copenhagen. After von Graefe's original investigations, observations were conducted with the perimeter and therefore, apart from the description of a scotoma by Landesberg (1869), they were confined to the awareness only of gross sectorial defects. This state of affairs persisted until Jannik Peterson Bjerrum [1851–1920] introduced the campimeter and founded quantitative perimetry. With this more efficient technique he rediscovered the comet-defect now named eponymously after him as *Bjerrum's sign* (1889), an observation which attracted world-wide attention to the value of perimetry and was elaborated particularly by Meisling (1900) in France, Friedenwald (1902) in America, and Sinclair (1905) in Scotland. Shortly thereafter, Bjerrum's mantle was taken over by his pupil, Rønne (1909) who did much to further the subject. He described the ultimate fate of Bjerrum's comet scotoma to end in the horizontal raphe where it was delimited sharply in *Rønne's nasal step*. Further elaboration led Erich Seidel (1914) of Jena[1] to claim the earliest appearance of this peculiar scotoma as a prolongation upwards or downwards of the blind-spot (*Seidel's sickle scotoma*), a finding amplified by Elliot (1922) who described its feathery edges. For some considerable time thereafter it was the generally accepted opinion that the field-defect of glaucoma always began as an extension of the blind-spot but, working with still smaller visual angles, Traquair (1927) in Edinburgh and Luther Peter (1927) in Philadelphia discovered that the first scotomatous defect appeared as a small detached area above or below the blind-spot which later became merged with it. Such a scotoma is difficult to find since it is away from the blind-spot and isolated, relative in nature and frequently fleeting, and occurs in eyes not usually suspected of being pathological. More recently these defects were further amplified by the techniques of angioscotometry by Evans (1926–39), and of skiascotometry by Goldmann and his co-workers (Goldmann, 1947; Gafner and Goldmann, 1955; Gafner, 1957).[2]

Our debt in this connection to the two professors of the University Clinic in Copenhagen is immense. Bjerrum's portrait and biography are in a previous Volume of this series[3]; here we shall pay a tribute to Rønne.

[1] Vol. IV, Fig. 36.
[2] For the clinical application of these techniques, see Vol. VII, pp. 399 *et seq.*
[3] Vol. VII, Fig. 319.

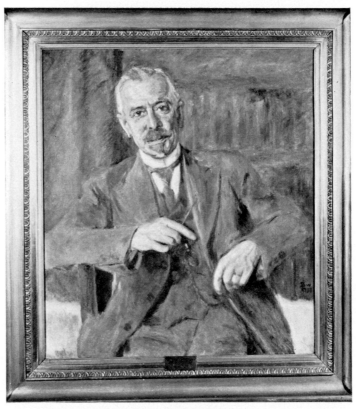

FIG. 492.—HENNING KRISTIAN TRAPPAUD RØNNE [1878–1947].
(A portrait by Sigurd Swane in the University Eye Clinic, Copenhagen; by courtesy of Prof. H. Ehlers.)

HENNING KRISTIAN TRAPPAUD RØNNE [1878–1947] (Fig. 492) was one of the most distinguished of all Danish ophthalmologists as well as one of the most industrious, a fact borne out by a study of his 216 publications between 1904 and 1945, which continued until nearly a year before his death when he had both hemiplegia and aphasia. Moreover, apart from his scientific attainments, his geniality and his sense of humour endeared him to his contemporaries.   Apart altogether from his work on the visual fields in glaucoma, his contributions to such subjects as toxic amblyopia, the colour sense, Weber's Law, adaptation, strabismus, choroiditis, the retinopathies, dyslexia and ocular histology, his greatest interest lay in the analysis of the ocular effects of lesions of the central visual pathways.

In simple glaucoma, especially in its earlier stages, the study of the visual fields is a most valuable method of investigation not only to establish the presence of the disease but also to measure its progress, estimate its prognosis, and assess the value of treatment.   The main features of the glaucomatous field are:

(1) The development of isolated scotomata around the fixation point which sooner or later coalesce with each other and with the blind-spot to form an arcuate scotoma.   The characteristic changes are nerve-fibre bundle defects, which in this disease attain a very high state of development.

(2) A general depression with peripheral contraction which is most pronounced on the nasal side and is frequently associated with a nasal step and at a later stage with wide sectorial defects.   The defects are at first relative but eventually become absolute.

(3) The retention of central vision until a late stage.

The initial defect in the visual field in cases of simple glaucoma varies in different patients.   An accentuation of the normal angioscotomata at the upper and lower poles of the blind-spot, originally demonstrated by Evans (1939), has been confirmed by subsequent workers[1] and is generally agreed to be the earliest change found in the visual field in co-operative patients. Similar changes may be produced by an artificial increase of ocular tension both in normal and glaucomatous subjects,[2] but the latter appear to be more sensitive to this artificial increase of tension.   A depression of the 1/2000 isopter, which is usually especially noticeable on the outer side of the blind-spot, is a further early sign while the peripheral field is still normal (Traquair, 1939; Blaxter, 1950); the isopter passes to the nasal instead of the temporal side of this landmark so that the *blind-spot is laid bare*, as it were, usually on its upper aspect (Fig. 493).   An enlargement of the blind-spot, originally described by Bjerrum (1889), is considered an early sign by several authors, including Grant (1947), Ferraris de Gaspare (1951) and Chrzanowska-Srzednicka (1965), but not by Blaxter (1950) nor by Aulhorn and Harms (1967).   These various changes are generally followed by constriction of the 1/2000 isopter and the development of a small nasal step (Fig. 494).   There-

[1] Humblet and Weekers (1948), Posner and Schlossman (1948), Dubois-Poulsen (1952), Abe (1965), and others.
[2] Gafner and Goldmann (1955), Drance (1962), Suda and Abe (1964), Abe (1965).

FIGS. 493 AND 494.—THE VISUAL FIELD IN EARLY SIMPLE GLAUCOMA
(Goldmann perimeter).

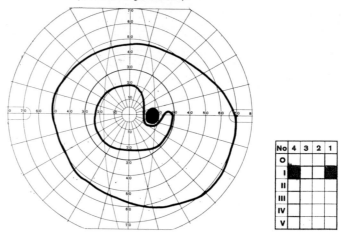

FIG. 493.—BARING OF THE BLIND-SPOT.

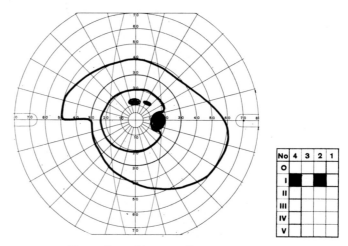

FIG. 494.—BARING OF THE BLIND-SPOT, ISOLATED SCOTOMATA AND NASAL STEP.

after this nasal step usually develops into a partial arcuate scotoma
advancing towards the blind-spot but not in contact with it. In it there
appears, sooner or later, one or more small blind areas forming an absolute
scotoma, at first usually unconnected with the blind-spot[1] (Fig. 494), but
eventually merging into it to form a *Seidel's sickle scotoma* (Fig. 495).
These early scotomata may be inconstant, demonstrable on some days and

[1] Peter (1927), Traquair (1931–39), Blaxter (1950), Kurz (1957), Aulhorn and Harms
(1967), and others.

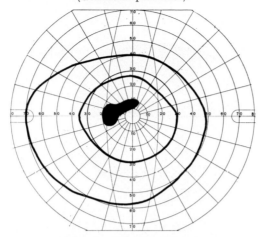

FIG. 495.—SEIDEL'S SCOTOMA.

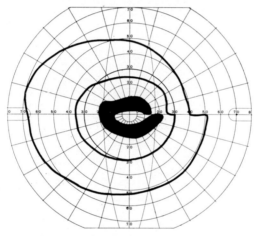

FIG. 496.—DOUBLE ARCUATE SCOTOMA WITH A NASAL STEP.

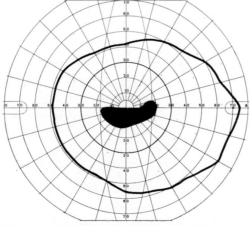

FIG. 497.—CENTRAL DEFECT WITHOUT PERIPHERAL CHANGE.

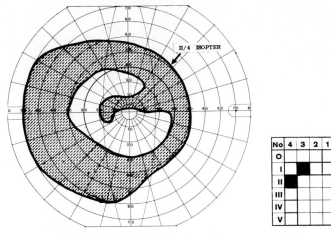

FIG. 498.—SEIDEL'S SCOTOMA AND PERIPHERAL CONTRACTION.

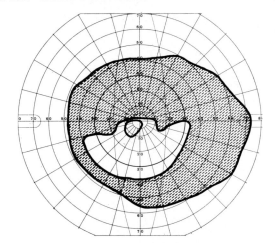

FIG. 499.—LOSS OF UPPER FIELD.

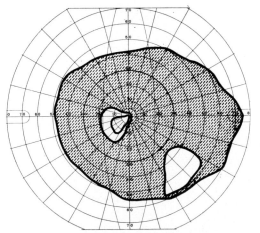

FIG. 500.—ALMOST COMPLETE LOSS OF THE FIELD.

not on others, and they may disappear after the use of miotics and may vary with the state of the eye, sometimes advancing and sometimes receding (Samojloff, 1924–26; Evans, 1930; Sloan, 1931; and others); moreover, they can be elicited only by the most careful quantitative methods, and can sometimes be demonstrated in reduced illumination while the field is normal in a good light (Haffmans, 1861; Marlow, 1932–47; Roll, 1938; Drance *et al.*, 1967), observations that have been confirmed by the techniques of mesopic and scotopic perimetry and campimetry.[1]

The more fully developed defect eventually forms *Bjerrum's comet scotoma* which arches from the blind-spot round the fixation area to end on the horizontal meridian where it forms the sharp *step of Rønne* (Fig. 498); sometimes both upper and lower sides are affected, in which case the fixation area may be almost or completely isolated by a *ring scotoma* (Fig. 496). Thereafter large sectorial defects may develop, the peripheral field failing more rapidly than the central, and the nasal field disappearing in advance of the temporal (Fig. 499); central vision is usually long preserved, but eventually it also succumbs, typically to be survived by a patch in the temporal periphery (Fig. 500). Occasionally the central part of the field fails early while the periphery remains intact, a small arcuate scotoma forming in the centro-cæcal area, or the whole central field or its upper or lower half is impaired or lost at a comparatively early stage of the disease (Fig. 497). Exceptionally, small spike-like scotomata appear in the peripheral field (D. P. Smith, 1925). It must not be forgotten, however, that miosis frequently results in an artificial contraction of the peripheral isopters and, in glaucomatous subjects, may also produce a central scotoma (Day and Scheie, 1953; Jayle *et al.*, 1959; Ourgaud and Étienne, 1961; and others). Lenticular changes, particularly in association with miosis, may also produce characteristically glaucomatous field changes which decrease on dilatation of the pupil or when the illumination is increased and disappear when the cataract is removed[2] (Day and Scheie, 1953; Forbes, 1966), while in myopic eyes the defects due to changes in the fundus may cause some confusion (Kurozumi *et al.*, 1966).

It is interesting that as a rule these changes, both peripheral and central, frequently tend to become remarkably symmetrical in the two fields. No definite sequence is followed and all types of variation occur, producing an infinite variety of different appearances, in all of which, however, the same basic tendencies can be found. It is to be remembered, especially in comparing the condition on different occasions as in an assessment of the progress of the disease or of the efficacy of treatment, that every care should be taken to maintain constancy in the conditions, such as the degree of illumination and the size of the pupil.

[1] Vol. VII, p. 419.
[2] p. 143.

Several workers have studied the critical fusion frequency[1] in simple glaucoma and have shown that depression of this frequency is nearly always found when defects in the visual fields can be demonstrated with the perimeter, and is often present before perimetric defects occur.[2]

The mode of the production of these defects in the visual fields has given rise to considerable controversy. It was originally thought that they were brought about by a pressure-atrophy of the nerve fibres largely determined by the anatomical conditions at the optic disc, the two massive bundles of nerve fibres entering the disc on the outer side of its upper and lower poles being first affected since here the fibres are most numerous; thereafter, successive fibres to the nasal side are involved and finally the macular fibres. A compression of the nerve fibres against the edge of the scleral foramen, however, cannot explain the characteristic nerve-bundle defects we have just studied; the arcuate defects do not begin at the edge of the blind-spot, nor do they creep outwards from it but to it and the spots of most intense blindness do not lie near the blind-spot. After the relief of tension the first area to recover is usually nearest to this landmark indicating it has been least affected. Moreover, a defect in the temporal field usually starts peripherally and the eventual functional remnant is near the blind-spot.

The evidence suggests that the primary damage is not to the nerve fibres but to their blood supply, depending on the obliteration of one or more of the arteriolar twigs supplying a bundle of fibres.[3] The absence of disproportion between the defects for white and colours indicates that when such a bundle becomes involved it is severely affected and the damage is often confined to a relatively narrow strand. The steepness of the edges of the scotomata indicates that one bundle is eliminated before the next is harmed and the groups of fibres in the neighbourhood of the vascular trunks are usually first involved; it is an angioscotoma which evolves into a Bjerrum scotoma. Moreover, the defects pathognomonic of glaucoma are mimicked by a wide variety of vascular lesions, particularly obliterative in nature, affecting the visual pathway anterior to the lateral geniculate body in the absence of raised intra-ocular pressure (Dubois-Poulsen, 1952). The initial glaucomatous defects are thus due to vascular insufficiency and may be reversible, but if the ischæmia persists degeneration of the nerve fibres leads to the development of permanent loss.

It is undoubtedly true that the defects in the field are generally related to the height of the ocular tension; but gross scotomata may occur when the tension has always been relatively low. There is also no doubt that on

[1] For technique see Vol. VII, p. 421.

[2] Weekers *et al.* (1949), Miles (1950), Campbell and Rittler (1959), Weinstein and Brooser (1962), Flachsmeyer (1964), Müller (1965), Müller *et al.* (1966), Pur and Pistelka (1966), and others.

[3] Lauber (1925), Reese and McGavic (1942), Traquair (1944), Gafner and Goldmann (1955), Harrington (1959–64), Drance *et al.* (1968).

lowering a high tension by medical or surgical treatment a considerable recession of the defects may occur particularly in their early stages. It may be that a vascular twig is compressed or occluded as it is stretched over the edge of the optic disc (Scott, 1957), or alternatively, that occlusion occurs in the peripheral part of the optic nerve affecting the arterial circle of Zinn-Haller or partial obstruction of the retinal arteries (Harrington, 1964). From this it follows that defects in the fields develop whenever vascular insufficiency occurs in the optic nerve whether this results from arterial occlusive disease, a raising of the intra-ocular pressure sufficient to overcome the diastolic pressure of the arterioles in the optic nerve-head, or a lowering of the diastolic pressure in the ophthalmic artery or in the local arterioles so that a slight increase in the intra-ocular pressure—or even a normal pressure—may induce the same ischæmic effect; anything, in fact, which upsets the balance between the intra-ocular pressure and the diastolic arteriolar pressure so that the flow of blood is decreased will be effective. It is interesting that in such cases a low diastolic pressure in the orbital arterioles is not uncommon (Johnson and Drance, 1968).

For this reason a glaucomatous bundle-scotoma may be induced or exaggerated by increasing the intra-ocular pressure (as by a dynamometer) if the diastolic blood pressure is low; an eye may resist the effects of high intra-ocular pressure for long periods provided the diastolic blood pressure is high, and if the latter is lowered by medication a Bjerrum scotoma may rapidly develop or become increased; while an eye with arterial disease will quickly show scotomatous defects with little or no rise in the intra-ocular pressure, and an eye without this may resist a raised ocular tension for a long time. These considerations, of course, have profound effects on the treatment necessary in such cases.

These defects are typically associated with both cupping of the disc and pallor of the nerve-head. When both are present the defects in the visual field are always found. If cupping is present without ischæmic pallor, the defects may be very slight or even absent. If pallor is present without or with only a trace of cupping, as may occur in elderly patients, the characteristic defects are present, but in these cases care should be taken to determine whether or not the disease is glaucomatous.

Abe. *Acta Soc. ophthal. jap.*, **69,** 105 (1965).

Aulhorn and Harms. *Glaucoma* (Tutzing Symp., ed Leydhecker), Basel, 151 (1967).

Bjerrum. *Nord. ophthal. T.*, **2,** 144 (1889); **5,** 71 (1892).

Blaxter. *Brit. J. Ophthal.*, **34,** 404 (1950).

Campbell and Rittler. *Trans. Amer. Acad. Ophthal.*, **63,** 89 (1959).

Chrzanowska-Srzednicka. *Klin. oczna,* **35,** 187 (1965).

Day and Scheie. *Arch. Ophthal.*, **50,** 418 (1953).

Drance. *Trans. ophthal. Soc. U.K.*, **82,** 73 (1962).

Drance. *Arch. Ophthal.*, **68,** 478 (1962).

Drance, Wheeler and Pattullo. *Canad. J. Ophthal.*, **2,** 249 (1967).

Amer. J. Ophthal., **65,** 891 (1968).

Dubois-Poulsen. *Le champ visuel*, Paris (1952).

Elliot. *Treatise on Glaucoma*, London (1922).

Evans. *Amer. J. Ophthal.*, **9,** 118, 489 (1926); **12,** 194 (1929); **14,** 772 (1931); **16,** 417 (1933).

Arch. Ophthal., **3,** 153 (1930); **22,** 410 (1939).

Clinical Scotometry, New Haven (1938).

Ferraris de Gaspare. *Boll. Oculist.*, **30,** 677 (1951).

Flachsmeyer. *Dtsch. GesundhWes.*, **19,** 2110 (1964).

Forbes. *Invest. Ophthal.*, **5,** 139 (1966).

Friedenwald, H. *Ann. Ophthal.*, **11,** 157 (1902).

Gafner. *Docum. ophthal.*, **11,** 1 (1957).

Gafner and Goldmann. *Ophthalmologica*, **130,** 357 (1955).

Goldmann. *Ophthalmologica*, **114,** 147 (1947).

von Graefe. *v. Graefes Arch. Ophthal.*, **1** (2), 299 (1855); **2** (2), 258, 291 (1856); **15** (3), 108 (1869).

Grant. *Amer. J. Ophthal.*, **30,** 1276 (1947).

Haffmans. *v. Graefes Arch. Ophthal.*, **8** (2), 124 (1861).

Harrington. *Amer. J. Ophthal.*, **47,** 177 (1959).
  The *Visual Fields*, 2nd ed., St. Louis (1964).

Humblet and Weekers. *Bull. Soc. belge Ophtal.*, No. 88, 305 (1948).

Jayle, Aubert, Boyer and Reboul (1959). *See* Ourgaud and Étienne (1961).

Johnson and Drance. *Canad. J. Ophthal.*, **3,** 149 (1968).

Kurozumi, Matsuno and Kani. *Acta Soc. ophthal. jap.*, **70,** 2238 (1966).

Kurz. *Acta med. orient.*, **16,** 139 (1957).

Landesberg. *v. Graefes Arch. Ophthal.*, **15** (1), 204 (1869).

Lauber. *Z. Augenheilk.*, **57,** 481 (1925).

Marlow. *Arch. Ophthal.*, **7,** 211 (1932); **38,** 43 (1947).

Meisling. *Ann. Oculist.* (Paris), **124,** 417 (1900).

Miles. *Arch. Ophthal.*, **43,** 661 (1950).

Müller, W. *v. Graefes Arch. Ophthal.*, **168,** 33 (1965).

Müller, W., Sack, Semm and Kössler. *Klin. Mbl. Augenheilk.*, **148,** 545 (1966).

Ourgaud and Étienne. *L'exploration fonctionnelle de l'oeil glaucomateux*, Paris, **2,** 1050 (1961).

Peter. *Arch. Ophthal.*, **56,** 337 (1927).

Posner and Schlossman. *Arch. Ophthal.*, **39,** 623 (1948).

Pur and Pistelka. *Cs. Oftal.*, **22,** 204 (1966).

Reese and McGavic. *Arch. Ophthal.*, **27,** 845 (1942).

Rønne. *Klin. Mbl. Augenheilk.*, **47** (1), 12 (1909).
  v. Graefes Arch. Ophthal., **71,** 52 (1909).

Roll. *Klin. Mbl. Augenheilk.*, **100,** 600 (1938).

Samojloff. *Klin. Mbl. Augenheilk.*, **69,** 59 (1922); **74,** 652 (1925).
  Ann. Oculist. (Paris), **161,** 523 (1924).
  Z. Augenheilk., **58,** 214, 282 (1926).

Scott. Traquair's *Clinical Perimetry*, 7th ed., London, 143 (1957).

Seidel. *v. Graefes Arch. Ophthal.*, **88,** 102 (1914).

Sinclair. *Trans. ophthal. Soc. U.K.*, **25,** 384 (1905).

Sloan. *Arch. Ophthal.*, **5,** 601 (1931).

Smith, D. P. *Brit. J. Ophthal.*, **9,** 233 (1925).

Suda and Abe. *Acta Soc. ophthal. jap.*, **68,** 1104 (1964).

Traquair. *Introduction to Clinical Perimetry*, London (1927).
  Trans. ophthal. Soc. U.K., **51,** 585 (1931); **64,** 3 (1944).
  Arch. Ophthal., **22,** 949 (1939).

Weekers, Roussel and Heintz. *Ophthalmologica*, **118,** 555 (1949).

Weinstein and Brooser. *Amer. J. Ophthal.*, **53,** 373 (1962).

THE LIGHT SENSE

It has long been recognized that the light sense suffers severely in simple glaucoma and patients remark constantly on their difficulties in adapting themselves on entering a dim illumination after a bright light or of their difficulties in reading by low artificial light.

The early investigators[1] thought that the light difference was first impaired, but that a fall in the perception of the light minimum was a late happening and indicative of optic atrophy. Henry (1920), however, concluded that at the earliest stages of the disease there was a rapid reduction of the light minimum but only a little change in the light difference, the reverse of the sequence in optic atrophy. The further observations of Ammann (1921), Tschenzow (1922) and Møller (1926) confirmed these findings to some extent, laying stress upon the influence of lowered visual acuity and field defects; and the question was largely clarified by the extended researches of Derby and his co-workers (Waite *et al.*, 1925; Derby

[1] Samelsohn (1885), Treitel (1890), Delorme (1912), Beauvieux and Delorme (1913).

et al., 1926–29). Using elaborate controls of the physical and physiological variables, they established that at low intensities of illumination the changes in the light difference were insignificant either in early or advanced simple glaucoma, but that the light minimum was considerably raised, and that the rate of dark adaptation was retarded (Fig. 501). In established glaucoma these tendencies may be marked, and these workers confirmed Henry's (1920) view that they were demonstrable in the earliest stages of the disease. At a later date, these conclusions were confirmed by several observers[1] (Fig. 502). Zanettin (1931) concluded that a reduction in the light sense of

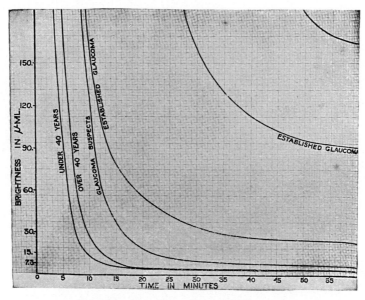

FIG. 501.—THE LIGHT SENSE IN GLAUCOMA.

Comparative curves of the light-minimum. The ordinate represents micro-millilamberts as units of intensity at the screen (J. H. Waite *et al.*).

the peripheral retina was a more constant feature of the disease, occurring even when the function of the central region is normal, affecting most markedly the temporal area, and thereafter, in order, the superior, inferior and nasal.

For these reasons the visual fields are constricted in glaucomatous subjects in subdued illumination, a fact first noted by Javal (1901) and confirmed by several others.[2] The visual acuity is also lowered in similar circumstances (Javal, 1901; Houssin, 1949).

[1] Feigenbaum (1928), Accardi (1933), Feldman (1936–39), Dashevskiy (1941), Mandelbaum (1941), Rubino and Pereyra (1948), Jayle *et al.* (1950–59).
[2] Møller (1926), Roll (1938), Mandelbaum (1941), Marlow (1947), Dubois-Poulsen (1952), and others.

Abnormalities in the adaptation curve in simple glaucoma[1] have been repeatedly confirmed by more recent workers,[2] but the value of adaptometry in the early diagnosis of this disease is less certain, for although it used to be claimed that the adaptation curve was abnormal, it is now believed to be within normal limits in the earliest stages (Ourgaud and Aubert, 1958; Ourgaud and Étienne, 1961). Similarly, the measurement of the light minimum, which is raised in established glaucoma, is within normal limits in early or suspected cases and its estimation is therefore of little value in the diagnosis, while the determination of the light difference appears to have little clinical applicability. These changes in sensitivity are not universal

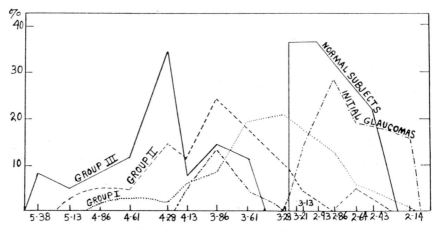

Fig. 502.—The Threshold for Light in Simple Glaucoma.

The ordinate shows the percentage of cases; the abscissa the thresholds in L.U. psb. The curves show the absolute light-threshold in normal subjects; in cases of initial glaucoma, showing only a slight contraction of the visual field and excavation but no pallor of the optic disc; in group II there is a classical nasal field-defect with a Bjerrum scotoma, excavation and pallor of the optic disc and a raised tension; group III show the same characteristics to a more marked degree with an elevation of the intra-ocular pressure not reducible by pilocarpine (after G. E. Jayle et al.).

in simple glaucoma and great individual variations occur with no constant relation to the height or duration of the ocular tension. The exploration of the light sense has, therefore, little diagnostic value, nor does it form a trustworthy basis for prognosis (Casten and Shaad, 1933; Feldman, 1939), but, as shown by Ourgaud and Étienne (1961), it yields important information for the interpretation of other tests of visual function.

THE COLOUR SENSE

Until recently there were a few scattered references in the literature to defects of colour vision in patients with glaucoma. Although red-green defects have been

[1] For clinical technique, see Vol. VII, p. 384.
[2] Jayle et al. (1949–59), Fabian (1950), Herbstein (1958), Ourgaud and Aubert (1958), Ourgaud and Étienne (1961), Peret (1961), Krzystkowa (1964), and many others.

described on several occasions,[1] François and Verriest (1958) found a blue-yellow defect in over 33% of glaucomatous patients, and only one case of red-green defect. Dubois-Poulsen and Magis (1960) demonstrated a glaucomatous tritanopia in an appreciable percentage of patients, and similar results were obtained by Ourgaud and Étienne (1961). The classical case of Javal, who suffered markedly from red-blindness long before he lost his sight completely from glaucoma, is therefore not typical of this disease.

Accardi. *Ann. Ottal.*, **61**, 561 (1933).

Ammann. *Klin. Mbl. Augenheilk.*, **67**, 564 (1921).

Beauvieux and Delorme. *Arch. Ophtal.*, **33**, 93 (1913).

Casten and Shaad. *Arch. Ophthal.*, **9**, 52 (1933).

Dashevskiy. *Vestn. Oftal.*, **18**, 241 (1941).

Delorme. *Du sens lumineux et du sens chromatique centraux dans le glaucome chronique* (Thèse), Toulouse (1912).

Derby, Chandler and O'Brien. *Arch. Ophthal.*, **1**, 692 (1929).

Derby, Chandler and Sloan. *Trans. Amer. ophthal. Soc.*, **27**, 110 (1929).

Derby, Waite and Kirk. *Arch. Ophthal.*, **55**, 575 (1926).

Dubois-Poulsen. *Le champ visuel*, Paris (1952).

Dubois-Poulsen and Magis. *Ophthalmologica*, **139**, 155 (1960).

Engelking. *v. Graefes Arch. Ophthal.*, **116**, 196 (1925).

Fabian. *Klin. oczna*, **20**, 56 (1950).

Feigenbaum. *Klin. Mbl. Augenheilk.*, **80**, 577, 596 (1928).

Feldman. *Arch. Ophthal.*, **15**, 1004 (1936); **19**, 882 (1938); **22**, 595 (1939).

François and Verriest. *Acta XVIII int. Cong. Ophthal.*, Brussels, **1**, 903 (1958).

Henry. *Brit. med. J.*, **2**, 111 (1920).

Herbstein. *Oftalmologia* (Buc.), **3**, 67 (1958).

Houssin. *Arch. Ophtal.*, **9**, 331 (1949).

Javal. *Ann. Oculist.* (Paris), **126**, 143, 161 (1901).

Jayle, Ourgaud, Baisinger and Holmes. *Night Vision*, Springfield, 220 (1959).

Jayle, Ourgaud, Benoit, Blet and Bérard. *La vision nocturne et ses troubles*, Paris (1950).

Jayle, Ourgaud and Bérard. *Bull. Soc. Ophtal. Fr.*, 153 (1949).

Koellner. *Hb. d. norm. u. path. Physiol.* (ed. Bethie *et al.*), Berlin, **12** (1), 517 (1929).

Krzystkowa. *Klin. oczna*, **34**, 125 (1964).

Mandelbaum. *Arch. Ophthal.*, **26**, 203 (1941).

Marlow. *Arch. Ophthal.*, **38**, 43 (1947).

Møller. *Acta ophthal.* (Kbh.), **3**, 170, 196 (1926).

Ourgaud and Aubert. *Acta XVIII int. Cong. Ophthal.*, Brussels, **1**, 893 (1958).

Ourgaud and Étienne. *L'exploration fonctionelle de l'œil glaucomateux*, Paris (1961).

Peret. *Rev. bras. Oftal.*, **20**, 5 (1961).

Roll. *Klin. Mbl. Augenheilk.*, **100**, 600 (1938).

Rubino and Pereyra. *Riv. oto-neuro-oftal.*, **23**, 227 (1948).

Samelsohn. *Cong. int. Sci. méd.*, *C.R. Sect. Ophtal.*, Copenhagen, **9** (1885).

Speciale-Piccichè. *Ann. Ottal.*, **55**, 884 (1927).

Szmyt. *Przegl. Lék.*, **9**, 338 (1951).

Treitel. *v. Graefes Arch. Ophthal.*, **36** (3), 99 (1890).

Tschenzow. *Russ. oftal. J.*, **1**, 235 (1922).

Waite, Derby and Kirk. *Trans. ophthal. Soc. U.K.*, **45**, 301 (1925).

Wessely. *Klin. Mbl. Augenheilk.*, **79**, 811 (1927).

Zanettin. *Ann. Ottal.*, **59**, 847 (1931).

Zimmermann. *Klin. Mbl. Augenheilk.*, **148**, 845 (1966).

OPHTHALMODYNAMOMETRY

We have already discussed in a previous Volume of this *System*[2] the theoretical basis and technique of ophthalmodynamometry, a simple and innocuous clinical test which gives a rough estimation of the lateral pressure in the ophthalmic artery. Within the past few years renewed interest has been shown in the results of this test in patients with simple glaucoma, particularly as a result of the studies of Lobstein and his co-workers (Lobstein *et al.*, 1960; Weigelin and Lobstein, 1961; Lobstein and Herr, 1966; Lobstein, 1968) who estimated the "efficient gradient", the mean pressure

---

[1] Engelking (1925), Speciale-Piccichè (1927), Wessely (1927), Koellner (1929), Szmyt (1951), Zimmermann (1966).

[2] Vol. VII, p. 355.

in the ophthalmic artery less the intra-ocular pressure. The greater this difference between the pressure in the ophthalmic artery and the intra-ocular pressure, the more copious is the blood-flow in the cribriform plate. A fall in the systemic blood-pressure, particularly its diastolic reading, in patients with simple glaucoma, and thus a reduction in the "efficient gradient", has been shown to result in deterioration in the visual field.[1]

THE ELECTROPHYSIOLOGICAL REACTIONS

THE ELECTRORETINOGRAM

It is generally accepted that the electroretinogram (ERG) is little affected in uncomplicated simple glaucoma,[2] although a few authors have described changes in this condition (Vanysek, 1955; Pilz and Grube, 1959; Alvis, 1966). It is generally believed, however, that changes in the ERG in simple glaucoma are due either to miosis or to concurrent retinal disease, such as vascular sclerosis, occlusion of the central retinal vein, or degenerative myopia, and the finding of an abnormal ERG should suggest such additional pathological changes. Even in absolute glaucoma when vision is lost, the ERG may be normal.[3]

THE ELECTRO-OCULOGRAM

The electro-oculogram is similarly unaffected except in absolute glaucoma wherein the base value is reduced (François et al., 1957), and when there is concurrent vascular sclerosis (Arden et al., 1962).

THE ELECTRO-ENCEPHALOGRAM

Changes in the electro-encephalogram, in particular a reduction of α activity and an increase in β activity, have been described in various types of glaucoma.[4] Such changes, however, are comparable with those found in many normal subjects, particularly as a result of anxiety or discomfort, are not necessarily indicative of any pathological process within the brain and therefore cannot be cited as evidence for a cerebral factor in the ætiology of glaucoma.

Alvis. *Amer. J. Ophthal.*, **61,** 121 (1966).

Arden, Barrada and Kelsey. *Brit. J. Ophthal.*, **46,** 499 (1962).

Belmonte González. *Arch. Soc. oftal. hisp.-amer.*, **22,** 1072 (1962).

Busti. *Boll. Oculist.*, **41,** 339 (1962).

Fois and Frezzotti. *G. ital. Oftal.*, **10,** 414 (1957).

Fradkin, Semenovskaya and Skvorchevskaya. *Helmholtz ophthal. Inst., Sci. Notes*, **6,** 18 (1961).

Franceschetti, Diéterlé and Monnier. *Rev. oto-neuro-ophtal.*, **27,** 381 (1955).

[1] McLean (1957), Harrington (1959), Lobstein et al. (1960–68), Belmonte González (1962), Pérez Llorca (1963), Johnson and Drance (1968), and others. See also p. 477.

[2] Karpe (1945), Leydhecker (1950), Henkes (1951), Rosenberg (1951), François (1952), Schmöger and Thieme (1955), Franceschetti et al. (1955), Straub (1957), François and DeRouck (1958–59), Ourgaud and Étienne (1961), Busti (1962), Ponte (1962), Jayle et al. (1965), and others.

[3] Leydhecker (1950), Rosenberg (1951), François (1952), François and DeRouck (1959).

[4] Levina and Neustadt (1951), Ségal and Majkowski (1953), Hartmann (1954), Fois and Frezzotti (1957), Salgado Gómez (1957), Moreau et al. (1958), Fradkin et al. (1961), Frasca and Scardovi (1961), Krejci and Krejcova (1962), Krejci et al. (1963).

François. *Bull. Soc. franç. Ophtal.*, **65**, 209 (1952).

François and DeRouck. *Acta XVIII int. Cong. Ophthal.*, Brussels, **1**, 899 (1958). *Ann. Oculist.* (Paris), **192**, 321 (1959).

François, Verriest and DeRouck. *Adv. Ophthal.*, **7**, 1 (1957).

Frasca and Scardovi. *Minerva oftal.*, **3**, 128 (1961).

Harrington. *Amer. J. Ophthal.*, **47** (2), 177 (1959).

Hartmann. *Acta XVII int. Cong. Ophthal.*, Montreal-N.Y., **2**, 937 (1954).

Henkes. *Ophthalmologica*, **121**, 44 (1951).

Jayle, Boyer and Saracco. *L'éléctrorétino-graphie*, Paris (1965).

Johnson and Drance. *Canad. J. Ophthal.*, **3**, 149 (1968).

Karpe. *Acta ophthal.* (Kbh.), Suppl. 25 (1945).

Krejci and Krejcova. *Cs. Oftal.*, **18**, 383 (1962).

Krejci, Polacek and Krejcova. *Cs. Oftal.*, **18**, 453 (1962); **19**, 171 (1963).

Levina and Neustadt. *Vestn. Oftal.*, **30** (5), 8 (1951).

Leydhecker. *Brit. J. Ophthal.*, **34**, 555 (1950).

Lobstein. *Mod. Prob. Ophthal.*, **6**, 73 (1968).

Lobstein, Bronner and Nordmann. *Ophthalmologica*, **139**, 271 (1960).

Lobstein and Herr. *Ann. Oculist.* (Paris), **199**, 38 (1966).

McLean. *Amer. J. Ophthal.*, **44**, 323 (1957).

Moreau, Ballivet and Boit. *Bull. Soc. Ophtal. Fr.*, 600 (1958).

Ourgaud and Étienne. *L'exploration fonctionnelle de l'œil glaucomateux*, Paris (1961).

Pérez Llorca. *Arch. Soc. oftal. hisp.-amer.*, **23** 966 (1963).

Pilz and Grube. *Ber. dtsch. ophthal. Ges.*, **62**, 195 (1959).

Ponte. *Boll. Oculist.*, **41**, 739 (1962).

Rosenberg. *Vestn. Oftal.*, **30** (5), 12 (1951).

Salgado Gómez. *Arch. Soc. oftal. hisp.-amer.*, **17**, 468 (1957).

Schmöger and Thieme. *Dtsch. Gesundh Wes.*, **10**, 1159 (1955).

Ségal and Majkowski. *Klin. oczna*, **23**, 101 (1953).

Straub. *Ophthalmologica*, Suppl. 48, 137 (1957).

Vanysek. *Klin. oczna*, **25**, 235 (1955).

Weigelin and Lobstein. *Ophthalmodynamometry*, Basel (1961).

Clinical Types of Simple Glaucoma

At this stage it might be useful to comment upon the various clinical pictures which may occur in simple glaucoma, particularly in its earlier stages, with special reference both to the different ways in which it may present and also to the various terminologies in current usage.

OCULAR HYPERTENSION

We have already noted[1] that cases exist characterized by the persistent presence of an intra-ocular pressure higher than is generally accepted as normal and yet show no typical signs of glaucoma as seen in the absence of anomalies at the optic disc or defects in the visual fields, associated with a normal facility of outflow as tonographically measured. Such a diagnosis, however, must be made with care and only after a lengthy period of observation, for the development of simple glaucoma may be a prolonged process. As has been so elegantly demonstrated by Leydhecker (1959), the interval of time between the onset of a raised ocular tension and the occurrence of defects in the visual field is on an average 18 years, thus indicating the desirability of diagnosing simple glaucoma before the onset of irreversible damage to the optic nerve-head. In those cases wherein there is a raised ocular tension with a reduced facility of outflow, in the absence of changes in the optic disc or visual field, a diagnosis of simple glaucoma should be made, for in these cases the concept of "hypertension without glaucoma" is out-dated (Leydhecker, 1966). It is more difficult, however, to assess those

[1] p. 379.

cases wherein the ocular tension is found repeatedly to be outside the normal range, yet the facility of outflow is within normal limits. Leydhecker (1967) has shown that 60% of eyes with an ocular tension of 22 mm. or more showed deterioration of their visual field within 7 years, yet Linnér and Stromberg (1967) found that in some subjects with a raised ocular tension and a normal facility of outflow, these parameters remained constant over 5 years. It appears, therefore, as Goldmann (1967) has suggested, that there are some individuals whose ocular tension is higher than 20·5 mm. but in whom it does not rise over several years, and there are others who, when first examined, have an ocular tension below 20·5 mm. but over the years develop a rise of tension above this figure. The former group may reasonably be considered to have OCULAR HYPERTENSION, for in the present state of our knowledge it is not yet possible to be certain of their eventual outcome. The latter group should be considered to be suspected cases of glaucoma.

The occurrence of eyes with a relatively high tension is not at all surprising. The concept of an upper limit of normal intra-ocular pressure at 21 or 22 mm. Hg is merely a convenient limit statistically imposed for clinical guidance. The distribution curve for the intra-ocular pressure in a population has shown a variation from low values to high with no definite line between those whom we have classified as "glaucoma suspects" and sufferers from simple glaucoma (Leydhecker et al., 1958; Leydhecker, 1959–60; Davanger and Holter, 1965; Bertelsen et al., 1965; and others). That such a curve shows skewness was interpreted by Leydhecker (1959–60) as statistical evidence that simple glaucoma was a pathological deviation from a normal distribution of tension, and was intriguingly explained by Davanger (1965) on the assumption of a normal distribution of the "effective" diameter of the trabecular pores in a population consisting of people both with and without the disease. Moreover, several observers have found the intra-ocular pressure to be considerably higher in families with cases of glaucoma than in those without (Kellerman and Posner, 1955; Becker et al., 1960; Miller and Paterson, 1962; and others). This would suggest that simple glaucoma has a multifactorial ætiology, corresponding to refractive errors the incidence of which may be interpreted as the chance combination of essentially normal elements.[1] A better analogy in this quantitative approach to disease is essential vascular hypertension which is most satisfactorily regarded not as a qualitative but as a quantitative deviation from the normal (Pickering, 1955–59; Platt, 1956–59; Oldham et al., 1960).[2]

LOW-TENSION GLAUCOMA

There is considerable confusion in the recent literature as to the use of the terms "low-tension glaucoma" and "pseudo-glaucoma". We have already mentioned on several occasions the condition of optic atrophy

[1] Vol. V.   [2] Vol. X, p. 315.

occurring in the presence of a normal ocular tension and a normal facility of aqueous outflow; such cases are believed to be due to sclerotic vascular disease within the optic nerve, and should be termed ISCHÆMIC OPTIC NEUROPATHY. Such a condition is usually bilateral but one-sided cases have been recorded (Morax, 1916; Kayser, 1921; vom Hofe, 1929; Magitot, 1938; and others), and a familial incidence has been noted (R. Weekers, 1942). The ischæmic atrophy may be associated with lesions outside the optic nerve itself, such as calcification of the adjacent cerebral arteries and tumours and calcifications in the hypophyseal region[1] (Thiel, 1930; Knapp, 1932; and others), but this occurrence is by no means invariable and probably acts through parallel sclerotic changes within the nerve. Similar changes may occur in the brain as lacunar atrophy when the cerebral circulation is impaired[2] (Sjøgren, 1946).

There is, in addition, a well-recognized, albeit uncommon group of cases wherein a normal ocular tension is associated with a reduced facility of aqueous outflow, glaucomatous cupping of the optic disc, and characteristic defects in the visual fields; for this group the term LOW-TENSION GLAUCOMA appears justified. It must be admitted, however, that the distinction between some cases of ischæmic optic neuropathy and others of low-tension glaucoma may not be clear-cut.

A type of low-tension glaucoma may possibly be due to a depression of secretion (*hyposecretory glaucoma*). In such cases, despite tonographic evidence of a decreased facility of outflow, the tension may remain normal but often shows fluctuations; damage to the optic nerve and loss of the visual field are often delayed but may occur in the absence of a diagnosis of the disease owing to the normality of the tension at the times of examination. The nature of this condition is unknown but hyposecretion is a common occurrence in advanced stages of glaucoma, caused presumably by degenerative changes in the ciliary body. It may also complicate tonographic records owing to the suppression of the formation of aqueous by a homeostatic mechanism[3] when the pressure is raised.

HYPERSECRETORY GLAUCOMA

There is a further rare group of cases, originally described by Becker and his co-workers (1956), wherein a raised ocular tension is associated with a normal facility of aqueous outflow and a raised aqueous minute-volume, occurring usually in females aged 40 to 60 suffering from vascular hypertension; similar cases have been described by Böck and Stepanik (1959) in myopic eyes, and by Mertens (1966). The rises of tension are usually intermittent reaching the tonometric value of the upper 20's or lower 30's, and probably because of their intermittency, damage to the optic nerve or defects in the visual fields are minimal and slow in developing. It is significant that these cases of HYPERSECRETORY GLAUCOMA may eventually

[1] Vol. XII.   [2] p. 440.   [3] Vol. IV, p. 330.

develop the characteristics of classical simple glaucoma with impaired drainage facilities (Becker and Shaffer, 1965).

The existence of such a condition is doubted by many observers and it must be admitted that the evidence in favour of it is sparse. Thus in his extensive tonographic surveys, Grant (1951) concluded that no case of glaucoma could be traced to hypersecretion and all to increased resistance to outflow. Moreover, evidence based solely on tonography with all its potential sources of error is suspicious. In such estimations it is essential to rule out a high episcleral venous pressure, an elevated ocular rigidity (by applanation tonometry), and the possibility of an intermittently closed angle which opens when the tonometer is applied. If the occurrence of such cases is accepted, miotics are of little value in relieving the raised tension which is rationally undertaken by diminishing the secretion of aqueous by topical adrenaline or, failing that, by carbonic anhydrase inhibitors.

PIGMENTARY GLAUCOMA

A migration of uveal pigment from the iris and ciliary body to the back of the cornea is a very common senile and degenerative phenomenon which occurs more frequently and at an earlier age in certain atrophic and inflammatory conditions, including glaucoma.[1] Although it has been suggested that the deposition of pigment at the filtration angle might be an ætiological factor in this disease, its absence in many cases of simple glaucoma and its frequent presence in normotensive eyes indicate that it is probably a concomitant of age.[2]

Many of the earlier observers noted that the deposition of pigment in the trabecular meshwork is a frequent occurrence in glaucomatous eyes.[3] In 1949, however, Sugar and Barbour described two cases of glaucoma which had several features in common, and since then over 100 cases of the condition they called *pigmentary glaucoma* have been reported.[4] Most of the patients have been young men (76·6%—Sugar, 1966) who were slightly or moderately myopic and who showed evidence of the dispersion of uveal pigment. This is indicated by a loss of the pigmentary epithelium at the periphery of the iris seen most clearly by transilluminating the iris (Scheie and Fleischhauer, 1958), and a deposition of pigment on the posterior surface

---

[1] Vol. VIII, p. 979.   [2] p. 448.

[3] von Hippel (1901), Levinsohn (1908–22), Salzmann (1914), Koeppe (1916–20), Schieck (1918), Gradle (1921), Trantas (1928–34), Barkan *et al.* (1936–54), Bangerter and Goldmann (1941), Sugar *et al.* (1941–51), Kronfeld and McGarry (1944), Sheppard and Romejko (1947), Troncoso (1947), François (1948–55), Löhlein (1949), and others.

[4] Calhoun (1952), Riffenburgh (1953), van Beuningen (1954–9), Bick (1957–62), Étienne and Pommier (1957), J. Malbrán (1957), Lebas (1958), Manna (1959), Oppel and Mrodzinsky (1959), Étienne (1960), Heinzen and Luder (1960), J. and E. Malbran (1960), Orzalesi and Verdi (1960), Perkins and Jay (1960), Bitrán and Garcés (1961), Cavka (1961), Dayal (1961), Kjer (1961), Legrand *et al.* (1961), Luder (1961), Perdriel and de Troyes (1961), Petersen (1961), Pietruschka (1961), Simón-Tor (1961), Stanković (1961), Gärtner (1964), Reboul (1964), Viñas *et al.* (1964), Perdriel *et al.* (1966), Sugar (1966), Zuege *et al.* (1967).

PLATE VI
PIGMENTARY GLAUCOMA
In a man aged 36 (Inst. Ophthal.)

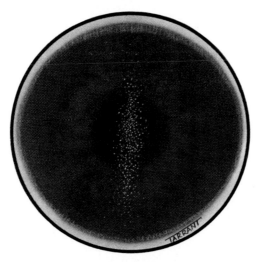

FIG. 1.—KRUKENBERG'S SPINDLE.

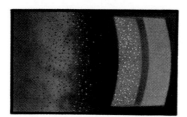

FIG. 2.—PIGMENT ON THE ENDO-
THELIAL SURFACE OF THE CORNEA.

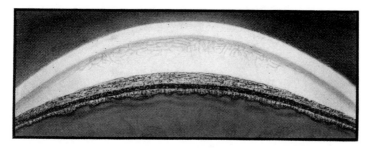

FIG. 3.—PIGMENT IN THE ANGLE OF THE ANTERIOR CHAMBER.

Figs. 503 and 504.—Pigmentary Glaucoma (N. Ashton).

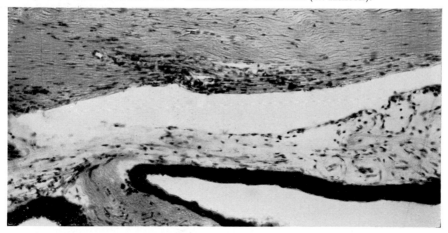

Fig. 503.—To show the accumulation of pigment granules in the drainage channels.

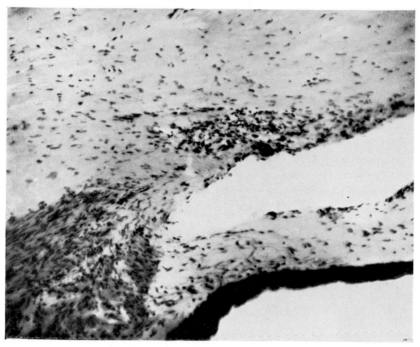

Fig. 504.—Both the drainage channels and the trabeculæ are heavily laden with pigment granules.

of the cornea, typically in the form of a Krukenberg spindle, on the trabecular meshwork of a gonioscopically open angle, on the anterior surface of the iris, on the zonular fibres, and on the surfaces of the lens (Plate VI; Figs. 503–4). The glaucoma appears similar to simple glaucoma although blurring of vision and headaches occasionally occur. Haloes around lights are common in the presence of an open angle and sometimes with a normal ocular tension; in these cases they are caused by the pigment on the posterior surface of the cornea. In some cases there is a rise in the ocular tension on dilating the pupil, even although the angle of the anterior chamber remains open, an effect explained by Sugar (1966) as being due to a mechanical narrowing of the already partly plugged trabecular spaces by the angle-crowding effect of pupillary dilatation.

There are various theories regarding the ætiology of pigmentary glaucoma. Bick (1957) and Scheie and Fleischhauer (1958) considered that concentric atrophy of the pigmentary epithelium of the iris was the primary lesion, while Sugar (1966) suggested that this atrophy resulted in the pigment-dispersion syndrome, the elevation of the ocular tension being a late-appearing component of the full syndrome. Other workers[1] do not believe that the pigmentation bears any relation to the glaucoma for which they postulate a developmental defect in the angle of the anterior chamber. Becker and his co-workers (Becker and Shaffer, 1965; Becker and Podos, 1966) considered that pigmentary glaucoma is only a variant of simple glaucoma and cited as evidence the occurrence of pigmentary glaucoma in the families of patients with simple glaucoma, the positive corticosteroid response in all members of the families of patients with pigmentary glaucoma, and the high incidence of a positive corticosteroid response in patients with Krukenberg spindles but without glaucoma.

The evidence so far available thus supports the concept that pigmentary glaucoma, like the glaucoma associated with pseudo-exfoliation of the lens capsule, is a variety of simple glaucoma and that the pigmentary disturbance is not the cause of the raised ocular tension.

Bangerter and Goldmann. *Ophthalmologica,* **102,** 321 (1941).

Barkan. *Amer. J. Ophthal.,* **37,** 504 (1954).

Barkan, Boyle and Maisler. *Amer. J. Ophthal.,* **19,** 209 (1936).

Becker, Keskey and Christensen. *Arch. Ophthal.,* **56,** 180 (1956).

Becker, Kolker and Roth. *Amer. J. Ophthal.,* **50,** 557 (1960).

Becker and Podos. *Arch. Ophthal.,* **76,** 635 (1966).

Becker and Shaffer. *Diagnosis and Treatment of the Glaucomas,* 2nd ed., St. Louis (1965).

Bertelsen, Davanger, Kolstad *et al. T. norske Lægeforen.,* **85,** 449 (1965).

van Beuningen. *v. Graefes Arch. Ophthal.,* **156,** 35 (1954).

Klin. Mbl. Augenheilk., **135,** 796 (1959).

Bick. *Arch. Ophthal.,* **58,** 483 (1957).

Amer. J. Ophthal., **54,** 831 (1962).

Bitrán and Garcés. *Arch. chil. Oftal.,* **18,** 43 (1961).

Böck and Stepanik. *v. Graefes Arch. Ophthal.,* **160,** 564 (1959).

Calhoun. *Trans. Amer. ophthal. Soc.,* **50,** 103 (1952).

Cavka. *Amer. J. Ophthal.,* **52,** 880 (1961).

Davanger. *Acta ophthal.* (Kbh.), **43,** 362 (1965).

Davanger and Holter. *Acta ophthal.* (Kbh.), **43,** 314 (1965).

[1] Calhoun (1952), Étienne and Pommier (1957), Malbrán (1957), van Beuningen (1959), Perkins (1960), Cavka (1961).

Dayal. *Amer. J. Ophthal.*, **51**, 324 (1961).
Étienne. *Ann. Oculist.* (Paris), **193**, 97, 224 (1960).
Étienne and Pommier. *Ann. Oculist.* (Paris.), **190**, 491 (1957).
François. *Bull. Soc. belge Ophtal.*, No. 88, 2 (1948).
  Adv. Ophthal., **4**, 19, 71 (1955).
Gärtner. *Ophthalmologica*, **147**, 393 (1964).
Goldmann. *Glaucoma* (Tutzing Symp., ed. Leydhecker), Basel, 213 (1967).
Gradle. *Amer. J. Ophthal.*, **4**, 427, 672 (1921).
Grant. *Arch. Ophthal.*, **46**, 113 (1951).
Heinzen and Luder. *Ophthalmologica*, **139**, 244 (1960).
von Hippel. *v. Graefes Arch. Ophthal.*, **52**, 498 (1901).
vom Hofe. *Arch. Augenheilk.*, **100–1**, 414 (1929).
Kayser. *Klin. Mbl. Augenheilk.*, **66**, 923 (1921).
Kellerman and Posner. *Amer. J. Ophthal.*, **40**, 681 (1955).
Kjer. *Acta ophthal.* (Kbh.), **39**, 993 (1961).
Knapp, A. *Arch. Ophthal.*, **8**, 637 (1932).
Koeppe. *Ber. dtsch. ophthal. Ges.*, **40**, 478 (1916); **42**, 87 (1920).
Kronfeld and McGarry. *Amer. J. Ophthal.*, **27**, 147 (1944).
Lebas. *Bull. Soc. belge Ophtal.*, No. 120, 628 (1958).
Legrand, Hervouët and Chevannes. *Bull. Soc. Ophtal. Fr.*, 807 (1961).
Levinsohn. *Arch. Augenheilk.*, **62**, 131 (1908).
  Klin. Mbl. Augenheilk., **68**, 471 (1922).
Leydhecker. *Trans. ophthal. Soc. U.K.*, **78**, 553 (1958).
  Docum. ophthal., **13**, 359 (1959).
  Glaukom: ein Handbuch, Berlin (1960).
  Glaucoma in Ophthalmic Practice, London (1966).
  Glaucoma (Tutzing Symp., ed. Leydhecker), Basel, 195 (1967).
Leydhecker, Akiyama and Neumann. *Klin. Mbl. Augenheilk.*, **133**, 662 (1958).
Linnér and Stromberg. *Glaucoma* (Tutzing Symp., ed. Leydhecker), Basel, 187 (1967).
Löhlein. *Wien. klin. Wschr.*, **61**, 698 (1949).
Luder. *Ophthalmologica*, **141**, 136 (1961).
Magitot. *Ann. Oculist.* (Paris), **175**, 349 (1938).
Malbrán, J. *Mod. Probl. Ophthal.*, **1**, 132 (1957).
Malbrán, J. and E. *Maroc méd.*, **39**, 430 (1960).
Manna. *Klin. oczna*, **29**, 233 (1959).

Mertens. *Klin. Mbl. Augenheilk.*, **148**, 175 (1966).
Miller and Paterson. *Brit. J. Ophthal.*, **46**, 513 (1962).
Morax. *Ann. Oculist.* (Paris), **153**, 25 (1916).
Oldham, Pickering, Roberts and Sowry. *Lancet*, **1**, 1085 (1960).
Opel and Mrodzinsky. *Med. Bild.*, **2**, 109 (1959).
Orzalesi and Verdi. *Ann. Ottal.*, **86**, 546 (1960).
Perdriel, Raynard, Joseph et al. *Bull. Soc. Ophtal. Fr.*, **66**, 260 (1966).
Perdriel and de Troyes. *Bull. Soc. Ophtal. Fr.*, 803 (1961).
Perkins. *Arch. Ophthal.*, **64**, 882 (1960).
Perkins and Jay. *Trans. ophthal. Soc. U.K.*, **80**, 153 (1960).
Petersen. *Acta ophthal.* (Kbh.), **39**, 688 (1961).
Pickering. *High Blood Pressure*, London (1955).
  Significant Trends in Medical Research (Ciba Fdn. Symp.), London (1959).
Pietruschka. *Wien. med. Wschr.*, **111**, 873 (1961).
Platt. *Trans. ophthal. Soc. U.K.*, **76**, 501 (1956); **79**, 559 (1959).
Reboul. *Bull. Soc. Ophtal. Fr.*, **64**, 852 (1964).
Riffenburgh. *Arch. Ophthal.*, **49**, 341 (1953).
Salzmann. *Z. Augenheilk.*, **31**, 1 (1914).
Scheie and Fleischhauer. *Arch. Ophthal.*, **59**, 216 (1958).
Schieck. *Klin. Mbl. Augenheilk.*, **61**, 332 (1918).
Sheppard and Romejko. *Amer. J. Ophthal.*, **30**, 159 (1947).
Simón-Tor. *Arch. Soc. oftal. hisp.-amer.*, **21**, 121 (1961).
Sjøgren. *Acta ophthal.* (Kbh.), **24**, 239 (1946).
Stanković. *Klin. Mbl. Augenheilk.*, **139**, 165 (1961).
Sugar. *Arch. Ophthal.*, **25**, 674 (1941).
  The Glaucomas, St. Louis, 300 (1951).
  Amer. J. Ophthal., **62**, 499 (1966).
Sugar and Barbour. *Amer. J. Ophthal.*, **32**, 90 (1949).
Thiel. *Ber. dtsch. ophthal. Ges.*, **48**, 133 (1930).
Trantas. *Arch. Ophtal.*, **45**, 617 (1928).
  Arch. Ottal., **41**, 39 (1934).
Troncoso. *A Treatise on Gonioscopy*, Phila., 306 (1947).
Viñas, Menezo and Quintana. *Arch. Soc. oftal. hisp.-amer.*, **24**, 407 (1964).
Weekers. *Ophthalmologica*, **104**, 316 (1942).
Zuege, Boyd and Stewart. *Canad. J. Ophthal.*, **2**, 271 (1967).

Ætiology

Our study of the pathology and clinical features of simple glaucoma has placed us in a position to assess what is known of its ætiology; unfortunately, our knowledge is not yet sufficient to allow us to dogmatize, particularly when we seek ultimate causes. It has now been established that one factor dominates the development of the disease—*an obstruction to the outflow of aqueous in the presence of an open angle*. This obstruction to outflow has been demonstrated by fluorometry (Goldmann, 1950), by tonography (Grant, 1951), and by the pressure-cup technique (Langham and Maumenee, 1964), but the site of the obstruction has not yet been finally decided. One fact is clear: that Priestley Smith's (1891) classical view that drainage was impeded by a large lens in a small eye is refuted by the gonioscopic finding that in simple glaucoma the angle is open.

THE SITE OF OBSTRUCTION TO THE OUTFLOW OF AQUEOUS

Over the past 30 years a considerable amount of research has been undertaken in order to determine the site of obstruction to the outflow of aqueous in simple glaucoma. At one time or another every tissue from the trabecular meshwork to the episcleral veins has been implicated; the various possible sites of obstruction will be discussed in turn.

1. THE TRABECULAR MESHWORK. Although some earlier workers such as Henderson (1910) and Verhoeff (1915) described a primary sclerosis and thickening of the trabecular meshwork in simple glaucoma, it was not until the pioneer work of Barkan (1936–54), when primary glaucoma had been divided into the narrow-angle and open-angle types, that gonioscopic changes in the trabeculæ were first adequately described. He found that in 65% of cases of simple glaucoma there was visible trabecular sclerosis and pigmentation, while in a further 25% there was trabecular sclerosis as indicated by a reduced permeability of the trabeculæ to direct light or to transillumination. Following this observation, some authors described gonioscopically visible changes attributable to trabecular sclerosis (Bangerter and Goldmann, 1941; Troncoso, 1947; van Beuningen, 1950; Vannini, 1952); van Beuningen (1950), for example, measured the optical density of the trabecular meshwork in simple glaucoma and found that in some patients there was a relationship between this and the ocular tension. On the other hand, most authors now believe that there are no gonioscopically pathognomonic signs of trabecular sclerosis.[1]

We have already seen[2] that the deposition of pigment in the trabecular meshwork is a frequent occurrence in glaucomatous eyes, but it must be remembered that pigmentary deposits of this nature are a constant occurrence in senile eyes[3] and are frequently observed in such conditions as diabetes, pigmentary retinal dystrophy and retinal detachments without affecting the ocular tension (Trantas, 1934). Since pigmentation of the trabecular meshwork is no more frequent in simple glaucoma than in normal

---

[1] Busacca (1945), François (1948–55), Kronfeld and McGarry (1948), Bottoni (1949), v. Fieandt (1949), Löhlein (1949), Hobbs (1950), Sugar (1951), Weekers and Prijot (1953), and many others.

[2] p. 486.   [3] Vol. IX, p. 750.

eyes of people over the age of 50, there is no substantial evidence that it contributes to the obstruction to the outflow of the aqueous.

The histological appearance of the trabecular meshwork in simple glaucoma has already been described[1] and it was concluded that although pathological changes can be demonstrated in the meshwork, it has not yet been conclusively determined that these changes are the cause of the raised tension rather than the result of it.

2. THE CANAL OF SCHLEMM. Seidel (1927) suggested that abnormalities in the endothelium of the canal of Schlemm rendered it relatively impermeable, but this observation has not been confirmed by subsequent workers although, as we have seen,[2] its narrowing and partial obstruction have been described.

One gonioscopic observation that has been widely reported in most cases of simple glaucoma is the absence of blood in the canal of Schlemm,[3] although Hobbs (1950), by compressing the episcleral tissues with a modified gonioprism, observed that blood entered the canal in a high proportion of cases. Blood is commonly seen in the canal of Schlemm in normal eyes and two possible explanations would account for its apparent absence with the normal methods of examination in simple glaucoma : either there is a marked pressure-gradient between the canal and the episcleral veins preventing the passage of blood into the canal, or the trabecular meshwork is less translucent than normal so that the view of the blood-filled canal is obscured.

3. THE COLLECTOR CHANNELS. Ascher (1942–53 ; Ascher and Spurgeon, 1949) has been a staunch champion of the concept that the collector channels are partially obstructed in simple glaucoma and that this was the cause of the reduction in the facility of outflow of aqueous ; his views have been supported by Gába (1949–51) but vigorously opposed by Goldmann (1946–55). It is agreed that in simple glaucoma, if a recipient vein is occluded just distal to its junction with an aqueous vein, blood flows from the recipient vein into the aqueous vein (the negative glass rod effect ; the blood influx phenomenon[4]). When this occurs, Ascher (1949) found that blood was rarely seen gonioscopically in the canal of Schlemm, and concluded that these observations indicated an obstruction in the collector channels ; on the other hand, Goldmann (1948–55) interpreted these observations as indicating a reduced flow in the canal of Schlemm due to an obstruction to the aqueous in the trabecular meshwork.

We have already mentioned the histological changes that have been described in the collector channels in simple glaucoma which in advanced cases may progress to complete obliteration of the episcleral veins due, presumably, to degenerative changes in the scleral collagen.[5] Although a

---

[1] p. 413.   [2] p. 415.
[3] Trantas (1934), Barkan *et al.* (1936), Bangerter and Goldmann (1941), Kronfeld (1947), François (1948), Bottoni (1949), Vannini (1952), Sugar (1957), Becker and Shaffer (1965), and others.
[4] Vol. II, p. 200.   [5] p. 419.

raised pressure in the episcleral veins has been associated with the diurnal variation in intra-ocular pressure in both normal and glaucomatous eyes,[1] it has been shown that there is no overall significant difference in this venous pressure between the normal and the pathological state (Goldmann, 1951; Linnér, 1956; Leith, 1963).

The great disadvantage of deducing the ætiology of the disease from histological evidence is the difficulty in ascribing the cause of the initial rise in tension to the appearances of tissue in the advanced stages when the eyes usually become available for microscopic study. Even in early cases, however, the occurrence of a decrease in the facility of outflow has been amply demonstrated clinically, but whether the obstruction lies in the trabecular region or in the outflow channels through the sclera or in both is a matter of debate. Possibly the evidence is in favour of the former being usually the more important.

On the other hand, more subtle factors may be operative. The size of the pores in the trabecular meshwork may be of importance for, according to Poiseuille's law, the flow should vary directly as the fourth power of their diameter. Davanger (1964–65) has shown that, assuming there is a reduction in their diameter averaging 5% from youth to old age, eyes which had initially a small pore-diameter and a relatively high normal intra-ocular pressure will tend to develop simple glaucoma, a process which would be hastened by the early occurrence of sclerotic changes. Such a suggestion accounts for an increase of simple glaucoma not proportionately but approximately exponentially with age. Again, the failure of the capacity of the endothelial cells of the trabecular wall of Schlemm's canal to aid the drainage of aqueous by the development of cytoplasmic vesicles[2] might contribute to similar difficulties.

Whatever the cause of the obstruction may be, it would seem to be an exaggeration of the sclerotic processes characteristic of age which, of course, show a hereditary tendency, and are frequently associated with anoxia of the tissues owing to vascular insufficiency as occurs in the optic nerve.

It has been suggested that the vasosclerosis undoubtedly seen in eyes with advanced glaucoma, whether this is causal or consequential, is a degenerative condition associated with widespread arteriosclerosis throughout the body, or is the result of neuro-vegetative or endocrine imbalance. We have seen,[3] however, that although simple glaucoma and generalized arteriosclerosis frequently occur in the same patient, the evidence for a direct association between the two conditions is far from strong, that a disturbance of the neuro-vegetative system probably plays no part in the ætiology of the disease, and that any association between certain endocrine disturbances and simple glaucoma needs further clarification.

HYPERSECRETION

von Graefe (1855) first assumed that glaucoma was due to the hypersecretion of the intra-ocular fluid owing to a serous choroiditis, a view modified by Donders (1862) who held that the cause of the excessive secretion was nervous irritation of the choroid.

[1] p. 456.   [2] p. 419.   [3] p. 408.

Following his teaching several observers attributed glaucoma to an over-secretion by ciliary "glands" under the stimulus of the trigeminal nerve (v. Hippel and Grünhagen, 1868–70; Mooren 1882) or sympathetic irritation (Abadie, 1897–1923; and others), or owing to general influences (Hill and Flack, 1912). Recently Becker and his co-workers (1956) have described a rare type of open-angle glaucoma characterized by an elevated ocular tension associated with an increased production of aqueous and a normal facility of aqueous outflow, occurring particularly in middle-aged women with systemic hypertension. Some of these cases have progressed to a clinical picture indistinguishable from simple glaucoma (Becker and Shaffer, 1965), but the evidence for the existence of this type of glaucoma is far from satisfying.[1]

SWELLING OF THE VITREOUS BODY. Many investigators in the past have considered that swelling of the vitreous body may be a determining factor in the ætiology of glaucoma. M. H. Fischer (1908–9) and Thomas and Fischer (1910) immersed excised eyes in acids and generated a pressure sufficient to burst the sclera; this Fischer explained as an œdematous swelling of the vitreous, but subsequent workers[2] demonstrated that the high pressures were due to swelling of all the other ocular tissues by exposure to concentrations of acids far in excess of physiological variations. It was then demonstrated that both the isolated proteins of the vitreous (Duke-Elder, 1930), and the vitreous gel *in vitro*[3] show a decrease of volume with an acid and an increase with an alkaline reaction, a result confirmed in the perfused experimental animal (Duke-Elder, 1931). Although it has been shown that swelling of the vitreous does occur to a small extent with alkaline reactions, we have already seen that the reaction of the blood and the calcium-potassium quotient of glaucomatous patients are within normal limits[4]; moreover, any change in the swelling-pressure is so small both in the normal and glaucomatous eye as to rule out any influence of the vitreous in the ætiology of pathological rises of tension (Duke-Elder *et al.*, 1935–36).

Other suggestions as to the possible mechanism of a swelling of the vitreous have been made—an alteration of the permeability of the hyaloid membrane, an increase in its protein content (Raeder, 1924; Nordenson, 1924–26), or a retention of mucin (Verhoeff, 1925); but these are equally unsubstantiated.

OSMOTIC THEORIES. The general osmotic concentration of the body was assumed to be at fault in glaucoma by Cantonnet (1904) and Hertel (1913), but as we have already seen,[5] the blood of glaucomatous patients shows no constant osmolar deviation. Osmotic changes in the intra-ocular fluid have also been associated with rises of tension, particularly a rise in the protein content, but these occurred in cases of glaucoma secondary to intra-ocular inflammations or of primary closed-angle glaucoma; indeed, it has been shown that in simple glaucoma there is no significant alteration in the molar concentration of the intra-ocular fluid (Benham *et al.*, 1938).

TOXÆMIA. That glaucoma is the expression of a general toxæmia has been suggested by several authors without any satisfying evidence.[6]

LOSS OF ELASTICITY OF THE SCLERA. Sclerosis of the sclera has been cited as an important factor in the determination of simple glaucoma (Kuschel, 1908), but the elasticity of this structure is so small that it cannot exert any great influence.

In summary, therefore, it may be said that the immediate cause of simple glaucoma is an obstruction to the drainage of the aqueous at the

---

[1] p. 485.

[2] Knape (1909), v. Fürth and Hanke (1913), Ruben (1913), Nakamura (1925), Heesch (1926), and F. P. Fischer (1929).

[3] Meesmann (1924), Redslob and Reiss (1928), Lobeck (1929), Duke-Elder (1930).

[4] p. 405.   [5] p. 406.

[6] Bjerrum (1912), Orr (1914), Sattler (1915), Kerry (1925), Davis (1928), and others.

angle of the anterior chamber in some—or all—of the channels of outflow. The evidence at present indicates that the trabecular meshwork is most probably the principal site of the lesion, particularly near the inner wall of the canal of Schlemm, but the intimate nature of the changes therein and their determining cause are not yet fully clarified. For practical purposes the several other ætiological theories which have been advanced can be neglected.

Abadie. *Arch. Ophtal.*, **17**, 375 (1897).
  Clin. Ophtal., **12**, 303 (1923).
Ascher. *Amer. J. Ophthal.*, **25**, 1174 (1942).
  Arch. Ophthal., **42**, 66 (1949); **49**, 438 (1953).
Ascher and Spurgeon. *Amer. J. Ophthal.*, **32** (2), 239 (1949).
Bangerter and Goldmann. *Ophthalmologica*, **102**, 321 (1941).
Barkan. *Arch. Ophthal.*, **15**, 101 (1936).
  Amer. J. Ophthal., **21**, 1099 (1938); **37**, 724 (1954).
Barkan, Boyle and Maisler. *Amer. J. Ophthal.*, **19**, 209 (1936).
Becker, Keskey and Christensen. *Arch. Ophthal.*, **56**, 180 (1956).
Becker and Shaffer. *Diagnosis and Therapy of the Glaucomas*, St. Louis (1965).
Benham, Duke-Elder and Hodgson. *J. Physiol.*, **92**, 355 (1938).
van Beuningen. *Ber. dtsch. ophthal. Ges.*, **56**, 132 (1950).
Bjerrum. *Klin. Mbl. Augenheilk.*, **50** (1), 42 (1912).
Bottoni. *Ann. Ottal.*, **75**, 279 (1949).
Busacca. *Éléments de gonioscopie*, São Paulo (1945).
Cantonnet. *Arch. Ophtal.*, **24**, 193 (1904).
Davanger. *Acta ophthal.* (Kbh.), **42**, 753, 764, 773 (1964); **43**, 362 (1965).
Davis. *Virginia med. Mthly.*, **54**, 628 (1928).
Donders. See Haffmanns. *v. Graefes Arch. Ophthal.*, **8** (2), 160 (1862).
Duke-Elder. *The Nature of the Vitreous Body* (*Brit. J. Ophthal.*, Monog. Suppl. 4), London (1930).
Duke-Elder and Davson. *Biochem. J.*, **29**, 1121 (1935).
  Brit. J. Ophthal., **19**, 433 (1935).
Duke-Elder, Davson and Benham. *Brit. J. Ophthal.*, **20**, 520 (1936).
Duke-Elder, W. S. and P. M. *J. Physiol.*, **71**, 268 (1931).
  Proc. roy. Soc. B, **109**, 19 (1931).
von Fieandt. *Acta ophthal.* (Kbh.), Suppl. 34 (1949).
Fischer, F. P. *Arch. Augenheilk.*, **100–1**, 146, 480 (1929).
Fischer, M. H. *Pflügers Arch. ges. Physiol.*, **124**, 69; **125**, 99, 396 (1908); **127**, 1, 46 (1909).
François. *La gonioscopie*, Louvain (1948).
  Glaucoma: a Symposium (ed. Duke-Elder), Oxon., 169 (1955).
von Fürth and Hanke. *Z. Augenheilk.*, **29**, 252 (1913).

Gába. *Cs. Oftal.*, **5**, 168 (1949); **7**, 251 (1951).
Goldmann. *Ophthalmologica*, **111**, 146 (1946); **119**, 65 (1950).
  Lhb. d. Augenheilk. (ed. Amsler *et al.*), Basel, 391 (1948).
  Ann. Oculist. (Paris), **184**, 1086 (1951).
  Glaucoma: a Symposium (ed. Duke-Elder), Oxon., 105 (1955).
von Graefe. *v. Graefes Arch. Ophthal.*, **2** (1), 248 (1855).
Grant. *Arch. Ophthal.*, **46**, 113 (1951).
Heesch. *Arch. Augenheilk.*, **97**, 546 (1926).
Henderson. *Glaucoma*, London (1910).
Hertel. *Klin. Mbl. Augenheilk.*, **51** (2), 351 (1913).
Hill and Flack. *Proc. roy. Soc. B.*, **85**, 439 (1912).
von Hippel and Grünhagen. *v. Graefes Arch. Ophthal.*, **14** (3), 219 (1868); **15** (1), 265 (1869); **16** (1), 27 (1870).
Hobbs. *Brit. J. Ophthal.*, **34**, 489 (1950).
Kerry. *Trans. ophthal. Soc. U.K.*, **45**, 355 (1925).
Knape. *Skand. Arch. Physiol.*, **23**, 162 (1909).
Kronfeld. *Arch. Ophthal.*, **38**, 400 (1947).
Kronfeld and McGarry. *J. Amer. med. Ass.*, **136**, 957 (1948).
Kuschel. *Z. Augenheilk.*, **19**, 97, 193, 426; Erg., 45; **20**, 423 (1908).
Langham and Maumenee. *Trans. Amer. Acad. Ophthal.*, **68**, 277 (1964).
Leith. *Brit. J. Ophthal.*, **47**, 271 (1963).
Linnér. *Amer. J. Ophthal.*, **41**, 646 (1956).
Lobeck. *v. Graefes Arch. Ophthal.*, **122**, 668 (1929).
Löhlein. *Wien. klin. Wschr.*, **61**, 698 (1949).
Meesmann. *Arch. Augenheilk.*, **94**, 115 (1924).
Mooren. *Ueber d. Verbreitung d. sympathischen Störungen*, Wiesbaden (1882).
Nakamura. *Arch. Augenheilk.*, **96**, 131 (1925).
Nordenson. *Upsala Läk.-Fören. Förh.*, **29**, 1 (1924); **31**, 289 (1926).
Orr. *Ophthal. Rev.*, **33**, 33 (1914).
Raeder. *T. norske Laegeforen.*, No. 14 (1924); see *Zbl. ges. Ophthal.*, **14**, 239 (1925).
Redslob and Reiss. *Ann. Oculist.* (Paris), **165**, 641 (1928); **166**, 1 (1929).
Ruben. *v. Graefes Arch. Ophthal.*, **86**, 258 (1913).
Sattler. *Trans. Amer. ophthal. Soc.*, **14**, 38 (1915).
Seidel. Abderhalden's *Hb. d. biol. Arbeitsmethoden*, Berlin, **5** (6), 1019 (1927).

Smith, Priestley. *The Pathology and Treatment of Glaucoma*, London (1891).

Sugar. *The Glaucomas*, St. Louis (1951); 2nd ed. (1957).

Thomas and Fischer. *Ann. Ophthal.*, **19,** 40 (1910).

Trantas. *Arch. Ottal.*, **41,** 39 (1934).

Troncoso. *Treatise on Gonioscopy*, Phila. (1947).

Vannini. *Rass. ital. Ottal.*, **21,** 65 (1952).

Verhoeff. *Arch. Ophthal.*, **44,** 129 (1915); **54,** 20 (1925).

Weekers and Prijot. *Ann. Oculist.* (Paris), **186,** 596 (1953).

Diagnosis

An eye which presents the classical features of simple glaucoma—a cupped and atrophic optic disc, typical defects in the visual fields, a raised ocular tension, and a reduced facility of outflow with a gonioscopically open angle, all in the absence of other ocular disease—offers no difficulty in diagnosis.

From the clinical point of view, the one sign on which doubt may arise is the cupping of the disc, for slight or atypical cases occur in which differentiation may be difficult or impossible on this sign alone. In any case, however, it is dangerous to make a diagnosis solely on this feature, but in forming a judgement the evidence which it supplies should be correlated with that from every available source; and this is sometimes only possible after repeated observations maintained over some time. In such observations a deepening of the cup is of importance and in making successive examinations reliance should be placed not on memory but on repeated drawings or preferably repeated photography.

The following conditions may be mistaken for a glaucomatous cup:

1. *A Physiological Cup.* Here the depression is rarely deep and usually does not involve the entire area of the disc; the portion which is excavated is white in colour but the other areas appear pink. The cup does not show an overhanging edge and the vessels can usually be traced from their first appearance without interruption until they reach the fundus and, although the nasal vessels may show a distinct bend, they show no abnormal pulsation (Fig. 505); moreover the physiological disc shows fluorescence throughout on fluorescein angiography while a glaucomatous disc does not (Fig. 506 compared with Figs. 470–5). The glaucomatous cup, on the other hand, although it may start on one side, usually the lower temporal quadrant, eventually involves the entire circumference and the whole area of the disc, so that its sides are steep and not shelving. Difficult cases, of course, arise, particularly when a physiological passes into a pathological cup, in which case ophthalmoscopic differentiation may be impossible.

2. *An atrophic cup* is usually very shallow without the steeply overhanging edge, and the vessels are normal: a differentiation is usually possible by the visual fields, and particularly the colour fields which are disproportionately affected in atrophic and not in glaucomatous states. Moreover, in glaucoma the light-minimum is affected and the light-difference not, while in atrophy the reverse is usually the case.

3. *A colobomatous cup* is usually larger than the area of a normal disc and generally gives the impression of an irregular funnel in emerging from which the vessels rarely show regular kinking. In most of these congenital conditions there are some congenital deformities elsewhere in the eye or its fellow, and the vessels on the floor of the coloboma are frequently veiled with neuroglial tissue. Moreover, if a peripapillary halo is present, it is irregular and usually heavily pigmented in a colobomatous eye (Stood, 1884;

Zade, 1907; Rønne, 1921; A. Fuchs, 1924–28). It is to be noted also that an obliquely inserted nerve-head may produce an apparent bending of the vessels at the margin of the disc (A. Fuchs, 1924).

4. The conditions of *ischæmic optic neuropathy* and *atrophy due to sclerosis of the cerebral arteries* frequently present many difficulties. As we have seen, in the former condition some help may be obtained from the fact that the field for red is disproportionately constricted and the photochromatic interval is greater than 5°. In most cases, however, reliance must be placed on the constant absence of abnormal tension and the presence of a normal facility of outflow, and this can only be safely assumed

FIGS. 505 AND 506.—PHYSIOLOGICAL CUPPING OF THE OPTIC DISC.

In a woman aged 44 with an intra-ocular pressure of 15 to 17 mm. Hg and normal visual fields (J. A. Oosterhuis).

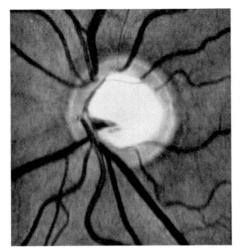
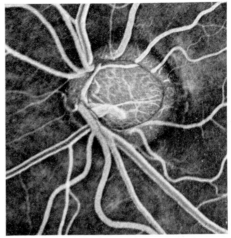

FIG. 505.—Photograph of the optic disc.

FIG. 506.—Fluorescence angiogram showing filling of all the small vessels on the disc (*cf.* Figs. 470 to 475).

after the demonstration of a normal diurnal tension-curve over a period of a few days and the ability of the eye to withstand more than one provocative tension-test. These questions will be discussed immediately.

The *diagnosis of early glaucoma*, however, is a much more difficult task and an important necessity in a disease the onset of which is usually insidious and often not realized by the patient, and the treatment of which is frequently effective in the initial stages but very problematical when much damage has been done to the function of the eye. Its importance is to be stressed in view of the length of time of the pre-glaucomatous stage; we have already seen that on the average the interval between the occurrence of a raised tension and the development of a deterioration in function is probably 18 years (Leydhecker, 1959), a period during which hypotensive measures can often be successfully undertaken. It is to be noted that *cupping of the optic disc and gross defects in the visual fields are signs of established glaucoma which has reached a stage at which considerable and irremediable functional damage has already occurred.*

In doubtful cases the estimation of the *ocular tension* is of the greatest importance. It is to be remembered that applanation tonometric recording is always preferable and that readings with an indentation tonometer should always be corrected for ocular rigidity particularly in myopic eyes wherein this factor may be low. Moreover, it cannot be stated too strongly that *in the diagnosis of early simple glaucoma the finding of a normal—or even subnormal—tension on one or more occasions is no criterion that glaucoma does not exist.* In suspicious cases an investigation of the *diurnal variations* in tension should be undertaken over a period of two or three days while the patient maintains a regular mode of life, measurements being taken several times a day, the first before the patient stirs in the morning. Even although the tension never rises above the "normal" limits, a variation of more than 5 mm. Hg indicates the presence of latent glaucoma.

The *visual fields* show changes only when the disease has become established but although they may only confirm and not initiate the diagnosis the detection of the earliest manifestations are of importance, particularly when other signs of the disease are equivocal. The examination should be made with the greatest care with campimetry in a low illumination and is best conducted at a distance of 2 metres using an object of 1/2,000, or with the use of the Goldmann perimeter. When the conditions for these standard methods are not available, small portable campimeters can be used, such as the projection scotopter of Ben-Tovim (1967). The earliest signs are a baring of the blind-spot, a depression of the upper portion of the central field, a step-defect on the horizontal meridian on the nasal side, and small isolated scotomata on the 15° circle between the blind-spot and the vertical meridian. The presence of the last characteristic is indicative of the occurrence of actual damage to the nerve fibres and its absence in no sense proves the absence of glaucoma.

PROVOCATIVE TESTS

The object of provocative tests is to elicit any lack of control of the ocular tension, for the normal eye has the capacity to maintain its pressure in equilibrium despite considerable stress, an adaptability which the glaucomatous eye tends to lose. Several of these have been suggested but it is to be remembered that, while fairly conclusive if positive, a negative result means little for they are not universally effective nor is there a uniform response with the same patient at different times; their value lies in the corroborative evidence they bear in conjunction with other factors.

The water-drinking test of Marx (1925–28) applied to the eye by Schmidt (1928–31) is probably the most useful in simple glaucoma. The patient is asked to undertake the distinctly unpleasant task of drinking 1 litre of water before breakfast as rapidly as possible and the ocular tension is then taken every 15 minutes for 1 or preferably 2 hours (Fig. 507). The earlier reports in the literature are difficult to evaluate[1] but more recently a rise of ocular tension of 7–10 mm. is generally considered to be pathological.[2] Leydhecker (1954) found that the test was positive in only 17% of patients with simple glaucoma when the initial ocular tension was normal, and in 62% when the initial tension was over 30 mm., although other workers have claimed a considerably higher percentage of positive results in this disease (82%—Bloomfield and Kellerman, 1947; 94·7%—Agarwal and Sharma, 1953; 70%—Swanljung and Blodi, 1956).

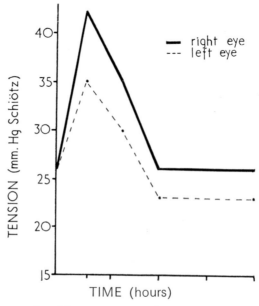

FIG. 507.—THE WATER-DRINKING TEST IN SIMPLE GLAUCOMA
(Ɖ. A. Campbell *et al.*).

A refinement of the water-drinking test is to perform tonography 1 hour after the ingestion of 1 litre of water and then to calculate the ratio P_0/C. Becker and Christensen (1956) found that, in these circumstances, P_0/C was greater than 100 in 97% of patients with simple glaucoma, and Leydhecker (1958) also found this combined test of particular value. This last worker recommended that tonography should be performed for 7 minutes but that only the results obtained in the last 4 minutes should be used to calculate the ratio P_3/C_{3-7}, a ratio which he considered more sensitive than

[1] Schmidt (1928–31), de Decker (1929), Poos (1930), Wegner (1930), Gradle (1931), Heegaard-Larsen (1931), Larsen (1932), Ohm (1936), Spadavecchia (1936–37), Evans (1942), and others.
[2] Sugar (1948), Leydhecker (1950–60), Agarwal and Sharma (1953), Campbell *et al.* (1955), Kronfeld (1955), Becker and Christensen (1956), Ourgaud and Junod (1959), and many others.

P_0/C_{0-4}.   More recent workers have confirmed the value of this combined test in the early diagnosis of the disease.[1]

BULBAR PRESSURE TESTS.   It has been known for some considerable time that massage of the globe or the resting of a weight upon the closed lid, should lower the ocular tension in the normal eye, and that this reduction in tension is less or does not occur in the glaucomatous eye.   This observation was the basis of the *massage test* of P. Knapp (1912) practised by Dieter (1928) and Gradle (1931), and has resulted in the development of tonography,[2] of Suda's compression test, and of Blaxter's bulbar pressure test.

FIGS. 508 AND 509.—BLAXTER'S BULBAR PRESSURE TEST.

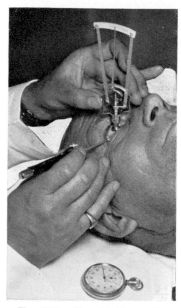

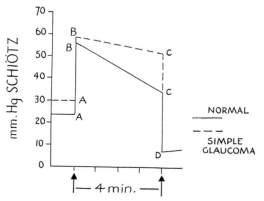

FIG. 508.—Showing the application of the ophthalmodynamometer and the Schiøtz tonometer (P. Blaxter).

FIG. 509.—The reaction in Blaxter's bulbar pressure test. A dynamometric pressure of 50 G. is applied at the first arrow and removed at the second. The initial tension is shown at A. The readings at B are taken 15 sec. later to allow the ocular tension to stabilize. After 4 min. the readings C are taken; on the release of pressure the reading D is taken. The outflow fraction is represented by $\dfrac{(B - C)\,100}{B}$.

Suda and his co-workers (1951–65) have demonstrated that after compressing the globe with a 50 G. weight for 10 minutes the ocular tension falls to very low levels in most normal eyes and falls to a less extent in glaucomatous eyes.   If the tension after compression is below 4 mm. Hg the eye can be considered free from glaucoma, while if the tension is over 8 mm. glaucoma is almost certainly present.

Blaxter (1953) described a test whereby a weight of 50 G. is applied by a dynamometer to the globe for 4 minutes while a tonometer is resting on

[1] Greinecker (1963), Becker and Shaffer (1965), Chandler and Grant (1965), Suda *et al.* (1965), Leydhecker (1966), Pollack (1967), and others.
[2] p. 461.

the cornea. This test depends upon the change of ocular tension during compression, and from this change an "outflow fraction" is calculated. If this fraction is below 30, an obstruction to the outflow of aqueous is considered to be present (Figs. 508–9). This test is simple to perform and has been considered by many workers to be useful in the early diagnosis of simple glaucoma[1] but does not replace tonography as a diagnostic method when the necessary equipment is available.

A similar test using a suction cup instead of a dynamometer was introduced by Evans and Klein (1959); the results in normal eyes and those with simple glaucoma are seen in Fig. 510.

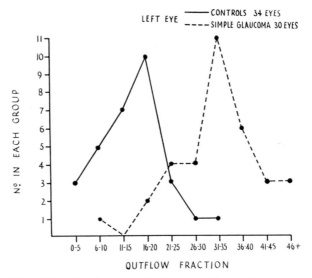

FIG. 510.—THE OUTFLOW FRACTION IN SIMPLE GLAUCOMA.

The outflow fraction (see Fig. 509) in normal eyes (continuous line) and eyes with simple glaucoma (broken line) (E. M. Evans and M. Klein).

BLOOD-PRESSURE TESTS. The *caffeine test*. In its simplest form the patient drinks 150 ml. water containing 45 G. caffeine: in the normal eye there is little change in the ocular tension; in the glaucomatous eye a rise of tension may occur in from 20 to 60 minutes.[2] A similar response follows the intravenous[3] or subcutaneous (Sallmann and Deutsch, 1930; Federici, 1932; Sugar, 1948) injection of 0·2 G. caffeine. In these tests Leydhecker and Niesel (1954) considered that a rise of 6 mm. Hg was probably, and one of 9 mm. definitely diagnostic of glaucoma, but the test is positive in only

[1] Andreani (1954), Ourgaud and Étienne (1961), Tulevech and Berens (1962), Reddy *et al.* (1966), and others.
[2] Thiel (1925), Gradle (1931), Ohm (1936), Gilde (1937), Brinke (1950), Schmidt (1950), Kolb (1952), Leydhecker (1955), Kern (1964), and others.
[3] Wegner (1925), Stein (1933), Evans (1942), Leydhecker (1955).

about 15% of eyes with simple glaucoma and is therefore considered unreliable. Wegner (1925–30) and Löhlein (1926) performed a similar test
by giving the patient two cups of strong black coffee to drink; a rise of
tension of 15–25 mm. Hg may occur after 20–40 minutes in glaucomatous
eyes.

The Vasculat Test. The subconjunctival injection of the vasodilator,
Vasculat (*p*-oxyphenyl-butamino-ethanol), was found to produce a rise of
ocular tension of more than 12 mm. Hg in a high proportion of eyes with
simple glaucoma (Leydhecker, 1953). It produces, however, a red and
painful eye and is therefore not suitable as a provocative test.

The Priscol Test. The subconjunctival injection of Priscol, however,
is well tolerated by the eye, and produces a rise of tension of 9 mm. Hg or
more in about 50% of eyes with simple glaucoma.[1]

The Amyl Nitrite Test. The inhalation of amyl nitrite was found by
Cristini and Pagliarani (1953) to cause little or no change in eyes with normal
intra-ocular pressure but a considerable fall in patients with simple glaucoma,
particularly those showing extensive diurnal variations.

The Jugular Compression Test. By constricting the neck so that venous congestion is produced, a rise of ocular tension has been reported in glaucomatous eyes
(Thiel, 1925; Bloomfield and Lambert, 1945; Agarwal and Sharma, 1953). Thomassen
and Leydhecker (1950), however, showed the very limited value of this test for they
found it positive in only 14% of patients with simple glaucoma.

In order to improve the selectivity of the jugular compression test, Bloomfield
and Lambert (1945) combined it with the *cold pressor test* of Hines and Brown (1933)
wherein one of the patient's hands is immersed in ice-cold water. Although several
workers have found this combined test (*the lability test*) of value in the early diagnosis
of simple glaucoma,[2] Thomassen and Leydhecker (1950) demonstrated that the cold
pressor test has little or no effect on the ocular tension so that the lability test should
be assessed solely as the effect of jugular compression and is thus of little value in the
diagnosis of simple glaucoma.

In this connection it is interesting that the increase in systemic venous pressure
induced by the Valsalva manœuvre (Rosen and Johnston, 1959) or by pressure-
breathing with the aid of an oxygen-inhalation apparatus (Segal *et al.*, 1967) has not
been found to raise the intra-ocular pressure in glaucomatous eyes more than in
normal controls.

Bodily Position. Changes in the position of the body from the vertical to the
horizontal normally cause little alteration in the intra-ocular pressure, averaging 1 to
6 mm. Hg (Bain and Maurice, 1959; Armaly and Salamoun, 1963), although a considerable rise may occur if the head is dramatically lowered (a rise of 19 to 21 mm. Hg
in the 75° head-down position, Tarkkanen and Leikola, 1967). In cases of simple
glaucoma, a slight tilting downwards (8 in. below the feet) may induce a higher rise of
ocular tension (av. 5·29 mm. Hg) than normal (av. 0·42 mm. Hg), a differentiation
increased when combined with the water-drinking test. This change in pressure is
probably due to a rise in the venous pressure.

[1] Leydhecker (1954–55), Cramer *et al.* (1955), Sugar and Santos (1955), Swanljung and
Blodi (1956), Primrose (1962), and others.
[2] Bloomfield *et al.* (1945–49), Stine (1948), Sugar (1948), Symowski (1948), Esente (1949).
Weinstein (1950), Imai and Shimizu (1951), and others.

Agarwal and Sharma. *Brit. J. Ophthal.*, **37**, 330 (1953).
Andreani. *Ann. Ottal.*, **80**, 261 (1954).
Armaly and Salamoun. *Arch. Ophthal.*, **70**, 603 (1963).
Bain and Maurice. *Trans. ophthal. Soc. U.K.*, **79**, 249 (1959).
Becker and Christensen. *Arch. Ophthal.*, **56**, 321 (1956).
Becker and Shaffer. *Diagnosis and Therapy of the Glaucomas*, St. Louis (1965).
Ben-Tovim. *Amer. J. Ophthal.*, **64**, 780 (1967).
Blaxter. *Brit. J. Ophthal.*, **37**, 641 (1953).
Bloomfield. *Arch. Ophthal.*, **38**, 368 (1947). *N.Y. St. J. Med.*, **49**, 659 (1949).
Bloomfield and Kellerman. *Amer. J. Ophthal.*, **30**, 869 (1947).
Bloomfield and Lambert. *Arch. Ophthal.*, **34**, 83 (1945).
Brinke. *Untersuch. ü d. Verwertbarkeit d. Coffeinbelastung als Frühdiagnose d. Glaukoms* (Diss.), Münster (1950).
Campbell, Gloster and Tonks. *Brit. J. Ophthal.*, **39**, 193 (1955).
Chandler and Grant. *Lectures on Glaucoma*, London (1965).
Cramer, Iribarren, Sampaolesi *et al. Arch. Oftal. B. Aires*, **30**, 347 (1955).
Cristini and Pagliarani. *Brit. J. Ophthal.*, **37**, 741 (1953).
de Decker. *Arch. Augenheilk.*, **100–1**, 180 (1929).
Dieter. *Arch. Augenheilk.*, **99**, 678 (1928).
Esente. *Boll. Oculist.*, **28**, 77 (1949).
Evans, E. M. and Klein. *Brit. J. Ophthal.*, **43**, 494 (1959).
Evans, J. N. *Arch. Ophthal.*, **27**, 1177 (1942).
Federici. *Boll. Oculist.*, **11**, 752 (1932).
Fuchs, A. *Amer. J. Ophthal.*, **7**, 425 (1924). *Brit. J. Ophthal.*, **12**, 65 (1928).
Gartner and Beck. *Amer. J. Ophthal.*, **59**, 1040 (1965).
Gilde. *Untersuch. ü. d. Wirkung d. Pilocarpins, Homatropins u. Kaffees a. d. intraokularen Druck . . .* (Diss.), Königsberg (1937).
Gradle. *Amer. J. Ophthal.*, **14**, 936 (1931).
Greinecker. *Klin. Mbl. Augenheilk.*, **142**, 634 (1963).
Heegaard-Larsen. *Acta ophthal.* (Kbh.), **9**, 302 (1931).
Hines and Brown. *Ann. intern. Med.*, **7**, 209 (1933).
Imai and Shimizu. *Acta Soc. ophthal. jap.*, **55**, 160 (1951).
Kern. *Ophthalmologica*, **147**, 93 (1964).
Knapp, P. *Klin. Mbl. Augenheilk*, **50** (1), 691 (1912).
Kolb. *Klin. Mbl. Augenheilk.*, **121**, 524 (1952).
Kronfeld. *Glaucoma: a Symposium* (ed. Duke-Elder), Oxon., 226 (1955).
Larsen. *Nord. Med.*, **4**, 318 (1932).
Leydhecker. *Brit. J. Ophthal.*, **34**, 456 (1950); **38**, 290 (1954).

Leydhecker. *Klin. Mbl. Augenheilk.*, **123**, 568 (1953); **125**, 57 (1954); **132**, 77 (1958). *Glaucoma: a Symposium* (ed. Duke-Elder), Oxon., 205 (1955). *Amer. J. Ophthal.*, **39**, 700 (1955). *Docum. ophthal.*, **13**, 357 (1959). *Glaukom: ein Handbuch*, Berlin (1960). *Glaucoma in Ophthalmic Practice*, London (1966).
Leydhecker and Niesel. *Klin. Mbl. Augenheilk.*, **125**, 458 (1954).
Löhlein. *Klin. Mbl. Augenheilk.*, **77**, Beil., 1 (1926).
Marx. *Klin. Wschr.*, **4**, 2339 (1925); **5**, 92 (1926); **6**, 1750 (1927). *Dtsch. Arch. klin. Med.*, **152**, 354; **153**, 358 (1926); **158**, 149 (1928).
Ohm. *v. Graefes Arch. Ophthal.*, **135**, 537 (1936).
Ourgaud and Étienne. *L'exploration fonctionnelle de l'œil glaucomateux*, Paris (1961).
Ourgaud and Junod. *Bull. Soc. Ophtal. Fr.*, 331 (1959).
Pollack. *Symposium on Glaucoma* (Trans. N. Orleans Acad. Ophthal.), St. Louis, 31 (1967).
Poos. *Klin. Mbl. Augenheilk.*, **84**, 340 (1930).
Primrose. *Brit. J. Ophthal.*, **46**, 129 (1962).
Reddy, Satapathy and Krishnamurthy. *Orient. Arch. Ophthal.*, **4**, 13 (1966).
Rønne. *v. Graefes Arch. Ophthal.*, **105**, 465 (1921).
Rosen and Johnston. *Arch. Ophthal.*, **62**, 810 (1959).
Sallmann and Deutsch. *v. Graefes Arch. Ophthal.*, **124**, 624 (1930).
Schmidt. *Med. Klin.*, **24**, 859 (1928). *Arch. Augenheilk.*, **104**, 102 (1931). *Klin. Mbl. Augenheilk.*, **116**, 614 (1950).
Segal, Gebicki, Janiszewski and Skwierczyńska. *Amer. J. Ophthal.*, **64**, 956, 965 (1967).
Spadavecchia. *Ann. Ottal.*, **64**, 611, 696 (1936); **65**, 194 (1937).
Stein. *Med. Klin.*, **29**, 1235 (1933).
Stine. *Amer. J. Ophthal.*, **31**, 1203 (1948).
Stood. *Klin. Mbl. Augenheilk.*, **22**, 285 (1884).
Suda and Kamao. *Kumamoto med. J.*, **4**, 15 (1951).
Suda, Sawada and Gyotoku. *Acta Soc. ophthal. jap.*, **69**, 480 (1965).
Sugar. *Amer. J. Ophthal.*, **31**, 1193 (1948).
Sugar and Santos. *Amer. J. Ophthal.*, **40**, 510 (1955).
Swanljung and Blodi. *Amer. J. Ophthal.*, **41**, 187 (1956).
Symowski. *Amer. J. Ophthal.*, **31**, 1305 (1948).
Tarkkanen and Leikola. *Acta ophthal.* (Kbh.), **45**, 569 (1967).
Thiel. *Arch. Augenheilk.*, **96**, 34, 331 (1925).
Thomassen and Leydhecker. *Brit. J. Ophthal.*, **34**, 169 (1950).
Tulevech and Berens. *Amer. J. Ophthal.*, **54**, 421 (1962).

Wegner. *Z. Augenheilk.*, **55**, 381; **56**, 48 (1925).
   Arch. Augenheilk., **102**, 1; **103**, 303, 511
   (1930).
   Zbl. ges. Ophthal., **24**, 1 (1931).

Weinstein.   *Amer. J. Ophthal.*, **33**, 1442
   (1950).
Zade.   *Klin. Mbl. Augenheilk.*, **45** (2), 435
   (1907).

Treatment

GENERAL PRINCIPLES OF TREATMENT

Since any rational system of treatment should be directed primarily against the cause of the disease and secondarily against the manifestations of its symptoms, the treatment of simple glaucoma must still be considered unsatisfactory, although a similar criticism may be levelled against the management of other degenerative disorders elsewhere in the body. It is true that we have progressed far beyond the state of affairs obtaining before the introduction of iridectomy by von Graefe (1857), when a diagnosis of glaucoma was tantamount to a sentence of blindness, and have even advanced considerably in the past 30 years since the division of primary glaucoma into the simple and closed-angle types has become universally accepted; but we still have a long journey to travel. In summarizing the ætiology of simple glaucoma[1] we concluded that an impairment to the outflow of aqueous was the major factor in the disease and that this resulted in an increase in the ocular tension which in turn could damage the optic nerve by its effect on the vascular supply. We also noted that the susceptibility of the optic nerve to such damage depended largely on the state of the vessels, for if these were impaired by sclerosis the nerve fell a readier victim to the effects of a raised ocular tension. This vascular factor can be attacked only by flank movements in vague and indefinite ways, since we are up against problems of great complexity the intimate mechanism of which is little understood, and although sometimes susceptible to amelioration and occasionally to relief, such a condition is not yet amenable to cure. The immediate causal factor (insufficient drainage) and its result (a raised ocular tension) can both be tackled seriously and to these the treatment of simple glaucoma is essentially confined; but the fundamental cause of the impairment to the outflow of aqueous is still unknown and is therefore not amenable to rational therapy, nor are we aware of any measures to increase the resistance of the important ocular tissues such as the optic nerve to the effects of pressure.

In general terms, therefore, it may be said that the available treatment of simple glaucoma devolves into an attempt to maintain the tension of the eye within normal limits by medical means. If these fail and the tension remains sufficiently high to cause damage or shows a dangerous instability, or if a deterioration of function persists despite our therapeutic endeavours, operative measures must be undertaken for its relief. On the different methods of treatment there is a confusing diversity of views, and it would

[1] p. 490.

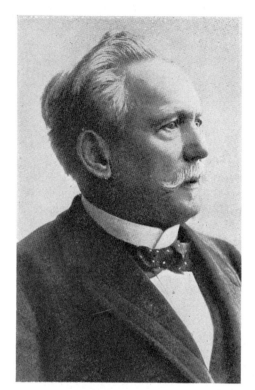

FIG. 511.—ADOLF WEBER
[1829–1915].

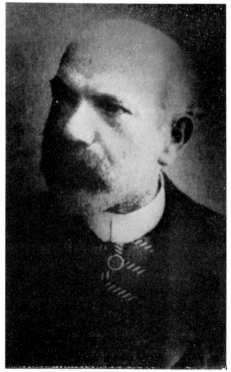

FIG. 512.—LUDWIG LAQUEUR
[1839–1909].
(By courtesy of A. Brini, Strasbourg.)

seem most economical in space first to summarize the more important of these, and then to give a logical and workable scheme suitable for the various clinical pictures which may present themselves.

Medical Treatment

HISTORY

In olden days the medical treatment of simple glaucoma was confined to the chronic and absolute phases of the disease when the therapeusis consisted of bathing the eyes with vegetable derivatives combined with the usual antiphlogistic methods of depletion—purging, cupping, emesis, blood-letting and leeches. The introduction of adequate treatment by drugs dates from the second half of the 19th century when almost simultaneously Adolf Weber (1876) of Darmstadt advocated the use of the extract of jaborandi (pilocarpine) and Ludwig Laqueur (1876–77) of Strasbourg that of the Calabar bean (physostigmine, eserine). In later years, particularly towards the middle of the present century, many cholinergic drugs and cholinesterase inhibitors have been synthesized so that today a wide range of miotics has been introduced into the pharmacological armamentarium.

A note of these two masters of ophthalmology is of interest.

ADOLF WEBER [1829–1915] (Fig. 511) was one of the most celebrated German ophthalmologists of his time. He studied at Giessen and Berlin where he was the pupil of Albrecht von Graefe who, at his death, left him all his surgical instruments; thereafter he went to Darmstadt where he practised for the remainder of his life. On the subject of glaucoma his two great contributions were in its pathology by demonstrating, contemporaneously with Max Knies, the obstruction to the drainage of the aqueous at the angle of the anterior chamber owing to the formation of peripheral synechiæ, and in its therapeutics by the discovery of the efficacy of pilocarpine as a hypotensive agent. Apart from glaucoma, his most outstanding contributions to ophthalmology were the introduction of the suction method of treating detachment of the retina, and his work on the lacrimal passages.

LUDWIG LAQUEUR [1839–1909] (Fig. 512), born in Silesia, was of German extraction and, after studying medicine in Breslau, in Berlin under von Graefe and in Paris, he spent his professional life in France, practising first in Lyons and becoming the first professor in Strasbourg (1872–1907). He himself was a sufferer from subacute attacks of closed-angle glaucoma from the early age of 35 when episodes of misty vision and the tell-tale haloes began to appear, to be noticed first when he lit a match. The following year (1876) he learned to control the attacks of which he suffered many, and obtained relief by the instillation of physostigmine; two years later the disease was permanently cured by a bilateral iridectomy carried out by Horner of Zürich, but the subsequent photophobia and his sensitiveness to the appearance of the colobomata tainted his whole life so that he constantly wore dark glasses and, casting his eyes downwards, rarely looked anyone in the face. He wrote a detailed account of the prodromal symptoms of glaucoma in von *Graefes Archiv* (**26** (3), 149, 1877) and a description of his symptoms in 1902 which was posthumously published.[1]

While the use of miotics has always remained the sheet-anchor in the medical treatment of simple glaucoma, other methods have been employed: the instillation of sympathomimetic drugs, initially by Darier (1900) and strongly advocated by Hamburger (1923–24); sympatholytic drugs introduced with compounds of ergot by Thiel

---

[1] *Klin. Mbl. Augenheilk.*, **2**, 639 (1909).

(1924); osmotic therapy, first by Cantonnet (1904) who administered sodium chloride by mouth and later by Hertel (1913–15) who gave intravenous injections of saline, a technique followed by the use of more effective substances such as sorbitol or urea intravenously or glycerol by mouth; and carbonic anhydrase inhibitors, initially acetazolamide by Becker (1954).

It is convenient to divide the various drugs employed in the treatment of glaucoma into 5 main classes: (1) parasympathomimetic (cholinergic and anticholinesterase) drugs with a primary action upon the musculature of the iris and ciliary body; (2) sympathomimetic drugs that diminish the formation of the aqueous humour and increase the facility of its outflow; (3) sympathetic blocking agents, the action of which on the ocular tension is incompletely understood; (4) drugs that diminish the formation of the aqueous humour such as the carbonic anhydrase inhibitors and the cardiac glycosides; and (5) osmotic agents, that raise the osmolarity of the plasma and thus abstract fluid from the eye.

The pharmacological action of most of these drugs has already been discussed in a previous Volume of this *System*,[1] but it is relevant to summarize the findings here and to discuss their use in the treatment of simple glaucoma.

1. PARASYMPATHOMIMETIC DRUGS

Cholinergic drugs act by simulating the effect of the acetylcholine naturally released at the autonomic synapses or the neuro-effector junctions of the parasympathetic system,[2] while *anticholinesterase drugs* by inhibiting cholinesterases, the enzymes capable of hydrolysing acetylcholine, produce the whole series of cholinergic effects by sensitizing the receptor mechanism to parasympathetic stimulation.[3] These two groups of parasympathomimetic drugs therefore produce similar effects on the eye and their particular therapeutic value in the treatment of simple glaucoma results from their increasing the facility of outflow of the aqueous humour (Figs. 513–14). This increase in the outflow of aqueous has been demonstrated for most of these drugs in clinical use[4] although the exact mechanism of their activity is still not clearly understood. The most widely held explanation is that contraction of the ciliary muscle exerts a pull on the scleral spur and thus opens up the trabecular meshwork and the canal of Schlemm (Figs. 515–16). It has also been suggested that contraction of the sphincter pupillæ has a similar effect on the trabecular meshwork, but this is less likely to be a factor in simple glaucoma since it has been demonstrated that the increase in the facility of aqueous outflow is unaffected by the absence of pupillary constriction (Armaly, 1959; Bárány, 1962). Bárány (1962) postulated that pilocarpine

[1] Vol. VII, Chap. XIX.   [2] Vol. VII, pp. 537, 556.   [3] Vol. VII, p. 563.
[4] Pilocarpine (Prijot and Weekers, 1952; Kronfeld, 1964; Bárány, 1966), physostigmine (Weekers, 1955; Kronfeld, 1964–66), DFP (Weekers, 1955; Kronfeld, 1966), echothiophate (Becker *et al.*, 1959; Drance, 1960; Kronfeld, 1966), demecarium (Becker and Gage, 1960; Kronfeld, 1966), Mintacol (Kronfeld, 1966), and many others.

FIGS. 513 AND 514.—PILOCARPINE AND AQUEOUS FLOW IN SIMPLE GLAUCOMA
(T. H. Hodgson and R. K. MacDonald).

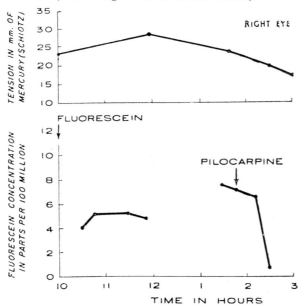

FIG. 513.—To show the drop in concentration of fluorescein in the aqueous after its instillation into the conjunctival sac. Usually the effect of pilocarpine is to cause a fall in ocular tension and in the concentration of fluorescein.

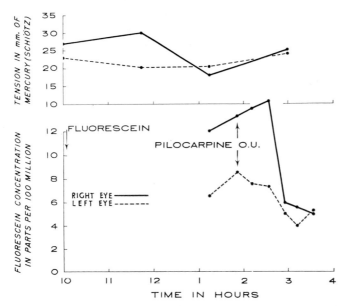

FIG. 514.—The fall in the concentration of fluorescein may occur even with a rise in ocular tension.

FIGS. 515 AND 516.—THE CILIARY MUSCLE AND PILOCARPINE.

In the vervet monkey. The drug was injected intracamerally to reach preferentially one segment of the ciliary muscle (E. H. Bárány).

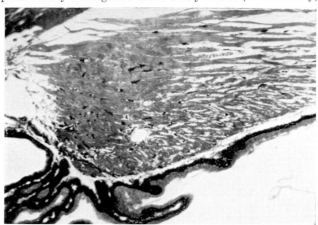

FIG. 515.—Showing the muscle contracted.

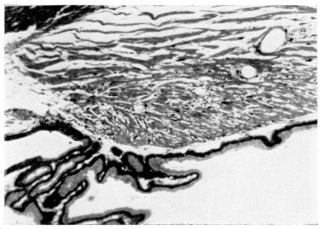

FIG. 516.—The diametrically opposite part of the same eye, showing the muscle relaxed. Note the disappearance of the intrafascicular spaces in the contracted portion and that the contraction is not propagated backwards but only into the circular portion of the muscle.

might have a direct effect on the endothelium of the canal of Schlemm, although in a later paper he doubted this possibility (Bárány, 1966).

The effects of these drugs on the ocular tension are complicated by the observation that contraction of the ciliary muscle by pilocarpine reduces the uveo-scleral outflow thus tending to increase the ocular tension (Bárány, 1966; Bill and Wålinder, 1966), while it has been suggested that pilocarpine might even stimulate the formation of aqueous (Bárány, 1966). Any possible increase of ocular tension by these two effects, however, is probably of little therapeutic importance. It is interesting that pilocarpine reduces the depth of the anterior chamber by an average amount of 0·16 mm. (Heim, 1941; Rosengren, 1950), an effect which is more dramatic with the more powerful cholinesterase inhibitors.[1]

Parasympathomimetic drugs also cause a vasodilatation of the conjunctival and the smaller intra-ocular blood vessels as well as an increase in the permeability of their walls, thus producing an initial transient rise of ocular tension (Colle *et al.*, 1931; Cristini, 1949; Leopold and Krishna, 1963), but the importance of these vascular effects is slight and has probably been over-stressed in the past.

(a) CHOLINERGIC DRUGS

Those which have been used in the treatment of simple glaucoma include the naturally occurring alkaloids, pilocarpine and arecoline, and several synthetic choline derivatives, methacholine, carbachol, bethanechol chloride, iricoline, furmethide and aceclydine. Some of these synthetic compounds are more active than pilocarpine and are useful when an allergic irritation to pilocarpine develops.

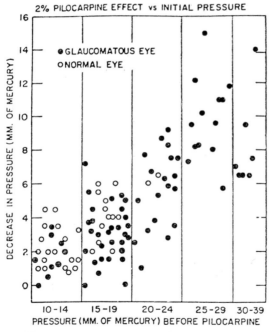

FIG. 517.—THE EFFECT OF PILOCARPINE ON THE OCULAR TENSION.

To show the difference between the average ocular tension for each eye before and after the instillation of 2% pilocarpine at a constant test-time. Note that the reduction in tension is proportionate to the average tension before pilocarpine and of the same order in normal and glaucomatous eyes (A. E. Krill and F. W. Newell).

[1] p. 511.

PILOCARPINE, which was first introduced into ophthalmic practice by Weber (1876), is an alkaloid obtained from the leaves of a South American plant, the jaborandi (*Pilocarpus pennatifolius*).[1] It acts by stimulating the neuro-effector junctions of parasympathetic nerves and is the most widely used of the miotics. It tends to lower the ocular tension of almost any eye with simple glaucoma to some degree although not necessarily sufficiently (Löhlein, 1926), and in addition lessens the amplitude of variations in the tension (R. Thiel, 1928; Odinzow and Nejman, 1929; Krill and Newell,

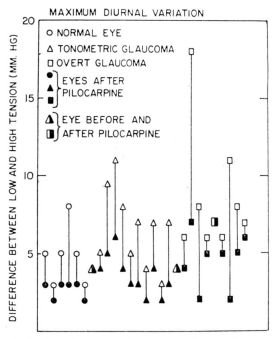

FIG. 518.—THE DIURNAL VARIATION IN SIMPLE GLAUCOMA.

A comparison of the maximal diurnal variation for each eye before and after pilocarpine. Note that the variation is less after the instillation of pilocarpine for 24 out of 27 eyes (A. E. Krill and F. W. Newell).

1964) (Figs. 517–18). The decrease in tension following its use is usually a linear function of the initial ocular tension (Linnér, 1958; Krill and Newell, 1964).

The drug may be given over long periods with little intolerance or irritation, although an allergic conjunctival reaction may eventually occur. It is usually given as drops, as pilocarpine nitrate or more usually the hydrochloride, in concentrations of 0·5 to 10% although those of over 4% appear to have little advantage over weaker solutions (Becker and Shaffer, 1965). Its effect lasts about 6 hours and the action may be prolonged by

[1] Vol. VII, Plate X, Fig. 1.

prescribing it as oily drops in parolein, in a methylcellulose base, or as an ointment in a base of soft yellow paraffin. In solution the optimum pH is 7 which can be maintained with a boric acid buffer (de Grosz and Kedvessy, 1951).

ARECOLINE (methyl tetrahydromethyl nicotinate) is the alkaloid of the betel nut, *Areca catechu*. On instillation into the eye, which, incidentally, causes a considerable degree of smarting, it induces a strong miosis beginning in 5 minutes, reaching its maximum in 15 to 30 minutes, while the pupil returns to normal in 70 minutes (Lavagna, 1895–97). It has no place in the modern treatment of simple glaucoma.

METHACHOLINE (*Mecholyl, Hypotan*) (acetyl-β-methyl choline), when instilled into the eye as drops (5 to 20%), produces a marked vasodilatation and a strong miosis[1] as well as an increased permeability of the blood-aqueous barrier (Swan and Hart, 1940). Although it is effective in reducing the ocular tension in simple glaucoma its vasodilatory effect precludes its long-continued use in this disease.

CARBACHOL (*Doryl*) (carbamylcholine chloride) is a still more powerful miotic which, when instilled into the conjunctival sac as drops or an ointment (0·75 to 3%), brings about a miosis which is established within 10 minutes and lasts more than 2 hours,[2] although only a 3% solution achieves an effect beyond 4 hours. Occasionally symptoms of intolerance appear after its instillation, manifested as giddiness, palpitation and profuse sweating (van Beuningen, 1952).

IRICOLINE (carbaminoyl-methyl choline), used as drops (1 to 2%), has been claimed to be a still more active product.

BETHANECHOL CHLORIDE (*Urecholine*) (urethane of β-methylcholine chloride) is claimed to be the longest acting and most potent of the choline series of derivatives in its miotic effect and has been employed ophthalmologically as 1% drops (Frisch and Leopold, 1953).

FURTRETHONIUM IODIDE (*Furmethide*) (furfuryl trimethyl ammonium iodide) is a potent miotic with an action more prolonged than most cholinergic esters. When instilled into the eye as 10% drops its hypotensive effect lasts 24 hours.[3] It produces, however, dacryostenosis in 71% of cases as compared with pilocarpine and eserine with which lacrimal obstruction occurs in only 2·5% (Shaffer and Ridgway, 1951), and is therefore no longer used as a therapeutic agent.

ACECLYDINE (*Glaucostat*) (3-acetoxy quinuclidine) is a recently synthesized parasympathomimetic drug which has been employed in the treatment of simple glaucoma as a 1 to 3% solution.[4] It is a powerful miotic which reduces the ocular tension to a similar extent as does 2% pilocarpine. Its mode of action has not, however, been completely elucidated for its effect on the facility of aqueous outflow has been variously reported as negligible (Lieberman and Leopold, 1967), as less than that of pilocarpine (Riegel and Leydhecker, 1967) or as similar to that of pilocarpine (Étienne *et al.*, 1967).

(*b*) ANTICHOLINESTERASE DRUGS

These may be divided into three main classes:

(1) *Carbamates*, such as the naturally occurring alkaloid, physostigmine,

---

[1] Villaret *et al.* (1931), Onfray *et al.* (1934), Myerson and Thau (1937), Wirth (1951).

[2] Velhagen (1934–36), Miloro (1935), de Sanctis (1937), Schoenberg (1938), Swan (1943–53), Kravitz (1944), Niemeyer (1968).

[3] Myerson and Thau (1940), Uhler (1943), Owens and Woods (1946–47), Esente (1948), Weinstein (1949), Goodwin (1951).

[4] Étienne *et al.* (1967), Kamilov and Arustamova (1967), Lieberman and Leopold (1967), Riegel and Leydhecker (1967), Mangouritsas and Koliopoulos (1967), Bastide *et al.* (1968).

and the related synthetic compounds, neostigmine and pyridostigmine. These drugs have the general structure

$$X-\underset{\underset{O}{\|}}{C}-N\begin{matrix} R_1 \\ \\ R_2 \end{matrix}$$

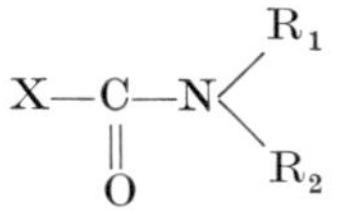

and react in a reversible manner with cholinesterase (E) to form a carbamylated enzyme (Fig. 519).

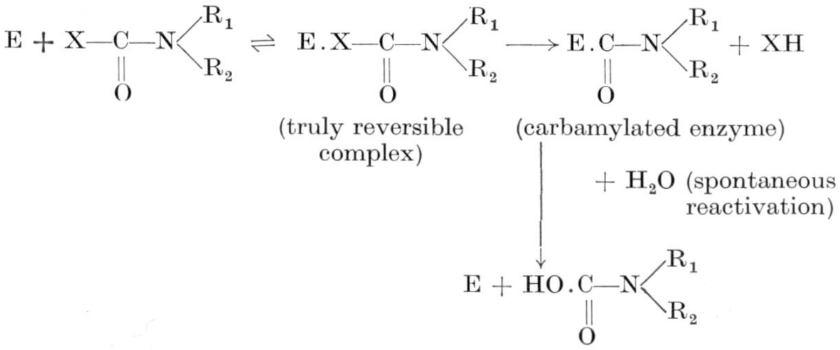

$$E + X-\underset{\underset{O}{\|}}{C}-N\begin{matrix} R_1 \\ \\ R_2 \end{matrix} \rightleftharpoons E.X-\underset{\underset{O}{\|}}{C}-N\begin{matrix} R_1 \\ \\ R_2 \end{matrix} \longrightarrow E.\underset{\underset{O}{\|}}{C}-N\begin{matrix} R_1 \\ \\ R_2 \end{matrix} + XH$$

(truly reversible complex)   (carbamylated enzyme)

$+ H_2O$ (spontaneous reactivation)

$$E + HO.\underset{\underset{O}{\|}}{C}-N\begin{matrix} R_1 \\ \\ R_2 \end{matrix}$$

FIG. 519.—THE REACTION OF CARBAMATES WITH CHOLINESTERASE.

The carbamylated enzyme and the reversible complex between carbamate and enzyme have a half-life of less than 1 hour (Wilson *et al.*, 1961) resulting in a gradual return of enzymic activity when the inhibited enzyme is exposed to acetylcholine. Demecarium, another synthetic drug in this group, is an exception to this, forming a much more stable, though still reversible, inhibited enzyme.

(2) *Organophosphates*, such as DFP, TEPP, echothiophate and Mintacol, have the general structure

$$X-\underset{\underset{O \text{ (or S)}}{\|}}{P}\begin{matrix} R_1 \\ \\ R_2 \end{matrix}$$

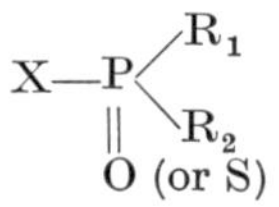

and react with cholinesterase to form a phosphorylated enzyme (Fig. 520).

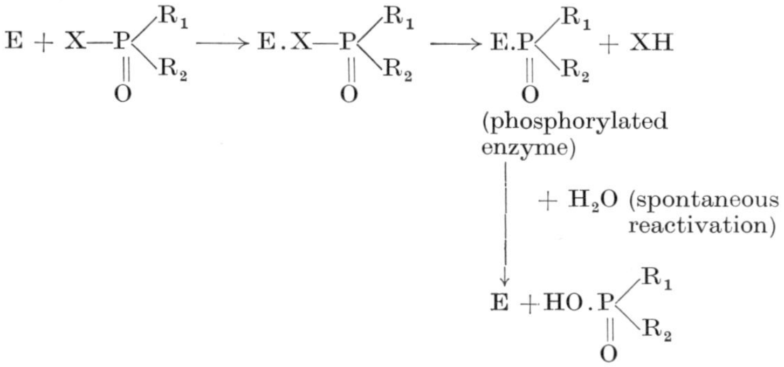

$$E + X-\underset{\underset{O}{\|}}{P}\begin{matrix} R_1 \\ \\ R_2 \end{matrix} \longrightarrow E.X-\underset{\underset{O}{\|}}{P}\begin{matrix} R_1 \\ \\ R_2 \end{matrix} \longrightarrow E.\underset{\underset{O}{\|}}{P}\begin{matrix} R_1 \\ \\ R_2 \end{matrix} + XH$$

(phosphorylated enzyme)

$+ H_2O$ (spontaneous reactivation)

$$E + HO.\underset{\underset{O}{\|}}{P}\begin{matrix} R_1 \\ \\ R_2 \end{matrix}$$

FIG. 520.—THE REACTION OF ORGANOPHOSPHATES WITH CHOLINESTERASE.

When diethoxy groups are present in the phosphorylated enzyme (as with TEPP, echothiophate and Mintacol) slow spontaneous reactivation takes place, amounting to less than 50% in 24 hours, while in cases wherein di-isopropoxy groups are involved (as with DFP) no spontaneous reactivation is detectable and any return of enzymic activity *in vivo* is due to the synthesis of new enzyme. These phosphorylated enzymes can, however, be speedily reactivated by the oximes (such as P_2AM and TMB).

(3) *Simple quaternary ammonium bases* and edrophonium (Tensilon) combine in a readily reversible manner with acetylcholinesterase and thus have a relatively short inhibitory effect on the enzyme and are of no therapeutic value in the treatment of simple glaucoma.

PHYSOSTIGMINE (ESERINE)[1] is an alkaloid obtained from the seed of the Calabar bean (*Physostigma venenosum*)[2] and was first used as a therapeutic agent in glaucoma by Ludwig Laqueur (1876–77). It inhibits the action of acetylcholinesterase by forming a reversible compound with this enzyme, thus enhancing the action of acetylcholine liberated at the neuro-effector junctions. Its therapeutic effect in simple glaucoma results from increasing the facility of outflow of aqueous, an effect similar to that of pilocarpine except that the action of physostigmine is considerably stronger and lasts longer than that of the latter drug. After the instillation of the drug in the eye, miosis begins in 10 minutes, reaches its maximum in 30 to 50 minutes, is fully effective for 3 to 4 hours and disappears gradually during the following 3 to 4 days. The continued use of physostigmine may result in the development of an allergic irritation of the conjunctiva, while the prolonged use of this drug may induce the condition of "rigidity of the iris" and cause the formation of cysts of the pigmentary epithelium at the pupillary margin, complications that may occasionally follow the prolonged use of pilocarpine.

Physostigmine is usually prescribed as drops of the salicylate (0·25 to 1·0%). Increasing the concentration to 2% appears to result in little increase in efficacy (Kronfeld, 1964), but it has been demonstrated that 0·5% physostigmine produces a much more marked hypotensive effect than a 0·25% solution of the drug; a longer reaction results from the use of the alkaloid in oil (0·5 to 1·0%). Aqueous solutions of the drug oxidize under the influence of light, air or the alkali of glass containers; this decomposition is retarded by the addition of boric acid and prevented by 0·1% potassium or sodium metabisulphite (Rae, 1946; Hind and Goyan, 1947). Since physostigmine supplements the action of pilocarpine, the instillation of both drugs is effective (O. Lowenstein and Loewenfeld, 1953), but the popularity of the prolonged use of physostigmine has waned in recent years since the advent of more powerful and stable anticholinesterases.

---

[1] Vol. VII, p. 563.
[2] Vol. VII, Plate X, Fig. 4.

NEOSTIGMINE (PROSTIGMINE) is a synthetic anticholinesterase drug, less potent than physostigmine, but more stable and with fewer side-effects. It has been employed as drops (3 to 5%) in the treatment of glaucoma (Myerson and Thau, 1937; Clarke, 1939; Simonelli, 1947).

DEMECARIUM BROMIDE (BC 48; *Humorsol, Tosmilen*), a more powerful miotic than physostigmine and comparable in its action to the organo-phosphates, has been investigated by a number of workers and found to be a valuable therapeutic agent in the treatment of simple glaucoma.[1] It is water-soluble and stable at room temperature and is used as drops in con-centrations of 0·06 to 0·5%. Because of its long action, demecarium bromide need never be used more than twice a day, and in some patients its instillation twice a week is all that may be required. The side-effects are similar to those of the organophosphates to be presently discussed.

DFP (*Floropryl, Dyflos*) (di-isopropyl phosphorofluoridate) was the first organophosphate anticholinesterase used in the treatment of glaucoma, having a more potent and longer-lasting action than physostigmine.[2] Quilliam (1947) considered that 0·1% DFP had a comparable action to 1% physostigmine, although Kronfeld (1966) found that its effect on ocular tension and resistance to outflow was greater than that of physostigmine and considerably more prolonged. Leopold and Cleveland (1953) observed that the therapeutic effect of 0·01% DFP was similar to that of 0·5 to 1% pilo-carpine. DFP has to be prepared in an oily medium for it is rapidly hydro-lysed and inactivated, a reaction particularly liable to occur if the drops are contaminated with tears. Its liability to contamination and to produce frequent sensitivity reactions has resulted in it being superseded as a therapeutic agent by other organophosphates.

ECHOTHIOPHATE (IODIDE) (*Phospholine*) is a water-soluble organo-phosphate, stable at 4° C but not at room temperature. It is long-acting and slow-acting, reaching its maximal effect between 10 and 28 hours after instillation (Kronfeld, 1966). It has been shown by many workers to be an effective drug in reducing the ocular tension in simple glaucoma and is used in concentrations of 0·06 to 0·25%,[3] producing a mean drop in ocular

[1] Gittler and Pillat (1956), Gerhard and Ketter (1958), Drance (1959), Drance and Carr (1959–60), Gittler (1959), Stepanik and Stelzer (1959), Becker and Gage (1960), Krishna and Leopold (1960), Lawlor and Lee (1960), Miller (1960), Terner *et al.* (1961), Lloyd (1963), Drance (1966), Bitrán and Weibel (1966), and others.
[2] Leopold and Comroe (1946), Weekers (1947), Marr (1947), Quilliam (1947), Haas (1948), Leopold and McDonald (1948), Böck and Veitl (1949), Raiford (1949), Stone (1950), Ourgaud (1951), Leopold and Cleveland (1953), Westsmith and Abernethy (1954), Callahan (1957), and others.
[3] Leopold *et al.* (1957), Maggi Zavalía *et al.* (1958), Becker *et al.* (1959), Drance (1959–66), Giardini and Paliaga (1959), Krishna and Leopold (1959), Becker and Gage (1960), Drance and Carr (1960), Gray and Robinson (1960), Lawlor and Lee (1960), Coyle *et al.* (1961), A. and E. Sacks-Wilner (1961), Klayman and Taffet (1963), Klendshoj and Olmsted (1963), Lloyd (1963), Hirsch-Hoffmann (1964–66), Levene (1964), Pratt-Johnson *et al.* (1964), Romano and Jackson (1964), Fisher *et al.* (1965), Levene and Friedman (1965), Blanton and Pollack (1966), Kellerman and King (1966), de Roetth (1966), and others.

tension of about 50% and an increase in the facility of aqueous outflow of 120% (Drance, 1960). Levene (1964) has shown that 0·125% echothiophate twice a day is more effective than 2% pilocarpine four times a day, while Pratt-Johnson and his co-workers (1964) found that 0·06% echothiophate twice a day was more effective than 4% pilocarpine four times a day. In common with other organophosphates, echothiophate tends to become less effective in reducing the ocular tension when used for a considerable period of time.

DIETHYL-*p*-NITROPHENYL PHOSPHATE (*Mintacol*) is an organophosphate that was popular on the continent of Europe for the treatment of simple glaucoma.[1] Like so many of these compounds it has tended to be replaced by demecarium and echothiophate.

Other organophosphates that have been used for a short period in the treatment of simple glaucoma include:

TETRAETHYL PYROPHOSPHATE (TEPP) (Grant, 1948; Grob and Harvey, 1949; Upholt *et al.*, 1956).
HEXA-ETHYL TETRAPHOSPHATE (HEPT; HEPP) (R. Thiel, 1954).
DIETHYL-*p*-NITROPHENYL THIOPHOSPHATE (DPP; DNTP) (*Parathion*) (R. Thiel, 1954).
TETRA-ISOPROPYL PYROPHOSPHATE (TIPP) (R. Thiel, 1954).
DIETHYL-CHLORMETHYL-COUMARINYL PHOSPHORO-THIONATE (*Coralox*) (Kadin, 1960).

Side-effects of Anticholinesterase Drugs

The anticholinesterase drugs, and in particular demecarium and the organophosphates, tend to produce local and systemic side-effects which limit their use in some patients. The local effects include ocular pain and frontal headache due to ciliary spasm, blurring of vision due to myopia induced by the ciliary spasm or to miosis in association with central lens opacities, dilatation of the conjunctival vessels, the formation of a plasmoid aqueous or even the development of an anterior uveitis (Dunphy, 1949), the formation of cysts of the pigmentary epithelium of the iris[2] (Abraham, 1954; Swan, 1954; Christensen *et al.*, 1956), and occasionally a retinal detachment.[3] A transient rise of ocular tension may occur when these drugs are first used, due apparently to swelling of the ciliary body, and attacks of closed-angle glaucoma have been precipitated in patients with narrow angles of their anterior chambers. Even when the drainage angle is open, the anterior chamber is made more shallow and an iris bombé may result[4]; moreover, Romano (1968) found that Phospholine iodide failed to control the tension if the anterior chamber was less than 2·2 mm. in depth before

[1] Glees and Wüstenberg (1949), H. L. Thiel (1949), Huerkamp and Wagner (1950), Gittler (1950), Neuenschwander (1950), Quintieri (1951), Rotter (1951), Caselli (1953), and others.
[2] Vol. IX, p. 769.
[3] Marr (1947), Butler (1952), Zekman and Snydacker (1953), Westsmith and Abernethy (1954), Weekers and Lavergne (1955), and others.
[4] Barkan (1954), Sugar (1957), Swan (1959), Grant (1962), Romano and Jackson (1964), Romano (1968).

its use. After the prolonged use of anticholinesterases, the frequent development of opacities of the lens has been noted.[1]

Systemic side-effects produced by these drugs include nausea and vomiting, diarrhœa, abdominal pain, bronchial constriction, hypotension, salivation and hyperhidrosis, and generalized weakness. These effects appear to be unrelated to the depression of plasma and red blood cell cholinesterase which occurs in some patients after the prolonged use of anticholinesterases.[2] It should be noted that Birks and his associates (1968) found that a patient treated with echothiophate iodide during the first 32 weeks of a pregnancy gave birth to a child with depressed pseudocholinesterase which rose rapidly afterwards, a circumstance which suggested that the drug had traversed the placenta. If this is confirmed, it would imply that it should not be used in the treatment of glaucoma in pregnancy.

2. SYMPATHOMIMETIC DRUGS

The SYMPATHOMIMETIC (ADRENERGIC) DRUGS simulate in their action the effects of stimulation of the post-ganglionic sympathetic nerves, the various effects of which on the eye have already been studied.[3]

The topical application of these drugs in normal subjects and in patients with simple glaucoma results in a reduction in the ocular tension; the exact mechanism of their action, although not yet completely elucidated, appears to depend upon their effects on the α and β receptors in the outflow channels and in the ciliary body, and possibly also on the blood vessels in the anterior segment of the eye. It will be recalled that Ahlquist (1948) divided adrenergic receptors into these two main groups depending upon their relative sensitivity to various amines and upon the specificity of blockade with two groups of agents. Noradrenaline is most active at α receptors, isoprenaline at β receptors, while adrenaline has high activity at both groups.

There is a growing body of evidence that α receptors are present in the outflow channels of the eye and that their stimulation results in an increase in the facility of the outflow of aqueous.[4] The presence of β receptors in the outflow channels, however, is more controversial; Eakins (1963), for example, found that the intravitreal injection of isoprenaline, a stimulator of β receptors, had no effect on the facility of the outflow of aqueous, while Bárány (1966) demonstrated that stimulation of β receptors in the outflow channels of rabbits resulted in an increase of this facility.

The sympathomimetic drugs also reduce the rate of aqueous secretion,

[1] p. 232. *See* Harrison (1960), Axelsson and Holmberg (1966), de Roetth (1966), Shaffer and Hetherington (1966), Shaffer (1967), Axelsson (1968), and others.
[2] Leopold and Comroe (1946), Leopold *et al.* (1959), Leopold (1961), Humphreys and Holmes (1963), Klendshoj and Olmsted (1963), and others.
[3] Vol. VII, pp. 537, 570.
[4] Sears and Bárány (1960), Eakins (1963), Eakins and Ryan (1964), Sears and Sherk (1964), Paterson (1966), Sears (1966), and others.

probably by stimulating β receptors (Eakins, 1963; Langham, 1965), but the site of their action is still not completely understood. This reduction in aqueous secretion may result from the reduced blood-flow to the ciliary processes which is known to occur on sympathetic stimulation (Linner, 1952; Langham, 1955), but it might also depend upon a direct action on the ciliary processes since Weekers and his co-workers (1966) have demonstrated that it can be produced by those sympathomimetic drugs which have no vasoconstrictor effect.

Of the several naturally occurring and synthetic amines with sympathomimetic effects, only adrenaline has so far been found useful in the treatment of simple glaucoma, although several other of these amines are known to reduce the ocular tension.

ADRENALINE (EPINEPHRINE) has been widely used in the treatment of simple glaucoma[1]; its action in reducing the ocular tension appears to result from a combination of the following factors:

(1) A decrease in the rate of production of the aqueous[2]; Becker and Ley (1958), for example, demonstrated a decrease of 37% in the rate of production following the topical administration of adrenaline.

(2) An immediate increase in the facility of the outflow of aqueous,[3] an increase which appears to be minimal when the facility is greatly reduced (Galin et al., 1966).

(3) A late and progressive increase in the facility of the outflow of aqueous.[4] Thus Becker and his co-workers (1961) demonstrated that in 62% of patients on topical adrenaline for 6 months or longer the facility increased by 50%; but the mechanism of this late increase is not understood.

Adrenaline is usually given as drops, as l-adrenaline bitartrate, hydrochloride or borate, in concentrations of 1 to 2%. The fall in ocular tension following its topical administration starts in under an hour, reaches its maximum in about 6 to 12 hours, and remains appreciable for over 48 hours (Fig. 521). In simple glaucoma it is usually used once or twice a day, and has been successfully combined with pilocarpine, the actions of the two being additive (Kronfeld, 1967; Duzanec and Leydhecker, 1967).

Adrenaline eye-drops tend to produce local and systemic side-effects in an appreciable percentage of patients when used for 6 months or longer.

---

[1] Kollner (1918–20), Knapp (1921), Hamburger (1923–24), Gradle (1924), Gifford (1928), Duke-Elder and Law (1929), Weekers et al. (1954–61), Becker and Ley (1958), Garner et al. (1959), Tittarelli (1960), Ballintine and Garner (1961), Becker et al. (1961), Vaughan et al. (1961), Byakov and Stroganov (1962), Kronfeld (1963), Menezo and Quintana (1963), Spiers (1963), Étienne and Barut (1965), Krill et al. (1965), Fechner (1966), Galin et al. (1966), Sears (1966), Richards and Drance (1967), Tarkkanen and Karjalainen (1967), and many others.

[2] Goldmann (1951), Becker and Friedenwald (1953), Weekers et al. (1954–55), Becker and Ley (1958), Ballintine and Garner (1961), Sears (1966).

[3] Weekers et al. (1954), Kronfeld (1963–64), Krill et al. (1965), Sears (1966), Richards and Drance (1967).

[4] Garner et al. (1959), Ballintine and Garner (1961), Becker et al. (1961), Étienne and Barut (1965), Sears (1966).

Conjunctival irritation, hyperæmia and an allergic blepharo-conjunctivitis
are often sufficiently severe to necessitate cessation of the drug although in
some patients these side-effects may be reduced by the simultaneous use of
topical corticosteroids, such as hydroxymethyl-progesterone (Medrysone) and
tetrahydrotriamcinolone, which have an anti-inflammatory activity but do
not cause a significant rise of ocular tension (Spaeth, 1966; Becker, 1967;
Dorsch and Thygeson, 1968; Drance and Scott, 1968).   In patients on long-
term therapy, black deposits formed by the oxidation of adrenaline to
melanin[1] are frequently found on the lid margins and conjunctiva but these
have no clinical significance.[2]   Occasional cases of corneal œdema and
macular changes (œdema, hæmorrhages and cysts) have also been reported
after its topical prolonged use (Becker, 1967).

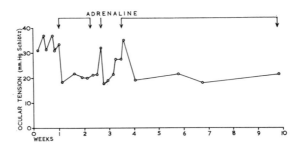

FIG. 521. ADRENALINE IN SIMPLE GLAUCOMA.

The hypotensive effect of repeated instillations of adrenaline for several weeks
in cases of simple glaucoma (R. Weekers *et al.*).

Tachycardia and extra-systoles due to the systemic absorption of
topically-applied adrenaline occur in a few patients, while an acute rise in
the blood pressure is a rare complication (Lansche, 1966).   The production
of an acute rise in ocular tension is exceptional.[3]

NORADRENALINE (NOREPINEPHRINE : ARTERENOL), the essential neuro-transmitter
of sympathetic activity in the periphery, is less effective than adrenaline in reducing
the ocular tension when instilled as drops into the conjunctival sac and is therefore of
no clinical value (Hofmann, 1954; Owe-Larsson, 1956; Weekers *et al.*, 1966).

PHENYLEPHRINE HYDROCHLORIDE (*Neosynephrine*), although it has been used in
the treatment of simple glaucoma, has an action so fleeting that its clinical use is small
(Heath, 1936; Posner, 1948; Heath and Geiter, 1949; Becker *et al.*, 1959).   As a 5%
solution, however, it may be of value in combination with pilocarpine (Demailly and
Kérisel, 1967).

ISOPRENALINE (ISOPROPYLARTERENOL) (*Aludrine*) is highly effective in reducing
the ocular tension when instilled into the conjunctival sac, and has neither mydriatic
nor vasoconstrictor action but unfortunately it causes an intense tachycardia in the
majority of patients (Weekers *et al.*, 1966).

[1] Vol. VIII, p. 597.
[2] A. Löwenstein (1927), Bietti (1938), Marchesani and Ullerich (1950), Corwin and Spencer
(1963), Veirs and McGrew (1963), Hansen (1964), Ferry and Zimmerman (1964), Spiers and
Eldrup-Jørgensen (1966), and others.
[3] p. 703.

3. SYMPATHETIC BLOCKING DRUGS

The SYMPATHETIC BLOCKING (SYMPATHOLYTIC) DRUGS block some or all of the effects of sympathetic stimulation. Although many of this diverse group of drugs have been used in the treatment of simple glaucoma, only guanethidine has been found to be of any clinical value although several others are of interest in elucidating the part played by the sympathetic nerves in the control of the ocular tension.

ERGOTAMINE TARTRATE (*Gynergen*) which blocks α receptors was employed by R. Thiel (1924) in the treatment of simple glaucoma. Since then, several other reports have appeared in the literature,[1] but Posner (1950) found it had no effect on the ocular tension in simple glaucoma.

DIHYDROERGOTAMINE has an action similar to ergotamine and, although it reduces the ocular tension temporarily (Pereyra, 1948; Persichetti, 1950; Shah *et al.*, 1955), it has no place in the treatment of simple glaucoma.

HYDERGINE, a mixture of three related ergot alkaloids, has a similar temporary effect on the ocular tension (Agarwal, 1954; Orbán, 1954; Mishra and Goel, 1962).

DIBENAMINE (dibenzyl chlorethylamine) is a powerful sympatholytic drug which acts by forming an irreversible union with α receptors. It must be administered intravenously and lowers the ocular tension probably by reducing the secretion of aqueous humour (DeLong and Scheie, 1953). It has no place in the treatment of simple glaucoma.

PHENOXYBENZAMINE (*Dibenyline*) has an action similar to that of dibenamine, and although it reduces the ocular tension in acute closed-angle glaucoma, it appears to have no effect on the ocular tension in simple glaucoma (Primrose, 1955).

PROPRANOLOL, a sympathetic blocking agent specific for β receptors, produces a fall of ocular tension when administered intravenously or orally to patients with simple glaucoma (Phillips *et al.*, 1967; Coté and Drance, 1968). Its exact mode of action is unknown.

GUANETHIDINE (*Ismelin*) blocks the release of noradrenaline at adrenergic nerve terminals and also causes some depletion of the store of noradrenaline, thus producing a sympathomimetic effect. When instilled into the con-junctival sac as 5% or 10% eye-drops it reduces the ocular tension in patients with simple glaucoma.[2] Its main action appears to result from reducing the production of the aqueous (Bonomi and di Comite, 1963–67; Verdi and de Molfetta, 1964), an effect due to its sympathetic blocking action. It also produces a transitory increase in the facility of outflow of aqueous, probably the result of its sympathomimetic effect (Stepanik, 1961; Bonomi and di Comite, 1963–67). The maximal lowering of the ocular tension occurs 6 to 8 hours after its instillation, and the effect lasts about 24 hours. Its action is comparable to that of 1% pilocarpine with which it has an additive effect (Castrén *et al.*, 1968). Conjunctival vaso-dilatation, slight ptosis and slight miosis are side-effects that occur in all

---

[1] Heim (1927), Hanssen (1928), Gifford (1928), Poos and Santori (1929), Barrenechea *et al.* (1944).

[2] Küchle (1961), Kutschera (1961–62), Stepanik (1961), Castrén and Pohjola (1962), Oosterhuis (1962), Stirpe and Bucci (1962), Bonomi and di Comite (1963–67), Grande (1963), Peyret (1963), Malik *et al.* (1964), Verdi and de Molfetta (1964), and others.

patients on guanethidine eye-drops; occasionally these prove troublesome and necessitate the cessation of this drug.

BRETYLIUM also blocks the release of noradrenaline at adrenergic nerve terminals and, when instilled into the conjunctival sac as 10% eye-drops, it causes a reduction in the ocular tension in patients with simple glaucoma (Bonomi and di Comite, 1963).

4. SECRETORY INHIBITORS

(a) CARBONIC ANHYDRASE INHIBITORS

The CARBONIC ANHYDRASE INHIBITORS, which act by inhibiting the formation of the aqueous humour, have already been discussed at length in previous Volumes of this *System*[1] where it was pointed out that their mode of action is unknown. The facts that no reduction of the ocular tension follows their instillation into the conjunctival sac or their subconjunctival or intracameral injection and that they are effective only after systemic administration suggest that a mechanism depending on changes in the blood is the responsible factor. Nevertheless, no evidence has been adduced that this is so. It is probably significant that injection into a carotid artery in experimental animals lowers the intra-ocular pressure of the ipsilateral eye (Wistrand, 1957); moreover, after intravenous injection the drugs reach the ciliary processes in a concentration sufficient to inhibit the carbonic anhydrase of that tissue (Ballintine and Maren, 1955), while the secretory activity of the isolated ciliary processes can be inhibited by their local application (Berggren, 1964). It would therefore seem likely that these agents exert their effect only when they reach a secretory tissue through the blood stream. However that may be, they probably act by reducing the secretory activity of the ciliary body by an unknown mechanism, an action not limited to the eye but effective on other secretions and on the cerebro-spinal fluid.

ACETAZOLAMIDE (*Diamox*), the first carbonic anhydrase inhibitor to be used therapeutically for the eye, is of great clinical value in lowering the ocular tension in simple glaucoma[2] (Fig. 522). It is usually given orally in doses of 125 to 500 mg. one to four times a day and after a single dose its action is apparent in from 60 to 90 minutes, reaches a maximum in 3 to 5 hours, and has worn off in about 12 hours. Sustained-action capsules of the drug have a more prolonged effect and need not be given more than twice a day.[3] Acetazolamide reduces the production of aqueous by about 50%

---

[1] Vol. IV, p. 316; Vol. VII, p. 623.

[2] Becker (1954–55), Breinin and Görtz (1954), Espíldora-Luque *et al.* (1954), Grant and Trotter (1954), Kleinert (1954), Purcell and Schane (1954), Agarwal and Saxena (1955), Balassanian and de Soldati (1955), Becker and Middleton (1955), Berggren and Wistrand (1955), Drance (1955–61), Gloster and Perkins (1955), Gonzalez-Pola *et al.* (1955), Kupfer *et al.* (1955), Rintelen and Jenny (1955), Campbell *et al.* (1956–57), Duke-Elder *et al.* (1956), Leopold and Carmichael (1956), Chandler (1957), Becker and Ley (1958), Görtz (1958), Kalfa *et al.* (1961), Libman (1961), Garner *et al.* (1963), Suda *et al.* (1963), Stepanik (1965), and many others.

[3] Drance (1961), Garner *et al.* (1963), Suda *et al.* (1963), Stepanik (1965), and others.

(Becker and Ley, 1958) and was originally recommended for the short-term treatment of various forms of glaucoma. It soon became apparent, however, that in spite of its side-effects, it was a particularly valuable addition to the available therapy for the long-term treatment of simple glaucoma, particularly when combined with miotics and adrenaline, and enabled many patients previously uncontrolled on medical therapy to avoid surgery.[1] Its efficacy has been reported to be increased, and its side-effects reduced, by prescribing it with oral doses of potassium bicarbonate or chloride (Campbell *et al.*, 1956–57; Draeger *et al.*, 1963), but this has not been universally accepted even for long-term therapy (Spaeth, 1967).

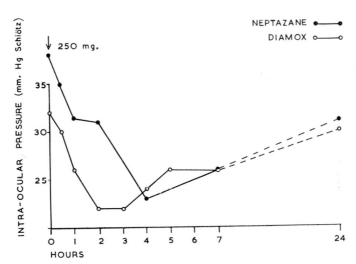

FIG. 522.—CARBONIC ANHYDRASE INHIBITORS IN SIMPLE GLAUCOMA.
The hypotensive effect of Neptazane and Diamox (Dorothy A. Campbell).

METHAZOLAMIDE (*Neptazane*) is said to be two or three times more potent than acetazolamide and causes fewer side-effects, particularly renal calculi since it does not depress urinary citrate. It is given orally in the treatment of simple glaucoma in doses of 50 to 100 mg. two to four times a day[2] (Fig. 522).

DICHLORPHENAMIDE (*Daranide*) is several times more potent than acetazolamide and is used in the treatment of simple glaucoma in doses of 50 to 100 mg. two to four times a day.[3]

ETHOXZOLAMIDE (*Cardrase*) is said to be twice as potent as acetazolamide as an ocular hypotensive agent (50 to 250 mg. two to four times a day).[4]

[1] Becker and Middleton (1955), Kupfer *et al.* (1955), Duke-Elder *et al.* (1956), Leopold and Carmichael (1956), de Carvalho *et al.* (1958), Becker and Shaffer (1965), Chandler and Grant (1965), Spaeth (1967), and many others.
[2] Becker (1957–60), Langham (1958), Coop (1959), Campbell (1960), Kandori *et al.* (1960), Suchat (1960), Mirande (1962), Agarwal *et al.* (1963), and others.
[3] Gonzales-Jimenez and Leopold (1958), Harris *et al.* (1958), Tanner and Harris (1958), Slezak (1959), Baron and Rozan (1960), Grande (1960), Schimek *et al.* (1960), Viallefont *et al.* (1960), Luntz (1961), Veronneau *et al.* (1961), Menezo and Quintana (1963), and others.
[4] D. M. Gordon (1958), Posner (1958), Drance (1959–60), Eliezer and de Carvalho (1959).

Systemic side-effects occur in a high percentage of patients, particularly when on long-term therapy with carbonic anhydrase inhibitors (Becker and Middleton, 1955; Leopold *et al.*, 1955). Many of these, such as general malaise, fatigue, paræsthesiæ, anorexia, nausea and vomiting, although relatively minor, require discontinuance of the drug. More serious is the renal colic due to depression of urinary citrate which has been reported on several occasions.[1] Exfoliative dermatitis and leucopenia have been reported as complications (C. and A. Turtz, 1958), as well as agranulocytosis (Pearson *et al.*, 1955; Underwood, 1956) and thrombocytopenia (Reisner and Morgan, 1956; Bertino *et al.*, 1957), both of which may be fatal. A fatal case of hepatic coma has also been recorded (Kristinsson, 1967).

(*b*) THE CARDIAC GLYCOSIDES

The CARDIAC GLYCOSIDES act by specifically inhibiting sodium-potassium-activated adenosine triphosphatase (NA-K-ATPase), an enzyme which is to some extent responsible for the secretion of the aqueous.[2] Among these substances the best known is *digoxin*. When given in full doses (1·0 mg. daily) this was found by Simon and Bonting (1962) to suppress the production of the aqueous by 45% and to cause a fall in the intra-ocular pressure averaging 14% in simple glaucoma; acetazolamide reduced the production by 45% and a combination of the two drugs by 65%. Awasthi and Saxena (1964) concluded that the drug acted most effectively in combination with pilocarpine and acetazolamide within a range of tension from 31 to 35 mm. Hg. In patients with simple glaucoma, however, who were inadequately controlled by standard methods of treatment, the additional fall in the ocular tension has been found to be small and occasional (Peczon, 1964; Pilz, 1967). Smith and Mickatavage (1963) found a slight lowering of the intra-ocular pressure by 4 to 5 mm. Hg when given topically either as drops or an ointment, but a digitalis keratopathy readily resulted.

It is obvious from the small experience hitherto reported that the glycosides are not generally effective in the treatment of simple glaucoma; moreover, the patient should be carefully evaluated lest any cardiac indication exists suggesting a danger in association with digitalization, while the toxicity of these drugs through chronic accumulation requires careful regulation of the dosage. Moreover, the deleterious effect of another cardiac glycoside, ouabain, on the function of the retina with extinction of the ERG after intravitreal injection in rabbits should be remembered (Langham *et al.*, 1967).

5. OSMOTIC AGENTS

The various hypertonic solutions of urea, mannitol, glycerol and isosorbide which when administered orally or intravenously produce a sudden change in the osmolarity of the plasma and thus a marked fall in ocular tension, have little place in the management of simple glaucoma except as a pre-operative measure in cases wherein the ocular tension is high. They are, however, of particular value in reducing the ocular tension in acute closed-angle and some types of secondary glaucoma and will therefore be discussed later in this Volume.[3]

[1] Kupfer *et al.* (1955), Glushien and Fisher (1956), Persky *et al.* (1956), Abeshouse and Applefeld (1956), E. E. Gordon and Sheps (1957), Barraquer and Escribano (1957), Yates-Bell (1958), Davies (1959), Mackenzie (1960), Zewi and Marjanen (1961).
[2] Vol. IV, p. 324.　　　　　　　　　[3] p. 610.

Of the many other drugs that have been advocated for the treatment of simple glaucoma, the following deserve brief mention:

(a) VASODILATORS. On the assumption that the defects in the visual fields of patients with simple glaucoma are the result of vascular changes within the optic nerve, various vasodilators have been recommended for the treatment of this disease. These include: nicotinic acid,[1] tolazoline (Priscol),[2] and Vasculat (Leydhecker (1952), which have been claimed to produce an improvement in the visual fields of some patients. All may cause a rise of ocular tension if the angle of the anterior chamber is narrow.

(b) BISHYDROXYCOUMARIN (*Dicumarol*) has been claimed to improve the field of vision (McGuire, 1948–53; Morpurgo, 1952) although these authors and McLean (1953) considered it too dangerous to use because of the risk of producing hæmorrhages throughout the body.

(c) HYALURONIDASE. The subconjunctival injection of this enzyme, or its passage into the anterior chamber by iontophoresis, has been said to increase the facility of the outflow of aqueous in simple glaucoma and thus reduce the ocular tension (Landesberg, 1959; Vanni and Lepri, 1959; Vanni and Palagi, 1959).

(d) ETHYL ALCOHOL. Ricklefs (1962–68) demonstrated the (delightfully welcome) fact that wine or brandy reduced the ocular tension of many patients with simple glaucoma, the reduction being frequently preceded by a small rise of tension. Peczon and Grant (1965) confirmed these findings with whisky or beer and showed that the tension-reducing effect lasted 4 or 5 hours.

Abeshouse and Applefeld. *Sinai Hosp. J.*, **5**, 73 (1956).
Abraham. *Amer. J. Ophthal.*, **37**, 327 (1954).
Agarwal. *Ophthalmologica*, **127**, 25 (1954).
Agarwal, Malik and Gupta. *Proc. All-India ophthal. Soc.*, **19**, 292 (1963).
Agarwal and Saxena. *Ophthalmologica*, **130**, 164 (1955).
Ahlquist. *Amer. J. Physiol.*, **153**, 586 (1948).
Armaly. *Amer. J. Ophthal.*, **47**, 879 (1959).
Awasthi and Saxena. *Orient. Arch. Ophthal.*, **2**, 151 (1964).
Axelsson. *Acta ophthal.* (Kbh.), **46**, 83, 99 (1968).
Axelsson and Holmberg. *Acta ophthal.* (Kbh.), **44**, 421 (1966).
Balassanian and de Soldati. *Dia méd.*, **27**, 599 (1955).
Ballintine and Garner. *Arch. Ophthal.*, **66**, 314 (1961).
Ballintine and Maren. *Amer. J. Ophthal.*, **40** (2), 148 (1955).
Bárány. *Invest. Ophthal.*, **1**, 712 (1962).
Drug Mechanisms in Glaucoma (ed. Paterson *et al.*), London, 41, 275 (1966).
Barkan. *Amer. J. Ophthal.*, **37**, 332 (1954).
Baron and Rozan. *Bull. Soc. Ophtal. Fr.*, 302 (1960).
Barraquer and Escribano. *Rev. clin. esp.*, **64**, 310 (1957).
Barrenechea, Contardo, Jarpa and Arentsen. *Arch. Oftal. B. Aires*, **19**, 246 (1944).
Bastide, Tronche and Rouher. *Arzneim.-Forsch.*, **18**, 322 (1968).

Becker. *Acta XVII int. Cong. Ophthal.*, Montreal-N.Y., **2**, 1109 (1954).
Amer. J. Ophthal., **39** (2), 177; **40** (2), 129 (1955); **49**, 1307 (1960).
Arch. Ophthal., **58**, 862 (1957).
Symposium on Glaucoma (trans. N. Orleans Acad. Ophthal.), St. Louis, 152, 170 (1967).
Becker and Friedenwald. *Arch. Ophthal.*, **50**, 557 (1953).
Becker and Gage. *Arch. Ophthal.*, **63**, 102 (1960).
Becker, Gage, Kolker and Gay. *Amer. J. Ophthal.*, **48**, 313 (1959).
Becker and Ley. *Amer. J. Ophthal.*, **45**, 639 (1958).
Becker and Middleton. *Arch. Ophthal.*, **54**, 187 (1955).
Becker, Pettit and Gay. *Arch. Ophthal.*, **66**, 219 (1961).
Becker, Pyle and Drews. *Amer. J. Ophthal.*, **47**, 635 (1959).
Becker and Shaffer. *Diagnosis and Therapy of the Glaucomas*, St. Louis (1965).
Berggren. *Invest. Ophthal.*, **3**, 266 (1964).
Berggren and Wistrand. *Svenska Läk.-T.*, **52**, 572 (1955).
Bertino, Rodman and Myerson. *Arch. intern. Med.*, **99**, 1006 (1957).
van Beuningen. *Klin. Mbl. Augenheilk.*, **121**, 345 (1952).
Bietti. *Boll. Oculist.*, **17**, 65 (1938).
Bill and Wålinder. *Invest. Ophthal.*, **5**, 170 (1966).

[1] R. Thiel (1943), Gallois (1945–50), Monfette (1948), Verrey (1948), Zaveroucha (1952).
[2] R. Thiel (1943), Gallois (1946–47), Zarrabi (1951).

Birks, Prior, Silk and Whittaker. *Arch. Ophthal.*, **79**, 283 (1968).

Bitrán and Weibel. *Arch. chil. Oftal.*, **23**, 108 (1966).

Blanton and Pollack. *Arch. Ophthal.*, **75**, 763 (1966).

Böck and Veitl. *Ber. dtsch. ophthal. Ges.*, **55**, 185 (1949).

Bonomi and di Comite. *Ann. Ottal.*, **89**, 135, 281 (1963).
  Boll. Oculist., **45**, 338 (1966).
  Arch. Ophthal., **78**, 337 (1967).

Breinin and Görtz. *Arch. Ophthal.*, **52**, 333 (1954).

Butler. *Amer. J. Ophthal.*, **35**, 1031 (1952).

Byakov and Stroganov. *Vestn. Oftal.*, **75** (3), 47 (1962).

Callahan. *Amer. J. Ophthal.*, **43**, 281 (1957).

Campbell. *Brit. J. Ophthal.*, **44**, 415 (1960).

Campbell, Jones, Renner and Tonks. *Brit. J. Ophthal.*, **41**, 746 (1957).

Campbell, Tonks and Jones. *Brit. J. Ophthal.*, **40**, 283 (1956).

Cantonnet. *Arch. Ophtal.*, **24**, 1 (1904).

de Carvalho, Lawrence and Stone. *Arch. Ophthal.*, **59**, 840 (1958).

Caselli. *Arch. Ottal.*, **57**, 413 (1953).

Castrén and Pohjola. *Acta ophthal.* (Kbh.), **40**, 359 (1962).

Castrén, Pohjola, Pakarinen and Karjalainen. *Ophthalmologica*, **155**, 194 (1968).

Chandler. *Arch. Ophthal.*, **57**, 639 (1957).

Chandler and Grant. *Lectures on Glaucoma*, Phila. (1965).

Christensen, Swan and Huggins. *Arch. Ophthal.*, **55**, 666 (1956).

Clarke. *Amer. J. Ophthal.*, **22**, 249 (1939).

Colle, Duke-Elder, W. S. and P. M. *J. Physiol.*, **71**, 1 (1931).

Coop. *Brit. J. Ophthal.*, **43**, 602 (1959).

Corwin and Spencer. *Arch. Ophthal.*, **69**, 317 (1963).

Coté and Drance. *Canad. J. Ophthal.*, **3**, 207 (1968).

Coyle, Weiner, Frank and Leonard. *Amer. J. Ophthal.*, **52**, 867 (1961).

Cristini. *Brit. J. Ophthal.*, **33**, 228 (1949).

Darier. *Clin. Ophtal.*, **6**, 141 (1900).

Davies. *Brit. med. J.*, **1**, 214 (1959).

DeLong and Scheie. *Arch. Ophthal.*, **50**, 289 (1953).

Demailly and Kérisel. *Arch. Ophtal.*, **27**, 683 (1967).

Dorsch and Thygeson. *Amer. J. Ophthal.*, **65**, 74 (1968).

Draeger, Grüttner and Theilmann. *Brit. J. Ophthal.*, **47**, 457 (1963).

Drance. *Brit. J. Ophthal.*, **39**, 659 (1955).
  Arch. Ophthal., **62**, 679 (1959); **64**, 433 (1960).
  Trans. Canad. ophthal. Soc., **21–2**, 84 (1959); **24**, 112 (1961).
  Trans. ophthal. Soc. U.K., **80**, 387 (1960).
  Drug Mechanisms in Glaucoma (ed. Paterson *et al.*), London, 301 (1966).

Drance and Carr. *Arch. Ophthal.*, **62**, 673 (1959).
  Amer. J. Ophthal., **49**, 470 (1960).

Drance and Scott. *Canad. J. Ophthal.*, **3**, 159 (1968).

Duke-Elder and Law. *Brit. med. J.*, **1**, 590 (1929).

Duke-Elder, Perkins and Langham. *Arch. Soc. oftal. hisp.-amer.*, **16**, 259 (1956).

Dunphy. *Amer. J. Ophthal.*, **32**, 1403 (1949).

Duzanec and Leydhecker. *Klin. Mbl. Augenheilk.*, **151**, 877 (1967).

Eakins. *J. Pharm. exp. Ther.*, **140**, 79 (1963).

Eakins and Ryan. *Brit. J. Pharm.*, **23**, 374 (1964).

Eliezer and de Carvalho. *Rev. bras. Oftal.*, **18**, 199 (1959).

Esente. *G. ital. Oftal.*, **1**, 274 (1948).

Espíldora-Luque, Thierry and Espíldora-Couso. *Arch. chil. Oftal.*, **11**, 106 (1954).

Étienne and Barut. *Ann. Oculist.* (Paris), **198**, 472 (1965).

Étienne, Barut and Gonzalès-Bouchon. *Ann. Oculist.* (Paris), **200**, 287 (1967).

Fechner. *Klin. Mbl. Augenheilk.*, **148**, 64 (1966).

Ferry and Zimmerman. *Amer. J. Ophthal.*, **58**, 205 (1964).

Fisher, Smith and Wheeler. *Brit. J. Ophthal.*, **49**, 369 (1965).

Frisch and Leopold. *Amer. J. Ophthal.*, **36**, 442 (1953).

Galin, Baras and Glenn. *Invest. Ophthal.*, **5**, 120 (1966).

Gallois. *Bull. Soc. franç. Ophtal.*, **59**, 224 (1940–46).
  Arch. Ophtal., **5**, 197 (1945).
  Ann. Oculist. (Paris), **180**, 20 (1947).
  Presse méd., **58**, 1399 (1950).

Garner, Carl and Ferwerda. *Amer. J. Ophthal.*, **55**, 323 (1963).

Garner, Johnstone, Ballintine and Carroll. *Arch. Ophthal.*, **62**, 230 (1959).

Gerhard and Ketter. *Bull. Soc. Ophtal. Fr.*, 549 (1958).

Giardini and Paliaga. *Boll. Oculist.*, **38**, 683 (1959).

Gifford. *Arch. Ophthal.*, **57**, 612 (1928).

Gittler. *Wien. klin. Wschr.*, **62**, 379 (1950).
  Österr. ophthal. Ges., **2**, 26 (1959).

Gittler and Pillat. *v. Graefes Arch. Ophthal.*, **157**, 473 (1956).

Glees and Wüstenberg. *Klin. Mbl. Augenheilk.*, **114**, 455 (1949).

Gloster and Perkins. *J. Physiol.*, **130**, 665 (1955).
  Brit. J. Ophthal., **39**, 647 (1955).

Glushien and Fisher. *J. Amer. med. Ass.*, **160**, 204 (1956).

Görtz. *Klin. Mbl. Augenheilk.*, **133**, 203 (1958).

Goldmann. *Ann. Oculist.* (Paris), **184**, 1086 (1951).

Gonzales-Jimenez and Leopold. *Arch. Ophthal.*, **60**, 427 (1958).

Gonzalez-Pola, Sanchez Salorio and Garcia Lopez. *Arch. Soc. oftal. hisp.-amer.*, **15**, 306 (1955).

Goodwin. *Amer. J. Ophthal.*, **34**, 1139 (1951).

Gordon, D. M. *Amer. J. Ophthal.*, **46**, 41 (1958).

Gordon, E. E. and Sheps. *New Engl. J. Med.*, **256**, 1215 (1957).

Gradle. *Amer. J. Ophthal.*, **7**, 851 (1924).

von Graefe. *v. Graefes Arch. Ophthal.*, **3** (2), 456 (1857).

Grande. *G. ital. Oftal.*, **13**, 125 (1960). *Minerva oftal.*, **5**, 61 (1963).

Grant. *Arch. Ophthal.*, **39**, 579 (1948). *Toxicology of the Eye*, Springfield, Ill., 368 (1962).

Grant and Trotter. *Arch. Ophthal.*, **51**, 735 (1954).

Gray and Robinson. *Amer. J. Ophthal.*, **49**, 1162 (1960).

Grob and Harvey. *Bull. Johns Hopk. Hosp.*, **84**, 532 (1949).

de Grosz and Kedvessy. *Arch. Ophtal.*, **11**, 155 (1951).

Haas. *Amer. J. Ophthal.*, **31**, 227 (1948).

Hamburger. *Med. Klin.*, **19**, 1224 (1923). *Klin. Mbl. Augenheilk.*, **72**, 47 (1924).

Hansen. *T. norske Lœgeforen.*, **8**, 678 (1964).

Hanssen. *Klin. Mbl. Augenheilk.*, **80**, 690 (1928).

Harris, Beaudreau and Hoskinson. *Amer. J. Ophthal.*, **45**, 120 (1958).

Harrison. *Amer. J. Ophthal.*, **50**, 153 (1960).

Heath. *Arch. Ophthal.*, **16**, 839 (1936).

Heath and Geiter. *Arch. Ophthal.*, **41**, 172 (1949).

Heim. *Klin. Mbl. Augenheilk.*, **79**, 345 (1927). *Ophthalmologica*, **102**, 193 (1941).

Hertel. *Klin. Mbl. Augenheilk.*, **51** (2), 351 (1913). *v. Graefes Arch. Ophthal.*, **90**, 309 (1915).

Hind and Goyan. *J. Amer. pharm. Ass.*, **36**, 33 (1947).

Hirsch-Hoffmann. *Ophthalmologica*, **147**, 96 (1964); **152**, 291 (1966).

Hofmann. *Klin. Mbl. Augenheilk.*, **124**, 63 (1954).

Huerkamp and Wagner. *Klin. Mbl. Augenheilk.*, **117**, 586 (1950).

Humphreys and Holmes. *Arch. Ophthal.*, **69**, 737 (1963).

Kadin. *Amer. J. Ophthal.*, **50**, 115 (1960).

Kalfa, Rozovskaya and Shekhtman. *Oftal. Zh.*, **16**, 259 (1961).

Kamilov and Arustamova. *Oftal. Zh.*, **22**, 3 (1967).

Kandori, Kurose and Kurimoto. *Amer. J. Ophthal.*, **49**, 1396 (1960).

Kellerman and King. *Amer. J. Ophthal.*, **62**, 278 (1966).

Klayman and Taffet. *Amer. J. Ophthal.*, **55**, 1233 (1963).

Kleinert. *Klin. Mbl. Augenheilk.*, **125**, 271 (1954).

Klendshoj and Olmsted. *Amer. J. Ophthal.*, **56**, 247 (1933).

Knapp. *Arch. Ophthal.*, **50**, 556 (1921).

Köllner. *Münch. med. Wschr.*, **65**, 229 (1918). *Z. Augenheilk.*, **43**, 381 (1920).

Kravitz. *Arch. Ophthal.*, **32**, 283 (1944).

Krill and Newell. *Amer. J. Ophthal.*, **57**, 34 (1964).

Krill, Newell and Novak. *Amer. J. Ophthal.*, **59**, 833 (1965).

Krishna and Leopold. *Amer. J. Ophthal.*, **49**, 554 (1960).

Kristinsson. *Brit. J. Ophthal.*, **51**, 348 (1967).

Kronfeld. *Amer. J. Ophthal.*, **55**, 829 (1963); **61**, 1198 (1966). *Invest. Ophthal.*, **3**, 258 (1964). *Arch. Ophthal.*, **78**, 140 (1967).

Küchle. *Klin. Mbl. Augenheilk.*, **139**, 224 (1961).

Kupfer, Lawrence and Linnér. *Amer. J. Ophthal.*, **40**, 673 (1955).

Kutschera. *Klin. Mbl. Augenheilk.*, **139**, 234 (1961). *Wien. med. Wschr.*, **112**, 704 (1962).

Landesberg. *Amer. J. Ophthal.*, **48**, 81 (1959).

Langham. *J. Physiol.*, **130**, 1 (1955). *Brit. J. Ophthal.*, **42**, 577 (1958). *Exp. Eye Res.*, **4**, 381 (1965).

Langham, Ryan and Kostelnik. *Life Sciences*, **6**, 2037 (1967).

Lansche. *Amer. J. Ophthal.*, **61**, 95 (1966).

Laqueur. *Zbl. med. Wiss.*, No. 24, 421 (1876). *v. Graefes Arch. Ophthal.*, **23** (3), 149 (1877).

Lavagna. *Ann. Ottal.*, Suppl. to Fasc. 4, 36 (1895). *Clin. Ophtal.*, **3**, 229 (1897).

Lawlor and Lee. *Amer. J. Ophthal.*, **49**, 808 (1960).

Leopold. *Amer. J. Ophthal.*, **51**, 885 (1961).

Leopold and Carmichael. *Trans. Amer. Acad. Ophthal.*, **60**, 210 (1956).

Leopold and Cleveland. *Amer. J. Ophthal.*, **36**, 226 (1953).

Leopold and Comroe. *Arch. Ophthal.*, **36**, 1, 17 (1946).

Leopold, Eisenberg and Yasuna. *Amer. J. Ophthal.*, **39**, 885 (1955).

Leopold, Gold, P. and D. *Arch. Ophthal.*, **58**, 363 (1957).

Leopold and Krishna. *Hb. d. experimentellen Pharmakologie* (ed. Eichler and Farah), Berlin, Erganz., **15**, 1051 (1963).

Leopold, Krishna and Lehman. *Trans. Amer. ophthal. Soc.*, **57**, 63 (1959).

Leopold and McDonald. *Arch. Ophthal.*, **40**, 176 (1948).

Levene. *Amer. J. Ophthal.*, **57**, 429 (1964).

Levene and Friedman. *Amer. J. Ophthal.*, **60**, 719 (1965).

Leydhecker. *Klin. Mbl. Augenheilk.*, **121**, 513 (1952).

Libman. *Vestn. Oftal.*, **74** (4), 17 (1961).

Lieberman and Leopold. *Amer. J. Ophthal.*, **64**, 405 (1967).

Linnér. *Acta physiol. scand.*, **26**, 70 (1952). *Brit. J. Ophthal.*, **42**, 38 (1958).

Lloyd. *Brit. J. Ophthal.*, **47**, 469 (1963).

Löhlein. *Klin. Mbl. Augenheilk.*, **77**, Beil., 1 (1926).

Löwenstein, A. *Ber. dtsch. ophthal. Ges.*, **46**, 439 (1927).

Lowenstein, O. and Loewenfeld. *Arch. Ophthal.*, **50**, 311 (1953).

Luntz. *Brit. J. Ophthal.*, **45**, 125 (1961).

McGuire. *Trans. Amer. ophthal. Soc.*, **46**, 96 (1948); **51**, 67 (1953).

Mackenzie. *J. Urol.* (Baltimore), **84**, 453 (1960).

McLean. *Trans. Amer. ophthal. Soc.*, **51**, 73 (1953).

Maggi Zavalía, Garibay Zurbriggen and Narvaja. *Arch. Soc. oftal. Litoral*, **11**, 95 (1958).

Malik, Sood, Jain and Gupta. *Orient. Arch. Ophthal.*, **2**, 162 (1964).

Mangouritsas and Koliopoulos. *Bull. Soc. hellén. Ophtal.*, **35**, 361 (1967).

Marchesani and Ullerich. *Ber. dtsch. ophthal. Ges.*, **56**, 312 (1950).

Marr. *Amer. J. Ophthal.*, **30**, 1423 (1947).

Menezo and Quintana. *Arch. Soc. oftal. hisp.-amer.*, **23**, 265, 830 (1963).

Miller. *Acta XVIII int. Cong. Ophthal.*, Brussels, **2**, 1489 (1960).

Miloro. *Ann. Ottal.*, **63**, 780 (1935).

Mirande. *Gaz. méd. Fr.*, **69**, 2747 (1962).

Mishra and Goel. *Antiseptic*, **59**, 861 (1962).

Monfette. *L'Union méd. Canad.*, **77**, 1433 (1948).

Morpurgo. *Ann. Ottal.*, **78**, 109 (1952).

Myerson and Thau. *Arch. Ophthal.*, **18**, 78 (1937); **24**, 758 (1940).

Neuenschwander. *Ophthalmologica*, **120**, 104 (1950).

Niemeyer. *Ophthalmologica*, **156**, 161 (1968).

Odinzow and Nejman. *Tr. Inst. vser. S-ezda glasn. Vrac.*, 51 (1929). *See Zbl. ges. Ophthal.*, **22**, 210 (1930).

Onfray, Abeloos and Suys. *Bull. Soc. franç. Ophtal.*, **47**, 297 (1934).

Oosterhuis. *Arch. Ophthal.*, **67**, 802 (1962).

Orbán. *Szemészet*, **91**, 35 (1954).

Ourgaud. *L'année thér. en ophtal.*, **2**, 248 (1951).

Owe-Larsson. *Acta ophthal.* (Kbh.), **34**, 27 (1956).

Owens and Woods. *Amer. J. Ophthal.*, **29**, 447 (1946); **30**, 995 (1947).

Paterson. *Drug Mechanisms in Glaucoma* (ed. Paterson *et al.*), London, 3 (1966).

Pearson, Binder and Neber. *J. Amer. med. Ass.*, **157**, 339 (1955).

Peczon. *Arch. Ophthal.*, **71**, 500 (1964).

Peczon and Grant. *Arch. Ophthal.*, **73**, 495 (1965).

Pereyra. *G. ital. Oftal.*, **1**, 165 (1948).

Persichetti. *Boll. Oculist.*, **29**, 234 (1950).

Persky, Chambers and Potts. *J. Amer. med. Ass.*, **161**, 1625 (1956).

Peyret. *Sem. méd.* (B. Aires), **123**, 1181 (1963).

Phillips, Howitt and Rowlands. *Brit. J. Ophthal.*, **51**, 222 (1967).

Pilz. *Klin. Mbl. Augenheilk.*, **151**, 492 (1967).

Poos and Santori. *v. Graefes Arch. Ophthal.*, **121**, 443 (1929).

Posner. *Amer. J. Ophthal.*, **31**, 222 (1948); **33**, 1551 (1950); **45**, 225 (1958).

Pratt-Johnson, Drance and Innes. *Arch. Ophthal.*, **72**. 485 (1964).

Prijot and Weckers. *Ophthalmologica*, **124**, 12 (1952).

Primrose. *Brit. J. Ophthal.*, **39**, 307 (1955).

Purcell and Schane. *Kresge Eye Inst. Bull.*, **5**, 64 (1954).

Quilliam. *Postgrad. med. J.*, **23**, 280 (1947).

Quintieri. *Boll. Oculist.*, **30**, 726 (1951).

Rae. *Pharm. J.*, **156**, 329 (1946).

Raiford. *Amer. J. Ophthal.*, **32**, 1399 (1949).

Reisner and Morgan. *J. Amer. med. Ass.*, **160**, 206 (1956).

Richards and Drance. *Canad. J. Ophthal.*, **2**, 259 (1967).

Ricklefs. *Öst. ophthal. Ges.*, **7**, 116 (1962). *Docum. ophthal.*, **25**, 43 (1968).

Riegel and Leydhecker. *Klin. Mbl. Augenheilk.*, **151**, 882 (1967).

Rintelen and Jenny. *Ophthalmologica*, **130**, 171 (1955).

de Roetth. *Amer. J. Ophthal.*, **62**, 619 (1966). *Trans. ophthal. Soc. U.K.*, **86**, 89 (1966).

Romano. *Brit. J. Ophthal.*, **52**, 361 (1968).

Romano and Jackson. *Brit. J. Ophthal.*, **48**, 480 (1964).

Rosengren. *Arch. Ophthal.*, **44**, 523 (1950).

Rotter. *Wien. klin. Wschr.*, **63**, 683 (1951).

Sacks-Wilner, A. and E. *Amer. J. Ophthal.*, **51**, 695 (1961).

de Sanctis. *Ann. Ottal.*, **65**, 25 (1937).

Schimek, Balian, Lepley *et al.* *Acta XVIII int. Cong. Ophthal.*, Brussels, **2**, 1466 (1960).

Schoenberg. *Brit. J. Ophthal.*, **22**, 417 (1938).

Sears. *Invest. Ophthal.*, **5**, 115 (1966).

Sears and Bárány. *Arch. Ophthal.*, **64**, 839 (1960).

Sears and Sherk. *Invest. Ophthal.*, **3**, 157 (1964).

Shaffer. *Symposium on Glaucoma* (Trans. N. Orleans Acad. Ophthal.), St. Louis, 129 (1967).

Shaffer and Hetherington. *Amer. J. Ophthal.*, **62**, 613 (1966).

Shaffer and Ridgway. *Amer. J. Ophthal.*, **34**, 718 (1951).

Shah, Wahia and Soomro. *Medicus* (Karachi), **10**, 189 (1955).

Simon and Bonting. *Arch. Ophthal.*, **68**, 227 (1962).

Simonelli. *Riv. Oftal.*, **2**, 119 (1947).

Slezak. *Klin. Mbl. Augenheilk.*, **134**, 829 (1959).

Smith, J. L., and Mickatavage. *Amer. J. Ophthal.*, **56**, 889 (1963).

Spaeth. *Arch. Ophthal.*, **75**, 783 (1966); **78**, 578 (1967).

Spiers. *Acta ophthal.* (Kbh.), **41**, 247 (1963).

Spiers and Eldrup-Jørgensen. *Trans. ophthal. Soc. U.K.*, **86**, 255 (1966).

Stepanik. *Klin. Mbl. Augenheilk.*, **139**, 174 (1961); **146**, 376 (1965).
   v. Graefes Arch. Ophthal., **164**, 6 (1961).

Stepanik and Stelzer. *v. Graefes Arch. Ophthal.*, **161**, 159 (1959).

Stirpe and Bucci. *Boll. Oculist.*, **41**, 862 (1962).

Stone. *Arch. Ophthal.*, **43**, 36 (1950).

Suchat. *Milit. Med.*, **125**, 489 (1960).

Suda, Sawada, Muto *et al. Rinsho Ganka*, **17**, 623 (1963).

Sugar. *The Glaucomas*, 2nd ed., N.Y., 120 (1967).

Swan. *Arch. Ophthal.*, **30**, 591 (1943); **49**, 419 (1953).
   Amer. J. Ophthal., **37**, 886 (1954).
   Symposium on Glaucoma (ed. Clark), St. Louis, 159 (1959).

Swan and Hart. *Amer. J. Ophthal.*, **23**, 1311 (1940).

Tanner and Harris. *Amer. J. Ophthal.*, **45**, 121 (1958).

Tarkkanen and Karjalainen. *v. Graefes Arch. Ophthal.*, **172**, 86 (1967).

Terner, Linn and Goldstrohm. *Amer. J. Ophthal.*, **52**, 553 (1961).

Thiel, H. L. *Klin. Mbl. Augenheilk.*, **114**, 454 (1949).

Thiel, R. *Ber. dtsch. ophthal. Ges.*, **44**, 118 (1924).
   Z. Augenheilk., **65**, 373 (1928).
   Klin. Mbl. Augenheilk., **109**, 433 (1943).
   Acta XVII int. Cong. Ophthal., Montreal-N.Y., **2**, 722 (1954).

Tittarelli. *Boll. Oculist.*, **39**, 873 (1960).

Turtz, C. and A. *Arch. Ophthal.*, **60**, 130 (1958).

Uhler. *Amer. J. Ophthal.*, **26**, 710 (1943).

Underwood. *J. Amer. med. Ass.*, **161**, 1477 (1956).

Upholt, Quinby, Batchelor and Thompson. *Arch. Ophthal.*, **56**, 128 (1956).

Vanni and Lepri. *Boll. Oculist.*, **38**, 114 (1959).

Vanni and Palagi. *Boll. Oculist.*, **38**, 373 (1959).

Vaughan, Shaffer and Riegelman. *Arch. Ophthal.*, **66**, 232 (1961).

Veirs and McGrew. *Eye, Ear, Nose, Thr. Mthly.*, **42**, 46 (1963).

Velhagen. *Klin. Mbl. Augenheilk.*, **92**, 472 (1934); **109**, 195 (1936).

Verdi and de Molfetta. *Minerva oftal.*, **6**, 69 (1964).

Veronneau, Rebouillat, Barut and Étienne. *Bull. Soc. Ophtal. Fr.*, 425 (1961).

Verrey. *Schweiz. med. Wschr.*, **78**, 887 (1948).

Viallefont, Boudet and Grandebarbe. *Bull. Soc. franç. Ophtal.*, **73**, 583 (1960).

Villaret, Besançon and Gallois. *Bull. Soc. franç. Ophtal.*, **44**, 532 (1931).

Weber. *Korresp.-Bl. med. Wiss.*, **14**, 986 (1876).

Weekers. *Bull. Soc. belge Ophtal.*, No. 86, 38 (1947).
   Glaucoma: a Symposium (ed. Duke-Elder), Oxon., 257 (1955).

Weekers, Collignon-Brach and Grieten. *Drug Mechanisms in Glaucoma* (ed. Paterson *et al.*), London, 51 (1966).

Weekers, Delmarcelle and Gustin. *Amer. J. Ophthal.*, **40**, 666 (1955).

Weekers, Gilson and Prijot. *Arch. Ophtal.*, **21**, 545 (1961).

Weekers and Lavergne. *Bull. Soc. belge Ophtal.*, No. 110, 273 (1955).

Weekers, Prijot and Gustin. *Brit. J. Ophthal.*, **38**, 742 (1954).

Weinstein. *Ophthalmologica*, **118**, 76 (1949).

Westsmith and Abernethy. *Arch. Ophthal.*, **52**, 779 (1954).

Wilson, Harrison and Ginsburg. *J. biol. Chem.*, **236**, 1498 (1961).

Wirth. *Aggiorn. terap. Oftal.*, **3**, Suppl. 4, 1 (1951).

Wistrand. *Acta pharmacol.*, **14**, 27 (1957).

Yates-Bell. *Brit. med. J.*, **2**, 1392 (1958).

Zarrabi. *Ophthalmologica*, **122**, 76 (1951).

Zaveroucha. *Vestn. Oftal.*, **31**, 31 (1952).

Zekman and Snydacker. *Amer. J. Ophthal.*, **36**, 1709 (1953).

Zewi and Marjanen. *Acta ophthal.* (Kbh.), **39**, 483 (1961).

Surgical Treatment

It must be recognized that surgical methods of treatment of simple glaucoma are confined merely to mechanical expedients to relieve the raised tension of the eye, and in this respect few fundamental advances have been made in the last quarter of a century. If it is accepted that the immediate cause of the rise of tension is an embarrassment of drainage, the obvious method of surgical treatment is to adopt measures to facilitate the outflow of aqueous; a less rational technique is to decrease the formation of aqueous. The latter is potentially dangerous from the physiological point of view, and cannot be said to rectify the cause; the former is in essence a matter of plumbing and, if it is possible, the ophthalmic surgeon should be more than a technician but rather a physician treating a patient with glaucoma. Particularly is this so in view of the fact that the loss of vision—the principal factor which we aim to avoid—although undoubtedly dependent on relative pressures, is essentially caused by vascular insufficiency in the optic nerve.

Any operation devised for the relief of glaucoma should ideally be such as to preserve the function of the eye, maintain its tension within normal limits, and retain the integrity of the globe. The number of operations advocated from time to time is evidence that this ideal has never been attained. This state of affairs will remain until our ideas regarding the ætiology of simple glaucoma are completely clarified, for the operative technique—if surgical interference is considered the ideal method of treatment—should restore the fluid dynamics of the eye to a normal equilibrium. All the surgical procedures at present available are imperfect since all of them are liable to affect the visual function and allow a return of hypertension, while most of them leave the integrity of the eye considerably impaired.

HISTORY

The effective surgical treatment of simple glaucoma was long delayed because it was not until the teaching of Pierre and Antoine-Pierre Demours was published in 1818 that the cardinal feature of a raised ocular tension was generally accepted. To WILLIAM MACKENZIE (1830) belongs the credit of the first suggestion for its surgical relief by a sclerotomy, and later by a paracentesis (1854) in the chronic stages of the disease. It is of interest that in cases of staphyloma " wherein the watery contents of the globe had increased ", James Wardrop (1808) had practised repeated paracenteses or even the formation of a permanent corneal fistula—sometimes with unpleasant results. A paracentesis, however, is obviously an unsatisfactory and temporary expedient; the first to attempt to make it permanent was GEORGE CRITCHETT (1857) (Fig. 523) of London, who, in his operation of *iridodesis*, drew a piece of iris with a blunt hook into the wound made at the limbus for a paracentesis, thus introducing the idea of drainage by an " iris inclusion ".

In the same year, Albrecht von Graefe, observing the recession of a staphyloma after an iridectomy presumably owing to the relief of raised tension, announced the effect of a basal iridectomy in the treatment of acute glaucoma but, while the effect in this type of the disease was acclaimed to be revolutionary and dramatic, equally good results were soon found to be absent in the more chronic forms unless, perhaps, the iris was incarcerated in the scar (Coccius, 1859–63; Bader, 1881; Parinaud, 1901). At the time of its introduction, the theoretical basis of von Graefe's iridectomy was vague but his pupil and ardent admirer, LOUIS DE WECKER (1869–71) (Fig. 526), devised an *anterior sclerotomy* with a view to increasing the drainage of the aqueous by the formation of a *filtering cicatrix*. In this procedure, after a puncture and counter-puncture had been made just behind the limbus, the knife cut up a short distance as in making an incision for cataract and then was slowly withdrawn leaving the upper pole of the limbus uncut. The operation was practised by Stellwag von Carion (1870) and Quaglino (1871) and at a later date was improved by de Wecker (1894) himself by making a dialysis in addition and subsequently by combining it with an iridectomy (1901); but the results remained unsatisfactory for the wound tended to close even although the operation was followed by prolonged massage (Dianoux, 1905).

A more dramatic attempt to improve drainage by a fistulous scar was made by Major H. HERBERT (1903) of Bombay in his *small-flap sclerotomy*. A small incision was made into the anterior chamber through the sclera behind and parallel to the limbus and at either end two cuts were made perpendicular to the corneal margin thus leaving a rectangular trap-door of sclera with its base attached to the cornea. In the operation he reverted to Critchett's idea of iris-inclusion by deliberately including a prolapse of the iris protected by a flap of conjunctiva in the scar. In a later suggestion, the *wedge-resection* of Herbert (1913), he isolated a wedge of sclera at the limbus attached to the conjunctiva only so that it shrivelled, a technique further amplified by Cruise (1921–47). These types of sclerotomy, however, are of little more than historical interest, but the principle of iris-inclusion was eventually popularized by SØREN HOLTH (1907) (Fig. 525) in his technique of *iridencleisis*.[1] As we shall presently see, several modifications of this technique have been introduced, but from the historical point of view the operation of *iridotasis*, introduced by Johan Borthen (1910) of Bergen, should be mentioned; he made the subconjunctival prolapse without an iridectomy, a technique which although now seldom used, has had its advocates (Harrower, 1918; Wilder, 1923; G. H. Bell, 1930; Dastoor, 1948).

The production of a filtering scar by *sclerectomy* was another expedient adopted to secure drainage. This idea was first introduced by DOUGLAS ARGYLL ROBERTSON (1876) of Edinburgh in his technique of *posterior trephining*; using a modification of the trephine devised by Bowman for operating on a conical cornea, he trephined the sclera at the junction of the pars plana and the ciliary body, reporting 4 cases with reasonably satisfactory results. This idea of draining the subchoroidal space was pursued by Freeland Fergus (1909–15) of Glasgow who improved upon it by introducing a spatula through the opening into the anterior chamber thus combining the trephining with a cyclodialysis. Such an operation has been practised in recalcitrant cases[2] but is not generally popular. George Young (1924) of Colchester, on the other hand, advised a double sclerectomy in this region, removing a portion of the muscle in so doing. With these procedures the results were not altogether satisfactory, but the concept was revolutionized by the operation of *corneo-scleral trephining* at the limbus introduced by Colonel ROBERT HENRY ELLIOT (1902–32) of Madras (Fig. 528), an operation still widely used.[3]

The operation of sclerectomy was further pursued by the great French surgeon, FÉLIX LAGRANGE (1906–7) of Bordeaux (Fig. 527), who finally achieved de Wecker's inspiration of establishing a filtering scar of a permanent nature. At a later date the fashioning of a similar type of drainage-scar by cauterizing the sclera was sought by Count Luigi Preziosi (1924) of Malta and elaborated by Harold Scheie (1958) of Philadelphia. These techniques will be subsequently described,[4] as well as various suggestions to maintain drainage by the insertion of a seton in the fistula.[5]

A further type of operation depends on the establishment of drainage channels within the eye. Such a procedure had been done incidentally in other techniques and was first conceived by LEOPOLD HEINE (1905) of Breslau as a primary operation in his technique of *cyclodialysis*[6] (Fig. 524). As with filtering operations, attempts have been made to maintain the patency of the cyclodialysis-cleft by the introduction of foreign materials, initially by Row (1934).[7]

Trabeculotomy is a further application of the same principle. Reasoning that glaucoma was caused by a failure of the aqueous to reach Schlemm's canal, the Italian surgeon, de Vincentiis (1893), conceived the rational idea of opening the canal by a knife introduced into the anterior chamber; the attempt was unsuccessful because he

---

[1] p. 538.

[2] Sallmann (1935), Ivanov (1937), Lauber (1939), Mügge (1947).

[3] p. 534.   [4] p. 536.

[5] p. 543.   [6] p. 544.   [7] p. 546.

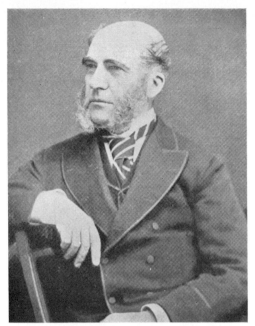

FIG. 523.—GEORGE CRITCHETT
[1817–1882].

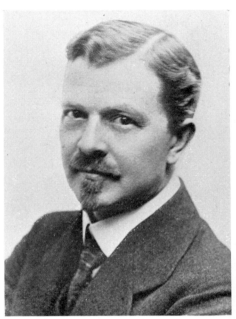

FIG. 524.—LEOPOLD HEINE
[1870–1940].
(By courtesy of Prof. H. Pau, Kiel.)

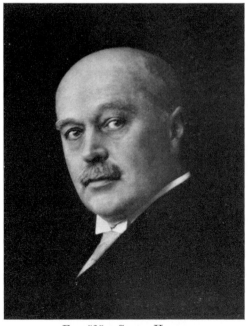

FIG. 525.—SOREN HOLTH
[1863–1937].
(By courtesy of Prof. T. L. Thomassen, Oslo.)

could not see where he was going. This feat was achieved by the ingenuity of Otto Barkan (1936–38) of San Francisco (Fig. 543) who, in his operation of trabeculotomy (or *goniotomy*), with the aid of a contact glass and intense transillumination, devised a technique by which the canal can be cut open from within. We have already seen that this is the most effective operation for those cases of congenital glaucoma which are due to anomalies in the development of the angle of the anterior chamber.[1] Somewhat similar in principle is the internalization of Schlemm's canal (R. Smith, 1960–62; Burian, 1960; and others) or its externalization (Krasnov, 1964–68; and others).

A final expedient recently adopted for the treatment of eyes with advanced glaucoma is the direct drainage of the anterior chamber into a vortex vein or the superficial temporal vein; these will be noted subsequently.

From the point of view of historical interest, other operations may be noted. Hancock (1860), believing that the action of the ciliary muscle was responsible for glaucoma, severed the ciliary body through a scleral incision (*intra-ocular ciliary myotomy*), an operation also practised by Solomon (1861). Abadie (1910) advised a somewhat similar *ciliarotomy*, cutting the ciliary body meridionally in order to section the ciliary nerve plexus. With a view to stopping nerve reflexes he also advised an *iridotomy*. Verhoeff (1924) recommended a *cyclectomy*, a small portion of the anterior part of the ciliary body being excised through a scleral incision after a buttonhole iridectomy.

Resection of the cervical sympathetic, suggested by Abadie (1897) and introduced by Jonnesco (1899), was practised to a considerable extent for some time thereafter[2]; the results, however, were irregular and disappointing (Elschnig, 1912).

Of those surgeons who pioneered these surgical techniques, the portraits of WILLIAM MACKENZIE of Glasgow[3] and DOUGLAS ARGYLL ROBERTSON of Edinburgh[4] appear elsewhere in this *System*; six others introduce this section.

GEORGE CRITCHETT [1817–82] (Fig. 523), whose medical school was The London Hospital, was one of the brilliant band of ophthalmologists constituting the staff of Moorfields Eye Hospital in the second half of the 19th century. He was a remarkable surgeon of great dexterity and introduced a number of operations into ophthalmic practice including the procedure of iris inclusion for glaucoma.

LOUIS DE WECKER [1832–1906] (Fig. 526) was one of the most famous European surgeons. Of German origin he was born in Frankfurt and studied at Würzburg, Berlin and Paris where he settled as an ophthalmologist in 1862. A devoted pupil of von Graefe (who left him all his surgical instruments), he strove to improve his master's iridectomy to attain drainage in simple glaucoma by introducing the operation of sclerotomy. An ophthalmologist of world fame, his *Traité des maladies des yeux* (Paris, 1863, 1869, 1870) is a masterpiece of scientific accuracy and literary style and his ingenuity as a surgeon is seen in the multitude of new techniques and instruments he devised; his name is still eponymously used for his iris-scissors.

FÉLIX LAGRANGE [1857–1928] (Fig. 527) of Bordeaux was one of the most prominent and personally delightful of the French ophthalmologists of his generation. His contributions to our specialty included fundamental work on refractive errors and strabismus and on intra- and extra-ocular tumours. In the latter connection his portrait in his official dress has appeared in a previous Volume[5]; but in view of his introduction of a fistulizing operation for glaucoma by combining a sclerectomy with an iridectomy, his photograph in his academic robes as a professor of medicine is included here.

[1] Vol. III, p. 562.
[2] Abadie (1899–1901), Ziehe and Axenfeld (1901), Rohmer (1902), Wilder (1904).
[3] Vol. IX, Fig. 400.   [4] Vol. XII.   [5] Vol. IX, Fig. 606.

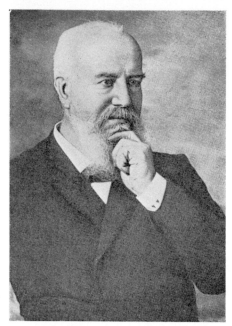

FIG. 526.—LOUIS DE WECKER
[1832–1906].

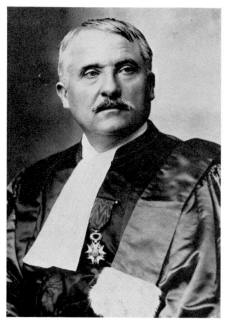

FIG. 527.—FÉLIX LAGRANGE
[1857–1928].

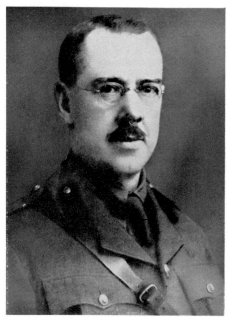

FIG. 528.—ROBERT HENRY ELLIOT
[1864–1936].
(By courtesy of Dr. T. T. Ramalingam, Madras.)

SØREN HOLTH [1863–1937] (Fig. 525), a Norwegian born in Naes, after working for 4 years at Drammen served his ophthalmological apprenticeship under Hjalmar Schiøtz at Oslo but declined the offer to follow him in the University Chair because of progressive otosclerosis. He was an enthusiastic worker and his 110 publications covered almost every branch of ophthalmology; but his primary interest was in surgery and the study of glaucoma wherein he introduced his operation of iridencleisis; he once performed a couching operation for cataract on a live lioness.

ROBERT HENRY ELLIOT [1864–1936] (Fig. 528) was born in Bombay, and after an unusually brilliant academic career at St. Bartholomew's Hospital in London he joined the Indian Medical Service (1892) in which he rose to the rank of Colonel and eventually became Superintendent of the Madras Ophthalmic Hospital; the new Ophthalmic Hospital and School at Madras are a lasting memorial to him. His health compelled him to return to England in 1913 where he was appointed ophthalmic surgeon to the Hospital for Tropical Diseases and lecturer and Vice-President at the London School of Hygiene; writing papers and books during the remainder of his life, his favourite subject was glaucoma in the treatment of which he introduced his operation of corneo-scleral trephining (1909), an innovation which brought him world fame. His vast experience in India made him an adept surgeon, and apart from glaucoma he made outstanding contributions to many branches of the subject, particularly the intracapsular extraction of cataract and the evils of couching based on a study of 550 cases. His textbook on *Tropical Ophthalmology*, the first to be published on this subject, was translated into many languages. His interests were not confined to ophthalmology; his first work in India was on snake venoms for which he received a D.Sc. degree from the University of Edinburgh (1904), while as a first-class conjurer and a student of illusions he became Chairman of the Occult Committee of the Magic Circle.

LEOPOLD HEINE [1870–1940] (Fig. 524), who was born in Dessau, became an assistant to Hess at Marburg and then to Uhthoff at Breslau before being called to the University Chair first at Greifswald and subsequently at Kiel where he worked until he retired in 1935. His early interests were concerned with physiological optics in such subjects as accommodation, myopia, binocular vision and the use of contact lenses in ametropia; but his greatest preoccupation was surgery, a subject in which his introduction of the operation of cyclodialysis has ensured that his memory will never be forgotten.

CONTEMPORARY SURGERY

The numerous operations that have been proposed for the relief of the raised ocular tension in simple glaucoma may be broadly classified into three groups: (1) operations to establish extra-ocular drainage; (2) operations to form paths for intra-ocular drainage; and (3) destructive procedures on the ciliary body or its blood supply aimed at reducing the production of the aqueous humour.

As is our custom in this *System*, we shall merely outline the various operative procedures presently employed, indicating their applicability, their advantages and disadvantages; details of operative technique will be found in the relevant works quoted in this Section and in standard textbooks on the operative surgery of the eye.[1]

The *pre-operative management* and *pre-operative medication* for an operation for simple glaucoma follow in general the lines indicated for

---

[1] E. B. Spaeth (1948), Böck (1950), Callahan (1956), Guillaumat *et al.* (1957), Foster (1961), Arruga (1962), Stallard (1965), J. M. McLean (1967), Harms and Mackensen (1967).

cataract surgery.[1] If the ocular tension is high, however, it is well to lower it before the operation, particularly if the visual field is grossly impaired in spite of the use of miotics; this may be accomplished by a retrobulbar injection of procaine (which also ensures anæsthetization of the inner eye if general anæsthesia is not employed) or, more effectively, by acetazolamide given over 24 or 48 hours before surgery, or by more dramatic measures such as osmotic therapy as indicated elsewhere.[2]

Immediately before the operation, especially when the upper part of the limbus is involved, it is well to ensure steadiness of the globe by a fixation (bridle) suture through the tendon of the superior rectus muscle and clamped to the head-towel by hæmostatic forceps.

The choice of operation for each type of case is indicated in the subsequent paragraphs. Most surgeons use the filtering operation of their choice; it is generally accepted that a cyclodialysis is peculiarly suitable for cases of aphakic glaucoma, while techniques designed to lower the secretion of the aqueous by the ciliary body are usually confined to advanced cases wherein other operations have failed, to cases of absolute glaucoma and when other surgical procedures are contra-indicated or are refused.

SCLERECTOMY

Drainage of a permanent nature is the aim of the operation of sclerectomy wherein a portion of the outer coat of the eye at the upper limbus is excised or cauterized, usually accompanied by an iridectomy. Credit for the introduction of a satisfactory operation of this type, designed to fulfil de Wecker's aspiration to establish a filtering scar of a permanent nature, belongs to Félix Lagrange (1906).

(1) LAGRANGE'S SCLERECTO-IRIDECTOMY (1906–7) consists of the cutting out of a small corneo-sclero-conjunctival flap at 12 o'clock with a knife, snipping away a piece of the scleral lip of the wound with scissors, performing a basal iridectomy and replacing and suturing the flap so that the aqueous drains freely into the subconjunctival tissues. In order to make a cleaner and more extensive aperture, Holth (1909) performed the sclerectomy on the corneal lip of the wound with punch forceps (*anterior lip sclerectomy*), while Iliff and Haas (1962) described a similar punch-sclerectomy but on the scleral side of the incision (*posterior lip sclerectomy*). Berens (1936) modified the anterior lip sclerectomy by making his incision with a keratome 2 mm. behind the limbus and then punching away the sclera forwards to the corneo-scleral junction along the whole length of the incision (*irido-corneo-sclerectomy*). A high percentage of successes has been claimed for these various types of sclerectomy (O'Brien, 1947—85% for Lagrange's sclerecto-iridectomy; Berens and Breakey, 1960—78% for Berens's irido-corneo-sclerectomy; Haas, 1967—85% for posterior lip sclerectomy).

(2) CORNEO-SCLERAL TREPHINING. The operation of trephining has

---

[1] p. 268.   [2] p. 610.

FIGS. 529 AND 530.—THE OPERATION OF TREPHINING.

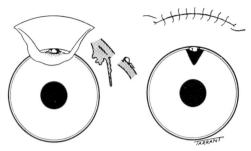

FIG. 529.—To show (on the left) the reflection of the conjunctival flap with the presentation of a knuckle of iris after removal of the trephine-disc and (on the right) the peripheral iridectomy and sutures of the conjunctival flap (after R. J. H. Smith).

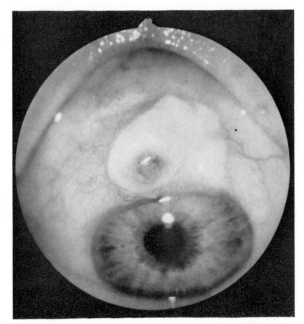

FIG. 530.—The filtering bleb (Inst. Ophthal.).

become popular through the corneo-scleral trephining of Elliot (1909–32). This operation consists of making a large flap of conjunctiva and the episcleral tissues down to the limbus when the superficial layers of the cornea beneath the epithelium are dissected for a distance of about 1 mm. A trephine-hole is then cut at the corneo-scleral margin, half over the cornea and half over the sclera, into the anterior chamber, a slight tilting movement being made before the perforation is complete so that the trephine-disc is left with a hinge on one side. A peripheral iridectomy is then made at the trephine-hole into which the iris usually prolapses, the disc is cut away, the iris, which usually springs back, is reposed to leave a round pupil, and the conjunctival flap sutured by a continuous suture of catgut preferably in two layers, one involving the forward extension of Tenon's capsule and the second the mucous membrane itself, in order to ensure as thick a covering as possible and to facilitate drainage beneath Tenon's capsule (Figs. 529–30). The principle is thus the same as in the operation of Lagrange and the operation has been used without serious modification, although some surgeons advise a limbo-scleral rather than a corneo-scleral trephining (Sugar, 1961; Scheie, 1962; Goodner, 1963).

Troublesome difficulties may arise during the operation. A film of tissue may be left at the bottom of the trephine-hole; this is best removed by raising it with a fine scleral hook and excising it with scissors. The disc may prolapse into the anterior chamber; if near the trephine-hole it may be coaxed out with a scleral hook, but if not it is best left. A buttonhole may be accidentally made in the conjunctival flap particularly when this membrane is thin; in this event the trephining should be made some 5 mm. to either side of the buttonhole or a large conjunctival hood-flap should be fashioned and securely sutured.

(3) CAUTERIZATION OF THE SCLERA is a third expedient for obtaining a fistulous scar. Such a technique was introduced in a simple procedure by Preziosi (1924) who inserted an electro-cautery at the limbus into the anterior chamber under a conjunctival flap and performed an iridectomy only if the iris prolapsed; this procedure has not gained much popularity, although good results have been claimed (Fankhauser and Schmidt, 1956; Colley, 1956). This idea was rendered much more practical in Scheie's (1958) simple operation of *cauterization of the sclera with a peripheral iridectomy*. Beneath a conjunctival flap the outer half of the limbus is gently cauterized along a line 6 mm. in length placed 1 mm. behind the corneo-scleral junction. An incision is made along this line with a scalpel extending down to the deeper layers of the sclera, and its lips, particularly the posterior lip, are again cauterized to induce their retraction. The incision is then completed to enter the anterior chamber and a basal iridectomy is performed, Tenon's capsule and the conjunctiva being finally sutured with catgut. The resulting filtration-bleb thus attained is usually more diffuse and substantial than after a trephine. The ocular tension is controlled by this procedure in 80 to 90% of patients with simple glaucoma,[1] and also in a high percentage of patients with juvenile glaucoma.

Although, like many other operations, these three types of sclerectomy are effective in a high percentage of cases of simple glaucoma, they differ in their complexity and in the incidence of post-operative complications Both Lagrange's and Elliot's operations are technically more difficult, involve more trauma to the eye, and probably tend more readily to the subsequent production of cataract than Scheie's operation. All may be

[1] Scheie (1958–64), Møller (1963), Nadel (1966), Malbran and Norbis (1968), and others.

followed by delay in the re-formation of the anterior chamber with its ultimate sequel of cataract or a recurrence of tension due to the formation of extensive peripheral anterior synechiæ,[1] while delayed re-formation after Elliot's operation has been followed by dense scarring with endothelial proliferation in the aperture (Collins, 1914), or its blockage by the anterior dislocation of the ciliary body (Fig. 531) (Troncoso and Reese, 1935) or of the lens capsule (Fig. 532) (Hobbs and Smith, 1954; Sugar, 1957). The development of cataract may also result from mechanical damage to the

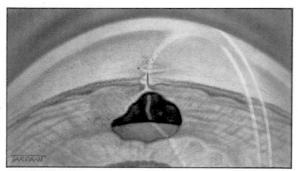

Fig. 531.—Blockage of a Trephine Hole by the Ciliary Body.
In a male aged 64 with simple glaucoma (Inst. Ophthal.).

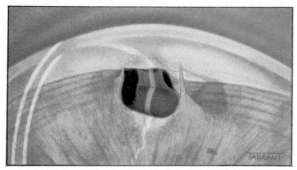

Fig. 532.—Prolapse of the Lens Capsule into a Trephine Hole.
In a male aged 53 with simple glaucoma (Inst. Ophthal.).

lens by the iris forceps or the trephine and is therefore less common after Scheie's operation wherein spontaneous prolapse of the iris more frequently occurs. The tragedy of the development of late infection, which usually appears some months to some years after operation, has already been discussed[2] and has been variously estimated.[3] It is now generally accepted that the incidence of infection following trephine operations is 1·7 to

[1] p. 714.   [2] Vol. IX, p. 51.
[3] Pillat (1921), 18·2%; Butler (1921), 3 in 150 cases; Davenport (1926–27), 14 in 536 cases; Wessely (1927), none in 134 cases; Duke-Elder (1940), 2 in 1,000 cases.

3·23%, higher than that following iridencleisis where the incidence is 0·27 to 1·4%,[1] and this complication has been one of the chief causes of a waning in enthusiasm for the trephine operation in recent years. In several series of cases of simple glaucoma, Elliot's operation has been successful in reducing the ocular tension to normal in an average of some 75% (Grom and van den Beld, 1964, 94·75%; Leydhecker, 1967, 58%; Rocha and Calixto, 1968, 72%), figures which compare unfavourably with those following Scheie's operation (80 to 90%).

IRIS INCLUSION

Following Critchett's introduction of the incarceration of the iris in a corneal incision in his operation of iridodesis and its elaboration by Herbert (1903), the first simple, practical and successful operation of this type for simple glaucoma was the *iridencleisis* designed by Holth (1906). Under a conjunctival flap reflected to the limbus, the anterior chamber is opened by a keratome which enters the sclera 2 mm. behind the limbus and is directed towards the filtration angle. The scleral lip of the section is depressed so that the iris prolapses into the wound; this tissue is then cut in the 12 o'clock meridian from the margin of the pupil to its root; the nasal pillar is drawn outwards over the sclera; the temporal pillar is reposed; and the conjunctival flap sutured (Fig. 534). Subsequent massage to the eye is usually considered necessary to ensure continued drainage because of the tendency to cicatrization.

In the modification described by L. and R. Weekers (1948) the iris is made to prolapse spontaneously and is then torn with iris forceps. Troutman (1954) demonstrated that the inclusion of two pillars of iris in the scleral wound was more effective than that of one pillar, the former procedure being successful in 90% and the latter in 69% of cases (Figs. 533, 535).

The advantages of iridencleisis are that it is easy to perform, it disturbs the eye only to a slight extent and involves little trauma, the anterior chamber re-forms rapidly and there is no sudden and acute fall in tension. Subsequent cataract formation is usually said to be rare and to occur less commonly than after a trephining (L. Weekers, 1959), although Leydhecker (1967) reversed the incidence (after iridencleisis: cataract in 8% after 1 year, 14% after 5 years; after Elliot's operation: 4% after 1 year, 9% after 5 years); late infections are statistically fewer than after sclerectomy.

For a considerable time after its introduction the operation did not achieve widespread popularity, largely because of the fear of the development of sympathetic ophthalmitis and late infection. Both of these undoubtedly occur; thus sympathetic ophthalmitis has been reported on several occasions (Trowbridge, 1937; Iliff, 1944; Mackie and Rubinstein, 1954) and late

---

[1] Scardapane (1926), Davenport (1926–27), Eerola (1934), Dellaporta (1948), Kalt and Loisillier (1958), Sugar and Zekman (1958).

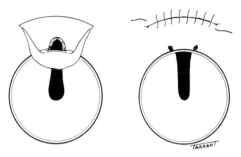

FIG. 533.—The reflection of the conjunctival flap (on the left) and the prolapse of the iris through the incision. On the right, the inclusion of the two pillars of the iris, and sutures of the conjunctival flap (after R. J. H. Smith).

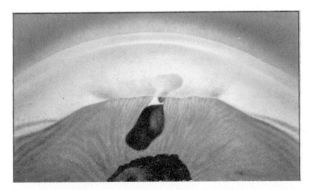

FIG. 534.—With the incorporation of one pillar of the iris (Inst. Ophthal.).

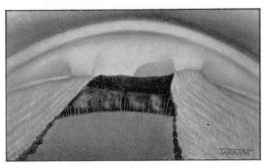

FIG. 535.—With the incorporation of both pillars (Inst. Ophthal.).

infections have been reported in from 0·27 to 1·4% of cases. As the long-term results of large series began to accrue, however, confidence has become greater and today it is undoubtedly and deservedly very popular. Thus many authors report a very satisfactory proportion of successes,[1] while numerous others speak highly of it.[2]

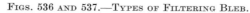

FIGS. 536 AND 537.—TYPES OF FILTERING BLEB.

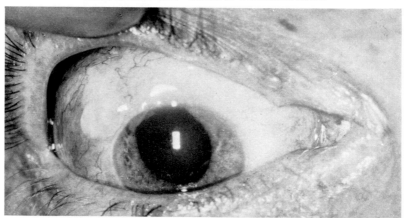

FIG. 536.—After an iris-inclusion with a flap sclerotomy
(S. H. J. Miller).

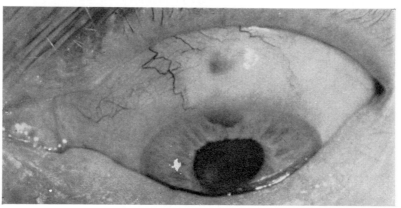

FIG. 537.—After an anterior flap sclerotomy with basal iridencleisis
(H. B. Stallard).

Several combinations of these filtering operations have been advocated in an attempt to eliminate failure in drainage. Thus an iridencleisis has been combined with

[1] 83% (Gjessing, 1923), 87% (Wilmer, 1927), 90% (Butler, 1932), 79·8% (Holst, 1947), 93% (Sourdille, 1950), 87% (Meyer, 1952), 90% (Paiva, 1955), 90% (Haye, 1955), 83% (Scheie, 1962), 70% after 1 year, 90% after 6 years (Leydhecker, 1966), 94% (Sampaolesi, 1968).
[2] Pillat (1928), Blaickner (1930), Holst (1931–34), Butler (1932–36), Goar and Schultz (1939), L. Weekers and Bonhomme (1940), L. and R. Weekers (1948), Dellaporta (1948), Reese (1952), Cassady (1959), Topalis and Roussos (1959), and many others.

the Lagrange sclerectomy (Syed, 1956), an Elliot trephining (Meesmann, 1956–60; Kapuściński, 1957; Kapuściński and Pacyńska, 1963; E. Mawas and Parizot, 1964; Baron and Michel, 1967) or a flap sclerotomy (Miller, 1963) (Fig. 536).

The *anterior flap sclerotomy with a basal iridencleisis* described by Stallard (1948–53) is a more elaborate extension of the same idea. Under a flap of conjunctiva and episcleral tissue, a scleral flap hinged to the limbus is cut, 1 mm. of its free edge being excised to form a sclerectomy if the ocular tension is high. An iris repositor is then introduced through the incision into the suprachoroidal space and is made to enter the anterior chamber to separate the attachment of the ciliary body to the scleral spur, thus effecting a small cyclodialysis. The stroma of the iris is then drawn through the wound, small incisions are made towards the root of the iris on both sides so that a tongue of iris based on its root remains protruding from the incision leaving the sphincter muscle and a round pupil intact. When the conjunctival incision is sutured, air is injected into the anterior chamber and beneath the conjunctival flap. For this somewhat complicated procedure Stallard (1953) claimed a success-rate of 97·7% (Fig. 537).

The Filtering Scar. In all these operations the object is to create a filtering scar which will remain a permanently open channel for drainage from the anterior chamber to the subconjunctival space. Such scars have received a considerable amount of pathological study, whether

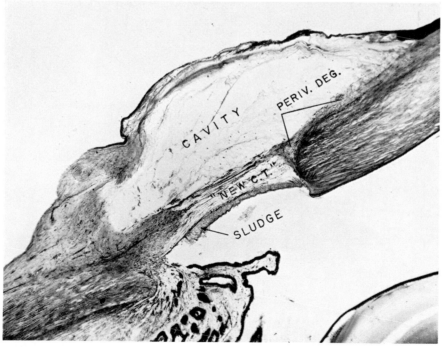

Fig. 538.—THE TREPHINE BLEB.

Twenty years after operation, showing the lining of the cavity composed of degenerated collagen with an amorphous substance in the centre. New connective tissue bridges the opening lined with sludge. Around the opening there is considerable perivascular degeneration (C. C. Teng *et al.*).

following trephining,[1] Lagrange's sclerectomy (Bachstez, 1914; Holth, 1931), peripheral iridectomy with scleral cautery (Regan, 1963), or iridencleisis (Holth, 1922–33; Teng *et al.*, 1959). Teng and his co-workers (1959) have demonstrated three main types of aqueous drainage produced by such procedures (Figs. 538–9): (1) the transconjunctival route, when aqueous produces degeneration of the collagen in the subconjunctival tissue which becomes more permeable so that the basement membrane and epithelium of the conjunctiva are also affected, resulting in oozing of aqueous through

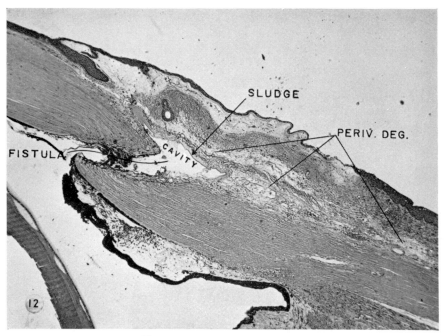

FIG. 539.—THE TREPHINE BLEB.

Thirty-three years after operation. There is much new-formed connective tissue in the subconjunctival region. The features are the same as in Fig. 538, with the presence of a fistula (C. C. Teng *et al.*).

the bleb; (2) the route through areas of perivascular degeneration when the aqueous causes degeneration of the collagen fibres around the sub-conjunctival blood vessels, thus creating a loose perivascular degeneration which facilitates filtration; and (3) direct new recanalization due to the development of endothelial-lined channels in the subconjunctival tissue. The transconjunctival route, which had previously been suggested by various workers,[2] results in a sharply outlined, anæmic, polycystic bleb consisting of multiple fluid-filled spaces, with a thin epithelial covering.

[1] Collins (1914), Verhoeff (1915), Greeves (1916), Elliot (1918), Holth (1922), Teng *et al.* (1959).

[2] Lagrange (1913), Verhoeff (1913), Herbert (1914), Seidel (1921), Elliot (1922).

This type of bleb, most frequently associated with trephines and sclerectomies, usually gives a positive fluorescein test indicating the transconjunctival escape of aqueous. The subconjunctival route, originally postulated by Verhoeff (1915), Holth (1922) and Gjessing (1923), results in a flat or slightly elevated area of succulence, opacity and anæmia of the conjunctiva which usually gives a negative fluorescein test; this type of bleb is most commonly seen after iridencleisis operations (Galin *et al.*, 1966). Teng and his associates (1959) suggested that when subconjunctival drainage resulted from direct new recanalization, a bleb may not be apparent. Failure to produce a filtering scar may result from post-operative scarring of the conjunctiva or from plugging of the fistula by uveal (Greeves, 1916) or lenticular tissue (Meek, 1948). Friedenwald (1950) suggested that the following factors may predispose to post-operative scarring of the conjunctiva: operative trauma, hæmorrhage, inflammation, operations done in previous operative sites, and racial and individual factors. Negroes, for example, are particularly prone to develop sufficient scar-tissue to block a filtration scar soon after surgery[1] (Friedenwald, 1950). When the fistula shows signs of ceasing to drain, Mittl and Galin (1967) suggested that the daily application of a suction-cup of 50 mm. Hg was more effective than the usual technique of digital massage.

The most useful clinical test to determine whether a scar is draining satisfactorily is the *fluorescein test* suggested by Seidel (1921) wherein a drop of this dye is placed on the bleb and slight pressure is applied to the globe, whereupon the flow of coloured fluid can be seen. If there is no bleb visible, tonography may provide evidence of the occurrence of drainage.

The interesting phenomenon of a *consensual hypotony* which may be evident for many months in the fellow eye when one has been operated on for glaucoma has been stressed by Blatt and Regenbogen (1960). In 100 eyes whereon a trephining operation was performed, the tension was unchanged in the fellow eye in 11%, it was lowered but not to the normal level in 9%, to the normal level in 71%, and rose in 3%. Similar results followed iridencleisis (85 cases) and cyclodialysis (60 cases). In the fellow eye also miotics were more effective after than before surgery. Such a reaction must be due to the consensual nervous regulation of the intra-ocular pressures[2] and may allow surgery on the second eye to be delayed or occasionally even omitted.

SETON OPERATIONS have been suggested to maintain the patency of a filtering scar in recalcitrant cases. Rollet (1907) inserted horse-hair through two corneal punctures in cases of absolute glaucoma, while others used silk threads (Zorab, 1912–13; Mayou, 1912–13; Wood, 1915; Vail, 1915; Wheelock, 1916), gold drains (L. Weekers, 1922; Stefansson, 1925) or a lacrimal cannula (in dogs) (Gibson, 1942). O. R. Wolfe and Blaess (1936) used a silk thread which could be remanipulated in a see-saw movement to encourage drainage if it subsequently failed. More recently, subconjunctival drainage has been attempted by a tantalum (Troncoso, 1949) or a glass tube (Böck, 1950), a platinum wire (Muldoon *et al.*, 1951), a protoplast loop (Habenberger, 1951), acrylic plates (Qadeer, 1954), absorbable gelatin (Gelfilm) (Laval, 1955; Lehman and McCaslin, 1959), a polythene tube (Epstein, 1959; Illig, 1959; La Rocca, 1962; Richards and van

[1] p. 554. [2] Vol. IV, p. 308.

Bijsterveld, 1965), a silicone tube (Ellis, 1960), or by Supramid, gold or stainless steel threads (Sampimon, 1966). In cases wherein a tube has been used, this eventually tends to become blocked, although in some instances the ocular tension has remained low, often without evidence of a filtering bleb, in which case it has been suggested that hypotension may have resulted from a localized detachment of the ciliary body (Richards and van Bijsterveld, 1965). None of these procedures, however, should be used except in recalcitrant cases or in eyes with absolute glaucoma when all other methods of surgery have failed to provide relief.

INTRA-OCULAR DRAINAGE

(a) CYCLODIALYSIS

This operation, initially conceived by Heine (1905), was based on a suggestion of Axenfeld that the good results of iridectomy were due to the frequently associated choroidal detachment. It depends on making a communication between the suprachoroidal space and the anterior chamber by breaking down the attachments of the pectinate ligament by a specially-shaped spatula introduced through an incision made in the sclera 5 mm. behind and concentric with the limbus and swept to either side in an arc so as to separate the attachment of the ciliary body to the scleral spur over about a quadrant of the eye (Figs. 540-1). Thereafter air may be injected along the track into the anterior chamber both to check any bleeding which may occur and to prevent rapid occlusion of the opening with fibrin. When an anterior ciliary artery is torn in the manipulations this hæmorrhage may occasionally be considerable; if the anterior chamber is filled with blood a paracentesis may be performed and the chamber washed out with urokinase (5,000 units in 5 ml. of saline).[1]

The action of cyclodialysis appears to depend on two factors: (a) the establishment of posterior drainage for the aqueous into the suprachoroidal space (Heine, 1905; Goldmann, 1951), and (b) the depression in the production of aqueous which occurs in the immediate post-operative period and which may continue thereafter for some considerable time (Goldmann, 1951). The influence of the former is suggested by the fact that closure of the cyclodialysis cleft can be seen gonioscopically in cases wherein the operation has failed,[2] while evidence for the latter has been provided both by the reduction of the volume of aqueous flow (Goldmann, 1951) and by histological examination which tends to confirm the presence to some degree of atrophy of the ciliary body (L. Weekers, 1907; von Grósz, 1924; Elschnig, 1932; Kronfeld, 1936).

The advantages of cyclodialysis are that it is easy to perform, it involves no cosmetic defect and no weakening of the globe, it can be repeated several times, and it can be followed by any other operation. Its disadvantages are that it is frequently followed by the development of cataract (12% of cases

[1] Vol. IX, p. 23.
[2] Barkan et al. (1936), Sugar (1941), Leydhecker (1964), Becker and Shaffer (1965), Chandler and Grant (1965), Sommer (1967), Gorin and Posner (1967).

FIGS. 540 and 541.—CYCLODIALYSIS.

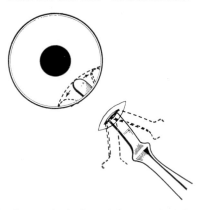

FIG. 540.—Showing the manipulation of the spatula (after R. J. H. Smith).

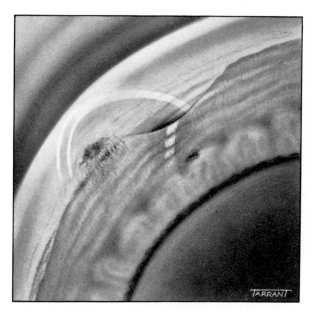

FIG. 541.—The cleft of cyclodialysis. In a case of simple glaucoma 8 years after the operation (Inst. Ophthal.).

after 1 year, 28% after 5 years, Leydhecker, 1967) and that closure of the cleft frequently results in a dramatic rise of ocular tension. For these reasons, although it has had many protagonists in the past,[1] it is tending to become less popular except in aphakic glaucoma for which it is peculiarly suitable.[2]

[1] Gradle (1931), Elschnig (1932), McPherson (1946), O'Brien and Weih (1949), Viikari and Tuovinen (1957), Haisten and Guyton (1958), Schultz et al. (1960), and others.
[2] p. 721.

To avoid the failure of a cyclodialysis, various combined procedures have been proposed.   Mauksch (1924) suggested tucking the iris into the suprachoroidal space, thus in a sense combining an iridotasis with a cyclodialysis (Raeder, 1928; Suker, 1931).   Cyclodialysis has also been combined with an iridectomy,[1] with cyclodiathermy (Dominguez, 1948; Cavka, 1954), with an iridencleisis (Scharf, 1949) and with a filtering cleft (Gauly, 1956).   O. R. Wolfe and his colleagues (1944) performed the cyclodialysis from an incision 1 mm. behind the limbus, directing the spatula posteriorly, a procedure, as we have seen, also used by Stallard (1948).   A further modification with some advantages was introduced by J. H. Allen (1951).   In this procedure, under a conjunctival flap extending over the limbus as in corneo-scleral trephining, a radial (instead of a circumferential) incision is made at the limbus and the attachment of the ciliary body to the scleral spur is separated without sweeping the spatula posteriorly; in this way damage to the anterior ciliary vessels (3 mm. posterior to the limbus) is avoided; thereafter a basal iridectomy may be performed, air is injected into the anterior chamber and the conjunctival flap sutured.

To ensure the permanent patency of the cleft of the cyclodialysis, foreign substances have been inserted into it.   The first such attempt was initiated by Row (1934) who introduced a loop of horse-hair into the suprachoroidal space and passed it into the anterior chamber, its ends being buried under Tenon's capsule.   Troncoso (1940) advanced the original idea of implanting a strip of magnesium in the wound between the ciliary body and the sclera; the metal is absorbed in about 20 days, giving off free bubbles of hydrogen, leaving a lacunar space between the anterior chamber and the suprachoroidal space, while its temporary presence and the bubbles of gas prevent an early re-attachment of the ciliary body to the sclera.   Bick (1947–49) and Troncoso (1949) inserted a tantalum implant in the cleft of the dialysis to retain its patency, Lösche (1952) a spatula of Supramid, Bietti (1952–55), Tamesis (1955), La Rocca (1962) and Gills (1966) polythene tubes, and Strampelli (1956) a Supramid thread in an operation he called *Cyclodiastasis.*

(b) TRABECULOTOMY

Reasoning that glaucoma was caused by a failure of the aqueous to reach the canal of Schlemm, the Italian surgeon de Vincentiis (1893) conceived the rational idea of opening the canal by a knife introduced into the anterior chamber; the attempt was unsuccessful because he could not see what he was doing.   This feat was achieved by the ingenuity of Otto Barkan (1936–38) of San Francisco who, in his operation of trabeculotomy (or *goniotomy*), with the aid of a contact glass and intense trans-illumination, devised a technique by which the canal can be cut open from within. Although this technique has proved successful in a high percentage of cases of congenital glaucoma, Barkan (1956) found it disappointing in adult simple glaucoma, but it appears to have a place in the treatment of some cases of juvenile glaucoma, particularly those which appear to be delayed forms of the congenital type.   Another operation that has proved successful in about 50% of cases of juvenile glaucoma is *gonio-puncture*, wherein the goniotomy knife is passed through the trabecular region into the subconjunctival tissue in order to produce a filtering track (Scheie, 1950–63;

---

[1] Czermak (1906), Torok (1923), Jervey (1927), Wootton (1932), Wheeler (1936), Lauber (1939), Cramer (1947).

Tyner and Swets, 1955). Sugar (1961) found that curettage of the trabecular meshwork or the excision of a small segment of meshwork and canal of Schlemm in cases of simple glaucoma resulted in a normal ocular tension which lasted for only a few days or weeks.

Several workers have performed a trabeculotomy via an *ab externo* approach. R. Smith (1960–62), using an operating microscope, inserted a nylon filament through two or more external incisions into Schlemm's canal so that it passed along the canal over a quadrant of the globe; it is then drawn taut, thus cutting through the inner wall of the canal and entering the anterior chamber anterior to Schwalbe's line and stretching across it like a bowstring, whereupon it is removed. Other surgeons have passed a probe or a knife through the canal of Schlemm into the anterior chamber (Burian, 1960; L. Allen and Burian, 1962; Walker and Kanagasundaram, 1964; Strachan, 1967); the short-term results of these procedures are encouraging. A trabeculectomy was proposed by Cairns (1968) by reflecting a corneo-scleral flap and excising a short length of Schlemm's canal with its trabecular adnexa.

EXTERNALIZATION OF THE CANAL OF SCHLEMM (*sinusotomy*) has also been described (Krasnov, 1964–68; Walker and Kanagasundaram, 1964; Postic and Stankov-Tomic, 1967); Krasnov (1968) achieved a success-rate of 83% in over 1,000 such operations in patients with simple glaucoma.

AQUEOUS-VENOUS SHUNTS

A final type of drainage operation recently suggested in otherwise recalcitrant cases is the connection of the anterior chamber with an extra-ocular vein. In experiments on normal and buphthalmic rabbits, Lee and Schepens (1966) introduced a polythene tube into the angle of the anterior chamber and connected it with a vortex vein, and Lee and his associates (1968) repeated the experiments on monkeys using a vein on the upper surface of the superior rectus muscle. The first operation of this type was undertaken in man by Strampelli and Valvo (1967).

The suggestion of connecting the anterior chamber with the *lacrimal sac* by means of a polythene tube was made by Mascati (1967) who reported 20 successful operations. The further expedient of similarly connecting the anterior chamber with the superior temporal vein was successfully performed by Sivayoham (1968) in a case of glaucoma secondary to orbital venous obstruction.[1]

DESTRUCTIVE PROCEDURES ON THE CILIARY BODY

(a) CYCLODIATHERMY

Following the observation of Weve (1932) that extensive surface diathermy over the ciliary body frequently resulted in ocular hypotension, Vogt (1936) proposed the operation of penetrating cyclodiathermy for various

[1] p. 678.

forms of glaucoma. Because of the frequent occurrence of post-operative complications, he modified his technique to one of partial penetrating cyclo-diathermy (Vogt, 1937–39), while others have suggested that non-penetrating diathermy is just as effective and is followed by fewer complications (Fig. 542).[1] It has been demonstrated that cyclodiathermy acts by reducing the formation of aqueous (R. Weekers and Prijot, 1952; Scheie *et al.*, 1955) and on histological examination partial atrophy of the ciliary body has been shown to occur in some cases (Scheie *et al.*, 1955).

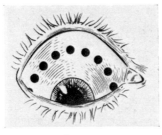

Fig. 542.—Cyclodiathermy.

A single row of trans-conjunctival applications of surface diathermy encircling the globe 7 mm. behind the limbus (P. D. Trevor-Roper).

(b) CYCLOCRYOSURGERY

The application of low temperatures to the region of the ciliary body also results in a reduction of the ocular tension, and this form of cryosurgery appears to be remarkably free from complications (Bietti, 1947–50; Krwawicz and Szwarc, 1965; de Roetth, 1966; Haye *et al.*, 1967).

(c) CYCLO-ELECTROLYSIS

Berens and his co-workers (1949) described the partial destruction of the ciliary body pro-duced at the cathode of a galvanic current by the chemical decomposition of the tissue by the liberation of sodium hydroxide. It has been claimed that this technique is safer and more effective than cyclodiathermy (Berens, 1955; Berens and Sheppard, 1960).

(d) ANGIODIATHERMY

The production of aqueous humour can also be reduced by diminishing the blood supply to the ciliary body. This can be attempted by performing diathermy over the site of the long ciliary arteries just posterior to the insertion of a horizontal rectus muscle, a procedure called *cyclo-anœmization* by Kettesy (1946).[2] The diathermy may be combined with a cyclodialysis (Schreck, 1949; Stumptner, 1953), while the performance of a temporary tenotomy of the four rectus muscles probably acts by cutting the anterior ciliary arteries; this may be combined with a retrociliary angiodiathermy (Streiff *et al.*, 1957; Streiff and Stucchi, 1966).

Because penetrating cyclodiathermy is sometimes complicated by the development of corneal ulceration, uveitis, peripheral anterior synechiæ and cataract, it has been replaced by partial penetrating and non-penetrating cyclodiathermy, particularly the latter. Even these procedures have a

[1] Albaugh and Dunphy (1942), L. and R. Weekers (1942), Villaseca (1947), Verrey (1949), Thomas *et al.* (1950), Goldsmith (1954), Scheie *et al.* (1955), Leydhecker (1967), and others.
[2] Arato (1948–53), Schreck (1949), Arruga (1950), Scheie *et al.* (1955), Paufique *et al.* (1956), and others.

higher incidence of complications than do filtering operations; Marr (1949), for example, found that phthisis bulbi developed in 12 out of 57 eyes while Berens and Sheppard (1960) reported an incidence of this disastrous complication in 15% of cases. Leydhecker (1967) noted that cataract developed in 20% of patients within a year of cyclodiathermy, and serious complications occurred more frequently than after iridencleisis, trephining or cyclodialysis. The percentage of successes as far as the ocular tension is concerned has varied considerably in different series,[1] while some authors have found the procedure relatively ineffective (Cristini, 1948; Marr, 1949; Berens, 1955). Cyclo-electrolysis and angiodiathermy are considered by some to be safer and more effective, while cyclocryosurgery appears to be the safest procedure of this type.

In view of the frequency and severity of post-operative complications, and also of the variable results achieved by these destructive procedures, they are probably best reserved for cases of simple glaucoma that have not responded to one or more filtering operations,[2] for cases of painful absolute glaucoma when enucleation is refused or contra-indicated, and for cases of secondary hæmorrhagic glaucoma wherein intra-ocular surgery is not indicated.

Specific Indications for Treatment

Having discussed the various medical and surgical methods available for the reduction of the ocular tension in simple glaucoma, it now remains for us to present a workable scheme for the treatment of the various clinical pictures that may be encountered. This must in no way be considered a didactic approach to the management of any one case; we shall present the principles of treatment accepting that each case must be assessed on its merits and that with the ever-increasing knowledge of this difficult subject the principles propounded today may become out-dated in the near future.

In the treatment of all cases of established glaucoma *the dangers of vascular hypotension* should always be remembered. We have already seen that the essential cause of the scotomata in the visual fields and the atrophy of the optic nerve is vascular insufficiency or obliteration, and that any factor which tends to approximate the capillary blood pressure to the intra-ocular pressure may have unfortunate consequences. This applies both to cases of low-tension glaucoma wherein the factor of vasosclerosis is often important and also to cases wherein the ocular tension is high. In this connection the danger of rapidly lowering the blood pressure in a patient with vascular hypertension should be remembered since too dramatic systemic treatment for the latter condition may result in a serious deterioration of the visual

---

[1] 72% (Wagner and Richner, 1939), 83% (Meyer, 1949), 68% (L. and R. Weekers, 1950), 50% (Leydhecker, 1967).
[2] Desvignes and Naudin (1948), Verrey (1949), Goldsmith (1954), Scheie *et al.* (1955), Becker and Shaffer (1965), and others.

fields, as great, indeed, as would a sudden increase in the intra-ocular pressure.

(a) *Ocular Hypertension*

In those cases characterized by the persistent presence of an ocular tension higher than is generally accepted as normal, in the absence of anomalies at the optic disc or defects in the visual fields, and with a normal facility of aqueous outflow, it is generally accepted that repeated examinations of the optic discs and the visual functions every few months are all that is required. This is certainly true when the ocular tension is under 30 mm.; when it is over this level it is probably more prudent to institute medical treatment in order to reduce the ocular tension to a safer level, for although the normal eye can often tolerate an elevated tension for many years without evidence of visual impairment, it must be assumed that few eyes can tolerate a very high tension for any considerable length of time. Notice should also be taken of the variations of the ocular tension at these routine examinations; if the tension shows gross diurnal variations and its base-level is increasing progressively over a period of months or years, this is an indication for considering the institution of treatment. Although the relationship between simple glaucoma and steroid-induced ocular hypertension appears to be indirect, it is our impression that patients with ocular hypertension who give a positive response to steroids should be considered for medical therapy, as should those patients with a family history of simple glaucoma, who have a raised tension irrespective of its height.

(b) *Suspected Cases of Simple Glaucoma*

In those cases wherein a raised ocular tension is associated with a borderline facility of aqueous outflow (between 0·18 and 0·13), yet with normal optic discs and full visual fields, the diagnosis of simple glaucoma may be difficult to confirm. If the ratio P_0/C is over 150, and particularly if it is over this level after the water-drinking test, the diagnosis can be made with some confidence. If, however, the diagnosis remains in some doubt, the same general principles of management as for ocular hypertension can be applied. Particularly in younger patients, however, treatment should be instituted at a lower level of ocular tension, for even when this is in the high 20s, a deterioration of the visual functions can be expected to occur with the passage of time.

(c) *Established Simple Glaucoma*

Once the diagnosis of simple glaucoma has been confirmed by an abnormally low facility of aqueous outflow (0·12 or below), by a P_0/C ratio of 150 or more, or by the presence of pathological cupping of the optic disc or of characteristic defects in the visual field associated with a reduced facility of outflow, it is mandatory to commence treatment in all but the most elderly patients.

The treatment of simple glaucoma is essentially medical and every effort should be made to control the ocular tension by this means. Only when full medical therapy has failed to prevent the progression of visual deterioration, or when the patient is unable to tolerate such a régime or is psychologically unsuited to maintain the discipline of the "miotic life", should surgery be undertaken; a further indication for surgery is when a patient proposes to remain in a part of the world where adequate supervision does not exist. The aim of medical therapy is to keep the ocular tension at a safe level *throughout the* 24 *hours of the day*. This level varies with each patient, but as a general rule a normal optic disc can tolerate an ocular tension rising at least to the mid-20s for a considerable period of time, a disc showing early pathological cupping cannot tolerate a tension of more than 20 mm., while one with advanced cupping will probably suffer further damage by a tension of over 15 mm.

Of the many topically-applied drugs now available, several have been recommended for the initial treatment of the disease. The most widely used is still pilocarpine, in concentrations of 1 to 4%, instilled at intervals which allow it to control the highest levels attained by the tension as brought out in its diurnal variations. Because its effect lasts about 6 hours, pilocarpine should seldom be prescribed at less than 6-hourly intervals, and may have to be instilled 4-hourly; it is also important that these instillations should be evenly spaced throughout the day. The anticholinesterase drugs, particularly demecarium bromide and echothiophate, have recently been advocated for the early stages of treatment[1]; for this purpose they are usually prescribed in low concentrations (demecarium bromide 0·06%; echothiophate 0·06%) and because of their prolonged action need only be instilled into the conjunctival sac once, or at the most, twice a day. These anticholinesterase drugs give rise to more side-effects than pilocarpine and the miosis they produce tends to be more marked making them unacceptable to many patients with lenticular changes; these disadvantages have to be weighed against the advantage of the infrequent instillation necessary to cause a satisfactory diurnal control of ocular tension. Adrenaline eye-drops (1 to 2%) are also suitable as a means of initial treatment and require to be instilled once or twice a day. This drug is of particular value in those patients with central lenticular changes in whom miotics produce a marked reduction in the visual acuity or an uncomfortable spasm of accommodation. Its great disadvantage is that conjunctival irritation and an allergic blepharo-conjunctivitis occur in a high percentage of patients on long-term treatment; these side-effects may be reduced by the simultaneous instillation of those topical steroids, such as hydroxymesterone and tetrahydrotriamcinolone, with an anti-inflammatory activity and without a tendency to raise the

[1] Drance (1960–66), Pratt-Johnson *et al.* (1964), Becker and Shaffer (1965), and others.

ocular tension. It must be remembered that anticholinesterase drugs and adrenaline are contra-indicated in patients with simple glaucoma and a narrow angle of the anterior chamber.

If the use of one topically-applied drug fails to control the ocular tension adequately, the effect of another should be ascertained before a combination of two is prescribed. Although pilocarpine has been popularly given with physostigmine for many years there is some evidence that such a combination of cholinergic and anticholinesterase drugs has no greater efficacy than its most potent component (Kronfeld, 1967). The addition of adrenaline, however, to the treatment of a patient already on pilocarpine results in a further increase in the facility of aqueous outflow and a reduction in the ocular tension, while an adrenaline-echothiophate combination is even more effective owing to the greater potency of the echothiophate.

The addition of a systemic carbonic anhydrase inhibitor is a further therapeutic measure which may be used in the long-term treatment of simple glaucoma (Becker and Middleton, 1955; G. L. Spaeth, 1967). The effect may be increased by the instillation of adrenaline eye-drops (Becker and Ley, 1958). The combination of an anticholinesterase drug, adrenaline and a carbonic anhydrase inhibitor therefore produces the maximal possible reduction of ocular tension that can be attained by medical means, and until such a combination has been tried it is incorrect to suggest that medical treatment has failed.

It must be remembered, however, that a *miotic life* demands a considerable amount of discipline on the part of the patient which must be rigorously maintained, and for this everyone is not suited; moreover, it is necessary that the case should be periodically and carefully controlled. If these desiderata cannot be guaranteed, some other method of therapeusis should be advised. Apart from visual impairment in patients with a central sclerosis of the lens, the miosis entails some disadvantages which, however, may be eliminated by the use of adrenaline; the small pupil restricts the entry of light, diminishing vision in subdued light, the darker shades of colour are missed and difficulties of accommodation may render prolonged reading awkward, particularly in dim illumination. Indeed, the patient's relief after successful surgery may be considerable with miosis no longer necessary and anxiety hopefully dispelled.[1]

It is now widely agreed that many cases of simple glaucoma can be controlled for a number of years by medical measures without an increase in ocular tension or a decrease in visual function.[2] It is wise to attempt to control simple glaucoma by these means, for the immediate hazards of an operation and the ultimate dangers to which it may expose the eye cannot legitimately be lightly accepted. There is no question, however,

[1] See an anonymous appreciation of the difficulties by an intelligent patient, *Brit. J. Ophthal.*, **48**, 354 (1964).

[2] Lawson (1913), Posey (1914–20), Fisher (1921), Young (1924–33), Becker and Shaffer (1965), Chandler and Grant (1965), and many others.

that if any deterioration of the visual fields occurs despite maximal medical therapy, operation should be undertaken in all but the most elderly patients; it is to be remembered that unjustified delay in operating has been responsible for more ultimate failures in results than have the risks of surgery.

If deterioration indicates that an operation should be performed, several choices are available, depending partly upon the personal preference of the surgeon. The consensus of opinion is growing that Scheie's operation is the most generally applicable for all types of simple glaucoma; the usual expedients adopted are a trephine, an iridencleisis or a sclerectomy; a cyclodialysis is best confined to aphakic eyes. A trephining operation is not advisable when the anterior chamber is shallow, but is usually indicated in an eye wherein the reduction of the tension to a level below the normal is desired. Resort should be made to destructive operations only when filtering operations have failed.

(d) *Absolute Glaucoma*

In absolute glaucoma the treatment of election is to enucleate the eye as soon as pain becomes distressing; in the degenerative stage no other treatment should be considered. Apart from the difficulty of controlling pain, it is important to remember that in a considerable proportion of such eyes there is an unsuspected malignant melanoma: thus Neame and Khan (1925) found that 10% of 402 eyes enucleated at Moorfields Eye Hospital over an 11-year period under the diagnosis of absolute glaucoma contained an unsuspected tumour of this kind. If, however, enucleation is contraindicated or refused, an attempt should be made to relieve the pain, and for this many expedients have been proposed.

Of the available non-surgical methods, x-rays have been used in the past but with little success. Of the surgical methods available for relieving the tension, none offers the prospect of invariable relief, and the drainage operations may be complicated by sympathetic ophthalmitis, a disastrous sequel that precludes their use in the treatment of this condition. Cyclodiathermy, or one of the other destructive procedures on the ciliary body, is the safest operation in these circumstances and, although if it is successful it tends to hasten the onset of degenerative changes in the eye, it is widely used. The other method of treatment widely practised is to make the eye insensitive, and this can be simply done by the retrobulbar injection of 90% alcohol (Grüter, 1918) which causes little trauma, even although it may produce a temporary ptosis and paresis of the extraocular muscles (Jaensch, 1926; Fejer, 1932); but its effects may not be prolonged. Other methods of rendering the eye insensitive, which are only of historical interest, include extirpation of the ciliary ganglion (Rohmer, 1902), and anæsthetization of the gasserian ganglion (Alexander, 1927–30).

It is relevant to comment here on the management of certain other clinical types of simple glaucoma.

Juvenile Glaucoma. This, as we have already seen,[1] is a mixture of various types of primary and secondary glaucoma. In those cases associated with gonioscopically visible abnormalities in the angle of the anterior chamber, treatment should be the same as for buphthalmos,[2] while in those that appear as simple glaucoma of early onset, the therapeusis should be similar to that of simple glaucoma. Because of the long life-expectancy of those affected, surgical treatment should be contemplated earlier than in older patients. Although they frequently respond to conventional drainage operations, an appreciable percentage responds satisfactorily to goniotomy (Barkan, 1956) or to gonio-puncture (Scheie, 1950–63).

Simple Glaucoma in the Aged. In patients whose life-expectancy is short a more conservative attitude may be taken towards the management of the raised ocular tension. Miotics are frequently not tolerated because of the co-existent lenticular changes, and the tension should, if possible, be controlled by adrenaline, if necessary with the addition of one of the carbonic anhydrase inhibitors. It is frequently unnecessary and unkind to demand the degree of control of ocular tension required in younger patients.

Low-tension Glaucoma. In patients with this type of glaucoma, the ocular tension must be reduced to considerably lower levels than is usually necessary in the more common forms of simple glaucoma. If these low levels of tension cannot be achieved by medical therapy, operative interference must be contemplated, and corneo-scleral trephining appears to give the best chance of achieving the hypotension required.

Hypersecretory Glaucoma. If the occurrence of this condition is accepted, and this is doubted by many authorities, the rational treatment would be to reduce the production of aqueous by the topical administration of adrenaline, or failing this, by carbonic anhydrase inhibitors.

Pigmentary Glaucoma. Patients with this condition should be managed in the same way as other cases of simple glaucoma. Medical treatment is successful in about 66% of cases, and the remainder responds to surgery (Scheie and Fleischhauer, 1958). It has been suggested that women with pigmentary glaucoma are more difficult to control than men (Becker and Shaffer, 1965).

Glaucoma in the Negro. Because of their tendency to produce excessive scar tissue, Negroes have been considered to respond badly to filtering operations.[3] It is now generally accepted that iridencleisis is the operation of choice in these patients,[4] although a peripheral iridectomy with scleral cauterization may also result in a satisfactory filtering bleb (Scheie, 1958; Nadel, 1966). Beta-radiation at the time of the operation has been recommended in order to reduce fibrosis (Cohen *et al.*, 1959; Tribin-Piedrahita, 1965).

---

[1] p. 397.   [2] Vol. III. p. 562.   [3] p. 543.
[4] McNair (1951), Scheie (1958), Cohen *et al.* (1959), Cassady (1959), Sédan (1964), and others.

SIMPLE GLAUCOMA AND CATARACT

The association of simple glaucoma with cataract, a relatively common combination, can be managed in a number of ways. If the glaucoma is medically controlled, the lens can be extracted first and any residual raised tension, which may not reappear for several months, should again be treated medically if this is possible.[1] If, on the other hand, the glaucoma cannot be medically controlled or if the miosis thus induced increases the visual disability caused by the cataract when the lenticular opacities are central, the alternative methods of treatment are to perform a drainage operation and then to remove the lens at a later date,[2] or to perform a combined cataract extraction and a drainage operation, often a sclerectomy with or without cauterization and sometimes with an iridencleisis.[3] This last choice, which has recently received much support, is not particularly difficult and is usually indicated, certainly in the elderly or frail patient on whom repeated operations may not be justified.

The best technique for the extraction of a cataract in a patient who has had a successful filtering operation—not an uncommon sequel—has excited considerable discussion. One method which may be employed if the subsequent development or worsening of a cataract is suspected at the time of surgery is to perform the filtering operation in the lower segment of the limbus so that the upper segment remains free for conventional cataract surgery. If, as is usual, the filtering bleb is in the upper segment, three courses are open all of which have had their advocates (see L. Weekers *et al.*, 1947); which course he prefers, each individual surgeon must choose. Some surgeons perform the conventional operation cutting through the bleb, neglecting the possibility of subsequent scarring of this area (Buffington, 1940; and others); indeed, it has been claimed that in cases treated in this manner 70% have a lower ocular tension after the operation than before and only 12% have a raised tension provided accurate closure of the wound has been attained and sutures are not inserted through the filtering area (Yasuna, 1964). The majority of surgeons, however, avoid the filtering area by performing a superior incision in the cornea anterior to the bleb (J. M. McLean, 1942; Gasteiger, 1949; Pillat, 1949; and others). A difficulty that may arise is that delivery of the lens may be difficult past the corneal shelf thus left and to avoid this Scheie (1956) suggested a technique of making the incision *ab externo*, cutting through the cornea in the region of the bleb perpendicularly with a knife; this, with modifications, has been successfully

[1] Chandler (1947), L. Weekers *et al.* (1947), Lee and Weih (1950), Leydhecker (1954–56), Mehra and Dutta (1963), Fronimopoulos (1964), and others.
[2] Chandler (1947), Thomas (1947), Sourdille (1950), Alagna (1954), Leydhecker (1954–56), Beauvieux *et al.* (1956), Mehra and Dutta (1963), and others.
[3] O'Brien (1947), Lee and Weih (1950), Birge (1952–66), O. D. Wolfe (1952), Wenaas and Stertzbach (1955), Hughes (1959), Chilaris (1960), Hauer (1960), Bessiere and Pelegris (1961), Mogilevskaya (1961), Küchle (1962), Bangerter (1963), Hughes *et al.* (1963), Harrison (1963), Verzella (1963), McLean (1964), Stocker (1964), L. G. Bell (1964), Nectoux *et al.* (1964), Boberg-Ans (1964), Nath and Shukla (1966), Labib and El-Guindi (1966), Harrington (1966), Pittar (1966), and others.

employed (Scheie and Muirhead, 1962; Kennedy, 1965). The third choice is to make the incision for the cataract extraction in an area separate from the filtering bleb, either temporally (Gifford, 1943) or infero-temporally (Callahan, 1952; Rizzuti, 1954; Dyson, 1968). This technique, however, is somewhat difficult since the surgeon must reverse his accustomed manipulations and it requires a peripheral iridectomy in an area not covered by the upper lid, difficulties which may be rendered greater if the pupil is drawn upwards as it may be after an iridencleisis. In all cases, whichever choice is made, suturing must be adequate and at the end of the operation air or saline should be injected into the anterior chamber in an endeavour to maintain its integrity and thus to prevent the occurrence of post-operative peripheral anterior synechiæ.

Abadie. *Arch. Ophtal.*, **17**, 375 (1897); **19**, 94 (1899); **30**, 262 (1910).
Ann. Oculist. (Paris), **125**, 194 (1901).
Alagna. *Atti Soc. oftal. ital.*, **14**, 46 (1954).
Albaugh and Dunphy. *Arch. Ophthal.*, **27**, 543 (1942).
Alexander. *Med. Klin.*, **23**, 1103 (1927).
Klin. Mbl. Augenheilk., **84**, 65 (1930).
Allen, J. H. *Sth. med. J.* (Bgham, Ala.), **44**, 931 (1951).
Allen, L. and Burian. *Amer. J. Ophthal.*, **53**, 19 (1962).
Arato. *Ophthalmologica*, **115**, 190 (1948); **120**, 325 (1950); **125**, 117 (1953).
Arruga. *Arch. Soc. oftal. hisp.-amer.*, **10**, 224 (1950).
Ocular Surgery (transl. 4th Spanish ed.), N.Y. (1962).
Bachstez. *Z. Augenheilk.*, **31**, 34 (1914).
Bader. *Trans. int. med. Cong.*, London, 7th Sess., **3**, 98 (1881).
Bangerter. *Ber. dtsch. ophthal. Ges.*, **65**, 84 (1963).
Barkan. *Amer. J. Ophthal.*, **19**, 951 (1936); **20**, 1237 (1937); **21**, 1099 (1938); **42**, 63 (1956).
Arch. Ophthal., **19**, 217 (1938); **21**, 331 (1939).
Barkan, Boyle and Maisler. *Amer. J. Ophthal.*, **19**, 21 (1936).
Baron and Michel. *Bull. Soc. franç. Ophtal.*, **80**, 704 (1967).
Beauvieux, Bessière and Chabot. *Bull. Soc. Ophtal. Fr.*, 178 (1956).
Becker and Ley. *Amer. J. Ophthal.*, **45**, 639 (1958).
Becker and Middleton. *Arch. Ophthal.*, **54**, 187 (1955).
Becker and Shaffer. *Diagnosis and Therapy of the Glaucomas*, St. Louis (1965).
Bell, G. H. *Arch. Ophthal.*, **3**, 194 (1930).
Bell, L. G. *Trans. ophthal. Soc. N.Z.*, **17**, 35 (1964).
Berens. *Amer. J. Ophthal.*, **19**, 470 (1936).
Arch. Ophthal., **54**, 548 (1955).
Berens and Breakey. *Amer. J. Ophthal.*, **50**, 45 (1960).

Berens and Sheppard. *Amer. J. Ophthal.*, **50**, 599 (1960).
Berens, Sheppard and Duel. *Trans. Amer. ophthal. Soc.*, **47**, 364 (1949).
Bessiere and Pelegris. *J. int. Coll. Surg.*, **35**, 77 (1961).
Bick. *Amer. J. Ophthal.*, **30**, 1033 (1947).
Arch. Ophthal., **42**, 373 (1949).
Bietti. *Atti Soc. oftal. ital.*, **36**, 64 (1947).
J. Amer. med. Ass., **142**, 889 (1950).
Ateneo parmense, **23**, 1 (1952).
Acta ophthal. (Kbh.), **33**, 337 (1955).
Birge. *Trans. Amer. ophthal. Soc.*, **50**, 241 (1952); **64**, 332 (1966).
Blaickner. *Z. Augenheilk.*, **72**, 265 (1930).
Blatt and Regenbogen. *Klin. Mbl. Augenheilk.*, **136**, 761 (1960).
Boberg-Ans. *Trans. ophthal. Soc. U.K.*, **84**, 113 (1964).
Bock. *Amer. J. Ophthal.*, **33**, 929 (1950).
Böck. Meller's *Augenärztliche Eingriffe*, 6th ed., Wien (1950).
Borthen. *Arch. Augenheilk.*, **65**, 42 (1910).
Buffington. *Texas St. J. Med.*, **35**, 700 (1940).
Burian. *Amer. J. Ophthal.*, **50**, 1187 (1960).
Butler. *Proc. roy. Soc. Med., Sect. Ophthal.*, **14**, 51 (1921).
Brit. J. Ophthal., **16**, 741 (1932).
Trans. ophthal. Soc. U.K., **56**, 194 (1936).
Cairns. *Amer. J. Ophthal.*, **66**, 673 (1968).
Callahan. *Arch. Ophthal.*, **47**, 132 (1952).
Surgery of the Eye: Diseases, Springfield, Ill. (1956).
Campbell, Jones, Renner and Tonks. *Brit. J. Ophthal.*, **41**, 746 (1957).
Cassady. *Arch. Ophthal.*, **62**, 239 (1959).
Cavka. *Acta XVII int. Cong. Ophthal.*, Montreal-N.Y., **2**, 1189 (1954).
Chandler. *Amer. J. Ophthal.*, **30**, 483 (1947).
Chandler and Grant. *Lectures on Glaucoma*, Phila. (1965).
Chilaris. *Bull. hellen. Soc. Ophthal.*, **28**, 69 (1960).
Coccius. *Ueber Glaukom*, Leipzig (1859).
v. Graefes Arch. Ophthal., **9** (1), 1 (1863).

Cohen, Graham and Fry. *Amer. J. Ophthal.*, **47**, 54 (1959).

Colley. *Brit. J. Ophthal.*, **40**, 436 (1956).

Collins. *Ophthalmoscope*, **12**, 589 (1914).

Cramer. *Arch. oftal. B. Aires*, **22**, 105 (1947).

Cristini. *G. ital. Oftal.*, **1**, 1 (1948).

Critchett. *Roy. Lond. ophthal. Hosp. Rep.*, **1**, 57 (1857).

Cruise. *Trans. ophthal. Soc. U.K.*, **41**, 248 (1921).
Brit. J. Ophthal., **31**, 64 (1947).

Czermak. *Prag. med. Wschr.*, **31**, 313 (1906).

Dastoor. *Proc. All-India ophthal. Soc.*, **9**, 58 (1948).

Davenport. *Brit. J. Ophthal.*, **10**, 474 (1926).
Trans. ophthal. Soc. U.K., **47**, 283 (1927).

Dellaporta. *Acta ophthal.* (Kbh.), **26**, 413 (1948).

Demours. *Traité des maladies de yeux*, Paris (1818).

Desvignes and Naudin. *Arch. Ophtal.*, **8**, 589 (1948).

Dianoux. *Ann. Oculist.* (Paris), **133**, 81 (1905).

Dominguez. *Arch. Soc. oftal. hisp.-amer.*, **8**, 117 (1948).

Drance. *Trans. ophthal. Soc. U.K.*, **80**, 387 (1960).
Drug Mechanisms in Glaucoma (ed. Paterson *et al.*), London, 301 (1966).

Duke-Elder. *Text-Book of Ophthalmology*, London, **3**, 2129 (1940).

Dyson. *Canad. J. Ophthal.*, **3**, 168 (1968).

Eerola. *Acta ophthal.* (Kbh.), **12**, 137 (1934).

Elliot. *Ophthalmoscope*, **7**, 804, 807 (1909); **8**, 482, 779 (1910).
Trans. ophthal. Soc. U.K., **38**, 227 (1918).
Treatise on Glaucoma, London (1922).
Amer. J. Ophthal., **14**, 999 (1931).
Arch. Ophthal., **8**, 797 (1932).

Ellis. *Amer. J. Ophthal.*, **50**, 733 (1960).

Elschnig. *Klin. Mbl. Augenheilk.*, **50** (1), 538 (1912); **70**, 667 (1923); **80**, 382 (1928).
Ber. dtsch. ophthal. Ges., **49**, 277, 353 (1932).

Epstein. *Brit. J. Ophthal.*, **43**, 641 (1959).

Fankhauser and Schmidt. *Ophthalmologica*, **131**, 342 (1956).

Fejer. *Amer. J. Ophthal.*, **15**, 135 (1932).

Fergus. *Brit. med. J.*, **2**, 983 (1909).
Ophthalmoscope, **8**, 74 (1910).
Ophthal. Rev., **34**, 129, 202 (1915).

Fisher. *Trans. ophthal. Soc. U.K.*, **41**, 264 (1921).

Foster. Philps's *Ophthalmic Operations*, 2nd ed., London (1961).

Friedenwald. *Amer. J. Ophthal.*, **33**, 1523 (1950).

Fronimopoulos. *Ann. Ophthal.* (Athens), **1**, 99 (1964).

Galin, Baras and McLean. *Amer. J. Ophthal.*, **61**, 63 (1966).

Gasteiger. *Klin. Mbl. Augenheilk.*, **114**, 370 (1949).

Gauly. *Klin. Mbl. Augenheilk.*, **129**, 67 (1956).

Gibson. *Trans. Amer. ophthal. Soc.*, **40**, 499 (1942).

Gifford. *Amer. J. Ophthal.*, **26**, 468 (1943).

Gills. *Amer. J. Ophthal.*, **61**, 841 (1966).

Gjessing. *Trans. ophthal. Soc. U.K.*, **43**, 616 (1923).

Goar and Schultz. *Arch. Ophthal.*, **22**, 1035 (1939).

Goldmann. *Ophthalmologica*, **121**, 94 (1951).
Ann. Oculist. (Paris), **184**, 1086 (1951).

Goldsmith. *Trans. ophthal. Soc. U.K.*, **74**, 41 (1954).

Goodner. *Int. Ophthal. Clin.*, **3**, 133 (1963).

Gorin and Posner. *Slit-lamp Gonioscopy*, 3rd ed., Baltimore (1967).

Gradle. *Amer. J. Ophthal.*, **7**, 851 (1924); **14**, 936 (1931).

von Graefe. *v. Graefes Arch. Ophthal.*, **3** (2), 456 (1857).

Greeves. *Trans. ophthal. Soc. U.K.*, **36**, 445 (1916).

Grom and van den Beld. *Arch. Soc. oftal. hisp.-amer.*, **24**, 931 (1964).

von Grósz. *Ber. dtsch. ophthal. Ges.*, **44**, 151 (1924).

Grüter. *Ber. dtsch. ophthal. Ges.*, **41**, 85 (1918).

Guillaumat, Paufique, de Saint-Martin, Schiff-Wertheimer and Sourdille. *Traitement chirurgical des affections oculaires*, Paris, **1** (1957).

Haas. *Symposium on Glaucoma* (Trans. N. Orleans Acad. Ophthal.), St. Louis, 175 (1967).

Habenberger. *Wien. klin. Wschr.*, **63**, 210 (1951).

Haisten and Guyton. *Arch. Ophthal.*, **59**, 507 (1958).

Hancock. *Roy. Lond. ophthal. Hosp. Rep.*, **3**, 13 (1860).

Harms and Mackensen. *Ocular Surgery under the Microscope* (Transl. Blodi), Chicago (1967).

Harrington. *Amer. J. Ophthal.*, **61**, 1134 (1966).

Harrison. *Arch. Ophthal.*, **70**, 842, 862 (1963).

Harrower. *Arch. Ophthal.*, **47**, 37 (1918).

Hauer. *Israel med. J.*, **19**, 254 (1960).

Haye. *Bull. Soc. ophthal. Fr.*, 615 (1955).

Haye, Haut and Mondon. *Bull. Soc. Ophtal. Fr.*, **67**, 383 (1967).

Heine. *Ber. dtsch. ophthal. Ges.*, **32**, 3 (1905).

Herbert. *Trans. ophthal. Soc. U.K.*, **23**, 324 (1903); **39**, 218 (1919); **41**, 239 (1921).
Ophthalmoscope, **5**, 292 (1907); **9**, 762 (1911); **11**, 398 (1913).
Proc. roy. Soc. Med., **7**, Sect. Ophthal., 127 (1914).
Brit. J. Ophthal., **4**, 216, 550 (1920); **5**, 183, 417 (1921); **14**, 433 (1930); **18**, 142 (1934).

Hobbs and Smith. *Brit. J. Ophthal.*, **38**, 279 (1954).

Holst. *Klin. Mbl. Augenheilk.*, **87**, 602 (1931).

Holst. *Acta ophthal.* (Kbh.), **12**, 348 (1934); **25**, 271 (1947).

Holth. *Ber. dtsch. ophthal. Ges.*, **33**, 123 (1906); **39**, 355 (1913).
Ann. Oculist. (Paris), **137**, 345 (1907); **142**, 1 (1909).
Ophthalmoscope, **9**, 487 (1911); **12**, 347 (1914).
Brit. J. Ophthal., **5**, 544 (1921); **6**, 10 (1922).
Arch. Ophthal., **4**, 803 (1930); **6**, 151 (1931); **9**, 913 (1933).
Trans. ophthal. Soc. U.K., **53**, 326 (1933).

Hughes. *Amer. J. Ophthal.*, **48**, 1 (1959).

Hughes, Kazdan, Brackup and Marinakos. *Amer. J. Ophthal.*, **56**, 391 (1963).

Iliff. *Amer. J. Ophthal.*, **27**, 731 (1944).

Iliff and Haas. *Amer. J. Ophthal.*, **54**, 688 (1962).

Illig. *Ophthalmologica*, **138**, 54 (1959).

Ivanov. *Vestn. Oftal.*, **11**, 519 (1937).

Jaensch. *Z. Augenheilk.*, **58**, 2 (1926).

Jervey. *Trans. Amer. ophthal. Soc.*, **25**, 160 (1927).

Jonnesco. *Wien. klin. Wschr.*, **12**, 483 (1899).

Kalt and Loisillier. *Ann. Oculist.* (Paris), **191**, 713 (1958).

Kapuściński. *Referat. XXV Zjazdu Okulist. Pols.*, **2**, 479 (1957).

Kapuściński and Pacyńska. *Klin. Mbl. Augenheilk.*, **143**, 625 (1963).

Kennedy. *Arch. Ophthal.*, **74**, 365 (1965).

Kettesy. *Brit. J. Ophthal.*, **30**, 643 (1946).

Krasnov. *Vestn. Oftal.*, **77**, 37 (1964).
Brit. J. Ophthal., **52**, 157 (1968).

Kronfeld. *Arch. Ophthal.*, **15**, 411 (1936); **78**, 140 (1967).

Krwawicz and Szwarc. *Klin. oczna*, **35**, 191 (1965).

Küchle. *Klin. Mbl. Augenheilk.*, **140**, 645, 769 (1962).

Labib and El-Guindi. *Bull. ophthal. Soc. Egypt*, **59**, 151 (1966).

Lagrange, F. *Bull. Soc. franç. Ophtal.*, **23**, 477 (1906).
Arch. Ophtal., **26**, 481 (1906); **27**, 439 (1907).
Ann. Oculist. (Paris), **137**, 89 (1907).
XVII int. Cong. Med., London, Sect. IX (1), 71 (1913).

La Rocca. *Brit. J. Ophthal.*, **46**, 404 (1962).

Lauber. *Trans. ophthal. Soc. U.K.*, **59**, 267 (1939).

Laval. *Arch. Ophthal.*, **54**, 677 (1955).

Lawson. *Trans. ophthal. Soc. U.K.*, **33**, 194 (1913).

Lee, Donovan and Schepens. *Canad. J. Ophthal.*, **3**, 22 (1968).

Lee and Schepens. *Invest. Ophthal.*, **5**, 59, 304 (1966).

Lee and Weih. *Arch. Ophthal.*, **44**, 275 (1950).

Lehman and McCaslin. *Amer. J. Ophthal.*, **47**, 690 (1959).

Leydhecker. *Acta XVII int. Cong. Ophthal.*, Montreal-N.Y., **1**, 233 (1954).
Docum. ophthal., **10**, 174 (1956).
Klin. Mbl. Augenheilk., **144**, 28 (1964); **148**, 818 (1966).
Glaucoma (Tutzing Symp., ed. Leydhecker), Basel, 224 (1967).

Löhlein. *Klin. Mbl. Augenheilk.*, **77**, Beil., 1 (1926).

Lösche. *Klin. Mbl. Augenheilk.*, **121**, 715 (1952).

Mackenzie. *A Practical Treatise on the Diseases of the Eye*, London, 1st ed. (1830); 2nd ed. (1835); 3rd ed. (1854).

Mackie and Rubinstein. *Brit. J. Ophthal.*, **38**, 641 (1954).

MacLean, A. L. *Arch. Ophthal.*, **71**, 653 (1964).

McLean, J. M. *Amer. J. Ophthal.*, **25**, 192 (1942).
Atlas of Glaucoma Surgery, St. Louis (1967).

McNair. *Amer. J. Ophthal.*, **34**, 70 (1951).

McPherson. *Amer. J. Ophthal.*, **29**, 848 (1946).

Malbran and Norbis. *Mod. Probl. Ophthal.*, **6**, 132 (1968).

Marr. *Amer. J. Ophthal.*, **32**, 241 (1949).

Mascati. *Int. Surg.* (Chic.), **47**, 10 (1967).

Mauksch. *Z. Augenheilk.*, **52**, 167 (1924).

Mawas and Parizot. *Trans. ophthal. Soc. U.K.*, **84**, 139 (1964).

Mayou. *Ophthalmoscope*, **10**, 254 (1912); **11**, 258 (1913).

Meek. *Amer. J. Ophthal.*, **31**, 1232 (1948).

Meesmann. *Ber. dtsch. ophthal. Ges.*, **60**, 307 (1956).
Klin. Mbl. Augenheilk., **136**, 774 (1960).

Mehra and Dutta. *J. All-India ophthal. Soc.*, **11**, 1 (1963).

Meyer. *Arch. Ophthal.*, **41**, 417 (1949).
Amer. J. Ophthal., **35**, 788 (1952).

Miller. *Brit. J. Ophthal.*, **47**, 211 (1963).

Mittl and Galin. *Klin. Mbl. Augenheilk.*, **151**, 485 (1967).

Møller. *Acta ophthal.* (Kbh.), **41**, 151 (1963).

Mogilevskaya. *Helmoholtz ophthal. Inst., Sci. Notes*, **6**, 303 (1961).

Mügge. *Klin. Mbl. Augenheilk.*, **112**, 104 (1947).

Muldoon, Ripple and Wilder. *Arch. Ophthal.*, **45**, 666 (1951).

Nadel. *Amer. J. Ophthal.*, **62**, 955 (1966).

Nath and Shukla. *J. All-India ophthal. Soc.*, **14**, 21 (1966).

Neame and Khan. *Brit. J. Ophthal.*, **9**, 618 (1925).

Nectoux, Chabat, Mawas and Parizot. *Bull. Soc. Ophtal. Fr.*, **64**, 377 (1964).

O'Brien. *Arch. Ophthal.*, **37**, 1 (1947).
Trans. ophthal. Soc. Aust., **7**, 87 (1947).

O'Brien and Weih. *Arch. Ophthal.*, **42**, 606 (1949).

Paiva. *Rev. bras. Oftal.*, **14**, 3 (1955).

Parinaud. *Bull. Soc. franç. Ophtal.*, **18**, 220 (1901).

Paufique, Rougier and Charleux. *Bull. Soc. Ophtal. Fr.*, 567 (1956).

Pillat. *Klin. Mbl. Augenheilk.*, **66**, 525 (1921).
Z. Augenheilk., Suppl. 9 (1928).
Arch. Ophthal., **42**, 567 (1949).

Pittar. *Trans. ophthal. Soc. Aust.*, **25**, 59 (1966).

Posey. *J. Amer. med. Ass.*, **63**, 219 (1914).
Arch. Ophthal., **49**, 293 (1920).

Postic and Stankov-Tomic. *Bull. Soc. franç. Ophtal.*, **80**, 716 (1967).

Pratt-Johnson, Drance and Innes. *Arch. Ophthal.*, **72**, 485 (1964).

Preziosi. *Brit. J. Ophthal.*, **8**, 414 (1924).

Qadeer. *Brit. J. Ophthal.*, **38**, 353 (1954).

Quaglino. *Ann. Ottal.*, **1**, 200 (1871).

Raeder. *Acta ophthal.* (Kbh.), **6**, 390 (1928).

Reese. *Trans. ophthal. Soc. Aust.*, **12**, 43 (1952).

Regan. *Trans. Amer. ophthal. Soc.*, **61**, 219 (1963).

Richards and van Bijsterveld. *Amer. J. Ophthal.*, **60**, 405 (1965).

Rizzuti. *Acta XVII int. Cong. Ophthal.*, Montreal-N.Y., **3**, 1831 (1954).

Robertson, Argyll. *Roy. Lond. ophthal. Hosp. Rep.*, **8**, 404 (1876).

Rocha and Calixto. *Mod. Probl. Ophthal.*, **6**, 180 (1968).

de Roetth. *Amer. J. Ophthal.*, **61**, 443 (1966).

Rohmer. *Ann. Oculist.* (Paris), **127**, 328; **128**, 1 (1902).

Rollet. *Rev. gén. Ophtal.*, **26**, 289 (1907).

Row. *Arch. Ophthal.*, **12**, 325 (1934).

Sallmann. *Z. Augenheilk.*, **86**, 111 (1935).

Sampaolesi. *Mod. Probl. Ophthal.*, **6**, 148 (1968).

Sampimon. *Ophthalmologica*, **151**, 637 (1966).

Scardapane. *Boll. Oculist.*, **4**, 866 (1926).

Scharf. *Klin. Mbl. Augenheilk.*, **115**, 500 (1949).

Scheie. *Arch. Ophthal.*, **44**, 761 (1950); **55**, 818 (1956).
Trans. Canad. ophthal. Soc., **10**, 31, 129 (1958).
Amer. J. Ophthal., **45** (2), 220 (1958); **53**, 571 (1962).
Trans. Amer. Acad. Ophthal., **67**, 458 (1963).
Trans. ophthal. Soc. U.K., **84**, 127 (1964).

Scheie and Fleischhauer. *Arch. Ophthal.*, **59**, 216 (1958).

Scheie, Frayer and Spencer. *Arch. Ophthal.*, **53**, 839 (1955).

Scheie and Muirhead. *Arch. Ophthal.*, **68**, 37 (1962).

Schreck. *v. Graefes Arch. Ophthal.*, **149**, 95 (1949).

Schultz, Watzke and Sawyer. *Arch. Ophthal.*, **64**, 408 (1960).

Sédan. *Ann. Oculist.* (Paris), **197**, 565 (1964).

Seidel. *v. Graefes Arch. Ophthal.*, **104**, 403 (1921).

Sivayoham. *Brit. J. Ophthal.*, **52**, 843 (1968).

Smith, R. *Brit. J. Ophthal.*, **44**, 370 (1960).

Smith, R. *Trans. ophthal. Soc. U.K.*, **82**, 439 (1962).

Solomon. *Med. Times Gaz.*, **1**, 54, 83, 141, 221, 327 (1861).

Sommer. *Klin. Mbl. Augenheilk.*, **151**, 47 (1967).

Sourdille. *Bull. Soc. franç. Ophtal.*, **63**, 242 (1950).
Brit. J. Ophthal., **34**, 428 (1950).

Spaeth, E. B. *Principles and Practice of Ophthalmic Surgery*, 4th ed., Phila. (1948).

Spaeth, G. L. *Arch. Ophthal.*, **78**, 578 (1967).

Stallard. *Brit. J. Ophthal.*, **32**, 753 (1948) **37**, 680 (1953).
Eye Surgery, 4th ed., Bristol (1965).

Stefansson. *Amer. J. Ophthal.*, **8**, 681 (1925).

Stellwag von Carion. *Lhb. d. praktischen Augenheilkunde*, Wien (1870).

Stocker. *Arch. Ophthal.*, **72**, 503 (1964).

Strachan. *Brit. J. Ophthal.*, **51**, 539 (1967).

Strampelli. *Ann. Ottal.*, **82**, 186 (1956).

Strampelli and Valvo. *Amer. J. Ophthal.*, **64**, 371 (1967).

Streiff, Bianchi and Stucchi. *Atti Soc. oftal. ital.*, **17**, 376 (1957).

Streiff and Stucchi. *Amer. J. Ophthal.*, **61**, 1325 (1966).

Stumptner. *Ber. dtsch. ophthal. Ges.*, **58**, 84 (1953).

Sugar. *Arch. Ophthal.*, **25**, 674 (1941).
The Glaucomas, 2nd ed., N.Y. (1957).
Amer. J. Ophthal., **51**, 623; **52**, 29 (1961).

Sugar and Zekman. *Amer. J. Ophthal.*, **46**, 155 (1958).

Suker. *Amer. J. Ophthal.*, **14**, 732 (1931).

Syed. *Medicus* (Karachi), **13**, 51 (1956).

Tamesis. *Philipp. J. Ophthal. Otol.*, **7**, 1 (1955).

Teng, Chi and Katzin. *Amer. J. Ophthal.*, **47**, 16 (1959).

Thomas. *Bull. Soc. Ophtal. Paris*, 497 (1947).

Thomas, Cordier and Algan. *Bull. Soc. belge Ophtal.*, No. 94, 249 (1950).

Topalis and Roussos. *Arch. Ophtal.*, **19**, 397 (1959).

Torok. *Arch. Ophthal.*, **52**, 574 (1923).

Tribin-Piedrahita. *Amer. J. Ophthal.*, **60**, 140 (1965).

Troncoso. *Arch. Ophthal.*, **14**, 557 (1935); **23**, 270 (1940).
Amer. J. Ophthal., **32**, 499 (1949).

Troncoso and Reese. *Amer. J. Ophthal.*, **18**, 103 (1935).

Troutman. *Acta XVII int. Cong. Ophthal.*, Montreal-N.Y., **2**, 674 (1954).

Trowbridge. *Amer. J. Ophthal.*, **20**, 135 (1937).

Tyner and Swets. *Arch. Ophthal.*, **54**, 59 (1955).

Vail. *Ophthal. Rec.*, **24**, 184 (1915).

Verhoeff. *Ophthalmoscope*, **11**, 220 (1913).
Arch. Ophthal., **44**, 129 (1915); **53**, 228 (1924).

Verrey. *Ophthalmologica*, **117**, 281 (1949).

Verzella. *Ann. Oculist.* (Paris), **196**, 688 (1963).

Viikari and Tuovinen. *Acta ophthal.* (Kbh.), **35**, 528 (1957).
Villaseca. *Arch. chil. Oftal.*, **4**, 425 (1947).
de Vincentiis. *Ann. Ottal.*, **22**, 540 (1893).
Vogt. *Arch. Ophtal.*, **1**, 856 (1937).
   Klin. Mbl. Augenheilk., **97**, 672 (1936); **99**, 9 (1937); **103**, 591 (1939).
Wagner and Richner. *Schweiz. med. Wschr.*, **69**, 1048 (1939).
Walker and Kanagasundaram. *Trans. ophthal. Soc. U.K.*, **84**, 427 (1964).
Wardrop. *Essays on the Morbid Anatomy of the Human Eye*, Edinb. (1808–18).
de Wecker. *Ber. dtsch. ophthal. Ges.* (1869).
   Klin. Mbl. Augenheilk., **9**, 305 (1871).
   Ann. Oculist. (Paris), **111**, 321 (1894).
   Bull. Soc. franç. Ophtal., **18**, 1 (1901).
Weekers, L. *Klin. Mbl. Augenheilk.*, **45** (2), 230 (1907).
   Arch. Ophtal., **39**, 279 (1922); **19**, 270 (1959).
Weekers, L., and Bonhomme. *Ophthalmologica*, **99**, 180 (1940).
Weekers, L. and R. *Ophthalmologica*, **104**, 1 (1942).
   Brit. J. Ophthal., **32**, 904 (1948).
   Acta XVI int. Cong. Ophthal., London, **2**, 950 (1950).
Weekers, L. and R., and Freson. *Bull. Soc. belge Ophtal.*, No. 88, 283 (1948).
Weekers, L. and R., and Thibert. *Bull. Soc. Ophtal. Paris*, 539 (1947).

Weekers, R. and Prijot. *Ophthalmologica*, **123**, 365 (1952).
Wenaas and Stertzbach. *Amer. J. Ophthal.*, **39**, 71 (1955).
Wessely. *Klin. Mbl. Augenheilk.*, **78**, 80 (1927).
Weve. *Ned. T. Geneesk.*, **76**, 5335 (1932).
Wheeler. *Arch. Ophthal.*, **16**, 569 (1936).
Wheelock. *Ophthal. Rec.*, **25**, 81 (1916).
Wilder. *Ann. Ophthal.*, **13**, 17 (1904).
   J. Amer. med. Ass., **81**, 2095 (1923).
Wilmer. *Trans. ophthal. Soc. U.K.*, **47**, 230 (1927).
Wolfe, O. D. *J. Iowa med. Soc.*, **42**, 522 (1952).
Wolfe, O. R. and Blaess. *Amer. J. Ophthal.*, **19**, 400 (1936).
Wolfe, O. R. and R. M., and Georgariou. *Amer. J. Ophthal.*, **27**, 1146 (1944).
Wood. *Ophthal. Rec.*, **24**, 179, 235 (1915).
Wootton. *Trans. Amer. ophthal. Soc.*, **30**, 64 (1932).
Yasuna. *Amer. J. Ophthal.*, **57**, 258 (1964).
Young. *Trans. ophthal. Soc. U.K.*, **44**, 338 (1924); **46**, 181 (1926); **53**, 348 (1933).
Ziehe and Axenfeld. *Samml. zwangl. Abhdl. Geb. Augenheilk.* (ed. Vossius), **4**, 1 (1901).
Zorab. *Ophthalmoscope*, **10**, 258 (1912); **11**, 211 (1913).

Prognosis

To make an assessment of the prognosis of any individual case of simple glaucoma is impossible. Uncontrolled, the disease is slowly progressive and eventually results in irremediable blindness—if the patient lives long enough ; and, as we have seen, it is bilateral. Fortunately, it usually affects patients in the latter half of life. With adequate treatment, however, in the majority of cases its progress can be stabilized or delayed so that useful vision remains until the death of the patient. This certainly applies if the diagnosis is made at an early stage or if resort is made to surgery if the ocular tension cannot be adequately controlled by medical means before serious functional deterioration has occurred. There is, however, a certain number of cases, often those wherein the tension is not particularly high but in which the circulation in the optic nerve is grossly impaired, that tends to progress gradually and imperceptibly despite much care ; these, essentially examples of ischæmic optic neuropathy, constitute a medical problem of considerable difficulty, frequently rendered less easy since such patients are often frail and are affected by generalized circulatory insufficiency. In a few cases the tension can be controlled only by repeated surgical interventions ; but these are rare.

The essential determinants in the prognosis of the disease are therefore the general condition of the patient, the earliness of the diagnosis, the adequacy of medical treatment, the resort to surgery before serious functional loss has occurred and the performance of more than one operation if a first has been or has become ineffective in maintaining the ocular tension at a level below that which damages the eye in question. It is always to be remembered that in the present state of our knowledge the disease cannot be cured but is only arrested; it demands constant observation and eternal vigilance maintained in a cat-and-mouse manner so that any exacerbation or deterioration can be combated by a change in medical treatment or by surgery, a vigilance that should be continued after an operation has been performed. In general terms it may be said that with adequate treatment some 70% of cases do well in so far as they become stabilized, 20% deteriorate so slowly that they maintain a useful amount of sight to the end, while some 10% are visually incapacitated. This is reflected in the statistics which show that glaucoma is the cause of approximately one-seventh of registered blindness in England (Sorsby, 1966) and the U.S.A. (Becker, 1967) and 10% in Canada (MacDonald, 1965). The entire prognosis, however, depends on early diagnosis and treatment. Thus if treated early as in the pre-scotoma period, Frühauf and his colleagues (1967) found that only 10% of patients suffered marked deterioration of vision over a period of 20 years, while 50% of those allowed to progress to a more advanced stage became blind in spite of adequate control of the ocular tension by medical or surgical means.

Becker. *Vision and its Disorders* (U.S. Publ. Hlth. Serv.), Bethesda, 110 (1967).

Frühauf, Müller and Sismuth. *Klin. Mbl. Augenheilk.*, **51**, 477 (1967).

MacDonald. *Canad. med. Ass. J.*, **92**, 264 (1965).

Sorsby. *The Incidence and Causes of Blindness in England and Wales* (1948–62), London (1966).

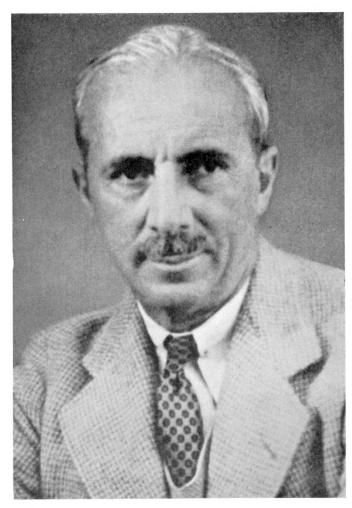

FIG. 543.—OTTO BARKAN
[1887–1958].

CHAPTER VIII

PRIMARY CLOSED-ANGLE GLAUCOMA

THE obvious introduction to this Chapter is the photograph of OTTO BARKAN [1887–1958] (Fig. 543), one of the great ophthalmologists of the West Coast of America who was essentially responsible for the classification of primary glaucoma into the two types, characterized by an open or closed angle. Of Hungarian descent, he studied in Oxford, London, Vienna and Munich, whereafter he returned to America in 1920 to Stanford University and San Francisco. His constant interest in the angle of the anterior chamber led him to contribute two other great advances in ophthalmology: the popularization of gonioscopy and the introduction of his operation of goniotomy which revolutionized the treatment of congenital glaucoma. An immensely enthusiastic character and a delightful companion, he was an ardent sportsman, rowing for Oxford University, and remaining an outstanding skier and alpinist throughout most of his life.

By PRIMARY CLOSED-ANGLE GLAUCOMA we mean a condition wherein the ocular tension is raised as a result of functional or organic obstruction to the outflow of the aqueous humour at the angle of the anterior chamber conse-quent upon the occurrence of irido-corneal contact, in the absence of any other disease of the eye. This condition, as we shall see, occurs in an eye with a particular anatomical configuration, the anterior chamber being shallow and its angle narrow. It may be divided into four stages:

(1) PRE-GLAUCOMA wherein the narrowness of the angle, although allowing adequate drainage, potentially leads to attacks of raised tension, which may be precipitated by the appropriate provocative stimuli;

(2) INTERMITTENT, when recurrent attacks of raised tension are separated by periods during which the ocular tension and the facility of the outflow of aqueous return to normal;

(3) ACUTE, during an acute phase of raised tension (the "acute con-gestive glaucoma" of older terminology); and

(4) CHRONIC closed-angle glaucoma wherein the drainage of aqueous is permanently impaired by the presence of peripheral anterior synechiæ.

An eye with a predisposition to primary closed-angle glaucoma (the stage of pre-glaucoma) may develop intermittent attacks, may develop an attack of acute glaucoma, or may pass imperceptibly into the stage of chronic closed-angle glaucoma, while an eye undergoing intermittent attacks may itself develop acute or chronic closed-angle glaucoma.

Incidence

Primary closed-angle glaucoma is a less common disease than simple glaucoma, although its true incidence is particularly difficult to assess from the literature. It is only since the advent of routine gonioscopic examinations that the diagnosis of closed-angle glaucoma has been made with any degree of certainty but, with few exceptions, this method of examination has not been performed in the numerous recent surveys from which the incidence of simple glaucoma has been ascertained. These surveys do not include cases of acute glaucoma, thus reducing the true incidence of primary closed-angle glaucoma, and in some instances secondary glaucomas have been included in the statistics. Even when these variations in presentation are taken into account, the incidence of primary closed-angle glaucoma shows a wide range in the various surveys.

	Incidence of simple glaucoma	Incidence of closed-angle glaucoma	Ratio of simple to closed-angle glaucoma
Gradle (1931) . . .	69%	13%	5·5 : 1
Carvill (1932) . . .	52%	46%	1·1 : 1
Lehrfeld and Reber (1937) .	72%	28%	2·6 : 1
Armstrong (1952) . .	62%	38%	1·6 : 1
Barkan (1954) . . .	55%	45%	1·2 : 1
Sveinsson (1956) . .	91%	9%	10 : 1
Kurland and Taub (1957) .	62%	7%	8·9 : 1
Sugar (1957) . . .	49%	12%	4·1 : 1
Klouman (1961) . .	85%	15%	5·7 : 1
Suda (1963) . . .	54%	46%	1·2 : 1
Gassler (1965) . . .	77%	23%	3·4 : 1
Hollows and Graham (1966)	51%	10%	5·1 : 1
Bankes et al. (1968) . .	76%	18%	4·2 : 1

The study by Hollows and Graham (1966) is particularly valuable, including as it does 92% of the population between the ages of 40 and 75 in three Welsh villages. Of the 4,231 inhabitants who were examined, 39 were found to have glaucoma; of these, 20 had simple glaucoma and 4 closed-angle glaucoma, the remainder being congenital or secondary in type. It appears, therefore, that in Great Britain and probably also in the United States of America, simple glaucoma is four to five times more common than the primary closed-angle type.

Race

We have already mentioned the difficulties inherent in attempting to assess the racial incidence of simple glaucoma,[1] although it was possible to conclude that this disease is rare in Australoids and Pacific Islanders and in Mongoloids, while it is common in Negroids and Caucasoids. Similar broad conclusions can be drawn for the racial incidence of primary closed-angle glaucoma, although these differ in many respects from the case of simple glaucoma.

[1] p. 396.

Primary closed-angle glaucoma is rare in Australoids and Pacific Islanders, in whom all forms of glaucoma are rare,[1] while it is much more common than simple glaucoma in most Mongoloids[2] except those of rural Malaya (Mann, 1966) where it is rare, and in American Indians among whom all forms of glaucoma are rare (Holmes, 1960–61 ; Mann, 1966). Acute closed-angle glaucoma seldom occurs in Negroids, whether African or American,[3] although the chronic type was frequently observed in American Negroids (Alper and Laubach, 1968). The position among Caucasoids needs further clarification for although, as we have seen, primary closed-angle glaucoma is four to five times less common than simple glaucoma in Britain and the United States, it appears to be over ten times less common in Iceland (Björnsson, 1955 ; Sveinsson, 1956–59), in Norway (Holst, 1947) and in Egypt (El-Arabi and Hosni, 1965), while it has been suggested that Australians of Greek and Italian origin also have a very low incidence of this type of the disease (Lowe, 1963).

Sex

In most of the reported series of closed-angle glaucoma the incidence of this disease in females is definitely higher than in males. Thus Priestley Smith (1879) found the "congestive" type in 346 females and 178 males, and Nelander (1933) reported twice as many females. This preponderance of females has been confirmed in more recent series. Holst (1947) found 64% females, Posner and Schlossman (1948) 73% females, Lemoine (1950) 70% females, Bennett (1956) about twice as many females as males, Bain (1957) 71% females, Smith (1958) three times as many females as males, Lowe (1963) 76% females, Suda (1963) 62·4% females and Alper and Laubach (1968) 80% females in Caucasoids but an equal sex-incidence in Negroids. Other authors have confirmed this predilection of the disease for the female sex,[4] although Törnquist (1956) reported an approximately equal distribution between the sexes. The increased incidence of this disease in females may be related to the decreased depth of the anterior chamber in this sex (Törnquist, 1956).

Age

Primary closed-angle glaucoma is a disease of late middle life, occurring preferentially a little earlier than simple glaucoma. Thus Lehrfeld and Reber (1937) found 11·5% in the fifth, 31·2% in the sixth, 36·2% in the seventh, 18·6% in the eighth, and 2·5% in the ninth decades. Lowe (1961) found that intermittent closed-angle glaucoma began most frequently

---

[1] Mann (1954–66), Loschdorfer (1955), Mann and Loschdorfer (1955), Ward (1955), Elliott (1959), Holmes (1961).

[2] Dansey-Browning (1958), Lim (1964), Mann (1966), Loh (1968).

[3] Venable (1952–58), Sarkies (1953), Rodger (1958), Neumann and Zauberman (1965), Avshalom et al. (1966), Alper and Laubach (1968).

[4] Lehrfeld and Reber (1937), Bonavolantà (1949), Armstrong (1952), Weekers et al. (1956), Sugar (1957), and others.

between 55 and 60 years of age, while acute closed-angle glaucoma began between 55 and 65 years.

Seasonal Incidence

There is general agreement in the earlier literature that acute glaucoma occurs more frequently in the winter months than in the summer.[1]   In India the peak occurrence is in June and July when solar radiation is at a minimum (Maynard, 1908).   This peculiarity has been associated with pupillary dilatation owing to diminished light.   There have also been reports of a definite relationship between acute glaucoma and meteorological conditions.[2]

Bilaterality

In the majority of cases primary closed-angle glaucoma eventually becomes bilateral.   Statistics on this subject are misleading since many cases which are unilateral at the time of examination become bilateral at a later date, and in many recent series involvement of the second eye has been prevented by prophylactic treatment.

In a series of 392 cases Lehrfeld and Reber (1937) found that 9 showed early, and 99 advanced unilateral glaucoma, 28 had early, 168 advanced, and 48 absolute bilateral glaucoma; of the whole, 42% were seen first when the condition was unilateral and 58% when it was bilateral.   Posner and Schlossman (1948) found that 31% of their cases were unilateral but considered that even uniocular cases probably represented a bilateral disturbance.   Winter (1955) reported that 32 out of 47 patients with acute glaucoma developed a similar condition in the second eye within 5 years, Adams (1956) found 43% within 6 years, and Rokitskaya (1964) 38% of patients usually within 4 years.   In 200 patients with unilateral acute closed-angle glaucoma Bain (1957) found that of the 7 on whom a prophylactic peripheral iridectomy was performed none developed symptoms in the fellow eye, while of the remaining 193, 53% developed symptoms of acute or intermittent closed-angle glaucoma on an average 4·25 years after their first attack.   In those patients treated prophylactically with miotics 39% developed closed-angle glaucoma, while in the untreated patients 78% developed acute attacks of tension.   Similar results were reported by Lowe (1962) who found that of 200 cases, 23 were bilateral, while of the remainder 64 had a prophylactic peripheral iridectomy performed on the second eye, one of which developed acute glaucoma, and of the 113 who were treated conservatively, 58 developed acute glaucoma.   Lim (1964) had similar results in the 37 out of 50 patients with unilateral glaucoma; 8 had a prophylactic peripheral iridectomy, none of whom developed the disease in the other eye, while of the 29 treated conservatively 17 developed acute glaucoma.

Heredity

Although by no means common, familial primary closed-angle glaucoma is a definite entity.   Most of the literature on this subject is difficult to assess

[1] Steindorff (1902), Bauer (1903), Büttner (1921), Rohner (1927), Pillat (1933), Weinstein (1934), Schorn (1947), Sobhy and Gohar (1952).
[2] Petersen and Milliken (1935), Brückner (1941), Schorn (1947), Fornaro (1948), Sobhy and Gohar (1952), Sautter and Daubert (1955), Brezowsky and Kästner (1958), Luner and Vasková (1964), Suda *et al.* (1964).

critically since it was produced prior to the advent of routine gonioscopy, but in most instances where a probable diagnosis of closed-angle glaucoma can be assumed, transmission occurred through two or more generations, signifying an autosomal dominant inheritance[1] (Fig. 544); in a few, however, an autosomal recessive inheritance has been postulated (Waardenburg, 1949–50; Biró, 1951) (Fig. 545).

The importance of a shallow anterior chamber in the ætiology of primary closed-angle glaucoma is now firmly established, and it has been demonstrated that the depth of the anterior chamber is inherited, probably as an autosomal dominant characteristic (Törnquist, 1953). It has also been demonstrated that shallow anterior chambers and narrow angles are

FIGS. 544 AND 545.—CLOSED-ANGLE GLAUCOMA.

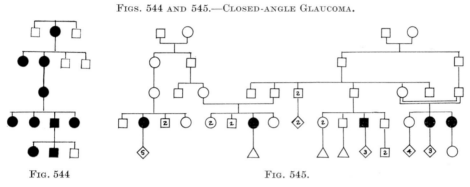

FIG. 544   FIG. 545.

FIG. 544.—Dominant inheritance (after J. Sédan and S. Sédan-Bauby, 1949).
FIG. 545.—Recessive inheritance (after P. J. Waardenburg, 1949).

significantly more frequent in relatives of patients with primary closed-angle glaucoma than in the normal population (Törnquist, 1953–56; Kellerman and Posner, 1955; Paterson, 1961).

The incidence of familial primary closed-angle glaucoma appears, however, to be considerably less common than that of simple glaucoma (Lowe, 1964) and it must therefore be assumed that several factors, not all necessarily influencing the depth of the anterior chamber, are concerned in the ætiology of this disease.

Adams. *Trans. Canad. ophthal. Soc.*, **7**, 227 (1956).

Allmaras. *Klin. Mbl. Augenheilk.*, **94**, 113 (1935).

Alper and Laubach. *Arch. Ophthal.*, **79**, 663 (1968).

Armstrong. *Med. Press*, **228**, 166 (1952).

Avshalom, Berson, Blumenthal *et al.* *Harefuah*, **70**, 250 (1966).

Bain. *Brit. J. Ophthal.*, **41**, 193 (1957).

Bankes, Perkins, Tsolakis and Wright. *Brit. med. J.*, **1**, 791 (1968).

[1] Pagenstecher (1861), von Graefe (1869), Howe (1887), Somya (1893), Rogman (1899), Harlan (1905), Haag (1915), Plocher (1918), Cantonnet (1924), James (1927), Werner (1929), Berg (1932), Allmaras (1935), Wolfsohn-Jaffé (1935), Biró (1939–51), Westerlund (1947), Holm-Pedersen (1948), Waardenburg (1948–50), Posner and Schlossman (1949), Sédan and Sédan-Bauby (1949), Ligorio and Toselli (1950), Probert (1952), Weekers *et al.* (1955–59), François (1958), Lowe (1964), and others.

Barkan. *Amer. J. Ophthal.*, **37**, 724 (1954).

Bauer. *Ueber d. Einfluss von Temperatur u. Jahreszeit a. d. Ausbruch d. akuten primären Glaukomfalles nach d. Material d. Klinik* (Diss.), Tübingen (1903).

Bennett. *Acta ophthal.* (Kbh.), **34**, 92 (1956).

Berg. *Acta ophthal.* (Kbh.), **10**, 568 (1932).

Biró. *Ophthalmologica*, **98**, 43 (1939); **122**, 228 (1951).

Björnsson. *Amer. J. Ophthal.*, **39**, 202 (1955).

Bonavolantà. *G. ital. Oftal.*, **2**, 108 (1949).

Brezowsky and Kästner. *Med. Mschr.*, **12**, 538 (1958).

Brückner. *Schweiz. med. Wschr.*, **71**, 1242 (1941).

Büttner. *Arch. Augenheilk.*, **88**, 204 (1921).

Cantonnet. *Bull. Soc. Ophtal. Paris*, 83 (1924).

Carvill. *Trans. Amer. ophthal. Soc.*, **30**, 71 (1932).

Dansey-Browning. *Brit. J. Ophthal.*, **42**, 394 (1958).

El-Arabi and Hosni. *Orient. Arch. Ophthal.*, **3**, 119 (1965).

Elliott. *Trans. ophthal. Soc. N.Z.*, **12**, 87 (1959).

Fornaro. *Arch. Ottal.*, **52**, 256 (1948).

François. *L'hérédité en ophtalmologie*, Paris (1958).

Gassler. *Klin. Mbl. Augenheilk.*, **146**, 362 (1965).

Gradle. *Amer. J. Ophthal.*, **14**, 140 (1931).

von Graefe. *v. Graefes Arch. Ophthal.*, **15** (3), 228 (1869).

Haag. *Klin. Mbl. Augenheilk.*, **54**, 133 (1915).

Harlan. *Trans. Amer. ophthal. Soc.*, **10**, 520 (1905).

Hollows and Graham. *Brit. J. Ophthal.*, **50**, 570 (1966).

Holmes. *VI Cong. Pan-Amer. Ophthal.*, Caracas, 129 (1960).
Amer. J. Ophthal., **51**, 253 (1961).

Holm-Pedersen. *Nord. Med.*, **39**, 1615 (1948).

Holst. *Amer. J. Ophthal.*, **30**, 1267 (1947).

Howe. *Arch. Ophthal.*, **16**, 72 (1887).

James. *Brit. J. Ophthal.*, **11**, 438 (1927).

Kellerman and Posner. *Amer. J. Ophthal.*, **40**, 681 (1955).

Klouman. *Acta ophthal.* (Kbh.), **39**, 614 (1961).

Kurland and Taub. *Amer. J. Ophthal.*, **43**, 539 (1957).

Lehrfeld and Reber. *Arch. Ophthal.*, **18**, 712 (1937).

Lemoine. *Amer. J. Ophthal.*, **33**, 1353 (1950).

Ligorio and Toselli. *Rass. ital. Ottal.*, **19**, 293 (1950).

Lim. *Singapore med. J.*, **5**, 82 (1964).
Trans. Asia-Pacif. Acad. Ophthal., **2**, 93 (1964).

Loh. *Singapore med. J.*, **9**, 76 (1968).

Loschdorfer. *Techn. inf. Circ.*, No. 13, S. Pacific Comm., Aug. (1955).

Lowe. *Trans. ophthal. Soc. Aust.*, **21**, 65 (1961).
Brit. J. Ophthal., **46**, 641 (1962); **47**, 721 (1963); **48**, 191 (1964).

Luner and Vasková. *Cs. Oftal.*, **20**, 469 (1964).

Mann. *Ophthalmic Survey of the Kimberley Division of Western Australia*, Perth (1954).
Ophthalmic Survey of the Estern Goldfields' Area of Western Australia, Perth (1954).
Culture, Race, Climate and Eye Disease, Springfield, Ill. (1966).

Mann and Loschdorfer. *Ophthalmic Surveys of the Territories of Papua and New Guinea*, Port Moresby (1955).

Maynard. *Brit. med. J.*, **2**, 744 (1908).

Nelander. *Acta ophthal.* (Kbh.), **11**, 370 (1933).

Neumann and Zauberman. *Amer. J. Ophthal.*, **59**, 8 (1965).

Pagenstecher. *Klinische Beobachtungen a. d. Augenheilanstalt in Wiesbaden*, Wiesbaden (1861).

Paterson. *Trans. ophthal. Soc. U.K.*, **81**, 561 (1961).

Petersen and Milliken. *The Patient and the Weather*, Ann Arbor, **4** (3) (1935).

Pillat. *v. Graefes Arch. Ophthal.*, **129**, 299 (1933).

Plocher. *Klin. Mbl. Augenheilk.*, **60**, 592 (1918).

Posner and Schlossman. *Amer. J. Ophthal.*, **31**, 915 (1948).
Arch. Ophthal., **41**, 125 (1949).

Probert. *Canad. med. Ass. J.*, **66**, 563 (1952).

Rodger. *Amer. J. Ophthal.*, **45**, 343 (1958).

Rogman. *Clin. Ophtal.*, **5**, 73 (1899).

Rohner. *Schweiz. med. Wschr.*, **57**, 780 (1927).

Rokitskaya. *Vestn. Oftal.*, **77**, 30 (1964).

Sarkies. *Brit. J. Ophthal.*, **37**, 615 (1953).

Sautter and Daubert. *Ophthalmologica*, **129**, 381 (1955).

Schorn. *v. Graefes Arch. Ophthal.*, **148**, 121 (1947).

Sédan and Sédan-Bauby. *Bull. Soc. Ophtal. Fr.*, 29 (1949).

Smith, Priestley. *Glaucoma*, London (1879).

Smith, R. *Trans. ophthal. Soc. U.K.*, **78**, 245 (1958).

Sobhy and Gohar. *Bull. ophthal. Soc. Égypt*, **42**, 173 (1952).

Somya. *Klin. Mbl. Augenheilk.*, **31**, 390 (1893).

Steindorff. *Dtsch. med. Wschr.*, **28**, 929 (1902).

Suda. *Kumamoto med. J.*, **16**, 145 (1963).

Suda, Abe and Okayama. *Acta Soc. ophthal. jap.*, **68**, 308, 450 (1964).

Sugar. *The Glaucomas*, 2nd ed., N.Y. (1957).

Sveinsson. *Lœknabladid*, **40**, 1 (1956).
Acta ophthal. (Kbh.), **37**, 191 (1959).

Törnquist. *Acta ophthal.* (Kbh.), Suppl. 39 (1953).
Nord. Med., **55**, 427 (1956).

Venable. *J. nat. med. Ass.* (N.Y.), **44**, 7 (1952); **50**, 79 (1958).

Waardenburg. *Ned. T. Geneesk.*, **92**, 2549 (1948); **93**, 1631, 3603 (1949). *Genetica*, **15**, 79 (1950).

Ward. *Ophthalmic Survey of Fiji* (Col. Off. Rep.), London (1955).

Weekers, Gougnard, C. and L., and Watillon. *Arch. Ophtal.*, **16**, 625 (1956).

Weekers, Gougnard-Rion and Gougnard, L. *Bull. Soc. belge Ophtal.*, No. 110, 255 (1955).

Weekers, Prijot, Delmarcelle *et al. Bull. Soc. belge Ophtal.*, No. 121, 1 (1959).

Weinstein. *Klin. Mbl. Augenheilk.*, **93**, 794 (1934).

Werner. *Acta ophthal.* (Kbh.), **7**, 162 (1929).

Westerlund. *Nord. Med.*, **36**, 2537 (1947).

Winter. *Amer. J. Ophthal.*, **40**, 557 (1955).

Wolfsohn-Jaffé. *Klin. Mbl. Augenheilk.*, **94**, 662 (1935).

Ætiology

Following the observations of Raeder (1923) and Rosengren (1930) that patients with acute glaucoma had shallow anterior chambers and those with simple glaucoma had anterior chambers of a normal depth, Barkan (1936–54) demonstrated that the primary forms of the disease could be divided by gonioscopic examination into two varieties, a narrow-angle (iris-block) type and an open-angle type, and that the axial depth of the anterior chamber was often an unreliable guide to the type of glaucoma. He suggested that in the narrow-angle (iris-block) type of primary glaucoma the local cause of the increased intra-ocular pressure was closure of the filtration angle by the root of the iris, while in the open-angle type closure of the angle did not occur and the obstruction which was the cause of the increased ocular tension was situated within the filtration apparatus including its emissaries. These observations have since been confirmed by numerous workers.[1]

The causes of a narrow filtration angle are several, the most important being the presence of a relatively large lens in a small eye. This idea was first suggested by Bowman (1862) although he proposed it for the ætiology of simple glaucoma, and was elaborated by Priestley Smith (1879) in much detail by statistical evidence of the gradual increase in the size of the lens with age and the smallness of the eye in glaucomatous subjects. There is no doubt that the lens increases in size almost throughout life[2] and that the depth of the anterior chamber decreases,[3] partly as a result of the growth of the lens and, to a smaller extent, because of a slight advance of the lens towards the cornea attributable to morphological changes in the ciliary muscle (Weale, 1962) (Fig. 546).

The *refractive condition* is also important since there is little doubt that a hypermetropic refractive error is particularly common in primary closed-angle glaucoma[4] although some authors have been unable to confirm

[1] Gradle and Sugar (1940), McLean (1940), Bangerter and Goldmann (1941), Kronfeld and Grossman (1941), Sugar (1941), Kronfeld and McGarry (1944), Troncoso (1947), François (1948–56), Vail (1948), Ogino (1951), Chandler (1952), Miller (1952), Smith (1954), Provotorova (1956), and many others.

[2] Smith (1883), Raeder (1922), Scammon and Hesdorffer (1937), Johansen (1947), Salmony (1961).

[3] Raeder (1922), Rosengren (1930), Berens (1943), Törnquist (1953).

[4] Gilbert (1912), Fuchs (1924), Hird (1933), Sugar (1941–57), Barkan (1954), Duke-Elder (1957), Chandler and Grant (1965), Becker and Shaffer (1965), Leydhecker (1966), and others.

this (Carvill, 1932; Lehrfeld and Reber, 1937; Posner and Schlossman, 1948). It has also been demonstrated that hypermetropia tends to be associated with a shallower anterior chamber than normal (Rosengren, 1930–50; Sugar, 1942; Sorsby *et al.*, 1957), and that higher degrees of hypermetropia tend to be associated with a reduced axial length of the eye and a flattening of the cornea (Tron, 1934; Stenström, 1946; Phillips, 1956; Sorsby *et al.*, 1957). On the other hand, Fuchs (1924) stated that highly

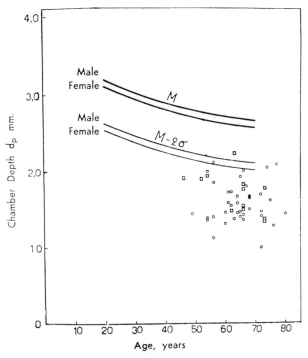

FIG. 546.—THE DEPTH OF THE ANTERIOR CHAMBER.

The upper curves (M) give the mean depth of the anterior chamber in normal individuals of both sexes; the chamber is shallower in females than in males. The lines below running parallel denote M–2σ. The squares (males) and circles (females) give the depth of the chamber in 49 patients aged between 46 and 80 with closed-angle glaucoma (after R. Törnquist).

myopic eyes may be regarded as having almost complete immunity against the disease. It appears, therefore, that several factors, almost certainly genetically determined, contribute to the particular anatomical configuration of an eye which is predisposed to develop primary closed-angle glaucoma.

While most eyes susceptible to primary closed-angle glaucoma have a shallow anterior chamber, a similar rise of tension may occur on mydriasis when the chamber is deep. In these eyes the iris is inserted into the ciliary body further forwards than is usual with the result that the entrance to the angle is narrow. In this rare condition wherein the iris instead of having a forward convexity takes the form of a flat plane, sometimes called *plateau iris* (Lowe, 1964; Chandler and Grant, 1965), when the pupil is dilated the periphery of the iris is bunched up and presses itself against the trabeculæ, closing the angle.

The concept that *primary closed-angle glaucoma occurs only in an eye with a gonioscopically narrow filtration angle* is now firmly established but, since this type of glaucoma is uncommon even in patients with narrow filtration angles, it would seem probable that several predisposing factors may be important in precipitating an attack.

PREDISPOSING FACTORS

PUPILLARY BLOCK

The concept that pupillary blockage is an important factor in the precipitation of attacks of primary closed-angle glaucoma was first proposed by Curran (1920–31), but it was not until Barkan's classification of primary

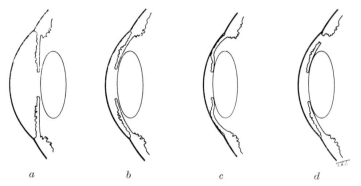

| a | b | c | d |

FIG. 547.—PUPILLARY BLOCKAGE IN CLOSED-ANGLE GLAUCOMA.

a. The configuration of the iris in a normal eye with a deep anterior chamber.
b. The configuration in an eye with a shallow anterior chamber. Note that the sphincter of the iris compresses it against the lens.
c. The configuration of the iris when the pupillary blockage becomes complete; there is an iris bombé with occlusion of the angle of the anterior chamber.
d. The relief of the condition seen in Fig. c by a peripheral iridectomy.

glaucomas into narrow-angle and open-angle types that this mechanism received much support. Barkan (1938–54) suggested that a major ætiological factor in determining the incidence of the disease was a relative pupillary blockage caused by a disproportionately large lens or by an anterior displacement of this structure (Fig. 547). This *relative pupillary blockage* results in an increased resistance to the flow of aqueous from the posterior to the anterior chamber so that an increased pressure builds up in the posterior chamber ballooning the iris forward and producing a peripheral iris bombé; this in turn will cause a narrowing of the filtration angle which, if already narrow, may be closed by irido-corneal contact thus producing an attack of raised tension (Fig. 548). The importance of pupillary blockage as a precipitating factor in primary closed-angle glaucoma has been confirmed by many authors in the past few years,[1] but its exact mechanism is still incompletely understood. It is generally assumed that in an eye with a relatively large lens and a shallow anterior chamber a greater area of the iris comes into contact with the lens than is usual (Chandler, 1952; Barkan, 1954) and that the sphincter muscle exerts a posteriorly directed vector of force pressing it against the lens (Sugar, 1964), while Mapstone (1968) stressed the importance of stretching of the iris by the contraction of the dilatator iridis. Barkan (1954) also suggested that relative pupillary blockage was aggravated by an

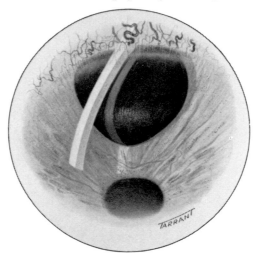

FIG. 548.—BALLOONING OF THE IRIS.

In a case of closed-angle glaucoma. A partial iridectomy was performed, leaving, however, the posterior pigmented layer of the iris untouched. This attenuated layer shows markedly the ballooning due to raised pressure in the posterior chamber. On a subsequent section of the pigmented layer the high tension resolved (S. J. H. Miller).

anterior displacement of the lens caused by a transmission to the vitreous of the increased pressure in the posterior chamber. In support of this theory was the observation that the lens becomes retro-placed following a peripheral iridectomy, an observation, however, refuted by several other observers (Törnquist, 1956; Weekers and Grieten, 1961; Lowe, 1964).

MYDRIASIS

Any factor which brings about a dilatation of the pupil may precipitate a glaucomatous attack in an eye with a narrow filtration angle. Such a rise of ocular tension may follow the use of mydriatics,[2] an observation

[1] Chandler (1952), Haas and Scheie (1952), Chandler and Trotter (1955), Sugar (1964), Chandler and Grant (1965), Becker and Shaffer (1965), Lowe (1966), Pollack (1967), and many others.

[2] p. 699.

which has led to the development of the mydriatic test used to provoke a rise of ocular tension in an eye suspected of being susceptible to the disease. A mydriasis may also be brought about by the exclusion of light from the eye (Grönholm, 1910) and, as we shall see presently, the rise of ocular tension on dark adaptation in an eye predisposed to closed-angle glaucoma forms the basis of another useful clinical method of diagnosis; an acute attack of glaucoma may also follow a cerebral lesion such as an extradural hæmorrhage causing a pupillary dilatation (Koeppen et al., 1967). This rise of ocular tension following mydriasis has been attributed in some cases to crowding of the angle of the anterior chamber with the retracted iris so that the drainage of the intra-ocular fluid is embarrassed.[1] Chandler (1952) and Chandler and Grant (1965), however, considered that the rise of tension occurs particularly when the pupil is dilated to a moderate degree so that the peripheral iris is relaxed and can then be pushed forwards by the increased pressure in the posterior chamber resulting from pupillary blockage. In eyes with a flat type of plateau iris, however, wherein the anterior chamber is of average depth, dilatation of the pupil pushes the periphery of the iris into the angle to close it (Lowe, 1964; Chandler and Grant, 1965).

Lowe (1966) studied the action of different mydriatics on eyes with narrow filtration angles and has demonstrated that parasympatholytic drugs, such as homatropine, tend to cause closure of the angle by bunching the peripheral iris into it, while sympathomimetic drugs, such as adrenaline, increase the tendency to pupillary blockage and thus to closed-angle glaucoma resulting from the increased pressure in the posterior chamber forcing the periphery of the iris into contact with the cornea.

MIOSIS

The stronger miotics, in particular the anticholinesterase drugs, are liable to precipitate attacks of acute closed-angle glaucoma in patients with narrow filtration angles, and there are many reports in the literature of this hazard being caused thereby.[2] The main action of these drugs in producing such a paradoxical rise in the ocular tension is their ability to cause pupillary blockage in susceptible eyes[3] and, in addition, they are liable to aggravate this effect by their vasodilatory action on the iris and ciliary body, and by their action on the ciliary muscle which results in relaxation of the zonule so that the lens tends to move forwards and the pupillary blockage is intensified. It is now generally agreed that these drugs are contra-indicated in patients with narrow filtration angles.

[1] Seidel (1920–27), Serr (1928), Barkan (1938), Lowe (1964–66), Pollack (1967), and others.
[2] DFP—Stone (1950), Butler (1952), Zekman and Snydacker (1953); echothiophate—Becker et al. (1959), Drance (1960); demecarium—Krishna and Leopold (1960), Deutsch and Rowlett (1963); and others.
[3] Becker and Shaffer (1965), Chandler and Grant (1965), Drance (1966), Leopold (1966–68), Shaffer (1967), and others.

ACCOMMODATION

In the normal young subject accommodation tends to decrease the depth of the anterior chamber, although in presbyopic people this effect is minimal. There are a few reports in the literature of an acute rise of ocular tension being precipitated by reading.[1] Higgitt and Smith (1955) suggested that the mechanism for the rise of ocular tension was a rotation of the ciliary body about the scleral spur resulting in closure of the filtration angle. In Törnquist's (1958) case the anterior chamber was of average depth but its angle was very narrow ("plateau iris").

VASOMOTOR INSTABILITY

In the earlier literature on glaucoma, considerable emphasis was placed on its vascular basis, and it was suggested that almost every case was associated with a disturbance of the capillaries, involving stasis. In simple glaucoma the disturbance was considered to be mild, involving either sclerosis or vaso-neurosis, while in acute congestive attacks the same mechanism was believed to occur and in these the functional derangements were especially stressed. We have already discussed the evidence for this in simple glaucoma and have concluded that disturbances of the capillary, neuro-vegetative and endocrine systems play little or no part in its ætiology.[2]

In acute glaucoma it was originally believed that disorganization of capillary function was followed by the spread of vascular disturbances throughout the entire uveal tract through the medium of axon reflexes which precipitated an acute attack by the liberation of histamine-like substances (Friedenwald, 1930; Duke-Elder, 1931). When the importance of a narrow filtration angle in the ætiology of closed-angle glaucoma became recognized, it was then suggested by protagonists of this hypothesis that congestion of the ciliary body induced by vasomotor disturbances resulted in a swelling of this structure and a bellying forwards of the iris together with an increased production of aqueous and consequent secondary closure of the filtration angle.[3] On the other hand, it has been argued that such vascular congestion was the result of an acute attack of raised tension rather than its cause.[4]

The evidence for the presence of vasomotor instability causing a dilatation of the vessels in the ciliary body in patients with closed-angle glaucoma is largely circumstantial. The diurnal variation in closed-angle glaucoma has been said to be abnormal, yet Miller (1953) demonstrated that in intermittent closed-angle glaucoma, during the intervals when the angle was open, the diurnal variation was normal in 20 and only slightly increased

[1] Leydhecker (1953), Miller (1953), Higgitt and Smith (1955), Törnquist (1958).
[2] p. 408.
[3] Friedenwald (1949), Duke-Elder (1949–57), Weinstein and Forgács (1951), Aoki (1952), Morpurgo (1953), François (1955–56), Weinstein (1960–63), and others.
[4] Chandler (1952), Barkan (1954), Maumenee (1959), Chandler and Grant (1965), and others.

in 5 patients; when the angle was closed the variations might become very great. The suggestion for the occurrence of vasomotor instability in this condition has been backed by the numerous reports of an association between closed-angle glaucoma and emotional instability; this question we shall now examine.

Psychic disturbances have frequently been said to determine the onset of an attack of acute closed-angle glaucoma—nerve-shock and strain, anxiety, overwork, sleeplessness or any surgical procedure,[1] while the ordeal of an operation on one eye may precipitate an attack on the other[2] (Fig. 581). The emotional and excitable temperament of glaucomatous subjects has, however, been recognized for over a century; at the beginning of the last century it was remarked on by Demours (1818), and was well known in the middle of the century to such astute observers as von Graefe (1854–55), Donders (1862) and de Wecker (1863); in the recent literature there are numerous references to this association providing a formidable amount of evidence in its favour.[3] This evidence is undoubtedly circumstantial, but in the absence of reports of more adequately controlled series it is difficult to assess the true significance of this association.

The influence of *menstruation* may also be mentioned here, for there are several reports in the literature that acute attacks of glaucoma tend to occur preferentially during the menstrual period.[4] Dalton (1967) found a definite time-relationship between menstruation and the ocular symptoms, 60% of which occurred during the paramenstruum; this observation might be related to the water-retention in the body occurring at this time.

Other Theories

We have already mentioned some of the ætiological hypotheses of historical interest when discussing simple glaucoma[5]; one is worthy of further mention, that of *swelling of the vitreous*. Barkan (1954) suggested that one of the factors producing an increasingly shallow anterior chamber was expansion of the vitreous compartment, possibly due to an increased formation of aqueous, while it has been demonstrated histologically that in acute closed-angle glaucoma the lens appeared to be displaced forwards by pressure from the vitreous, possibly as a result of pooling of aqueous into or behind the gel (Christensen, 1963; Christensen and Irvine, 1966).

In summary, therefore, it may be said that the immediate cause of primary closed-angle glaucoma is an obstruction to the drainage of the aqueous at the angle of the anterior chamber by the peripheral portion of

---

[1] Gartner and Billet (1958), Blancard (1960), M. and L. J. Croll (1960), Wang *et al.* (1961), Radnót (1962), Hugonnier and Charleux (1963), and others.
[2] Sonder (1906), Maiden (1917), Scalinci (1924), Besso (1924), Krasso (1930), and many others.
[3] Hibbeler (1947), Posner and Schlossman (1948), Sykes (1949), Ripley and Wolff (1950), van Alphen and Stokcis (1951), Hartmann (1952), Ourgaud *et al.* (1952), Böhringer *et al.* (1953), Duke-Elder (1957), Grom (1960), Hollwich (1963), Sédan (1964), Vasková and Blaták (1964), and many others.
[4] Marx (1923), Salvati (1923), Lagrange (1925), Costi (1930), Weinstein (1935).
[5] p. 493.

the iris, an occurrence possible only when the angle is narrow. This obstruction is precipitated by pupillary blockage and is sometimes increased by miosis or by a crowding of the angle by iris tissue as in mydriasis due to drugs or darkness. In some cases these mechanisms appear to be aggravated by accommodation or by emotional stresses.

van Alphen and Stokcis. *Ned. T. Geneesk.*, **95**, 2246 (1951).

Aoki. *Acta Soc. ophthal. jap.*, **56**, 890 (1952).

Bangerter and Goldmann. *Ophthalmologica*, **102**, 321 (1941).

Barkan. *Arch. Ophthal.*, **15**, 101 (1936).
Trans. Amer. Acad. Ophthal., **41**, 469 (1936).
Amer. J. Ophthal., **21**, 1099 (1938); **37**, 332, 724 (1954).

Barkan, Boyle and Maisler. *Amer. J. Ophthal.*, **19**, 209 (1936).

Becker, Pyle and Drews. *Amer. J. Ophthal.*, **47**, 635 (1959).

Becker and Shaffer. *Diagnosis and Therapy of the Glaucomas*, 2nd ed., St. Louis (1965).

Berens. *Arch. Ophthal.*, **29**, 171 (1943).

Besso. *Boll. Oculist.*, **3**, 683 (1924).

Blancard. *Ann. Oculist.* (Paris), **193**, 659 (1960).

Böhringer, Meerwein and Müller. *Klin. Mbl. Augenheilk.*, **123**, 283 (1953).

Bowman. *Brit. med. J.*, **2**, 377 (1862).

Butler. *Amer. J. Ophthal.*, **35**, 1031 (1952).

Carvill. *Trans. Amer. ophthal. Soc.*, **30**, 71 (1932).

Chandler. *Arch. Ophthal.*, **47**, 695 (1952).

Chandler and Grant. *Lectures on Glaucoma*, Phila. (1965).

Chandler and Trotter. *Arch. Ophthal.*, **53**, 305 (1955).

Christensen. *Trans. Amer. Acad. Ophthal.*, **67**, 71 (1963).

Christensen and Irvine. *Arch. Ophthal.*, **75**, 490 (1966).

Costi. *Arch. Oftal. hisp.-amer.*, **30**, 521 (1930).

Croll, M. and L. *Amer. J. Ophthal.*, **49**, 297 (1960).

Curran. *Arch. Ophthal.*, **49**, 131 (1920).
Trans. ophthal. Soc. U.K., **51**, 520 (1931).

Dalton. *Brit. J. Ophthal.*, **51**, 692 (1967).

Demours. *Traité des maladies des yeux*, Paris (1818).

Deutsch and Rowlett. *J. Tenn. med. Ass.*, **56**, 5 (1963).

Donders. *v. Graefes Arch. Ophthal.*, **8** (2), 124 (1862).

Drance. *Amer. J. Ophthal.*, **50**, 270 (1960).
Drug Mechanisms in Glaucoma (ed. Paterson *et al.*), London, 301 (1966).

Duke-Elder. *Arch. Ophthal.*, **6**, 1 (1931); **42**, 538 (1949).
Amer. J. Ophthal., **33**, 11 (1950).
Trans. ophthal. Soc. Aust., **17**, 12 (1957).

François. *La gonioscopie*, Louvain (1948).

François. *Glaucoma: a Symposium* (ed. Duke-Elder), Oxon., 169 (1955).
Trans. ophthal. Soc. Aust., **16**, 13 (1956).

Friedenwald. *Arch. Ophthal.*, **3**, 560 (1930).
Trans. Amer. Acad. Ophthal., **53**, 169 (1949).

Fuchs. *Textbook of Ophthalmology* (8th ed., transl. Duane), Phila., 787 (1924).

Gartner and Billet. *Amer. J. Ophthal.*, **45**, 668 (1958).

Gilbert. *v. Graefes Arch. Ophthal.*, **82**, 389 (1912).

Gradle and Sugar. *Amer. J. Ophthal.*, **23**, 1135 (1940).

von Graefe. *v. Graefes Arch. Ophthal.*, **1** (2), 299 (1854); **2** (1), 248 (1855).

Grönholm. *Arch. Augenheilk.*, **66**, 346; **67**, 136 (1910).

Grom. *Acta XVIII int. Cong. Ophthal.*, Brussels, **2**, 1419 (1960).

Haas and Scheie. *Trans. Amer. Acad. Ophthal.*, **56**, 589 (1952).

Hartmann. *Ann. Oculist.* (Paris), **185**, 438 (1952).

Hibbeler. *Amer. J. Ophthal.*, **30**, 181 (1947).

Higgitt and Smith. *Brit. J. Ophthal.*, **39**, 103 (1955).

Hird. *Bgham. med. Rev.*, **8**, 7 (1933).

Hollwich. *Dtsch. med. Wschr.*, **88**, 1141 (1963).

Hugonnier and Charleux. *Bull. Soc. Ophtal. Fr.*, **63**, 262 (1963).

Johansen. *Undersøgelser over det indbyrdes Størrelsesforhold mellem Cornea og Lens crystallina hos Mennesket*, Copenhagen (1947).

Koeppen, Madonick and Barest. *Amer. J. Ophthal.*, **63**, 1696 (1967).

Krasso. *Z. Augenheilk.*, **70**, 355 (1930).

Krishna and Leopold. *Amer. J. Ophthal.*, **49**, 554 (1960).

Kronfeld and Grossman. *Trans. Amer. Acad. Ophthal.*, **45**, 184 (1941).

Kronfeld and McGarry. *Amer. J. Ophthal.*, **27**, 147 (1944).

Lagrange. *Brit. J. Ophthal.*, **9**, 398 (1925).

Lehrfeld and Reber. *Arch. Ophthal.*, **18**, 712 (1937).

Leopold. *Drug Mechanisms in Glaucoma* (ed. Paterson *et al.*), London, 287 (1966).
Amer. J. Ophthal., **65**, 297 (1968).

Leydhecker. *Ber. dtsch. ophthal. Ges.*, **58**, 326 (1953).
Glaucoma in Ophthalmic Practice, London (1966).

Lowe. *Amer. J. Ophthal.*, **57**, 931 (1964); **61**, 642 (1966).

Lowe. *Brit. J. Ophthal.*, **50**, 385 (1966).
McLean. *Trans. Amer. Acad. Ophthal.*, **45**, 176 (1940).
Maiden. *Ophthal. Rec.*, **26**, 174 (1917).
Mapstone. *Brit. J. Ophthal.*, **52**, 19 (1968).
Marx. *Ann. Oculist.* (Paris), **160**, 873 (1923).
Maumenee. *Symposium on Glaucoma* (ed. Clark), St. Louis, 98 (1959).
Miller. *Brit. med. J.*, **1**, 456 (1952).
  Brit. J. Ophthal., **37**, 1 (1953).
Morpurgo. *Ann. Ottal.*, **79**, 377 (1953).
Ogino. *Acta Soc. ophthal. jap.*, **55**, 147 (1951).
Ourgaud, Cain and Bérard. *Bull. Soc. franç. Ophtal.*, **65**, 193 (1952).
Phillips. *Brit. J. Ophthal.*, **40**, 136 (1956).
Pollack. *Symposium on Glaucoma* (Trans. N. Orleans Acad. Ophthal.), St. Louis, 31 (1967).
Posner and Schlossman. *Amer. J. Ophthal.*, **31**, 915 (1948).
Provotorova. *Vestn. Oftal.*, **69** (3), 3 (1956).
Radnót. *Szemészet*, **99**, 1 (1962).
Raeder. *v. Graefes Arch. Ophthal.*, **110**, 73 (1922); **112**, 29 (1923).
Ripley and Wolff. *Psychosom. Med.*, **12**, 215 (1950).
Rosengren. *Acta ophthal.* (Kbh.), **8**, 99 (1930).
  Arch. Ophthal., **44**, 523 (1950).
Salmony (1961). Quoted by Weale, *The Aging Eye*, London, 70 (1963).
Salvati. *Ann. Oculist.* (Paris), **160**, 568 (1923).
Scalinci. *G. Oculist.*, **5**, 33 (1924).
Scammon and Hesdorffer. *Arch. Ophthal.*, **17**, 104 (1937).
Sédan. *Rev. oto-neuro-ophtal.*, **36**, 65 (1964).
Seidel. *v. Graefes Arch. Ophthal.*, **102**, 415 (1920); **119**, 15 (1927).
Serr. *v. Graefes Arch. Ophthal.*, **121**, 3 (1928).
Shaffer. *Symposium on Glaucoma* (Trans. N. Orleans Acad. Ophthal.), St. Louis, 129 (1967).

Smith, Priestley. *Glaucoma*, London (1879).
  Trans. ophthal. Soc. U.K., **3**, 79 (1883).
Smith, R. *Brit. J. Ophthal.*, **38**, 136 (1954).
Sonder. *Arch. Ophthal.*, **26**, 567 (1906).
Sorsby, Benjamin, Davey *et al.* *Emmetropia and its Aberrations* (M.R.C. Spec. Rep. Series, No. 293), London (1957).
Stenström. *Acta ophthal.* (Kbh.), Suppl. 26 (1946).
Stone. *Arch. Ophthal.*, **43**, 36 (1950).
Sugar. *Arch. Ophthal.*, **25**, 674 (1941).
  Amer. J. Ophthal., **24**, 851 (1941); **25**, 1230 (1942); **30**, 451 (1947).
  The Glaucomas, 2nd ed., N.Y. (1957).
Sorsby's *Modern Ophthalmology*, London, **4**, 567 (1964).
Sykes. *Dis. nerv. Syst.*, **10**, 104 (1949).
Törnquist. *Acta ophthal.* (Kbh.), Suppl. 39 (1953); **36**, 419 (1958).
  Brit. J. Ophthal., **40**, 421 (1956).
Tron. *v. Graefes Arch. Ophthal.*, **132**, 182 (1934).
Troncoso. *A Treatise on Gonioscopy*, Phila. (1947).
Vail. *Trans. Amer. Acad. Ophthal.*, **53**, 232 (1948).
Vasková and Blaták. *Cs. Oftal.*, **20**, 466 (1964).
Wang, Tannenbaum and Robertazzi. *J. Amer. med. Ass.*, **177**, 108 (1961).
Weale. *Brit. J. Ophthal.*, **46**, 660 (1962).
de Wecker. *Traité théorique et pratique des maladies des yeux*, Paris, **1** (1863).
Weekers and Grieten. *Bull. Soc. belge Ophtal.*, No. 129, 361 (1961).
Weinstein. *Arch. Ophthal.*, **13**, 181 (1935).
  Amer. J. Ophthal., **49**, 1032 (1960).
  Orient. Arch. Ophthal., **1**, 27 (1963).
Weinstein and Forgács. *Orv. Hetil.*, **92**, 539 (1951).
Zekman and Snydacker. *Amer. J. Ophthal.*, **36**, 1709 (1953).

Pathology

We have already discussed at length the pathological results of increased intra-ocular pressure,[1] changes which occur throughout the tissues of the eye as a consequence of long-standing simple glaucoma, of acute glaucoma and, to a particularly marked degree, of absolute glaucoma. There remain to discuss here the pathological changes in the angle of the anterior chamber that are characteristic of primary closed-angle glaucoma, and the changes within the eye that are peculiar to the early stages of the acute types of the disease.

The importance of occlusion of the filtration angle in the ætiology of glaucoma was first suggested by Knies (1876) and Weber (1877) and in the earlier literature there are numerous reports, particularly in cases of acute

[1] p. 423.

FIGS. 549 TO 551.—THE CONFIGURATION OF THE ANGLE OF THE ANTERIOR CHAMBER

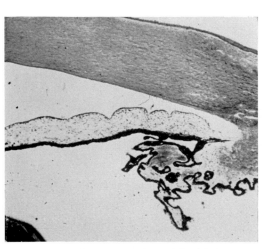

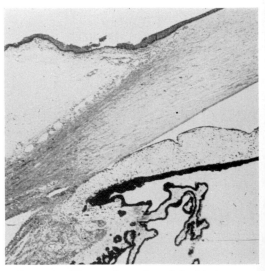

FIG. 549.—The configuration of the iris in an eye with a shallow anterior chamber but an open and functioning drainage angle (M. J. Reeh).

FIG. 550.—The configuration of the iris in an eye with a similarly shallow anterior chamber but with complete closure of the drainage angle by the apposition of the iris to the trabeculæ and the cornea (M. J. Reeh).

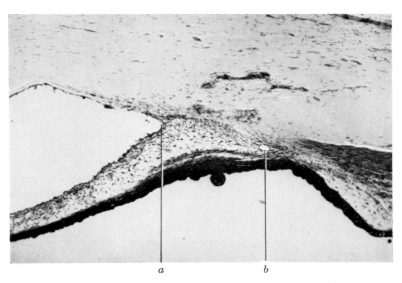

FIG. 551.—The angle is obliterated by peripheral anterior synechiæ. *a* shows the closed new angle thus formed, and *b* the position of the canal of Schlemm indicating the site of the original angle (N. Ashton).

FIGS. 552 AND 553.—THE OPTIC NERVE-HEAD IN ACUTE CLOSED-ANGLE GLAUCOMA
(L. E. Zimmerman).

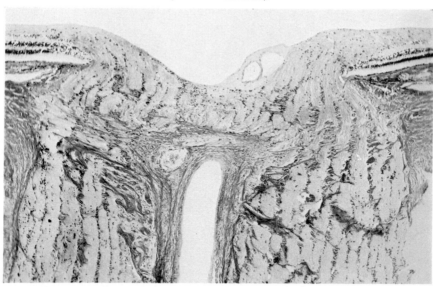

FIG. 552.—The optic disc in an elderly woman with an ocular tension of 80 mm. Hg for 24 hours before she died of a pulmonary embolus. The optic disc is normal without any obvious papillœdema or cupping (× 50).

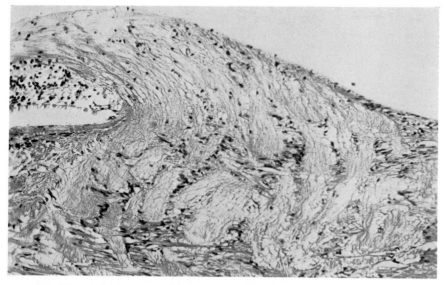

FIG. 553.—The same nerve-head as in Fig. 552, showing acute hydropic degeneration of the nerve fibres within and just anterior to the lamina cribrosa (× 145).

Figs. 554 and 555.—The Optic Nerve-head in Unrelieved Acute Glaucoma
(L. E. Zimmerman).

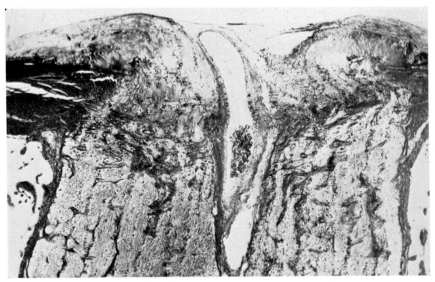

Fig. 554.—In a woman aged 70 who had the eye enucleated after an intra-ocular pressure above 90 mm. Hg for 6 days. There is distinct papilloedema and the swollen nerve fibres have displaced the retina laterally away from the margins of the optic disc obliterating the physiological cup (Masson).

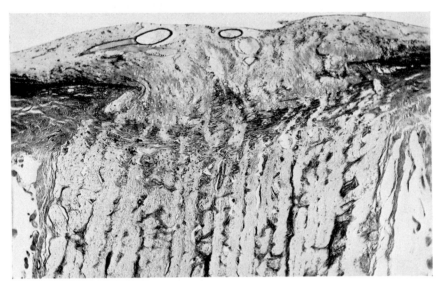

Fig. 555.—A higher magnification of the case seen in Fig. 554, showing axonal degeneration (towards the right) (PAS stain).

FIGS. 556 AND 557.—THE OPTIC NERVE IN ADVANCED CLOSED-ANGLE GLAUCOMA.

The tension was unrelieved by an operation and the eye was enucleated 2 months after the onset of the disease (L. E. Zimmerman).

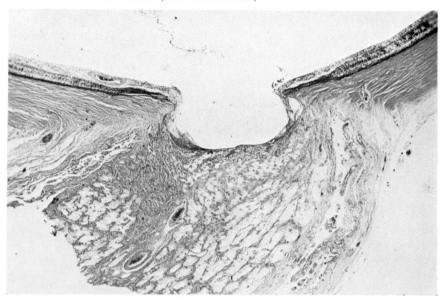

FIG. 556.—There is extensive cupping, almost no tissue remaining on either side of the cup. The peripheral portion of the nerve is completely riddled with cavernous spaces.

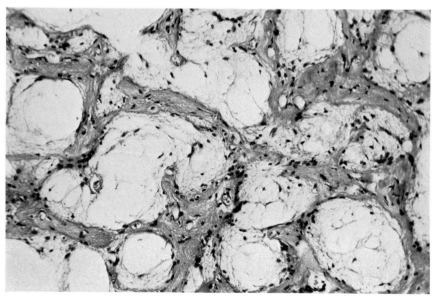

FIG. 557.—Transverse section of the optic nerve showing the cavernous spaces filled with acid mucopolysaccharide.

or absolute glaucoma, of a closed angle resulting from an adherence of the base of the iris to the posterior surface of the cornea. Many of these cases have had raised ocular tension of long standing, the type of which is frequently difficult to ascertain. Of the few eyes that reached histological investigation at an early stage, all showed narrowing or obliteration of the filtration angle (Birnbacher, 1890; Elschnig, 1896; Friedenwald, 1930), a

Figs. 558 and 559.—The Optic Nerve in Severe Unrelieved Acute Glaucoma.

A female patient had a high intra-ocular pressure for 7 days before the eye was enucleated (L. E. Zimmerman).

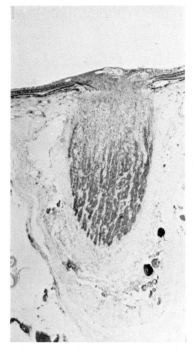

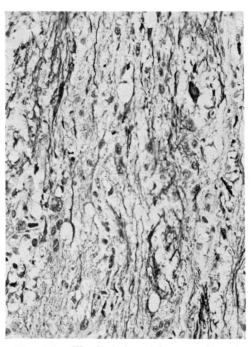

Fig. 558.—Demyelination of the nerve fibres is seen immediately posterior to the lamina cribrosa.

Fig. 559.—The depletion of the nerve fibres in the demyelinated area. Those that remain are irregular, vacuolated, swollen or fragmented.

picture confirmed by more recent observations, the angles in these cases being partially or completely occluded by irido-corneal contact or by peripheral anterior synechiæ[1] (Figs. 549–551); this appearance is in marked contrast to that in simple glaucoma where the angle remains open except in a few instances wherein absolute glaucoma has supervened. In the cases reported by Christensen and Irvine (1966) forward displacement of the lens-iris diaphragm was thought to have resulted from liquefaction of the posterior vitreous followed by gradual pooling of additional fluid (presumably aqueous)

[1] Focosi (1948), Kornzweig (1957), Reeh (1958), Christensen (1963), Christensen and Irvine (1966), Zimmerman (1967).

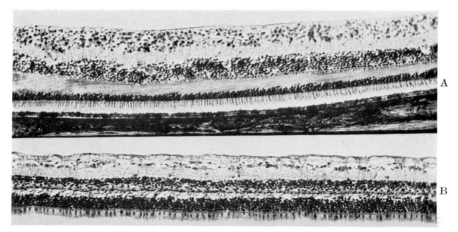

FIG. 560.—THE RETINA IN CLOSED-ANGLE GLAUCOMA.

A, the region of the macula; B, the peripheral retina. The retinal architecture is well preserved and there is only a spotty disappearance of ganglion cells (L. E. Zimmerman).

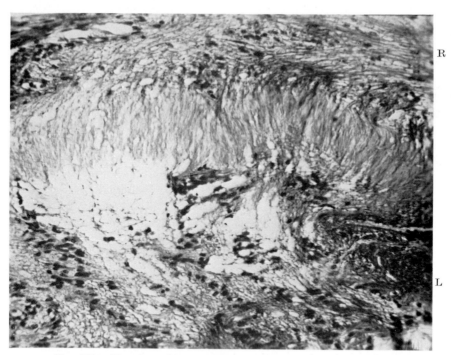

FIG. 561.—THE OPTIC NERVE-HEAD IN CLOSED-ANGLE GLAUCOMA.

From the same case as Fig. 555, showing swelling and hydropic degeneration of the axons of the nerve fibres passing from the retina, R, towards the lamina cribrosa, L (L. E. Zimmerman).

within the area of liquefaction; this caused forward displacement of the formed anterior vitreous which pressed upon the lens-iris diaphragm.

In the earlier cases reported above, all are singularly alike in their pathology; the essential feature in each case was a generalized œdema involving not only the vascularized tissues but also the cornea, the retina, and the optic nerve. The œdema seemed to be due to extreme vasodilatation and congestion, associated usually with a perivascular cellular infiltration and with a sero-fibrinous or hæmorrhagic extravasation. This was general over the uveal tract, but was centred particularly in the ciliary body which had become swollen. A common finding in several of the cases was an obliteration of one or more of the vortex veins by endo- or peri-phlebitis or thrombosis. These changes have not been observed in some of the more recent reports and were probably the result of the unrelieved high ocular tension, comparable to the clinical picture of ischæmia of the anterior segment seen in some cases of acute glaucoma (O'Day et al., 1966; Crock, 1967).

The pathological changes in the optic nerve that occur within the first few days of an attack of primary acute closed-angle glaucoma have been beautifully demonstrated by Zimmerman (1967). Twenty-four hours after the onset (Figs. 552–3) the nerve-head shows neither papillœdema nor cupping, but an acute hydropic degeneration of nerve fibres is present within and just anterior to the lamina cribrosa. Three days after the onset of the acute phase of tension the nerve-head shows a mild papillœdema as well as hydropic degeneration of the nerve fibres, while 6 days after the onset of unrelieved acute glaucoma there is marked papillœdema displacing the retina away from the disc margins, and areas of complete axonal disintegration are apparent within the nerve. After one week of unrelieved acute glaucoma the papillœdema subsides, while the nerve fibres anterior to the lamina cribrosa show hydropic degeneration and those immediately posterior to the lamina have become demyelinated. Two weeks after the onset of secondary acute glaucoma deep cupping of the optic disc is evident while the nerve shows commencing cavernous degeneration, the spaces being filled with an acid mucopolysaccharide, a change more marked after two months of unrelieved acute tension (Figs. 554–9).

In these same cases Zimmerman (1967) also described the early changes within the retina that result from acute glaucoma. After 3 days of un-relieved acute glaucoma there are minimal changes consisting of spotty disappearance of ganglion cells near the macula, the retinal architecture being preserved, while after one week the retina is still relatively unaffected (Figs. 560–1).

These changes in the optic nerve-head have been confirmed in experi-mentally produced acute glaucoma in owl monkeys by injecting α-chymo-trypsin into the posterior chamber followed by such substances as talcum powder and dental moulding or colloidal thorium dioxide (Kalvin et al., 1966; Hamasaki and Fujino, 1967; Zimmerman et al., 1967; Lampert

FIGS. 562 TO 564.—EXPERIMENTAL GLAUCOMA IN THE OWL MONKEY
(N. H. Kalvin *et al.*).

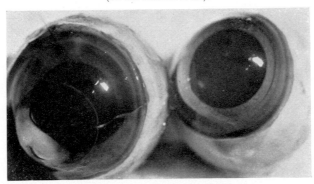

FIG. 562.—The eye to the left which shows buphthalmic changes in comparison
with the control (to the right) was injected intracamerally with alpha-chymotrypsin,
and the lens is dislocated into the anterior chamber.

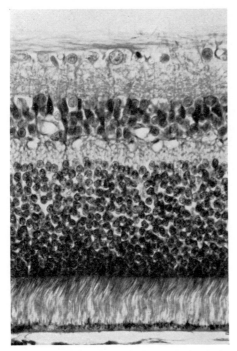

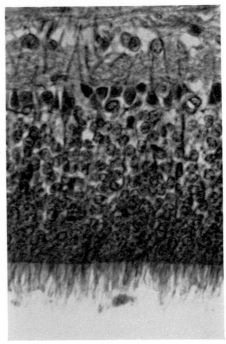

FIG. 563.—Section of the retina of the
control eye seen in Fig. 562.

FIG. 564.—Section of the retina of the
glaucomatous eye seen in Fig. 562. Note the
severe damage to the outer layers of the
retina.

FIGS. 565 AND 566.—THE OPTIC DISC IN EXPERIMENTAL GLAUCOMA
(N. H. Kalvin *et al.*).

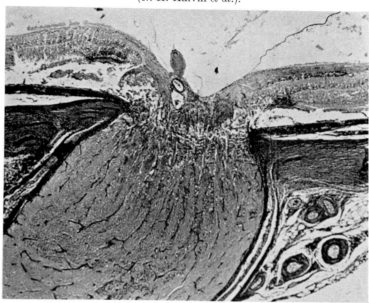

FIG. 565.—The appearance two days after the rise in intra-ocular pressure when the maximum was 76 mm. Hg six hours after the injection.

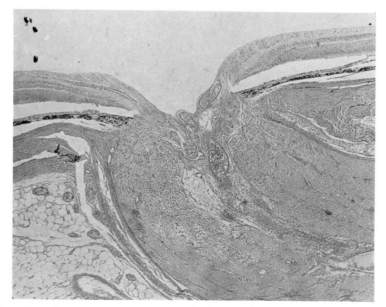

FIG. 566.—Seven days after the rise in intra-ocular pressure, the maximum being 94 mm. Hg.

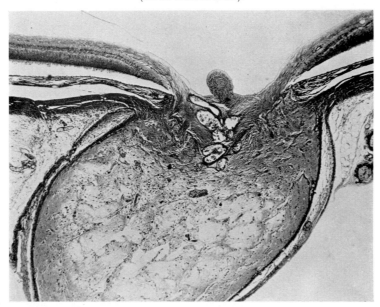

FIG. 567.—After the intracameral injection of alpha-chymotrypsin in the monkey, 14 days after the rise in intra-ocular pressure, the maximum being 72 mm. Hg on the third day. There is marked cavernous atrophy.

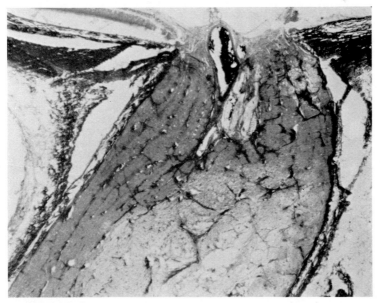

FIG. 568.—Seventeen days after the induction of a moderate glaucoma in the owl monkey following the intracameral injection of talcum powder. There is marked cavernous atrophy in the temporal portion of the nerve and close to the optic disc. The intravascular injection of Indian ink is seen only in the larger arteries and very few of the small vessels. The break in the temporal part of the disc and retina is artificial.

et al., 1968).   Within one week the intra-ocular pressure reached a height
sufficient to enlarge the globe to a considerable extent (Fig. 562).   In these
circumstances Kalvin and his co-workers (1966) found that the outer layers
of the retina were severely damaged (Figs. 563–4); within 2 days the
lamina cribrosa was bowed backwards and in 7 days had become cupped
(Figs. 565–6), while in 14 days necrosis of the nerve fibres and cavernous
degeneration had appeared (Fig. 567).   At the same time, an injection of
Indian ink into the left ventricle demonstrated the poor filling of the capillaries both of the retina and the optic nerve, suggesting that their collapse

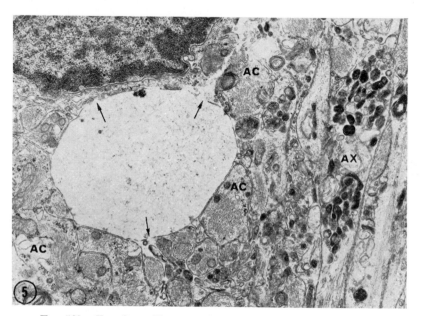

FIG. 569.—THE OPTIC NERVE IN ACUTE EXPERIMENTAL GLAUCOMA.

In the owl monkey, 24 hours after the induction of glaucoma with a maximum
intra-ocular pressure of 71 mm. Hg. The hydropic degeneration of an axon is seen;
the arrows point to areas where the axolemma is ruptured. AC, astrocytic processes
filled with glial filaments; AX, reactive axons filled with mitochondria and dense
bodies (electronmicrograph; × 13,500) (P. W. Lampert *et al.*).

caused the degenerative changes (Fig. 568).   Similarly, Zimmerman and his
colleagues (1967) and Lampert and his associates (1968) showed that in the
initial stages a hydropic degeneration of the nerve fibres occurred which was
followed after some days by cystic transformation of the necrotic tissue
causing its dissolution, thus producing extracellular cavernous spaces
containing hyaluronic acid, while the degenerated axons and debris were
removed by phagocytes some of which were derived from hæmatogenous
macrocytes (Fig. 569).

These pathological changes found in acute glaucoma of recent onset correlate well with the known gonioscopic appearances in this condition,[1] while the permanent visual deterioration which sometimes follows an attack of acute glaucoma can be explained by the changes which have been observed within the optic nerve.

Birnbacher. *Festsc'ir. der k.k. Universität in Graz*, **3** (1890).

Christensen. *Trans. Amer. Acad. Ophthal.*, **67**, 71 (1963).

Christensen and Irvine. *Arch. Ophthal.*, **75**, 490 (1966).

Crock. *Trans. ophthal. Soc. U.K.*, **87**, 513 (1967).

Elschnig. *Arch. Augenheilk.*, **33**, Erg., 187 (1896).

Focosi. *Boll. Oculist.*, **27**, 209 (1948).

Friedenwald. *Arch. Ophthal.*, **3**, 560 (1930).

Hamasaki and Fujino. *Arch. Ophthal.*, **78**, 369 (1967).

Kalvin, Hamasaki and Gass. *Arch. Ophthal.*, **76**, 82, 94 (1966).

Knies. *v. Graefes Arch. Ophthal.*, **22** (3), 163 (1876).

Kornzweig. *Ophthal. ibero amer.*, **19**, 290 (1957).

Lampert, Vogel and Zimmerman. *Invest. Ophthal.*, **7**, 199 (1968).

O'Day, Galbraith, Crock and Cairns. *Lancet*, **2**, 401 (1966).

Reeh. *Amer. J. Ophthal.*, **45**, 444 (1958).

Weber. *v. Graefes Arch. Ophthal.*, **23** (1), 1 (1877).

Zimmerman. *Symposium on Glaucoma* (Trans N. Orleans Acad. Ophthal.), St. Louis, 1 (1967).

Zimmerman, de Venecia and Hamasaki. *Invest. Ophthal.*, **6**, 109 (1967).

Clinical Features

Primary closed-angle glaucoma may develop in a variety of ways: an acute attack may appear without warning and with great suddenness in an eye apparently healthy in every way, although with a shallow anterior chamber; but more usually it is preceded from time to time by mild prodromal intermittent attacks, the significance of which may not have been realized so that their occurrence may only be admitted after careful questioning. The evolution of the disease is subject to considerable variations. The typical sequence involves five phases: (1) an initial phase of intermittent prodromal attacks, which culminate in (2) an acute attack which, if untreated, is followed by (3) a chronic congestive phase which terminates in (4) absolute glaucoma, the eye eventually undergoing (5) degenerative changes. These phases differ only in degree, the second consisting of a more severe replica of the first, and the third a persistence of the same state showing indefinite prolongation although decreased violence, to be followed by degenerative changes due to the long-continued raised tension. The first and second stages may occur alone and resolve, although rarely, and a chronic phase may develop gradually with no acute introduction. Although the disease is almost invariably bilateral, an acute attack in both eyes simultaneously is uncommon.

The PRODROMAL ATTACKS of INTERMITTENT CLOSED-ANGLE GLAUCOMA, which were first described by Demours (1821) with surprising accuracy, may occur intermittently for months or years before the final crisis arrives, and are viewed by some patients with interested amusement and by others with lively terror. They are commonly precipitated by situations resulting in a dilatation of the pupil and therefore usually occur in the evening,

[1] p. 596.

to be relieved by the miosis of sleep at night; a visit to the cinema is a typical precipitating incident with rapid relief if the patient comes out during daylight but not if he comes out in the dark.

They are less frequently induced by mydriatics, whether locally applied to the eye or systemically administered, and may also be precipitated by miotics and by emotional disturbances. The vision becomes temporarily misty, sometimes for a few minutes, sometimes for a few hours, rainbow-rings appear around lights, while complaint is usually made of a localized headache. Examination of the eye may reveal a circumcorneal flush with dilatation of the ciliary vessels although the globe is frequently white, a somewhat steamy cornea, usually a very shallow anterior chamber and a dilated pupil, a raised tension, but usually a normal optic disc. Each attack indicates functional closure of the angle of the anterior chamber and as time goes on the repeated attacks may result in the development of peripheral anterior synechiæ and permanent impairment of the drainage of the aqueous, so that the recurring crises become more frequent, last longer and are more severe. In the great majority of cases the condition passes almost imperceptibly into the phase of chronic closed-angle glaucoma or an acute crisis may develop with dramatic intensity.

An ACUTE ATTACK of CLOSED-ANGLE GLAUCOMA may be one of the more serious occurrences in medicine. It usually, but not invariably, starts suddenly and violently in one eye during the early hours of the morning. The two dominant groups of symptoms are, first, an excruciating pain in the eye together with profuse lacrimation and an intense trigeminal neuralgia radiating over the head and jaws and sometimes beyond, frequently associated with nausea and vomiting, and second, a rapid fall in vision which may involve complete loss of the perception of light within a few hours. The constitutional disturbance may be so great that the patient is prostrated with an irregular, intermittent pulse, pallid face and cold extremities, or is flushed and fevered with a raised temperature. The eye is intensely congested, the conjunctiva perhaps chemotic and the lids œdematous; the globe is extremely tender and the patient shrinks from the slightest touch, but it can be felt to be stony hard. The cornea is dull, steamy and insensitive, the pupil widely dilated and vertically oval in shape, the anterior chamber shallow and clouded, and the lens may have a peculiar greenish appearance. Ophthalmoscopic examination is usually impossible through the œdematous cornea, but if the optic disc can be seen it is œdematous and hyperæmic.

Such an acute attack, if untreated, may evolve in one of three ways. (1) Sometimes after a period varying from some hours to some days, the acute phase may spontaneously resolve, as a result either of the development of necrosis of the iris which relieves the pupillary block, or of the semi-dilated pupil which may have the same effect but, although to casual examination the eye may appear normal, it is permanently damaged. (2) More frequently, resolution may be partial and a condition of CHRONIC

CLOSED-ANGLE GLAUCOMA results. The tension remains above the normal level, usually considerably so, there is a permanent circumcorneal injection with dilatation of the ciliary vessels, the cornea is hypo-æsthetic, the anterior chamber shallow with its angle partially or completely obliterated, the pupil moderately or widely dilated, the iris sluggish and congested, or grey and atrophic and sometimes richly vascularized, while ophthalmoscopic examination reveals a cupped disc with a surrounding halo of atrophy, a tesselated fundus, congested veins and pulsating arteries. Meantime the visual acuity is markedly diminished, the fields constricted and the blind-spot enlarged. In this way the eye gradually deteriorates in structure and function, its downward course being hastened by periodic acute crises until it passes on to complete blindness and absolute glaucoma. (3) More rarely resolution may not occur but the attack ends in a permanently hard eye and involves swift and complete blindness—GLAUCOMA FULMINANS. Such an outcome is rare, however, in a first attack, which usually undergoes partial resolution.

CHRONIC CLOSED-ANGLE GLAUCOMA, which as we have just seen, may develop following an acute attack, results from partial obliteration of the angle of the anterior chamber by peripheral anterior synechiæ. A similar pathological process but without an antecedent history of acute glaucoma may develop more gradually in patients with narrow filtration angles, and may occur even in the absence of intermittent closed-angle attacks. In these latter cases, the signs of ocular congestion are absent and the condition may develop insidiously, the raised ocular tension eventually resulting in cupping of the optic disc and defects in the visual field. Such a presentation may be distinguished from that of simple glaucoma only by the presence of gonioscopically visible peripheral anterior synechiæ, the extent of which determines in large measure the base-pressure of the eye.

The final stages of unrelieved closed-angle glaucoma, ABSOLUTE GLAUCOMA and the occurrence of DEGENERATIVE CHANGES, are similar to those of simple glaucoma and have already been described in detail.[1]

EXTERNAL EXAMINATION

The CONJUNCTIVA may appear normal in the insidiously developing type of chronic closed-angle glaucoma, although if the ocular tension is above 60 mm. Hg the anterior ciliary arteries are nearly always dilated, while if it is below 40 mm. they usually appear normal (Dobree, 1954). Mild intermittent closed-angle attacks, while increasing the ocular congestion, usually involve the development of a ciliary flush; while in the more acute phases the general congestion and redness may be intense and confluent and provoke a massive chemotic œdema (Figs. 570–1). In absolute glaucoma the dilated anterior ciliary veins stand out prominently as a tortuous irregular circle of anastomoses, producing the appearance aptly known as the *caput medusæ* (Heerfordt, 1911).[2]

[1] p. 423.   [2] p. 442.

In the CORNEA, haziness and anæsthesia are characteristic signs of acute and intermittent closed-angle glaucoma. In addition to epithelial œdema which we have already described as an occasional occurrence in simple glaucoma,[1] the cornea may show stromal œdema and the endothelium may

FIGS. 570 AND 571.—CLOSED-ANGLE GLAUCOMA
(Inst. Ophthal.).

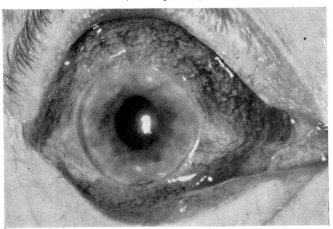

FIG. 570.—In the subacute stage.

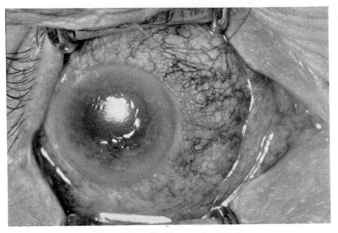

FIG. 571.—In the acute stage.

be spattered with small white dots, often partially pigmented, looking as though it has been sand-blasted (Jones, 1959). Following an acute attack when the ocular tension has become reduced either spontaneously or as a result of treatment, a gross striate keratopathy may supervene.

In the IRIS vascular dilatation and œdema occur in an acute attack of

[1] p. 423.

FIGS. 572 TO 574.—GLAUCOMATOUS ATROPHY OF THE IRIS
(J. Winstanley).

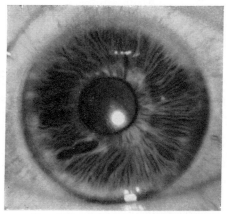

FIG. 572.—In the early stages.

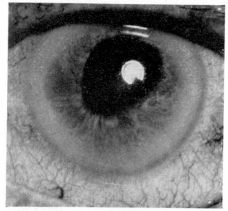

FIG. 573.—In the late stages with the typical eccentric pupillary dilatation.

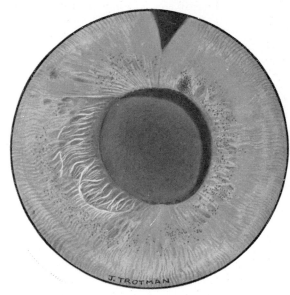

FIG. 574.—In a lightly pigmented eye. The anterior layer is very depigmented. In a patient aged 65 whose attack of closed-angle glaucoma lasted 18 hours before being brought under control.

closed-angle glaucoma, while some degree of atrophic change is evident provided the ocular tension has remained high for 12 hours or more (Riddell, 1946; Winstanley, 1961). The vascular changes, which were originally believed to be the main ætiological factor in the development of an acute attack and are now thought to result from the high ocular tension,[1] present

[1] Chandler (1952), Barkan (1954), Posner (1961), Winstanley (1961), Chandler and Grant (1965), and others.

as visibly dilated vessels and œdema of the stroma of the iris, which results in this structure losing its delicate architecture. The inflammatory response consequent upon these vascular changes and the necrosis of the tissue of the iris result in an outpouring of exudate and cells from the grossly dilated vessels into the aqueous, producing a clinical picture resembling an anterior uveitis (the *iritis glaucomatosa* of Jones, 1959). The atrophic changes, which have been discussed in a previous Volume,[1] are due to thinning and necrosis of the sphincter muscle followed by a tangential displacement of the radial stromal fibres in the segment in which the sphincter has been damaged so that there is a disturbance of the regular arrangement of the stromal

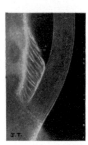

FIG. 575.—GLAUCOMATOUS IRIDOSCHISIS.

To show the formation of peripheral anterior synechiæ (J. Winstanley).

architecture and a bunching together of the tissues in the segment opposite the atrophy (Figs. 572–4). In cases in which the ocular hypertension has been prolonged this atrophic area may extend over more than half the iris. Less frequently, a type of iridoschisis develops wherein the anterior leaf of the iris becomes separated, sometimes in the middle of this tissue and sometimes at its root so that peripheral anterior synechiæ may form, thus blocking the filtration angle (Fig. 575). In addition, gross pigmentary disturbances may occur even at an early stage leading to the formation of lacunæ in the posterior epithelial layers which become visible on transillumination, and a powdering of pigment on the posterior surface of the cornea and in the trabeculæ (the *melano-hypostasis* of Vogt, 1942). In occasional cases this atrophy may involve all the layers of the iris, resulting in a spontaneous cure of an acute attack of closed-angle glaucoma by producing a communication between the posterior and anterior chambers and thus relieving the pupillary block.[2]

In the type of chronic closed-angle glaucoma that follows an unrelieved acute attack, the degree of atrophy of the entire uveal tract may be extreme, being similar to that described for absolute glaucoma wherein the iris loses its delicate architecture, develops patches of advanced atrophy and shows an extreme ectropion of its pigmented layer.[3]

The PUPIL has a typical appearance in acute closed-angle glaucoma, being dilated with a vertically oval shape, the dilatation tending to persist unless the tension falls spontaneously or after medical measures at an early stage (Figs. 576–7). This characteristically oval shape of the pupil is said to result from the increased shallowness of the angle of the anterior chamber superiorly (Phillips, 1956). Once segmental atrophy of the iris has developed

[1] Vol. IX, p. 681.
[2] Posner (1961), Winstanley (1961), Frayer and Scheie (1963), Tavolara (1965), and others.
[3] p. 426.

the pupil becomes distorted with a wide dilatation in the atrophic zone towards which it is displaced, while the inflammatory response which results from the vascular changes and necrosis within the iris may lead to the formation of posterior synechiæ and further distortion. After an acute attack such a pupil may remain fixed even after the instillation of miotics (Phillips, 1956) (Fig. 576).

The ANTERIOR CHAMBER in acute closed-angle glaucoma is usually very shallow, an observation known to von Graefe (1857) and Priestley Smith (1887) and confirmed by Raeder (1923) and Rosengren (1930). Measurements of the depth of the anterior chamber have produced varying results depending upon the method of estimation used. In acute glaucoma,

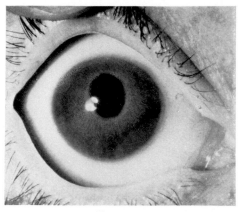
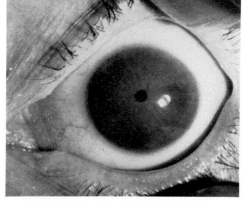

FIG. 576.   FIG. 577.

FIGS. 576 AND 577.—THE INFLUENCE OF MIOTICS AFTER AN ACUTE ATTACK OF CLOSED-ANGLE GLAUCOMA.

The pupil of the affected right eye (Fig. 576) shows little contraction, but the shortness of the iris at 12 o'clock has eliminated the pupillary blockage thus resolving the acute attack. The unaffected left eye (Fig. 577) shows marked miosis (C. I. Phillips).

for example, Barkan (1954) found that the depth was 1·5 mm. or less in 74% of cases, the normal figure by his method being 2·0 mm.; Törnquist's (1956) measurements were 1·70 mm. in males and 1·63 mm. in females with acute glaucoma, figures that were two-thirds of those found in a normal population; while Aizawa (1960) observed an average depth of 2·13 mm. in acute glaucoma, 2·44 mm. in chronic congestive glaucoma, and 3·04 mm. in simple glaucoma, the last being similar to that of the normal population. Rosengren (1953) calculated that with a depth of the anterior chamber of over 2·53 mm. the chances of developing acute glaucoma were 1 in 32,573, while below 2·53 mm. the chances were 1 in 152; Törnquist's figures are similar: with a depth from 2·50 to 2·00 mm. the chances were 1 in 180, from 2·00 to 1·50 mm. they were 1 in 10, while with a depth of anterior chamber of under 1·50 mm. the chances of developing acute glaucoma were

52 to 1. Although the above figures refer to acute closed-angle glaucoma, the anterior chamber is also more shallow than normal in intermittent and chronic closed-angle glaucoma. It is well-recognized, however, that a small but appreciable percentage of cases of gonioscopically-proven primary closed-angle glaucoma has a normal axial depth of the anterior chamber (Barkan, 1954), many of these cases being examples of " plateau iris " (Shaffer, 1956; Chandler, 1956; Törnquist, 1958; Lowe, 1964; Becker and Shaffer, 1965; Gorin and Posner, 1967).

It is an interesting observation that the upper segment of the angle of

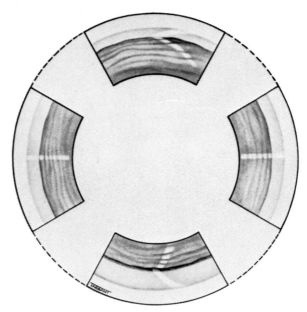

FIG. 578.—GONIOSCOPIC APPEARANCES IN PRE-GLAUCOMA.
Diagrammatic representation to show the angle of the anterior chamber closed above, open below, and extremely narrow if not closed nasally and temporally (C. I. Phillips).

the anterior chamber is usually the narrowest and that there goniosynechiæ usually tend to occur first (Fig. 578) (Barkan, 1936–38; François, 1955; Phillips, 1956; Törnquist, 1959). The reason for this is somewhat speculative but probably depends on the flattening of the cornea in this segment with age whereby the tendency to direct astigmatism " with the rule " is diminished or is converted into inverse astigmatism[1] (Hirsch, 1959); indeed, McLenachan and Loran (1967) found a significant correlation between the presence of inverse astigmatism and the occurrence of closed-angle glaucoma.

We have already made mention on several occasions of Barkan's

[1] Vol. V.

(1936–54) observation that in closed-angle glaucoma the immediate cause of the raised ocular tension is closure of the filtration angle by the root of the iris. The gonioscopic appearance of the angle of the anterior chamber in this condition is usually diagnostic and, although the different stages of the disease often show different appearances, they are all characterized by a very narrow filtration angle. In acute closed-angle glaucoma the angle is frequently difficult to examine because of the presence of corneal œdema, but if this can be cleared by the instillation of hypertonic glycerol, by reducing the tension by medical means, or by removing the œdematous epithelium, the angle will appear to be completely closed by contact between the peripheral iris and cornea, and iris bombé will be present; in many cases this contact will be visible even without a gonioscope. Although iris

FIGS. 579 AND 580.—THE ANGLE OF THE ANTERIOR CHAMBER IN CLOSED-ANGLE GLAUCOMA.

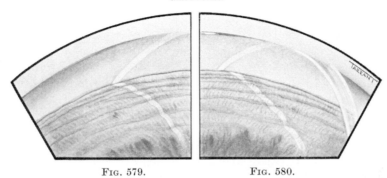

FIG. 579.   FIG. 580.

FIG. 579.—There is no displacement of the slit-beam if the angle is completely closed.

FIG. 580.—The parallactic displacement in the slit-beam when the angle is very narrow but open.

bombé due to relative pupillary block is a characteristic of most cases of primary closed-angle glaucoma, it is not present in the condition of " plateau iris ", wherein the iris is quite flat and runs directly towards the line of Schwalbe.[1]

In intermittent closed-angle glaucoma the angle will be closed, although not necessarily completely, when the ocular tension is raised, but will reopen but remain narrow when the tension returns to normal (Figs. 579–80).[2] In mild intermittent closed-angle attacks it may be difficult to be certain that the angle becomes closed because the miosis produced by the light results in its opening. If the widest part of the angle is examined and the light turned off for a few seconds and then switched on again, a change is frequently seen which in its most marked form looks like the rapid opening

[1] p. 571.

[2] Chandler (1952), Smith (1954), Chandler and Trotter (1955), Gorin (1957), Becker and Shaffer (1965), and many others.

of a previously closed angle (the " on-off " sign of Smith, 1954). In chronic
closed-angle glaucoma, the angle will be closed over a varying extent, most
frequently by broad peripheral anterior synechiæ where the peripheral iris
is in contact with the line of Schwalbe (Fig. 551). These usually extend
over more than half the circumference of the angle before the ocular tension
becomes raised. Another appearance in chronic closed-angle glaucoma is a
fusion of the root of the iris at first with the posterior part of the trabecular
meshwork, the synechia then slowly extending forwards towards the line of
Schwalbe. This condition of " shortening of the angle " produces a clinical
picture which can be distinguished from that of simple glaucoma only by
gonioscopy.[1]

It is important to emphasize that in all cases of primary closed-angle
glaucoma when the ocular tension is raised the angle of the anterior chamber
will be partially or completely occluded by contact between the iris and the
cornea, and that a firm diagnosis can be made only on gonioscopic
examination.

In the LENS in acute primary closed-angle glaucoma a characteristic
change occurs in the subcapsular region, first described by Vogt (1930–31)
as *cataracta disseminata subcapsularis glaucomatosa acuta* (*Glaukomflecken*)
and subsequently amply confirmed; the appearance and significance of
these subcapsular flecks have already been described.[2]

OPHTHALMOSCOPIC EXAMINATION

In acute closed-angle glaucoma examination of the fundus is usually
impossible owing to haziness of the media, but if it can be made out the
disc is usually seen to be œdematous and hyperæmic, and spontaneous
pulsation of the retinal arteries may be apparent. It is unusual to find
cupping of the optic disc, even after several attacks of acute or intermittent
closed-angle glaucoma, although this will eventually occur in the insidiously developing type of chronic closed-angle glaucoma, wherein the appearance becomes similar to that in simple glaucoma.[3]

THE OCULAR TENSION

In closed-angle glaucoma the ocular tension varies within the widest
limits depending on the phase of the disease so that any single reading may
be quite illusory. In the earlier stages when the angle is open the tension
and its diurnal variations are normal; when the angle is closed the tension
may be raised to almost any height up to that of the diastolic arterial
pressure to fall again as rapidly when it opens (Miller, 1953) (Figs. 581, 584).
As the disease progresses and attacks of raised tension tend to occur daily,
the ocular tension usually rises every evening to fall again during sleep at
night (Fig. 586); dozing or sleeping in the evening may produce the same

---

[1] Gorin (1960–61), Byron (1961), Lowe (1964), Gorin and Posner (1967).
[2] p. 40.   [3] p. 449.

FIGS. 581 TO 584.—THE TENSION IN CLOSED-ANGLE GLAUCOMA
(S. J. H. Miller).

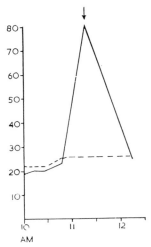

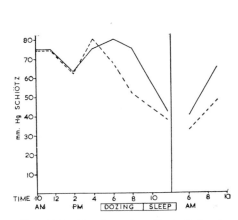

FIG. 581.—The spontaneous rise in tension in an untreated patient who was apprehensive at the time of examination. At the arrow miotics were instilled.

FIG. 582.—To show the effect of sleeping in an untreated case.

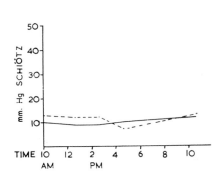

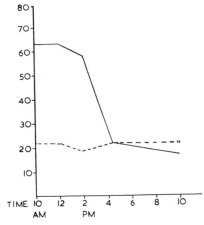

FIG. 583.—A normal diurnal variation in a quiet phase.

FIG. 584.—In the same patient as Fig. 583; the tension during an attack of closed-angle glaucoma; the fall was spontaneous.

hypotensive reaction (Fig. 582), but in still more established cases these ameliorating circumstances have less effect (Fig. 585).

THE FACILITY OF AQUEOUS OUTFLOW

As the rise of ocular tension in closed-angle glaucoma is due primarily to closure of the filtration angle either by irido-corneal contact or by the development of peripheral anterior synechiæ, it is not surprising that the

FIGS. 585 TO 587.—THE DIURNAL VARIATION IN CLOSED-ANGLE GLAUCOMA
(S. J. H. Miller).

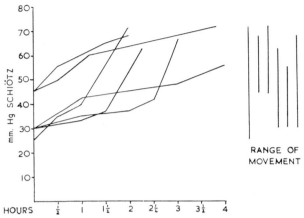

FIG. 585.—The rise in tension in 6 patients from whom miotics were withheld for
24 hours.

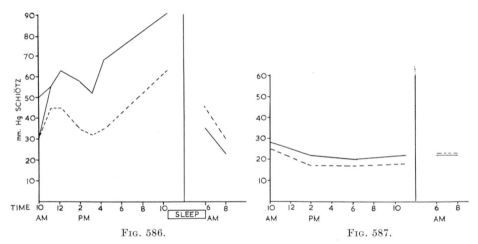

FIG. 586.

FIG. 587.

FIG. 586.—The variation in an untreated patient who saw haloes each night.

FIG. 587.—The effect of miotics on the same patient as Fig. 586.

raised tension is invariably associated with a reduced facility of aqueous
outflow. This association has been clearly established in the various stages
of the disease. In the acute attack, Grant (1951–55) demonstrated by
tonography that the facility of outflow[1] in the affected eye was greatly
diminished, being between 0·01 and 0·06, while in the fellow eye it was
normal, and this observation has been confirmed for both acute and intermittent closed-angle glaucoma.[2] These observations, while interesting, are

[1] p. 461.
[2] deRoetth and Knighton (1952), Weekers and Prijot (1952), Becker and Friedenwald
(1953), Chandler and Trotter (1955), Scheie *et al.* (1955), and many others.

of little clinical value as they do not contribute to the diagnosis or prognosis. Between acute or intermittent attacks, however, tonography may be useful in selected cases in order to assess the functional reserve of the filtration angle, although the results usually do no more than confirm the degree of obstruction to outflow that may be observed gonioscopically.[1] Similarly, in chronic closed-angle glaucoma, wherein the ocular tension is persistently raised owing to partial or complete closure of the filtration angle, the facility of aqueous outflow will be reduced.

VISUAL SYMPTOMS

The visual acuity in intermittent and acute closed-angle glaucoma is always affected, to a greater or less extent in the former, and usually severely in the latter form of the disease. In the intermittent form, definite attacks of indistinctness of vision appear during the periods of hypertension, the patient experiencing a feeling as of looking through a haze or mist. The phenomenon is due to corneal œdema, and the same anatomical change may produce the entoptic appearance of coloured haloes round lights owing to diffraction by droplets of fluid in the corneal epithelium. These attacks tend to come on in the evening when the dim lighting conditions result in dilatation of the pupil which, in a susceptible individual, is probably the main predisposing factor to an attack of closed-angle glaucoma. As a rule, in the early stages of the disease they are fleeting and the vision rapidly regains its normal standard; at a later stage they may easily be dissipated by a miotic; but in more prolonged periods of high tension they may be lasting and distressing. In attacks of acute closed-angle glaucoma the vision fades out suddenly and completely; if the tension is rapidly reduced vision may return almost as rapidly as it went and within 48 hours may be almost normal; but if the tension remains high for a sufficient time to allow degenerative changes to take place, some vision is permanently lost.

A *glaucomatous halo* is best seen when looking at a bright light from a distance in the dark: two coloured rings are always seen, an inner blue-violet and an outer yellow-red, the red tinge being on the outside, while a green ring may separate these. At times they are so faint that they have to be specially elicited, and at other times their prominence causes much worry and confusion to the patient. Their physical causation, the methods of testing for them, and their differentiation from haloes due to physiological and other pathological conditions have already been fully discussed.[2] It may be useful to demonstrate their appearance to the patient and, as von Fraunhofer (1823) first showed, this can be done by asking him to look at a light through a film of lycopodium powder pressed between two glass plates, a device which may be retained with the test-lenses ordinarily used

---

[1] Adams and Bourne (1953), Chandler and Trotter (1955), Espíldora-Couso and Eggers (1961).

[2] Vol. VII, p. 450.

(Foster, 1937). In diagnosis it will be remembered that the pathological haloes are distinguished from the physiological (due to the lens) by the fact that they are not partially eclipsed and broken up but only suffer a diminution of intensity if a straight edge (Druault, 1898–1923) or a stenopæic slit (Emsley and Fincham, 1923) is passed across the pupil. Haloes due to corneal œdema can further be differentiated from other pathological haloes by measuring their diameter[1]; the former have an angular diameter varying with the size of the œdematous droplets from 7° to 12°—that is, the linear diameter of the outer red ring measured on a wall, when the light is 10 ft. from the patient, is 15 to 25 in. While haloes due to conjunctival mucus or lacrimal secretion are larger (14°), those due to lenticular diffraction are smaller (6° to 7°) and those due to the corneal endothelium are smaller still (4°). It is to be noted, however, that a halo of the glaucomatous type is not pathognomonic of glaucoma, for it occurs in any condition of corneal œdema whether the pressure is raised or not (Duke-Elder, 1927).

THE VISUAL FIELDS

In acute closed-angle glaucoma the condition of the vision is such that a study of the visual fields is impossible, apart from rough tests to hand movements or light perception when the peripheral field is found to be greatly depressed, this frequently being most marked in the upper nasal quadrant, and central vision is lost at an early stage. After one short attack of acute glaucoma the visual field may be unaffected, but after repeated attacks of high tension there are usually a general depression of all isopters, the peripheral being more affected than the central, a particular depression of the upper nasal isopters, an enlargement of the blind-spot and a widening of angioscotomata (Harrington, 1956). In chronic closed-angle glaucoma, particularly when it develops insidiously, the fields may eventually be typically glaucomatous.[2]

ELECTROPHYSIOLOGICAL TESTS

As is the case in simple glaucoma,[3] the electroretinogram and electro-oculogram are little affected in closed-angle glaucoma, except in the absolute stage of the disease when the base-value of the electro-oculogram may be reduced. Similarly, the changes in the electro-encephalogram which have been described in the literature are found in many normal subjects, and little significance can be attached to their occurrence.

Adams and Bourne. *Trans. Canad. ophthal. Soc.*, **6**, 17 (1953).

Aizawa. *Acta Soc. ophthal. jap.*, **64**, 869 (1960).

Barkan. *Arch. Ophthal.*, **15**, 101 (1936). *Amer. J. Ophthal.*, **19**, 951 (1936); **21**, 1099 (1938); **37**, 724 (1954).

Becker and Friedenwald. *Arch. Ophthal.*, **50**, 557 (1953).

Becker and Shaffer. *Diagnosis and Therapy of the Glaucomas*, St. Louis (1965).

Byron. *Amer. J. Ophthal.*, **52**, 492 (1961).

Chandler. *Arch. Ophthal.*, **47**, 695 (1952). *Glaucoma* (Trans. 1st Macy Conf., ed. Newell), N.Y. (1956).

Chandler and Grant. *Lectures on Glaucoma*, Phila. (1965).

[1] Sheard (1919), Koeppe (1920), Elliot (1921–23), Druault (1923), Priestley Smith (1924).
[2] p. 469.   [3] p. 482.

Chandler and Trotter. *Arch. Ophthal.*, **53**, 305 (1955).

Demours. *Précis théorique et pratique sur les maladies des yeux*, Paris (1821).

Dobree. *Brit. J. Ophthal.*, **38**, 500 (1954).

Druault. *Arch. Ophtal.*, **18**, 312 (1898); **40**, 458, 536 (1923).

Duke-Elder. *Brit. J. Ophthal.*, **11**, 342 (1927).

Elliot. *Brit. J. Ophthal.*, **5**, 500 (1921).
 A Treatise on Glaucoma, London (1918; 1922).
 Amer. J. Ophthal., **6**, 1 (1923).

Emsley and Fincham. *Amer. J. physiol. Opt.*, **4**, 247 (1923).

Espíldora-Couso and Eggers. *Arch. chil. Oftal.*, **18**, 85 (1961).

Foster. *Trans. ophthal. Soc. U.K.*, **57**, 364 (1937).

François. *Glaucoma: a Symposium* (ed. Duke-Elder), Oxon., 169 (1955).

Fraunhofer. *Denkschr. kön. bayer. Akad.*, Munich, Bd. 8 (1823).

Frayer and Scheie. *Amer. J. Ophthal.*, **55**, 335 (1963).

Gorin. *Mod. Probl. Ophthal.*, **1**, 125 (1957).
 Amer. J. Ophthal., **49**, 141 (1960).
 Eye, Ear, Nose, Thr. Monthly, **40**, 469 (1961).

Gorin and Posner. *Slit-lamp Gonioscopy*, 3rd ed., Baltimore (1967).

von Graefe. *v. Graefes Arch. Ophthal.*, **3** (2), 456 (1857).

Grant. *Trans. Amer. Acad. Ophthal.*, **55**, 774 (1951).
 Glaucoma: a Symposium (ed. Duke-Elder), Oxon., 126 (1955).

Harrington. *The Visual Fields*, St. Louis (1956).

Heerfordt. *v. Graefes Arch. Ophthal.*, **78**, 413 (1911).

Hirsch. *Amer. J. Optom.*, **6**, 395 (1959).

Jones, B. R. *Trans. ophthal. Soc. U.K.*, **79**, 753 (1959).

Koeppe. *Klin. Mbl. Augenheilk.*, **65**, 556 (1920).

Lowe. *Amer. J. Ophthal.*, **57**, 931 (1964).
 Brit. J. Ophthal., **48**, 191 (1964).

McLenachan and Loran. *Brit. J. Ophthal.*, **51**, 441 (1967).

Miller. *Brit. J. Ophthal.*, **37**, 1 (1953).

Phillips. *Brit. J. Ophthal.*, **40**, 136 (1956).

Posner. *Eye, Ear, Nose, Thr. Monthly*, **40**, 352 (1961).

Raeder. *v. Graefes Arch. Ophthal.*, **112**, 29 (1923).

Riddell. *Brit. J. Ophthal.*, **30**, 74 (1946).

deRoetth and Knighton. *Arch. Ophthal.*, **48**, 148 (1952).

Rosengren. *Acta ophthal.* (Kbh.), **8**, 99 (1930).
 Amer. J. Ophthal., **36**, 488 (1953).

Scheie, Spencer and Helmick. *Trans. Amer. ophthal. Soc.*, **53**, 265 (1955).

Shaffer. *Glaucoma* (Trans. 1st Macy Conf., ed. Newell), N.Y. (1956).

Sheard. *Amer. J. Ophthal.*, **2**, 185 (1919).

Smith, Priestley. *Ophthal. Rev.*, **6**, 191 (1887).
 Brit. J. Ophthal., **8**, 145 (1924).

Smith, R. *Brit. J. Ophthal.*, **38**, 136 (1954).

Tavolara. *Ann. Ottal.*, **91**, 770 (1965).

Törnquist. *Brit. J. Ophthal.*, **40**, 421 (1956); **43**, 169 (1959).
 Acta ophthal. (Kbh.), **36**, 419 (1958).

Vogt. *Klin. Mbl. Augenheilk.*, **85**, 586 (1930).
 Lhb. u. Atlas d. Spaltlampenmikroskopie d. lebenden Auges, 2nd ed., Berlin, **2**, 565 (1931); **3**, 893 (1942).

Weekers and Prijot. *Brit. J. Ophthal.*, **36**, 511 (1952).

Winstanley. *Trans. ophthal. Soc. U.K.*, **81**, 23 (1961).

Diagnosis

The only disease which can give rise to difficulty in the diagnosis of acute closed-angle glaucoma is anterior uveitis: the differentiation between the two has already been discussed.[1] Apart from this there may arise doubts as to whether the glaucoma is primary or secondary, particularly to an intra-ocular tumour—a question which is frequently insoluble if the inner eye cannot be examined until the ocular tension has been reduced.

Occasionally the radiating headache and violent nausea and vomiting divert attention to the abdomen, the patient being in too unhappy a condition to observe that he has lost the sight of an eye; in this way the diagnosis has been missed altogether by the unwary.

In intermittent closed-angle glaucoma the patient is usually seen between the attacks of raised tension. If an acute attack of glaucoma has occurred in the fellow eye the diagnosis can seldom be in doubt, but in

[1] Vol. IX, p. 154.

most cases this has not occurred and recourse must be made to the history of blurring of vision associated with the characteristic haloes, the typically narrow appearance of the filtration angle, and the response to provocative tests.

In chronic closed-angle glaucoma the patient may present a clinical picture identical to that of simple glaucoma, the one distinguishing feature being the gonioscopic appearance of a narrow filtration angle partially occluded by irido-corneal contact. More frequently, however, occasional attacks of blurring of vision and haloes also occur in this form of the disease and alert the physician to the possibility of the presence of a closed angle.

PROVOCATIVE TESTS

The object of provocative tests in closed-angle glaucoma is to embarrass the filtration angle by dilating the pupil. In susceptible eyes this may result in crowding of the angle by the peripheral iris, thus producing a rise in the ocular tension. As mydriasis is only one of the predisposing factors in closed-angle glaucoma, it is not surprising that the dark-room and mydriatic tests are frequently unreliable and, although a positive result is significant, a negative response frequently occurs in an eye that eventually develops this form of the disease. It follows that a careful clinical history and gonioscopic examination are more reliable in diagnosis than provocative tests (Lowe, 1967).

The Dark-room Test of Seidel (1914–27). The patient, after having his tension taken, is put in a dark room for 60 to 90 minutes, at the end of which time the tension is taken again in a dim light, a difficult procedure when using the applanation tonometer. This is probably the safest provocative test for suspected closed-angle glaucoma, but it is positive in only 30% of cases (Foulds, 1956–59) (Figs. 588–9). The criteria for a positive test vary with different authors: a rise of 8 mm. or more is considered positive by Becker and Shaffer (1965), one of 9 mm. or more by Foulds (1957–59), while a rise of 10 mm. or more is considered necessary to make the diagnosis by Higgitt (1954), Leydhecker (1955) and Törnquist (1958). A pathological rise of tension should be accompanied by gonioscopic evidence of a partial or complete closure of the filtration angle, but this is difficult to observe since the use of a slit-lamp tends to produce miosis and thus open the angle and reduce the tension; it is also associated with a low facility of outflow in the eye before the test was taken, suggesting the presence of some degree of closure of the angle when the ocular tension was within normal limits (Foulds, 1959) (Fig. 590).

The dark-room test may be made more specific by performing a *tonography* both before and after the patient has been in the dark; a reduction in the facility of outflow of 30% or more is considered positive, and such a

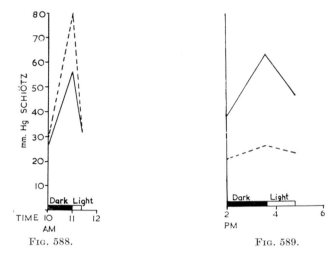

FIG. 588. FIG. 589.

FIGS. 588 AND 589.—THE DARK-ROOM TEST IN CLOSED-ANGLE GLAUCOMA.

To show the rapid rises of ocular tension during the dark and the sudden fall on exposure to light (S. J. H. Miller).

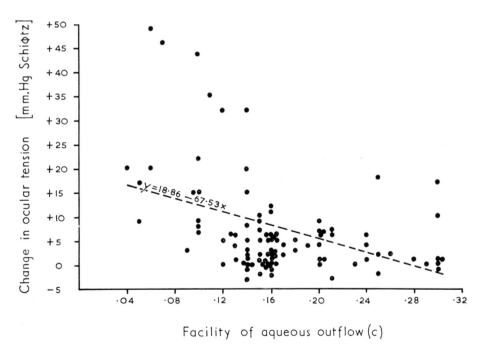

FIG. 590.—THE FACILITY OF AQUEOUS OUTFLOW IN CLOSED-ANGLE GLAUCOMA.

The relationship between the resting facility of aqueous outflow (C) and the rise in ocular tension occurring during the dark-room test. Low initial levels of outflow are associated with greater rises in ocular tension than are higher levels of outflow. The regression line is indicated (W. S. Foulds).

result has been found in 67% of patients with closed-angle glaucoma (Foulds, 1956–59).

The mydriatic test consists of dilating the pupil with a short-acting mydriatic such as homatropine,[1] euphthalmine,[2] paredrine (Sugar, 1941; Kronfeld *et al.*, 1943), phenylephrine (Sugar, 1948; Rose, 1951), or tropicamide (Becker and Shaffer, 1965; Pollack, 1967) and measuring the rise of tension when the pupil is dilated. A rise of 7 to 10 mm. is generally considered to be positive,[3] although Leydhecker (1952–66) required a rise of 12 mm. or more before establishing a certain diagnosis. The tension should be measured every 30 minutes after instilling the mydriatic and on the

FIGS. 591 AND 592.—THE EFFECT OF READING IN CLOSED-ANGLE GLAUCOMA
(S. J. H. Miller).

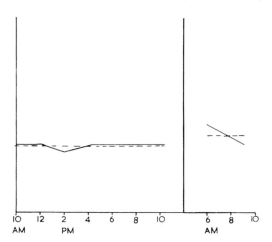
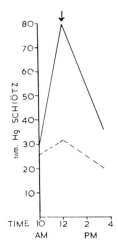

FIG. 591.—The diurnal variation curve showing a normal variation.

FIG. 592.—The same case showing a spontaneous rise after a period of reading. At the arrow miotics were instilled.

occurrence of a positive result a miotic must be instilled until the pupil has become small, the angle is open gonioscopically and the tension has fallen. If a precipitous rise of tension occurs, a carbonic anhydrase inhibitor and oral glycerol should be administered as well.

A refinement of the mydriatic test is to perform *tonography* before and after instillation of the mydriatic. A decrease in the facility of outflow of 25 to 30% is usually considered a positive result[4] and occurs in over 80%

[1] Gradle (1936), Sugar (1941–48), Kronfeld *et al.* (1943), Stine (1948), Leydhecker (1954–55), and others.
[2] Gradle (1936), Sugar (1941), Stine (1948), Becker and Shaffer (1965), and others.
[3] Gradle (1936), Stine (1948), Sugar (1948), Leydhecker (1951), Mills and Becker (1963). Becker and Shaffer (1965), Pollack (1967), and many others.
[4] Becker and Thompson (1958), Mills and Becker (1963), Becker and Shaffer (1965), Pollack (1967), and others.

of cases of closed-angle glaucoma, a considerably higher percentage of positive results than with the mydriatic test. Kristensen (1967) suggested a " triple-test " wherein mydriasis combined with a water-drinking test was followed by the instillation of pilocarpine; a rise of over 10 mm. Hg was considered suspicious.

The Reading Test. The tension is measured; the patient reads small print concentratedly for 45 minutes and in an eye with a predisposition to closed-angle glaucoma the tension may rise 10 to 15 mm. or more (Gradle, 1931; Miller, 1953; Higgitt and Smith, 1955) (Figs. 591–2).

Becker and Shaffer. *Diagnosis and Therapy of the Glaucomas*, St. Louis (1965).

Becker and Thompson. *Amer. J. Ophthal.*, **46**, 305 (1958).

Foulds. *Trans. ophthal. Soc. U.K.*, **76**, 83 (1956).
　Brit. J. Ophthal., **41**, 200 (1957); **43**, 613 (1959).

Gradle. *Amer. J. Ophthal.*, **14**, 936 (1931).
　Berens's *The Eye and its Diseases*, Phila., 699 (1936).

Higgitt. *Brit. J. Ophthal.*, **38**, 242 (1954).

Higgitt and Smith. *Brit. J. Ophthal.*, **39**, 103 (1955).

Kristensen. *Acta ophthal.* (Kbh.), **45**, 814 (1967).

Kronfeld, McGarry and Smith. *Amer. J. Ophthal.*, **26**, 245 (1943).

Leydhecker. *Ber. dtsch. ophthal. Ges.*, **57**, 199 (1951).
　Klin. Mbl. Augenheilk., **121**, 174 (1952).

Leydhecker. *v. Graefes Arch. Ophthal.*, **155**, 386 (1954).
　Glaucoma: a Symposium (ed. Duke-Elder), Oxon., 205 (1955).
　Glaucoma in Ophthalmic Practice, London (1966).

Lowe. *Brit. J. Ophthal.*, **51**, 727 (1967).

Miller. *Brit. J. Ophthal.*, **37**, 1 (1953).

Mills and Becker. *Trans. Canad. ophthal. Soc.*, **26**, 196 (1963).

Pollack. *Symposium on Glaucoma* (Trans. N. Orleans Acad. Ophthal.), St. Louis, 31 (1967).

Rose. *Trans. Canad. ophthal. Scc.*, **14**, 113 (1951).

Seidel. *v. Graefes Arch. Ophthal.*, **88**, 102 (1914); **119**, 15 (1927).

Stine. *Amer. J. Ophthal.*, **31**, 1203 (1948).

Sugar. *Amer. J. Ophthal.*, **24**, 851 (1941); **31**, 1193 (1948).

Törnquist. *Acta ophthal.* (Kbh.), **36**, 664 (1958).

Treatment

HISTORICALLY, apart from the transient relief obtained by a vitreous puncture or a paracentesis as suggested by Mackenzie (1835), until von Graefe introduced his surgical technique for the treatment of the acute crisis of closed-angle glaucoma in 1856 (von Graefe, 1857), a rational and effective means of treating the condition did not exist, and even this dramatic success was arrived at largely by chance with no understanding of the cause of the disease or the mechanism of the action of an iridectomy. Treatment had been on general humoral lines, consisting of bleeding and purging with the later addition of counter-irritation and inunction with mercury. The position was well summed up in the advice given by von Arlt (1853) both as a prophylactic and therapeutic measure: the causes of the disease were the struggle for a livelihood, grief, weeping, vexation, eye-strain and a damp dwelling (an early recognition of the ætiological factor of emotional stress), and its appropriate treatment (in which there is some sense but little joy) was said to be a life with few pleasures, no rich food, no luxurious living, no excess of alcohol and little sex.

GENERAL PRINCIPLES OF TREATMENT

Now that the ætiology of closed-angle glaucoma has become largely understood, its treatment can be discussed on a more rational basis than that of simple glaucoma. Although the underlying defect, the peculiar anatomical configuration of the anterior segment of the eye, is not amenable to any form of therapy, be it preventative or curative, the more important predisposing factors, particularly the pupillary block and mydriasis, can either be prevented from occurring or at least reduced to such an extent that their deleterious effects on the eye seldom occur. The major factor— that of pupillary block—is not amenable to cure as it depends upon pre-determined anatomical factors but its effects can be prevented, certainly in the earlier stages of the disease, by a relatively simple operative procedure.

The management of closed-angle glaucoma can logically be discussed in three parts: the prevention of the disease in susceptible eyes; the treat-ment of acute and intermittent attacks prior to the development of irre-versible changes at the filtration angle; and the treatment of the late stages of the disease once permanent impairment to the drainage of aqueous has occurred. In general terms the management of the disease is basically surgical, although medical means are essential as a pre-operative measure in the acute stage, and are complementary to surgical treatment in the chronic stages.

Before presenting a logical and workable scheme for the different clinical pictures, we shall summarize the various available means of treatment, many of which have already been discussed in the chapter on simple glaucoma.[1]

Medical Methods of Treatment

The various drugs employed in the treatment of closed-angle glaucoma can be conveniently divided into three main classes: (1) parasympatho-mimetic drugs; (2) secretory inhibitors; and (3) osmotic agents. Most of these drugs have already been discussed both in a previous Volume of this *System*[2] and in the chapter on simple glaucoma,[3] and all that remains for us to indicate here is their particular use in the closed-angle form of the disease.

1. PARASYMPATHOMIMETIC DRUGS

THE CHOLINERGIC DRUGS are of temporary value in preventing attacks of raised ocular tension both in susceptible eyes and in eyes already under-going intermittent attacks of closed-angle glaucoma; they are also useful in combination with other drugs in the immediate treatment of acute glaucoma. They act by producing a miosis which prevents both crowding of the angle by the peripheral iris and relaxation of this part of the iris thus making it less susceptible to being pushed forwards into contact with the cornea. It has also been suggested that miotics, other than the strong anti-cholinesterase drugs, tend to reduce pupillary blockage which is most liable to occur when the pupil is in a state of semi-dilatation.[4] These drugs, however, cannot be relied upon for the long-term prevention or treatment of

---

[1] p. 505. [2] Vol. VII. [3] p. 506.
[4] Chandler (1952), Sugar (1964), Lowe (1966), Mapstone (1968).

acute or intermittent rises in tension, since attacks are liable to develop in about 40 to 60% of patients in spite of medical treatment.[1]

THE ANTICHOLINESTERASE DRUGS, on the other hand, should not be used in most cases of closed-angle glaucoma. As a preventative measure in susceptible eyes and in eyes with intermittent hypertensive episodes they are certainly not justified, while in acute attacks, although the use of physostigmine is widespread as was initially practised by Laqueur (1876) on his own eyes,[2] the stronger anticholinesterases are contra-indicated.[3] These drugs tend to produce a paradoxical rise of ocular tension by their ability to cause pupillary block in susceptible eyes, an effect which may be aggravated by their vasodilatory action on the iris and ciliary body, and by their causing a relaxation of the ciliary muscle resulting in a forward movement of the lens.[4] Even the use of physostigmine is seldom justified in acute attacks, now that carbonic anhydrase inhibitors and osmotic agents are available to reduce the ocular tension, and in those cases wherein its use is considered necessary it should be administered sparingly; in addition, local steroids should be exhibited in order to suppress the inflammatory response that invariably accompanies the use of this drug.

It is relevant to mention here that adrenaline and guanethidine, which reduce the ocular tension in simple glaucoma, are also contra-indicated in acute and intermittent closed-angle glaucoma,[5] although their judicious use in chronic closed-angle glaucoma is sometimes necessary in order to control the ocular tension.

2. SECRETORY INHIBITORS

THE CARBONIC ANHYDRASE INHIBITORS[6] are particularly valuable additions to the therapy available for the treatment of acute closed-angle glaucoma.[7] Although these drugs may be administered orally, they are more effective and have a quicker action when given by intramuscular injection, a particularly valuable route of administration in patients with nausea and vomiting; they may also be useful in the management of patients with chronic closed-angle glaucoma wherein they are used as in cases of simple glaucoma.

[1] Winter (1955), S. T. Adams (1956), Bain (1957), Lowe (1962), Lim (1964), and others.
[2] p. 566.
[3] DFP—Scheie (1949), Stone (1950), Becker and Shaffer (1965); echothiophate—Becker et al. (1959), Drance (1960), Lloyd (1963), Becker and Shaffer (1965); demecarium—Krishna and Leopold (1960), Deutsch and Rowlett (1963), Becker and Shaffer (1965).
[4] p. 515.
[5] Adrenaline—Veirs and McGrew (1963), Etienne and Barut (1965), Lowe (1966); guanethidine—Kutschera (1962).
[6] p. 520.
[7] Becker (1954), Breinin and Görtz (1954), Posner (1954), Andreani and Lepri (1955), H. and A. Arruga (1955), Demers and Monfette (1955), Drance (1955), Lorente (1955), Moreu Gonzalez-Pola et al. (1955), Perkins (1955), Serpell (1955), Duke-Elder et al. (1956), Chandler (1957), Görtz (1958), Pletneva and Sakhieva (1958), Graham and Stevens (1960), Luntz (1961), and many others.

3. OSMOTIC AGENTS

THE OSMOTIC AGENTS raise the osmolarity of the plasma so that fluid is drawn out of the eye with a resultant fall in ocular tension.[1] Their effect is only temporary, becoming ineffective as soon as osmotic equilibrium is re-established between the aqueous and the plasma, and thus their therapeutic value is essentially an emergency measure to reduce the tension before surgery in an eye with dangerously high tension. This they do in almost every case of acute closed-angle glaucoma so that it has usually become unnecessary to operate in this condition until the tension has been reduced to within normal limits.

UREA (*Urevert; Ureaphil*) is a substance with a low molecular weight which penetrates the blood-aqueous barrier with some difficulty (Adler, 1933; Duke-Elder *et al.*, 1949). It is administered intravenously as a 30% solution in 10% invert sugar in a dosage of 0·5 to 2·0 G. per kg. bodyweight at a rate of about 60 drops a minute. It induces a marked ocular hypotony in 30 to 45 minutes which lasts about 4 to 6 hours, and has been widely used in the pre-operative management of acute closed-angle glaucoma.[2] It is irritating to the subcutaneous tissue if it escapes from a vein, producing a localized slough and a thrombophlebitis. Oral urea is also effective in lowering the ocular tension (Aizawa, 1962; de Ocampo and Pinzon, 1962) although since the advent of glycerol and isosorbide it is seldom administered by this route.

MANNITOL (*Osmitrol*) is a hexahydric alcohol with a higher molecular weight than urea. When administered intravenously it is confined to the extracellular fluid, produces a more profound dehydration, and penetrates the eye to a less extent than does urea. It is administered as a 20% solution in water in a dosage of 0·5 to 3·0 G. per kg. bodyweight at a rate of about 60 drops a minute. It produces a similar effect on the ocular tension to that of urea, but is less irritating to the subcutaneous tissue if it escapes from a vein. It is more effective in the presence of a grossly inflamed eye and is said to have fewer side-effects than urea. Its value as a hypotensive agent in acute closed-angle glaucoma has been confirmed by several authors.[3]

SODIUM ASCORBATE, administered intravenously as a 20% solution in a dosage of 0·4 to 1·0 G. per kg. bodyweight also lowers the intra-ocular pressure (Virno *et al.*, 1965; Hilsdorf, 1967), as does a glycerol-sodium ascorbate combination (the latter being used at 0·5 G. per kg. bodyweight)

[1] Vol. VII, p. 628.

[2] Galin *et al.* (1959–63), Klöti (1960), Ackerman (1961), Crews and Davidson (1961), Davis *et al.* (1961), Fink *et al.* (1961), Hill *et al.* (1961), Honegger (1961), Keith (1961), Tarter and Linn (1961), Verdaguer *et al.* (1961), Aizawa (1962), Krejčí (1962), Pur and Hrstka (1962), Chutko (1963), Protonotarios and Tyllianakis (1963), Liu (1964), Koltman (1965), Becker (1967), and others.

[3] Weiss *et al.* (1962), R. E. Adams *et al.* (1963), Cappelli and Lepri (1963), Galin *et al.* (1963), Hill (1964), Kishimoto *et al.* (1964), Seeger and Lewis (1964), Artifoni (1965), Okuda *et al.* (1965), Vergez and Solignac (1965), Cardoso de Melo (1966), Becker (1967), and others.

which is said to eliminate the danger of hæmaturia when ascorbate is used alone (Bietti and Bucci, 1966; Virno et al., 1966).

GLYCEROL has the great advantage over urea and mannitol in that it can be given orally in a dosage of 0·75 to 1·5 G. per kg. bodyweight as a 50% solution flavoured with fruit juice. It is probably the safest osmotic agent available, although it produces nausea and vomiting in some patients, and it penetrates the eye poorly. It is very effective in reducing the ocular tension in acute closed-angle glaucoma, although it takes about 1 hour to achieve its maximal effect.[1] It must be used with care in diabetic patients since, unlike urea and mannitol, it is metabolized by the body to sugar.

ISOSORBIDE (*Hydronol*) is a dihydric alcohol which can also be administered orally in a dosage of 1 to 2 G. per kg. bodyweight. It has the same effect as glycerol on the ocular tension but has the advantage that it is not metabolized by the body, thus being a safer osmotic agent to use in diabetic patients (Becker et al., 1967).

Of historical interest is the use of various other osmotic agents. These include: SALINE, at first administered orally (Cantonnet, 1904), then by mouth and rectum (H. G. Thomas, 1917), and most effectively intravenously[2]; GLUCOSE intravenously and rectally (Sansum, 1917); SUCROSE intravenously (Dyar and Matthew, 1937); SORBITOL (Bellows et al., 1938); and GUM ACACIA (Gifford, 1940).

Side-effects of Osmotic Agents

The osmotic agents in general, because they produce dehydration of the body, may cause headache, pain in the back, and mental confusion and disorientation (Tarter and Linn, 1961; d'Alena and Ferguson, 1966; Becker, 1967). A diuresis is inevitable, being most marked with mannitol, and in the elderly this may result in urinary retention or a metabolic acidosis secondary to the loss of potassium. They must be used with caution in patients with cardiac, renal or hepatic disease; mannitol is said to be safer than urea in these patients (Adams et al., 1963; Honegger, 1966). The intravenously-administered osmotic agents may produce congestive cardiac failure and pulmonary œdema, while with urea in particular, a thrombophlebitis may occur. Oral glycerol is a gastric irritant and may therefore produce nausea and vomiting, a complication which seldom occurs with isosorbide; in addition, glycerol is metabolized by the body to sugar and must be used with care in diabetic patients.

---

[1] Brick and Ferreira Cantador (1963), Borgmann et al. (1963), Casey and Trevor-Roper (1963), Mangouritsas and Palimeris (1963), L. Palmieri and Graziano (1963), Rubichi (1963), R. P. Thomas (1963), Vila Ortiz et al. (1963), Ardouin et al. (1964), Drance (1964), Espíldora et al. (1964), Hari-Charan and Sharma (1964), Holzhauer and Pilger (1964), Kecmanović and Daković (1964), Nörskov (1964), Consul et al. (1965–66), Kandori and Fukunaga (1965), Müller (1965), Segal and Smolarz-Dudarewicz (1965), Sood et al. (1965), Becker (1967), Hanisch et al. (1967), Krudysz (1967), and others.

[2] Hertel (1915), Weekers (1923), Duke-Elder (1926), Lambert and Wolff (1929), C. Palmieri (1936), and others.

Ricklefs (1967) found that ALCOHOL (42 ml. of 38%) frequently decreased the ocular tension in acute closed-angle glaucoma by some 20%. It might be considered as a useful (and comforting) adjunct to treatment.

Ackerman. *Amer. J. Ophthal.*, **52**, 875 (1961).

Adams, R. E., Kirschner and Leopold. *Arch. Ophthal.*, **69**, 55 (1963).

Adams, S. T. *Trans. Canad. ophthal. Soc.*, **7**, 227 (1926).

Adler. *Arch. Ophthal.*, **10**, 11 (1933).

Aizawa. *Rinsho Ganka*, **16**, 1037 (1962).

d'Alena and Ferguson. *Arch. Ophthal.*, **75**, 201 (1966).

Andreani and Lepri. *Ann. Ottal.*, **81**, 389 (1955).

Ardouin, Urvoy and Lefranc. *Bull. Soc. Ophtal. Fr.*, **64**, 330 (1964).

von Arlt. *Krankheiten d. Auges für praktische Ärzte*, Prag, **2** (1853).

Arruga, H. and A. *Bull. Soc. franç. Ophtal.*, **68**, 175 (1955).

Artifoni. *Aggiorn. Ter. oftal.*, **17**, 404 (1965).

Bain. *Brit. J. Ophthal.*, **41**, 193 (1957).

Becker. *Acta XVII int. Cong. Ophthal.*, Montreal-N.Y., **2**, 1109 (1954).
Symposium on Glaucoma (Trans. N. Orleans Acad. Ophthal.), St. Louis, 170 (1967).

Becker, Kolker and Krupin. *Arch. Ophthal.*, **78**, 147 (1967).

Becker, Pyle and Drews. *Amer. J. Ophthal.*, **47**, 635 (1959).

Becker and Shaffer. *Diagnosis and Therapy of the Glaucomas*, St. Louis (1965).

Bellows, Puntenney and Cowen. *Arch. Ophthal.*, **20**, 1036 (1938).

Bietti and Bucci. *Boll. Oculist.*, **45**, 735 (1966).

Borgmann, Schmack and Dardenne. *Ber. dtsch. ophthal. Ges.*, **65**, 107 (1963).

Breinin and Görtz. *Arch. Ophthal.*, **52**, 333 (1954).

Brick and Ferreira Cantador. *Arch. bras. Oftal.*, **26**, 204 (1963).

Cantonnet. *Arch. Ophtal.*, **24**, 1 (1904).

Cappelli and Lepri. *Atti Cong. Soc. oftal. ital.*, **21**, 223 (1963).

Cardoso de Melo. *Rev. bras. Oftal.*, **25**, 41 (1966).

Casey and Trevor-Roper. *Brit. med. J.*, **2**, 851 (1963).

Chandler. *Arch. Ophthal.*, **47**, 695 (1952); **57**, 639 (1957).

Chutko. *Vestn. Oftal.*, **76**, 82 (1963).

Consul and Kulshrestha. *Amer. J. Ophthal.*, **60**, 900 (1965).

Consul, Kulshrestha and Mehrotra. *Orient. Arch. Ophthal.*, **4**, 9 (1966).

Crews and Davidson. *Brit. J. Ophthal.*, **45**, 769 (1961).

Davis, Duehr and Javid. *Arch. Ophthal.*, **65**, 526 (1961).

Demers and Monfette. *Canad. med. Ass. J.*, **72**, 529 (1955).

Deutsch and Rowlett. *J. Tenn. med. Ass.*, **56**, 5 (1963).

Drance. *Brit. J. Ophthal.*, **39**, 659 (1955).
Trans. ophthal. Soc. U.K., **80**, 387 (1960).
Arch. Ophthal., **72**, 491 (1964).

Duke-Elder. *Brit. J. Ophthal.*, **10**, 1, 30 (1926).

Duke-Elder, Davson and Woodin. *Brit. J. Ophthal.*, **33**, 452 (1949).

Duke-Elder, Perkins and Langham. *Arch. Soc. oftal. hisp.-amer.*, **16**, 259 (1956).

Dyar and Matthew. *Arch. Ophthal.*, **18**, 57 (1937).

Espíldora, Eggers, Greiber and Covian. *Arch. chil. Oftal.*, **21**, 5 (1964).

Etienne and Barut. *Ann. Oculist.* (Paris), **198**, 472 (1965).

Fink, Binkhorst and Funahashi. *Amer. J. Ophthal.*, **52**, 872 (1961).

Galin, Aizawa and McLean. *Arch. Ophthal.*, **62**, 347, 1099 (1959); **63**, 281 (1960).
Amer. J. Ophthal., **50**, 379 (1960).

Galin, Davidson and Pasmanik. *Amer. J. Ophthal.*, **55**, 244 (1963).

Gifford. *Arch. Ophthal.*, **23**, 301 (1940).

Görtz. *Klin. Mbl. Augenheilk.*, **133**, 203 (1958).

von Graefe. *v. Graefes Arch. Ophthal.*, **3** (2), 456 (1857).

Graham and Stevens. *Brit. J. Ophthal.*, **44**, 357 (1960).

Hanisch, Orbán, Vereb and Hegedüs. *Klin. Mbl. Augenheilk.*, **151**, 87 (1967).

Hari-Charan and Sharma. *Orient. Arch. Ophthal.*, **2**, 177 (1964).

Hertel. *v. Graefes Arch. Ophthal.*, **90**, 309 (1915).

Hill. *Amer. J. Ophthal.*, **58**, 79 (1964).

Hill, Whitney and Trotter. *Arch. Ophthal.*, **65**, 497 (1961).

Hilsdorf. *Klin. Mbl. Augenheilk.*, **150**, 352 (1967).

Holzhauer and Pilger. *Trans. Pacif. Cst. oto-ophthal. Soc.*, **45**, 399 (1964).

Honegger. *Ber. dtsch. ophthal. Ges.*, **64**, 420 (1961).
Med. Klin., **61**, 1425 (1966).

Kandori and Fukunaga. *Rinsho Ganka*, **19**, 287 (1965).

Kecmanović and Daković. *Acta ophthal. iugos.*, **1**, 213 (1964).

Keith. *Brit. J. Ophthal.*, **45**, 307 (1961).

Kishimoto, Yamanouchi, Kakimoto et al. *Rinsho Ganka*, **18**, 1255 (1964).

Klöti. *Ophthalmologica*, **140**, 135 (1960).

Koltman. *Vestn. Oftal.*, **78**, 35 (1965).

Krejcí. *Cs. Oftal.*, **18**, 47 (1962).

Krishna and Leopold. *Amer. J. Ophthal.*, **49**, 554 (1960).

Krudysz. *Klin. oczna*, **37**, 645 (1967).

Kutschera. *Wien. med. Wschr.*, **112**, 704 (1962)

Lambert and Wolff. *Arch. Ophthal.*, **2**, 198 (1929).

Laqueur. *Zbl. med. Wiss.*, **14**, 421 (1876).

Lim. *Singapore med. J.*, **5**, 82 (1964).

Liu. *Trans. Soc. ophthal. Sin.*, **3**, 42 (1964).

Lloyd. *Brit. J. Ophthal.*, **47**, 469 (1963).

Lorente. *Arch. Soc. oftal. hisp.-amer.*, **15**, 355 (1955).

Lowe. *Brit. J. Ophthal.*, **46**, 641 (1962); **50**, 385 (1966).
Med. J. Aust., **2**, 1037 (1966).

Luntz. *Brit. J. Ophthal.*, **45**, 125 (1961).

Mackenzie. *A Practical Treatise on the Diseases of the Eye*, 2nd ed., London (1835).

Mangouritsas and Palimeris. *Bull. Soc. hellén. Ophtal.*, **31**, 198 (1963).

Mapstone. *Brit. J. Ophthal.*, **52**, 19 (1968).

Moreu Gonzalez-Pola, Sanchez Salorio and Garcia Lopez. *Arch. Soc. oftal. hisp.-amer.*, **15**, 306 (1955).

Müller. *Klin. Mbl. Augenheilk.*, **146**, 424 (1965).

Nörskov. *Nord. Med.*, **72**, 1145 (1964).

de Ocampo and Pinzon. *Philipp. J. Surg.*, **17**, 278 (1962).

Okuda, Ouchi and Yokota. *Folia ophthal. jap.*, **16**, 509 (1965).

Palmieri, C. *Ann. Ottal.*, **64**, 217 (1936).

Palmieri, L. and Graziano. *Ann. Ottal.*, **89**, 749 (1963).

Perkins. *Trans. ophthal. Soc. U.K.*, **75**, 207 (1955).

Pletneva and Sakhieva. *Vestn. Oftal.*, **72** (3), 3 (1958).

Posner. *Eye, Ear, Nose, Thr. Monthly*, **33**, 366 (1954).

Protonotarios and Tyllianakis. *Klin. Mbl. Augenheilk.*, **143**, 632 (1963).

Pur and Hrstka. *Cs. Oftal.*, **18**, 66 (1962).

Ricklefs. *Ber. dtsch. ophthal. Ges.*, **68**, 355 (1967).

Rubichi. *Romagna med.*, **15**, 651 (1963).

Sansum. *J. Amer. med. Ass.*, **68**, 1885 (1917).

Scheie. *Trans. Amer. Acad. Ophthal.*, **53**, 186 (1949).

Seeger and Lewis. *Arch. Ophthal.*, **72**, 219 (1964).

Segal and Smolarz-Dudarewicz. *Klin. oczna*, **35**, 199 (1965).

Serpell. *Med. J. Aust.*, **2**, 845 (1955).

Sood, Malik, Gupta and Seth. *Orient. Arch. Ophthal.*, **3**, 176 (1965).

Stone. *Arch. Ophthal.*, **43**, 36 (1950).

Sugar. *Sorsby's Modern Ophthalmology*, London, **4**, 567 (1964).

Tarter and Linn. *Amer. J. Ophthal.*, **52**, 323 (1961).

Thomas, H. G. *Ophthalmology*, **13**, 582 (1917).

Thomas, R. P. *Arch. Ophthal.*, **70**, 625 (1963).

Veirs and McGrew. *Eye, Ear, Nose, Thr. Monthly*, **42**, 46 (1963).

Verdaguer, Lira, Zambrano and Riveros. *Arch. chil. Oftal.*, **18**, 101 (1961).

Vergez and Solignac. *Arch. Ophtal.*, **25**, 171 (1965).

Vila Ortiz, Gallo, L., González del Cerro and Gallo, C. *Arch. Oftal. B. Aires*, **38**, 390 (1963).

Virno, Bucci, Pecori-Giraldi and Cantore. *Boll. Oculist.*, **44**, 542 (1965).
Amer. J. Ophthal., **62**, 824 (1966).

Weekers. *Arch. Ophtal.*, **40**, 513 (1923).

Weiss, Shaffer and Wise. *Arch. Ophthal.*, **68**, 341 (1962).

Winter. *Amer. J. Ophthal.*, **40**, 557 (1955).

Surgical Treatment

THE HISTORY of the surgical treatment of closed-angle glaucoma centres around FRIEDERICH WILHELM ERNST ALBRECHT VON GRAEFE [1828–1870]. Although he lived only a brief 42 years, he was undoubtedly the greatest ophthalmologist who ever existed. His professional achievements have been summarized in a previous Volume of this series where his portrait during his professional prime appears[1]; but in view of the fact that he was the first to introduce a surgical cure for this disease and thus transformed its prognosis from a condition sooner or later ending in blindness, he must certainly be commemorated again. On this occasion, however, our tribute is somewhat less orthodox. The son of Carl Ferdinand von Graefe, professor of surgery at the University of Berlin and also an ophthalmic surgeon, Albrecht received his early education at the French Gymnasium from which he was the youngest boy ever to graduate and, being too young to enter the University, he spent a year studying mathematics, physics and chemistry, and mountaineering (Fig. 593). At the University which he entered as the youngest student on record, he followed a gay life, founding a students' society, the Camellias (Fig. 594). After a year's part-time military service wherein he was banished from parades because he

[1] Vol. VII, p. 283, Fig. 134.

FIGS. 593 AND 594.—ALBRECHT VON GRAEFE IN HIS YOUTH.
Sketches by his sister Ottilie.

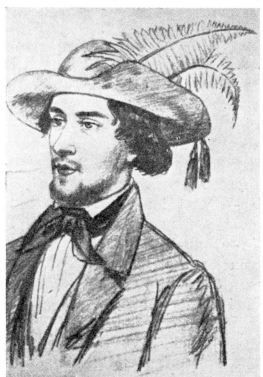

FIG. 593.—In the Harz Mountains, aged 16.

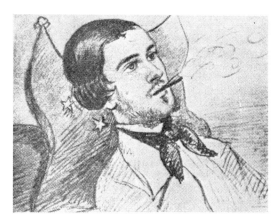

FIG. 594.—As a university student aged 17.

insisted on wearing a beard, he graduated in 1847. Thereafter he wandered for 3 years, watching, questioning and learning in Paris (where he studied under Sichel, Desmarres and Claude Bernard), Vienna (Jaeger, von Brücke), Prague (von Arlt), London (Bowman), Glasgow (William Mackenzie) and Dublin (Sir William Wilde). In 1850, back in Berlin, after advertising the fact, he set up an Eye Clinic at which his first ophthalmoscope was introduced in 1851 and his life's work started whereby he was to create modern ophthalmology. His clinic was to become the most famous in the 19th century; to it ophthalmologists from all over the world came and were fascinated; and there he worked as few have worked before or since, writing a constant stream of revolutionary papers until Nature took revenge and he died slowly from tuberculosis after a long illness during which he continued to study and treat his patients. The last paper he wrote was on glaucoma in 1869.

Initially von Graefe, finding the usual treatment of acute glaucoma by purging, blood-letting and leeching useless, tried Mackenzie's suggestion of a paracentesis but was frustrated by its temporary effect. Noting the hypotensive effect of an iridectomy in cases of corneal staphyloma, he tried the same operation in acute glaucoma as an experiment, first on a 51-year-old woman in 1856. The immediate results of his early operations were "startlingly good", but he remained suspicious "until time proved that a lasting cure had been effected". At that time he was corresponding with most of the significant ophthalmologists in Europe and he told them of his results and, finally convinced of the permanency of cure, at the first International Congress in Brussels in 1857 he announced his discovery and received an astonishing ovation. Thereafter a large-sector iridectomy involving tearing away the iris from its base became the standard procedure for the disease until E. J. Curran (1920) of Kansas, noting the phenomenon of occlusion of the pupil, advocated a peripheral iridectomy, an idea consolidated by Otto Barkan (1938) of San Francisco. Today with few exceptions the latter is the preferred technique.

While it has been recognized that surgical methods of treatment of simple glaucoma are confined merely to mechanical expedients to relieve the raised tension of the eye, surgical methods of treatment of closed-angle glaucoma, particularly in its earlier stages, are concerned with the abolition of the deleterious effects of pupillary blockage. In suitably selected cases before the filtration angle has become embarrassed to a significant extent by the development of peripheral anterior synechiæ, iridectomy has become the treatment of choice. Once the drainage of aqueous has been impaired by organic adhesion between the iris and the cornea, an iridectomy is insufficient to restore the ocular tension to normal, and in these cases a drainage operation or an operation to reduce the secretion of aqueous will become necessary once the tension cannot be controlled by medical means. In these late cases, the problem, as with simple glaucoma, becomes one of plumbing, and the procedures previously described as being appropriate for cases of the simple type of the disease are equally applicable to those of chronic closed-angle glaucoma.

IRIDECTOMY

The classical broad iridectomy of von Graefe (1857–69), the introduction of which revolutionized the treatment of the disease, must always take pride of place in any discussion on the operative treatment of closed-angle glaucoma. In it a considerable sector of the iris is removed up to the root (Fig. 595). The rationale of the reduction of the ocular tension has been a matter of controversy for many years, and many theories have been advanced since von Graefe's original suggestion that removal of part of the iris diminished the secretion of the aqueous. For long the most universally accepted theory, suggested by Weber (1877) and illustrated anatomically by Collins (1894), ascribed its main effect to the mechanical opening up of a closed angle of the anterior chamber, and it was generally held that the operation was successful only in so far as it did this and therefore the iris was removed so completely that the angle could not be blocked again. Gonioscopic studies, however, show that this cannot be the entire explanation, for in many cases the base of the iris is left behind; if it is, the result may be good, and if it is totally removed, the result may be bad.[1]

FIGS. 595 AND 596.—IRIDECTOMY
(after R. J. H. Smith).

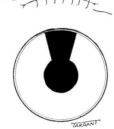

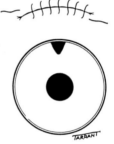

FIG. 595.—A complete sector iridectomy.

FIG. 596.—A peripheral iridectomy. The sewn conjunctival flap is seen above.

Other suggestions have been put forward: that a fresh absorbing surface is presented to the aqueous (Ulrich, 1884), which, since a wound in the iris does not cicatrize (Fuchs, 1896; Henderson, 1907; McBurney, 1914), remains permanently; that a filtering scar is formed accidentally with or without the incorporation of uveal tissue (de Wecker, 1867); or that vasomotor reflexes are cut and abolished (Abadie, 1910).

Although a number of authors had suggested that increased communication between posterior and anterior chambers was a factor in the action of iridectomy,[2] it was Curran (1920) who developed the theory of relative pupillary block and suggested that a peripheral iridectomy would prevent the iris being pushed towards the cornea by the increased pressure in the posterior chamber. This theory has since been elaborated, particularly by Barkan (1938–56) and Chandler (1952), and it is now widely accepted that a peripheral iridectomy is the procedure of choice in preventing closed-angle

[1] Troncoso (1933–35), Werner (1931), Puig Solanes (1937), Moreu (1943).
[2] Coccius (1859), Panas (1884), Knies (1893), Leber (1903), Czermak and Elschnig (1908).

attacks in susceptible eyes in which the filtration angle, although narrow, still remains open[1] (Fig. 596). To ensure that the iridectomy is performed at the base of the iris and to avoid the difficulty of cutting a section in an eye with a shallow anterior chamber, the best approach is an incision *ab externo* undertaken beneath a conjunctival flap. In acute closed-angle glaucoma, the classical broad iridectomy was, until recently, the treatment of choice. Since the advent of routine gonioscopy and the use of carbonic anhydrase inhibitors and osmotic agents, it has been possible to plan a more rational approach to the management of the disease by the performance of the simpler and less traumatic procedure, particularly as the rationale for performing a broad iridectomy, that of tearing the iris out of the closed angle, does not bear critical gonioscopic confirmation. It is now hardly ever necessary to operate in a case of acute closed-angle glaucoma while the ocular tension is abnormally high; it can usually be reduced by miotics and carbonic anhydrase inhibitors and, failing this, the addition of osmotic agents is almost invariably successful. Once the tension has been reduced to a normal level it is necessary to assess the state of the filtration angle, for if it has reopened, a peripheral iridectomy is all that is required to prevent further attacks, while if it remains predominantly closed, a formal drainage operation is necessary.

The successes claimed for broad iridectomy in the treatment of acute closed-angle glaucoma vary widely, although a good average is 60% (Wilmer, 1927; Ploman and Granström, 1932; and many others). These figures were produced, however, before the advent of routine gonioscopy, and more recent series have been divided into those treated with an iridectomy and those with a drainage operation. Goldberg (1951) claimed an 81% success-rate following iridectomy, while Dalgleish and Naylor (1965) found peripheral iridectomy successful in over 90% of early cases, and Williams and his colleagues (1968) in 100% of prophylactic operations, 92·5% of acute cases and 88·2% of chronic cases. The success-rate following iridencleisis or Scheie's procedure is between 80 and 90%.[2]

Specific Indications for Treatment

Having discussed both in this and in the previous Chapter[3] the various medical and surgical methods available for the treatment of closed-angle glaucoma, it now remains for us to present a workable scheme for the treatment of the various stages of this condition. It will be noted that in recent years the management of some of the phases in which it appears

[1] Haas and Scheie (1952), Reese (1952), Posner (1953), Chandler and Trotter (1955), Sternberg (1955), Bain (1957), Gorin (1957), McLean (1957), Sloan (1957), Becker and Thompson (1958), Foulds (1959), Blaxter and Chatterjee (1960), Luntz (1960), Primrose (1960), Lowe (1963), de Carvalho (1965), Dalgleish and Naylor (1965), Etienne (1965), Pintér (1966), and many others.

[2] Goldberg (1951), Günther and van Beuningen (1954), Mackie and Rubinstein (1954), Pillat and Nemetz (1958), Graham and Stevens (1960), Scheie (1964), and others.

[3] pp. 506, 608.

has become more logical and less controversial than that of simple glaucoma, an indication of our increasing knowledge and understanding of the basic ætiology of the former disease.

(a) PRE-GLAUCOMA

In patients who on routine examination are found to have extremely narrow filtration angles yet have not developed symptoms suggestive of intermittent or acute attacks of closed-angle glaucoma, the danger of such attacks developing spontaneously or being precipitated by mydriatics must always be borne in mind. It has been demonstrated by Törnquist (1956) that if the depth of the anterior chamber is between 2·0 and 1·5 mm. the chances of developing acute closed-angle glaucoma are 1 in 10, while if the depth is under 1·5 mm. the chances increase dramatically to 52 to 1. It is probably prudent to subject an eye with a depth of anterior chamber of less than 2 mm. to the dark-room and mydriatic provocative tests which if positive would indicate the desirability of recommending a prophylactic peripheral iridectomy. It must be remembered, however, that negative provocative tests do not preclude the possibility of developing an acute rise of tension so that patients with very narrow filtration angles but with negative provocative tests should be warned of the symptoms that might indicate an attack.

(b) INTERMITTENT CLOSED-ANGLE GLAUCOMA

Once the occurrence of intermittent attacks of closed-angle glaucoma has been established, it is widely agreed that peripheral iridectomy is the treatment of choice, so long as the ocular tension and the facility of aqueous outflow return to normal levels between attacks.[1] Although miotics will usually reduce the incidence of repeated attacks, it is important to remember that they will not prevent the recurrence of the intermittent or acute attacks which eventually occur in a high percentage of these patients. Long-term miotic therapy should therefore be reserved for those patients on whom surgery is refused or contra-indicated.

(c) ACUTE CLOSED-ANGLE GLAUCOMA

In acute glaucoma treatment must be instant and urgent. The ideal which can now be achieved in almost all patients is to reduce the tension by medical methods before operating. In the rare cases in which this cannot be accomplished within a few hours of starting treatment, operation should not be delayed beyond this interval; otherwise the function of the eye will probably be greatly and permanently impaired, and peripheral adhesions will almost certainly have formed in the angle of the anterior

---

[1] Haas and Scheie (1952), Reese (1952), Posner (1953–55), Barkan (1954), Chandler and Trotter (1955), Sternberg (1955), Gorin (1957), Blaxter and Chatterjee (1960), Kronfeld (1963), Lowe (1963), de Carvalho (1965), Dalgleish and Naylor (1965), and many others.

chamber. In these rare cases, although broad iridectomy is the procedure hallowed by age, iridencleisis is probably the best operation (Leydhecker, 1959).

Hypotensive medical treatment should include the immediate administration of sufficient analgesics to allay pain and anxiety, intensive miotic therapy, and the use of carbonic anhydrase inhibitors and osmotic agents. The frequent instillation of 2–4% pilocarpine, one drop per minute for 5 minutes, a drop every 5 minutes for 30 minutes, then quarter-hourly until the angle opens, is probably better than physostigmine which increases the congestion of the eye, tends to encourage the formation of posterior synechiæ, increases pupillary block and, with its liability to induce nausea, often provides a distressing experience for the patient. If physostigmine is used, steroid eye-drops should be instilled at the same time in order to lessen the inflammatory response.

The action of miotics is enhanced by a fall in the ocular tension produced by carbonic anhydrase inhibitors and osmotic agents, which should therefore be administered as soon as treatment is commenced. If the patient is able to tolerate oral therapy, 500 mg. acetazolamide should be given at the same time as oral glycerol or isosorbide; if he cannot, the acetazolamide should be given intramuscularly or intravenously and urea or mannitol given by intravenous drip. A fall of tension with medical treatment is nearly always heralded by a lessening of the pupillary dilatation. At first the pupil contracts slowly, and then as the tension approaches its normal height a sudden miosis develops. Simultaneously the anterior chamber deepens, the tension may fall to subnormal and vision returns; within 6 to 8 hours thereafter the congestion and other signs of the attack may have gone.

Although the retrobulbar injection of procaine, either alone or followed by alcohol, dramatically abolishes the pain and usually lowers the ocular tension, this form of therapy has now no place in the modern treatment of acute glaucoma, but may be employed if the other drugs are not immediately available. A further expedient which has been suggested but is not required if modern methods of lowering the tension are at hand is to operate on the patient after the systemic administration of one of the polymethonium compounds such as hexamethonium which act as vascular depressants by blocking the activity of the autonomic ganglia.[1] The dramatic fall in blood pressure lowers the intra-ocular pressure and reduces congestion (Barnett, 1951–52; Cameron and Burn, 1952; Leonardi, 1954). These drugs, however, are not without their dangers for the sudden cerebral anæmia may occasionally result in visual accidents such as hemianopia, or the collapse of the central artery of the retina may result in blindness. They should, therefore, be administered only after the patient has been overhauled by a physician and under the careful supervision of a competent anæsthetist.

Once the ocular tension has returned to normal, surgical treatment should be undertaken without too much delay, as the continued use of acetazolamide may mask the formation of peripheral anterior synechiæ

[1] Vol. VII, p. 554.

(Chandler, 1957). The choice of operation is open to some discussion. There is a growing body of opinion that peripheral iridectomy is the procedure of choice if the tension returns to normal within 24 to 36 hours, if peripheral anterior synechiæ are not extensive, leaving at least one-third to one-quarter of the angle open, and if the facility of aqueous outflow is not greatly reduced[1]; Forbes and Becker (1964), however, recommend this procedure even in long-standing and neglected cases, the raised tension then being controlled by medical means. Shaffer (1958) suggested performing a peripheral iridectomy in all cases and then examining the filtration angle gonioscopically after reformation of the anterior chamber; only if extensive peripheral anterior synechiæ are present should a cyclodialysis or a drainage operation then be performed. Others recommend a filtering operation, particularly an iridencleisis or a Scheie's procedure, either in all cases or more commonly in those in which peripheral anterior synechiæ are extensive and the outflow reduced[2]; in this respect Becker and Thompson (1958) recommended a peripheral iridectomy if the facility of outflow were greater than 0·10 and filtering procedures if it were less than this. On the other hand, Chandler (1952) and Barkan (1954) recommended a broad basal iridectomy accompanied by a cyclodialysis throughout the area to break the peripheral synechiæ in neglected cases. Although the operation of trephining has been occasionally recommended, it is probably safest to discourage its use in closed-angle glaucoma since there may be difficulties in the re-formation of the anterior chamber.

(d) CHRONIC CLOSED-ANGLE GLAUCOMA

In the chronic congestive or non-congestive phases attempts should be made to lower the ocular tension as much as possible on the lines already laid down; in this type, however, longer time can be taken over medical treatment than in the acute stage, although surgery should not be too long delayed lest the peripheral anterior synechiæ invariably present in this type of closed-angle glaucoma extend insidiously to close the whole extent of the filtration angle. Prior to surgery the anticholinesterase drugs and adrenaline are contra-indicated; the former increase pupillary blockage and so hasten the development of peripheral synechiæ; the latter, by dilating the pupil, encourage synechiæ by crowding the peripheral iris into the filtration angle.

The surgical procedures that have been recommended for this type of closed-angle glaucoma fall into two types: drainage operations, either

---

[1] Haas and Scheie (1952), Chandler (1952), Reese (1952), Chandler and Trotter (1955), Posner (1955), Sternberg (1955), Sloan (1957), Becker and Thompson (1958), Leydhecker (1959), Blaxter and Chatterjee (1960), Luntz (1960), Kronfeld (1963), Lowe (1963), de Carvalho (1965), Dalgleish and Naylor (1965), and many others.

[2] Reese (1952), Günther and van Beuningen (1954), Mackie and Rubinstein (1954), Chandler and Trotter (1955), Sternberg (1955), Bengisu and Ilday (1955), Becker and Thompson (1958), Pillat and Nemetz (1958), Scheie (1958–64), Gormaz and Eggers (1959), Tyner et al. (1960), Lowe (1963), Möller (1963), Bounds et al. (1964), Gordon (1964), Etienne (1965), and others.

iridencleisis or Scheie's procedure, and peripheral iridectomy usually followed by medical treatment. Drainage operations have been widely recommended and, particularly in those cases wherein the angle is almost totally occluded, have a high rate of success.[1] More recently, however, it has been suggested that it is safer to do a peripheral iridectomy in order to relieve pupillary blockage and then to treat the residual raised tension by medical means, including the strong miotics, adrenaline and carbonic anhydrase inhibitors[2]; a similar line of treatment has been recommended for the chronic closed-angle glaucoma due to peripheral synechiæ (Gorin, 1960).

In cases of *plateau iris*, whether it produces the clinical picture of acute, intermittent or chronic closed-angle glaucoma, a peripheral iridectomy has been recommended to relieve the mild degree of pupillary block usually present, followed by the long-term administration of weak miotics to prevent dilatation of the pupil (Becker and Shaffer, 1965; Chandler and Grant, 1965). Kronfeld (1963), however, considered iridectomy of limited value in this condition, while Etienne (1965) found it of no use; in these cases pupillary blockage plays only a minor role and a broad basal iridectomy may be preferable (Godel *et al.*, 1968).

(e) THE MANAGEMENT OF THE SECOND EYE

We have already seen that primary closed-angle glaucoma is a bilateral disease and that although symptoms usually start unilaterally, the second eye is eventually involved in a high percentage of cases within a period of 5 years, particularly if left untreated but even if treated prophylactically with miotics.[3] It is widely agreed, therefore, that a prophylactic peripheral iridectomy to the second eye is justified in almost every patient in whom closed-angle glaucoma has developed in one eye[4]; Posner (1960) is one of the few recent authors who did not recommend it as a routine as he considered that minor differences between filtration angles may be important in determining which eyes are predisposed to closed-angle attacks. Although the serious complications of sympathetic ophthalmitis, severe intra-ocular hæmorrhage and damage to the lens have been occasionally reported (Adams, 1955; Swan, 1959), it has been suggested that these can be prevented by correct surgical technique. In a study of 103 prophylactic peripheral iridectomies, for example, Douglas and Strachan (1967) observed complications of a relatively minor nature in 14 eyes, none of which reduced the visual acuity, while Williams and his colleagues (1968) reported 100% successes.

[1] Gorin (1957), Tyner *et al.* (1960), Leydhecker (1963), Chandler and Grant (1965), Dalgleish and Naylor (1965), Nadel (1966).
[2] Kronfeld (1963), Forbes and Becker (1964), Becker and Shaffer (1965), Pollack (1967).
[3] p. 566.
[4] Chandler (1952), Adams (1955), Winter (1955), Kronfeld (1956), Bain (1957), Foulds (1959), Lowe (1962), Becker and Shaffer (1965), Chandler and Grant (1965) Leydhecker (1966), Douglas and Strachan (1967), and others.

During an attack of acute glaucoma unusual care should always be given to the other eye in which miosis must be maintained; it is advisable, however, only to use weak miotics such as 1% pilocarpine, for the stronger drugs such as the organophosphates may themselves precipitate closed-angle glaucoma by increasing pupillary blockage.

MIXED GLAUCOMA

The combination of simple and closed-angle glaucoma in the same eye is an uncommon occurrence and one frequently difficult to diagnose with certainty although its existence can often be suspected.[1] In a study of 1,861 consecutive cases of glaucoma, Abrams (1961) found that only 3 cases could be diagnosed as mixed glaucoma although several others were doubtful possibilities, while Lowe (1966), in a study of 300 cases of closed-angle glaucoma, found only 2 patients with intermittent closed-angle attacks complicated by simple glaucoma. In order that the diagnosis should be made with some degree of certainty, the ocular tension must be raised and the facility of aqueous outflow reduced in the presence of a very narrow but open filtration angle. In addition, attacks of further increased tension must occur during which time the angle must be seen gonioscopically to be closed; these attacks may occur spontaneously or be precipitated by the dark-room or mydriatic provocative tests.

In patients with simple glaucoma and very narrow filtration angles the use of adrenaline or the strong miotics, such as the anticholinesterase drugs, may precipitate an attack of closed-angle glaucoma. In these patients, particularly if the dark-room test is positive, it may be necessary to perform a peripheral iridectomy before maximal medical therapy can be prescribed for the simple glaucoma. It is also possible, although it has never been proven, that repeated attacks of closed-angle glaucoma might damage the trabecular meshwork and result in an impaired facility of aqueous outflow in the absence of peripheral anterior synechiæ.

The importance of recognizing the possibility of the presence of a mixed glaucoma is to ensure that closed-angle attacks are not precipitated by the medical therapy required to control the raised ocular tension due to the simple glaucoma. If mixed glaucoma is suspected or confirmed, surgery will almost certainly be required at some stage in the disease. If the ocular tension can be controlled medically between the acute attacks, a peripheral iridectomy is indicated; if the tension is uncontrolled, a drainage operation will be required.

CLOSED-ANGLE GLAUCOMA AND CATARACT

If closed-angle glaucoma occurs together with a cataract the usual intracapsular extraction of the lens accompanied by a peripheral iridectomy

---

[1] Haas (1955), Sugar (1957), Abrams (1961), Becker and Shaffer (1965), Chandler and Grant (1965), Lowe (1966).

generally deals effectively with both conditions, the iridectomy sufficing to keep the glaucoma in check. In those instances wherein the intumescence of a cataractous lens is the cause of the raised tension, the extraction should, of course, be performed as soon as possible, and in every case precautions should be taken with adequate suturing and the injection of air to avoid a subsequent loss of the anterior chamber and the consequent formation of peripheral anterior synechiæ. On the other hand, if the tension is high and the eye is congested, the acute attack of glaucoma should be treated first and the cataract removed at a later date.

A cataract extraction following peripheral iridectomy for closed-angle glaucoma sometimes presents difficulties. After an acute attack the vitreous may be fluid, the anterior chamber may be unusually shallow, and synechiæ both posterior and anterior may be present. These, however, can usually be overcome. An extraction following a filtering operation presents the same problems as have already been considered with simple glaucoma.[1]

Abadie. *Arch. Ophtal.*, **30**, 262 (1910).

Abrams. *Brit. J. Ophthal.*, **45**, 503 (1961).

Adams. *Trans. Canad. ophthal. Soc.*, **7**, 227 (1955).

Bain. *Brit. J. Ophthal.*, **41**, 193 (1957).

Barkan. *Amer. J. Ophthal.*, **21**, 1099 (1938); **37**, 504 (1954); **41**, 964 (1956). *Arch. Ophthal.*, **19**, 217 (1938).

Barnett. *Lancet*, **1**, 1415 (1951). *Brit. J. Ophthal.*, **36**, 593 (1952).

Becker and Shaffer. *Diagnosis and Therapy of the Glaucomas*, St. Louis (1965).

Becker and Thompson. *Amer. J. Ophthal.*, **46**, 305 (1958).

Bengisu and Ilday. *Oto-nörö-oftal.*, **10**, 51 (1955).

Blaxter and Chatterjee. *Brit. J. Ophthal.*, **44**, 114 (1960).

Bounds, Minton and Lyle. *Amer. J. Ophthal.*, **58**, 84 (1964).

Cameron and Burn. *Brit. J. Ophthal.*, **36**, 482 (1952).

de Carvalho. *Rev. bras. Oftal.*, **24**, 5 (1965).

Chandler. *Arch. Ophthal.*, **47**, 695 (1952); **57**, 639 (1957).

Chandler and Grant. *Lectures on Glaucoma*, Phila. (1965).

Chandler and Trotter. *Arch. Ophthal.*, **53**, 305 (1955).

Coccius. *Ueber Glaukom*, Leipzig (1859).

Collins. *Lancet*, **2**, 1329, 1463 (1894).

Curran. *Arch. Ophthal.*, **49**, 131 (1920).

Czermak and Elschnig. *Die augenärztlichen Operationen*, 2nd ed., Wien (1908).

Dalgleish and Naylor. *Eye, Ear, Nose, Thr. Monthly*, **44**, 90 (1965).

Douglas and Strachan. *Brit. J. Ophthal.*, **51**, 459 (1967).

Etienne. *Ann. Oculist.* (Paris), **198**, 788 (1965).

Forbes and Becker. *Amer. J. Ophthal.*, **57**, 57 (1964).

Foulds. *Brit. J. Ophthal.*, **43**, 697 (1959).

Fuchs. *Ber. dtsch. ophthal. Ges.*, **25**, 179 (1896).

Godel, Stein and Feiler-Ofry. *Amer. J. Ophthal.*, **65**, 555 (1968).

Goldberg. *Amer. J. Ophthal.*, **34**, 1376 (1951).

Gordon. *Oftal. Zh.*, No. 7, 491 (1964).

Gorin. *Mod. Probl. Ophthal.*, **1**, 125 (1957). *Amer. J. Ophthal.*, **49**, 141 (1960).

Gormaz and Eggers. *Arch. chil. Oftal.*, **16**, 32 (1959).

von Graefe. *v. Graefes Arch. Ophthal.*, **3** (2), 456 (1857); **15** (3), 108 (1869).

Graham and Stevens. *Brit. J. Ophthal.*, **44**, 357 (1960).

Günther and van Beuningen. *v. Graefes Arch. Ophthal.*, **155**, 1 (1954).

Haas. *Trans. Indiana Acad. Ophthal.*, **38**, 60 (1955).

Haas and Scheie. *Trans. Amer. Acad. Ophthal.*, **56**, 589 (1952).

Henderson. *Ophthal. Rev.*, **26**, 191 (1907).

Knies. *Ber. dtsch. ophthal. Ges.*, **23**, 118 (1893).

Kronfeld. *Glaucoma* (Trans. 1st Macy Conf., ed. Newell), N.Y., 20 (1956). *Trans. Amer. Acad. Ophthal.*, **67**, 476 (1963).

Leber. *Graefe-Saemisch Hb. d. ges. Augenheilk.*, 2nd ed., Leipzig, **2** (2), Kap. XI (1903).

Leonardi. *Wien. klin. Wschr.*, **66**, 816 (1954).

Leydhecker. *Klin. Mbl. Augenheilk.*, **135**, 802 (1959); **142**, 260 (1963). *Glaucoma in Ophthalmic Practice*, London (1966).

Lowe. *Brit. J. Ophthal.*, **46**, 641 (1962). *Trans. ophthal. Soc. Aust.*, **23**, 71 (1963). *Med. J. Aust.*, **2**, 1037 (1966).

[1] p. 534.

Luntz. *Trans. ophthal. Soc. U.K.*, **80**, 169 (1960).

McBurney. *Arch. Ophthal.*, **43**, 12 (1914).

Mackie and Rubinstein. *Brit. J. Ophthal.*, **38**, 641 (1954).

McLean. *Amer. J. Ophthal.*, **44**, 323 (1957).

Möller. *Acta ophthal.* (Kbh.), **41**, 151 (1963).

Moreu. *Manual de gonioscopia*, Madrid (1943).

Nadel. *Amer. J. Ophthal.*, **62**, 955 (1966).

Panas. *Arch. Ophtal.*, **4**, 481 (1884).

Pillat and Nemetz. *Wien. klin. Wschr.*, **70**, 763 (1958).

Pintér. *Szemészet*, **103**, 20 (1966).

Ploman and Granström. *Acta ophthal.* (Kbh.), **10**, 54 (1932).

Pollack. *Symposium on Glaucoma* (Trans. N. Orleans Acad. Ophthal.), St. Louis, 31 (1967).

Posner. *Eye, Ear, Nose, Thr. Monthly*, **32**, 715 (1953); **34**, 193, 201 (1955); **39**, 657 (1960).

Primrose. *Trans. ophthal. Soc. U.K.*, **80**, 179 (1960).

Puig Solanes. *Amer. J. Ophthal.*, **20**, 731 (1937).

Reese. *Trans. ophthal. Soc. Aust.*, **12**, 43 (1952).

Scheie. *Amer. J. Ophthal.*, **45** (2), 220 (1958).

Trans. ophthal. Soc. U.K., **84**, 127 (1964).

Shaffer. *Arch. Ophthal.*, **59**, 532 (1958).

Sloan. *Henry Ford Hosp. med. Bull.*, **5**, 245 (1957).

Sternberg. *J. int. Coll. Surg.*, **23**, 777 (1955).

Sugar. *The Glaucomas*, 2nd ed., N.Y. (1957).

Swan. *Symposium on Glaucoma* (ed. Clark), St. Louis, 38 (1959).

Törnquist. *Brit. J. Ophthal.*, **40**, 421 (1956).

Troncoso. *XIV int. Cong. Ophthal.*, Madrid, **4**, 409 (1933).

Arch. Ophthal., **14**, 557 (1935).

Tyner, Laney, Eliff and Watts. *Arch. Ophthal.*, **64**, 268 (1960).

Ulrich. *v. Graefes Arch. Ophthal.*, **30** (4), 235 (1884).

Weber. *v. Graefes Arch. Ophthal.*, **23** (1), 1 (1877).

de Wecker. *Traité des maladies des yeux*, Paris, **2**, 571 (1867).

Werner. *Acta ophthal.* (Kbh.), **9**, 112, 275, 286 (1931).

Williams, Gills and Hall. *Amer. J. Ophthal.*, **65**, 548 (1968).

Wilmer. *Trans. ophthal. Soc. U.K.*, **47**, 230 (1927).

Winter. *Amer. J. Ophthal.*, **40**, 557 (1955).

Prognosis

Untreated, the prognosis of closed-angle glaucoma is as bleak as it was before the new era ushered in by von Graefe, and the eye progresses to the condition of absolute glaucoma with blindness[1]; but if adequately treated in its early stages before the formation of extensive peripheral anterior synechiæ—as it should be—the prognosis is good. A peripheral iridectomy, especially when carried out on an eye in a phase of low tension—as is almost always possible—is an operation causing little trauma and involving fewer complications than almost any other in surgery. The patient can certainly be assured of an excellent prognosis provided that before the operation when the tension is relieved the facility of outflow is not lower than 0·10. If, however, an acute attack is allowed to remain untreated for more than 24 or 36 hours, the vision may be permanently damaged even although the tension is controlled thereafter. The prognosis of an established case in the chronic phase, provided repeated acute attacks of raised tension have not seriously damaged the vision, is comparable to that of simple glaucoma.[2]

[1] p. 607.　　　[2] p. 560.

CHAPTER IX

SECONDARY GLAUCOMA

We are introducing this Chapter with the portrait of PRIESTLEY SMITH [1845–1933] (Fig. 597) which hangs in Queen's Hospital in Birmingham where he was a surgeon for 30 years. In his youth for 4 years he served an apprenticeship in mechanical engineering, a training which was of undoubted value to him in contriving ingenious types of apparatus in his subsequent experiments. To these classical experiments he devoted much of his life, pursuing them to within a few months of his death at the age of 88, despite a considerable disability with a partial paresis of his hands which he largely overcame by devising mechanical contrivances. In his researches he stressed particularly the growth of the lens in a small eye and obstruction to the drainage of the aqueous humour owing to abnormalities at the angle of the anterior chamber, a view which he applied especially to secondary glaucoma wherein such an obstruction is usually obvious. His theories, always lucid and logical, may often have been too mechanically simple, but upon his work has depended much subsequent thought on the subject. A delightful and modest individual of the highest integrity, a musician and an artist, he was one of the great figures in ophthalmology in his day, being President of the Ophthalmological Society and an Honorary Fellow of the Royal Colleges of Surgeons of England and Ireland, while he gave the Bowman Lecture and received the first Nettleship Medal in his own country, the Lucian Howe Medal from the American Society, the Gullstrand Medal from the Swedish Society, and was a member of the Imperial Society of Vienna, an unusual honour for a foreigner.

SECONDARY GLAUCOMA may be defined as a loosely-knit and unrelated clinical group of cases among which the only common denominator is the fact that some recognized pathological lesion is complicated by an increase in the intra-ocular pressure with attendant symptoms. Such an occurrence is not at all rare, and statistics vary widely with the care with which the precipitating disease is diagnosed; most statistics average between 20 and 40% of all cases of raised ocular tension (Carvill, 1932; Lehrfeld and Reber, 1937; Kurland and Taub, 1957; Hollows and Graham, 1966). The increase in tension and the symptoms to which it may give rise may be violent and acute or insidious and chronic, but in all cases the complication should be looked upon as serious, for the treatment frequently involves problems the solution of which requires much clinical judgement and in many cases, despite the greatest care and the largest experience, the end-results are bad.

The ætiological factors are many and various. It may be said in general terms that in almost all cases there is *an obstruction to the circulation of the intra-ocular fluids*, sometimes at the pupil, frequently at the drainage angle, and in many cases at both sites. This mechanical concept of the ætiology of secondary glaucoma was propounded particularly by Priestley Smith (1891).

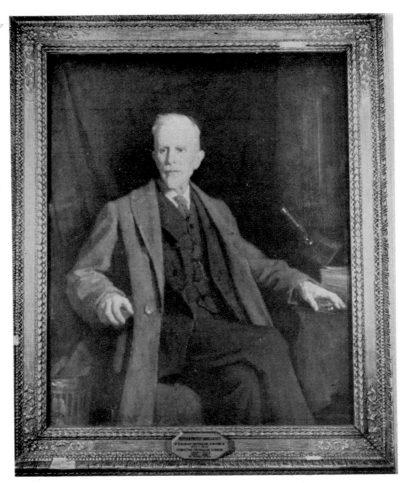

FIG. 597.—PRIESTLEY SMITH
[1845–1933].
(A portrait in Queen's Hospital, Birmingham, by courtesy of P. Jameson Evans.)

In so far as the conditions with which a secondary glaucoma is associated have all been discussed in detail in this and other Volumes of this *System*, it will be sufficient to recapitulate them briefly here; and in the following paragraphs attention will be focused on the ætiology and pathology of the causal factors with a note on the specific therapeutic measures advisable for each particular condition; a fuller discussion of the signs, symptoms, pathology and treatment of the hypertensive state has already been dealt with in the Chapters on primary glaucoma.

This heterogeneous collection may be classified as follows:

I. Glaucoma secondary to developmental anomalies.
    1. Simple buphthalmos.

    2. Associated with other ocular anomalies:

> anterior microphthalmos; cornea plana; aniridia; Axenfeld's and Rieger's anomalies; diffuse neurofibromatosis; the Sturge-Weber syndrome.

    3. In systemic syndromes:

> the Marfan syndrome; the Marchesani syndrome; homocystinuria; the Lowe syndrome; the Pierre-Robin syndrome; oculo-dento-digital dysplasia; the Hurler syndrome; the various forms of trisomy; the Ehlers-Danlos syndrome.

II. Glaucoma secondary to ocular inflammations.
    1. Hypertensive uveitis:

> acute anterior uveitis; cyclitis; glaucomato-cyclitic crises; heterochromic cyclitis.

    2. Post-inflammatory obstructive glaucoma:

> obstruction at the pupil; at the angle of the anterior chamber.

    3. Extra-ocular inflammations: trachoma.

III. Glaucoma secondary to changes in the lens.
    1. Deformities of the lens (microphakia).
    2. Displacements of the lens:

> subluxation; dislocation.

    3. Intumescence of the lens.
    4. Morgagnian cataract.
    5. Phacolytic glaucoma.

IV. Glaucoma secondary to vascular diseases.
    1. Hæmorrhagic glaucoma:

> venous occlusion; arterial occlusion; giant-cell arteritis; rubeosis in diabetes; sickle-cell disease; retinal detachment; the Coats syndrome; Eales's disease; following irradiation.

    2. With intra-ocular hæmorrhages.

3. With extra-ocular venous obstruction.

4. Due to scar-tissue associated with vascular anomalies:

retrolental fibroplasia; persistence of the vascular sheath of the lens.

V. Glaucoma secondary to hæmopoietic diseases:

leucæmia; polycythæmia; dysproteinæmia.

VI. Epidemic dropsy.

VII. Glaucoma secondary to degenerations and dystrophies:

essential atrophy of the iris; the Chandler syndrome; iridoschisis; pseudo-exfoliation; pigmentary dystrophy of the retina; primary familial amyloidosis.

VIII. Glaucoma secondary to cysts and tumours.

IX. Iatrogenic glaucoma:

after mydriatics, miotics, corticosteroids, sulphonamides.

X. Traumatic glaucoma.

1. Injuries:

concussion; perforation; retained foreign bodies.

2. Post-operative:

after glaucoma surgery; cataract extraction; air in the anterior chamber; displaced lenticulus; after keratoplasty; scleral shortening; light-coagulation.

Before describing these types of secondary glaucoma we shall first shortly note the various means of producing glaucoma experimentally; a full discussion of this subject is found in another Volume.[1]

Carvill.   *Trans. Amer. ophthal. Soc.*, **30,** 71 (1932).
Hollows and Graham.   *Brit. J. Ophthal.*, **50,** 570 (1966).
Kurland and Taub.   *Amer. J. Ophthal.*, **43,** 539 (1957).
Lehrfeld and Reber.   *Arch. Ophthal.*, **18,** 712 (1937).
Smith, Priestley.   *Glaucoma*, London (1891).

Experimental Ocular Hypertension

The difficult feat of producing an experimental glaucoma was first accomplished by ÄMILIAN ADAMÜK [1839–1906] (Fig. 598), a native of Lithuania, who became professor of ophthalmology in the University of Kasan. He was one of the great experimental ophthalmologists of Russia in the latter part of the last century and his work on raising the intra-ocular pressure by ligating the vortex veins was among the first he performed in his comparative youth (1867).

The experimental work which has been done to elucidate the cause of glaucoma has led to little pragmatic result. We have already seen[2] that the intra-ocular pressure may be raised by several methods—by increasing the general or local blood pressure, by inducing venous engorgement, by

[1] Vol. IV, Chap. IV.   [2] Vol. IV, Chap. IV.

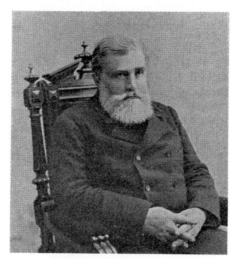

Fig. 598.—ÄMILIAN ADAMÜK
[1839–1906.]

bringing about capillary stasis, by exciting the local neuro-vascular axon reflexes, by varying the osmotic equilibrium between the blood and the intra-ocular fluid by lowering the osmolarity of the former or raising that of the latter, or by increasing the volume of the contents of the globe. A condition of established, long-standing glaucoma, however, is difficult to produce in experimental animals; it has only been accomplished by variations of two methods—the production of a permanent condition of vascular stasis and congestion, and a blockage of the circulation of the intra-ocular fluids. The resultant glaucoma is, of course, of the secondary type. The usual experimental animal has been the rabbit or monkey in which a condition somewhat akin to human buphthalmos can be produced provided a considerable rise of pressure has been maintained for a sufficient time (Fig. 562).

THE PRODUCTION OF CIRCULATORY STASIS

By ligating the vortex veins as they issue from the eye, intra-ocular pressures up to 80 or 90 mm. Hg can readily be produced.[1] The venous return from the eye has also been embarrassed by tying all the vessels at the posterior pole with the result that the ocular hypertension continued for several months (Huggert, 1957). Flocks and his co-workers (1959) produced a similar effect by encircling the eye with a tight rubber band situated at the equator and found the resulting decrease in the facility of aqueous outflow remained after the band was removed.

After ligating the anterior ciliary veins a similar acute glaucoma

[1] Adamük (1867), Leber (1873), Weber (1877), Schoeler (1879), v. Schultén (1884), Ulrich (1889), Koster (1895), v. Geuns (1899), Macri (1960), and others.

results (Bartels, 1905; Macri, 1960), and again the effect may last several months. Damage to the episcleral veins has given inconsistent results. Nikolaou (1963) failed to produce glaucoma by applying partially penetrating diathermo-coagulation behind the limbus in rabbits, while Huggert (1957) cauterized the episcleral veins and produced an ocular hypertension lasting from 2 to 20 days. The most successful technique has been that of Luntz (1962–66): he injected phenol subconjunctivally into all 4 quadrants of the rabbit's globe and produced a rise in ocular tension that persisted until the experiment was terminated; histological examination of the treated eyes demonstrated that the angle of the anterior chamber had remained open and that no inflammatory changes had been produced in the trabecular meshwork. A similar result is seen clinically in the secondary glaucoma following extensive corrosive burns of the sclera (Zade, 1909).

Obstruction to the venous return remote from the eye yields somewhat equivocal results possibly owing to the free venous anastomoses. This applies particularly to ligation of the jugular veins,[1] but ligation of the superior vena cava in the dog was found by Alfano (1965) to give rise to an increase in the ocular tension which returned to the normal level in a few minutes after the ligature was removed. When all the venous channels are successfully impeded, however, the rise in pressure is more marked, as on passing a ligature around the neck (Schulze, 1907; Wessely, 1908; Bonnefon, 1922), on compressing the thorax (Mazzei, 1919–20) or the abdomen (Comberg and Stoewer, 1926).

OBSTRUCTION TO THE CIRCULATION OF INTRA-OCULAR FLUID

The most usual method by which this has been achieved is by *obstructing the angle of the anterior chamber*. This has been done in several ways:

(i) By the injection of non-diffusible oils and colloids into the eye which embarrass the filtration channels mechanically and, if they are irritating in nature, intensify the obstruction by exciting an inflammatory reaction.[2] In some cases the rise in the intra-ocular pressure has been slight and transient, to some extent possibly because the formation of aqueous may have been inhibited by the hypertension itself in a physiological compensatory mechanism or by the pathological reaction to trauma. In other cases, however, the rise has been marked and prolonged; thus Langham (1959) found that the intra-ocular pressure rose to the height of the diastolic blood pressure in rabbits after the injection of mineral oil into the anterior chamber, while Kupfer (1961–62) implanted lengths of polythene tubing round the angle and thus obtained an intra-ocular pressure up to 50 or 60 mm. Hg for some months. Several experimenters on the owl monkey have produced

---

[1] Mimocky (1865), Adamük (1867), von Schultén (1884), Parsons (1903), Henderson and Starling (1904).

[2] Weber (1877), Heisrath (1879), Bentzen (1895), Geering (1896), Troncoso (1901–5), Schreiber and Wengler (1909), Seidel (1921), Voronina (1954), Huggert (1957–58), Peter *et al.* (1957), Samis (1962), Rohen (1963), Kalvin *et al.* (1966), Thomas (1968), and others.

acute attacks of glaucoma with ocular tensions rising above 90 mm. Hg by injecting alpha-chymotrypsin into the posterior chamber or the anterior vitreous followed by such substances as talcum powder, dental moulding cement or colloidal thorium dioxide (Kalvin *et al.*, 1966; Hamasaki and Fujino, 1967; Zimmerman *et al.*, 1967; Lampert *et al.*, 1968).[1]

(ii) By exciting an inflammatory reaction in the filtration angle with the ultimate production of synechiæ by punctures and scratches at the limbus (Bentzen, 1895) or cauterization (Schoeler, 1879; Bentzen, 1895; Kümmell, 1912; Lagrange, 1922). The hypertensive reaction produced in rabbits by nitrogen mustards instilled into the conjunctival sac (Davson and Huber, 1950; Wudka and Leopold, 1955) is probably also inflammatory in ætiology. The systemic administration of sanguinarine (Leach, 1955) and the intra-ocular injection of alpha-chymotrypsin alone (Hamasaki and Ellerman, 1965) are techniques which produce a rise of ocular tension in monkeys, the mechanisms of which are not yet understood.

(iii) By exciting a proliferative reaction of the endothelium at the filtration angle by the action of the electrolytic products of iron, either by introducing a steel needle as a positive pole into the anterior chamber, or by injecting therein the prepared electrolytic products (Erdmann, 1907; Schreiber and Wengler, 1909; Parisotti, 1911; Miyaki, 1923).

(iv) By blocking the outflow channels by applying the electro-cautery or diathermy to the aqueous-carrying vessels in the perilimbal region several experimenters have sought to produce a condition of glaucoma (Weekers and Prijot, 1950; Huggert, 1957; Gazala *et al.*, 1965); in some cases the rise in tension was evanescent and in others no hypertension resulted (Nikolaou, 1963).

(v) An experimental *obstruction at the pupil* was established by Rombolotti (1903) by the introduction of a celluloid disc; glaucoma supervened with a complicating iridocyclitis. Wortham (1952) inserted a grooved disc into the pupil, thus displacing the iris forwards; glaucoma resulted from mechanical obstruction of the angle of the anterior chamber which was also occluded by an inflammatory reaction

Adamük. *Zbl. med. Wiss.*, **5**, 433 (1867).
  Ann. Oculist. (Paris), **58**, 1 (1867).
Alfano. *Amer. J. Ophthal.*, **60**, 412 (1965).
Bartels. *Z. Augenheilk.*, **14**, 103, 258, 458 (1905).
Bentzen. *v. Graefes Arch. Ophthal.*, **41** (4), 42 (1895).
Bonnefon. *Ann. Oculist.* (Paris), **159**, 840 (1922).
Comberg and Stoewer. *Z. Augenheilk.*, **58**, 92 (1926).
Davson and Huber. *Brit. med. J.*, **1**, 939 (1950).
Erdmann. *v. Graefes Arch. Ophthal.*, **66**, 325, 391 (1907).

Flocks, Tsukahara and Miller. *Amer. J. Ophthal.*, **48** (2), 11 (1959).
Gazala, Geeraets and Guerry. *Amer. J. Ophthal.*, **60**, 247 (1965).
Geering. *Ueber d. Einfluss subkonjunktivaler Sublimat-Injektionen a. d. Verhalten d. vordern Kammerwinkels* (Diss.), Basel (1896).
von Geuns. *v. Graefes Arch. Ophthal.*, **47**, 249 (1899).
Hamasaki and Ellerman. *Arch. Ophthal.*, **73**, 843 (1965).
Hamasaki and Fujino. *Arch. Ophthal.*, **78**, 369 (1967).
Heisrath. *Zbl. med. Wiss.*, **17**, 769 (1879).

[1] p. 584.

Henderson and Starling. *J. Physiol.*, **31**, 305 (1904).

Huggert. *Acta ophthal.* (Kbh.), **35**, 1 (1957); **36**, 750 (1958).

Kalvin, Hamasaki and Gass. *Arch. Ophthal.*, **76**, 82, 94 (1966).

Koster. *v. Graefes Arch. Ophthal.*, **41** (2), 113; (4), 274 (1895).

Kümmell. *Arch. Augenheilk.*, **72**, 261 (1912).

Kupfer. *Arch. Ophthal.*, **65**, 565 (1961). *Invest. Ophthal.*, **1**, 474 (1962).

Lagrange. *Du glaucome et de l'hypotonie*, Paris (1922).

Lampert, Vogel and Zimmerman. *Invest. Ophthal.*, **7**, 199 (1968).

Langham. *J. Physiol.*, **147**, 29P (1959).

Leach. *Trans. ophthal. Soc. U.K.*, **75**, 425 (1955).

Leber. *v. Graefes Arch. Ophthal.*, **19** (2), 87 (1873).

Luntz. *Trans. ophthal. Soc. U.K.*, **82**, 271 (1962). *Amer. J. Ophthal.*, **61**, 665 (1966).

Macri. *Arch. Ophthal.*, **63**, 953 (1960); **65**, 571 (1961).

Mazzei. *Arch. Ottal.*, **26**, 163 (1919); **27**, 83 (1920).

Mimocky. *v. Graefes Arch. Ophthal.*, **11** (2), 84 (1865).

Miyaki. *Jap. ophthal. Cong.*, Kioto (1922). See *Zbl. ges. Ophthal.*, **9**, 87 (1923).

Nikolaou. *Bull. Soc. franç. Ophtal.*, **76**, 604 (1963).

Parisotti. *Bull. Soc. franç. Ophtal.*, **28**, 340 (1911).

Parsons. *The Ocular Circulation*, London (1903).

Peter, Lyda and Krishna. *Amer. J. Ophthal.*, **44** (2), 198 (1957).

Rohen. *Arch. Ophthal.*, **69**, 335 (1963).

Rombolotti. *Arch. Augenheilk.*, **46**, 297 (1903).

Samis. *Amer. J. Ophthal.*, **54**, 1089 (1962).

Schoeler. *v. Graefes Arch. Ophthal.*, **25** (4), 63 (1879).

Schreiber and Wengler. *v. Graefes Arch. Ophthal.*, **71**, 99 (1909).

von Schultén. *v. Graefes Arch. Ophthal.*, **30** (3), 1 (1884).

Schulze. *Z. Augenheilk.*, **17**, 222 (1907).

Seidel. *v. Graefes Arch. Ophthal.*, **104**, 357 (1921).

Thomas. *Amer. J. Ophthal.*, **65**, 729 (1968).

Troncoso. *Ann. Oculist.* (Paris), **126**, 401 (1901); **133**, 5 (1905).

Ulrich. *Arch. Augenheilk.*, **20**, 270 (1889).

Voronina. *Biull. eksp. biol. med.*, **37**, 30 (1954).

Weber. *v. Graefes Arch. Ophthal.*, **23** (1), 1 (1877).

Weekers and Prijot. *Ophthalmologica*, **119**, 321 (1950).

Wessely. *Arch. Augenheilk.*, **60**, 1, 97 (1908).

Wortham. *Amer. J. Ophthal.*, **35**, 477 (1952).

Wudka and Leopold. *Arch. Ophthal.*, **53**, 487 (1955).

Zade. *v. Graefes Arch. Ophthal.*, **72**, 507 (1909).

Zimmerman, de Venecia and Hamasaki. *Invest. Ophthal.*, **6**, 109 (1967).

Glaucoma Secondary to Developmental Deformities

Many developmental anomalies are complicated by a secondary glaucoma which in all cases is essentially based on structural deformations in the angle of the anterior chamber resulting in an obstructive rise in the ocular tension. All have been described in a previous Volume of this *System*[1] so that for purposes of reference a short note is all that is required here.

BUPHTHALMOS

This relatively common condition, its clinical features, symptoms, diagnosis and treatment, have already been studied[2] when it was pointed out that the essential cause was a congenital dysplasia of the tissues of the irido-corneal angle (Fig. 599; Plate VII, Fig. 1). It may become evident at birth, in early childhood or a raised tension may appear later in life when it is known as JUVENILE GLAUCOMA. The same clinical picture arises whether the hypertension is due to an isolated congenital anomaly (simple buphthalmos), or is associated with other anomalies in the globe or elsewhere (associated buphthalmos), or is secondary to foetal or infantile inflammation

---

[1] Vol. III.   [2] Vol. III, p. 548.

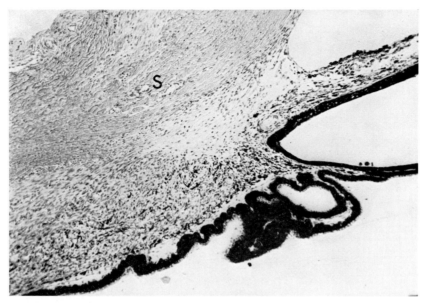

Fig. 599.—Buphthalmos.

The angle of the anterior chamber showing incomplete cleavage and forward attachment of the meridional ciliary fibres onto the trabecular face. S indicates the canal of Schlemm (M. J. Reeh).

such as that arising from inherited syphilis or maternal rubella, or to neoplasic processes (secondary buphthalmos).

GLAUCOMA WITH OCULAR ANOMALIES

In ANTERIOR MICROPHTHALMOS (MICROCORNEA)[1] and CORNEA PLANA,[2] an obstructive glaucoma may result as a sequel to the smallness and impaired development of the anterior segment (Friede, 1921–39; Sweet, 1924; Barkan and Borley, 1936; François and Neetens, 1955; Meyer-Schwickerath and Grüterich, 1957).

ANIRIDIA

We have already seen that a recalcitrant buphthalmos or juvenile glaucoma develops in about 30% of cases of aniridia.[3] In some instances the rudimentary iris is adherent to the posterior surface of the cornea (Treacher Collins, 1891; Callahan, 1949), while in others the angle of the anterior chamber is found on gonioscopic examination to be filled with mesodermal tissue (Figs. 600–1). The raised tension should, if possible, be controlled by medical means as surgical treatment is unsatisfactory in most cases. Barkan (1953), however, found that goniotomy was sometimes effective if performed early, before the canal of Schlemm had become obliterated.

[1] Vol. III, p. 503.   [2] Vol. III, p. 505.   [3] Vol. III, p. 567.

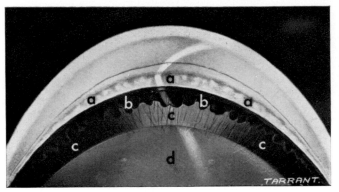

FIG. 600.—ANIRIDIA.

Gonioscopic view showing the mesodermal tissue filling the angle of the anterior chamber, *a*; a small stump of iris behind which are the ciliary processes, *b*; the exposed zonular fibres, *c*; and a cataractous lens, *d* (H. E. Hobbs, Inst. Ophthal.).

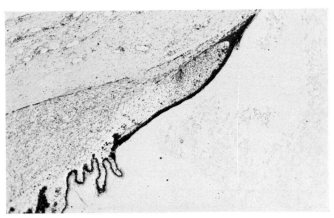

FIG. 601.—ANIRIDIA.

The rudimentary iris is adherent to the trabeculæ and the peripheral cornea, completely obliterating the angle of the anterior chamber (M. J. Hogan and L. E. Zimmerman, *Atlas of Ophthalmic Pathology*, Saunders, Philadelphia).

AXENFELD'S AND RIEGER'S ANOMALIES

Posterior embryotoxon, an accentuation of the ring of Schwalbe, is present in 15 to 30% of individuals and usually occurs as an isolated anomaly in an otherwise normal eye. It may be associated with pectinate strands running from the anterior surface of the iris across the angle of the anterior chamber to find insertion into the line of Schwalbe (*Axenfeld's anomaly*)[1] and is occasionally part of a more extensive mesodermal dysgenesis of the anterior segment (*Rieger's anomaly*)[2] where there is faulty differentiation of the angle of the anterior chamber. Posterior embryotoxon and Axenfeld's and Rieger's anomalies appear, therefore, to present a continuous spectrum

[1] Vol. III, p. 521.   [2] Vol. III, p. 543.

of congenital abnormalities of the angle of the anterior chamber, each increasing in severity. Although Streiff (1949) considered that posterior embryotoxon may predispose to glaucoma, it is in the more grossly abnormal

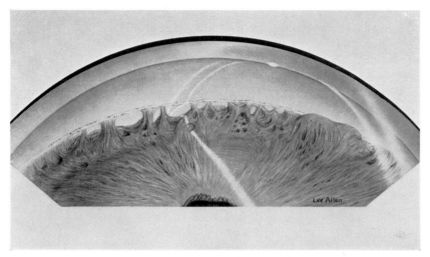

FIG. 602.—AXENFELD'S ANOMALY.

The lower quadrant of the eye, showing massive iris processes adhering to a prominent Schwalbe's ring. Note that the corneal wedge disappears behind the tissues of the iris (H. M. Burian, A. E. Braley and L. Allen).

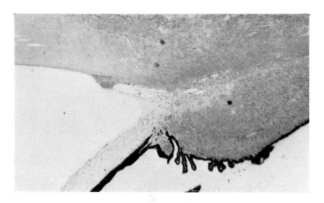

FIG. 603.—AXENFELD'S ANOMALY.

The trabeculæ are inserted directly into the prominent border ring of Schwalbe (H. S. Sugar).

Axenfeld's and Rieger's anomalies that buphthalmos and juvenile glaucoma are particularly liable to develop (Fig. 602).

Glaucoma is said to occur in about one-half of the cases of Axenfeld's anomaly (Bartolozzi et al., 1964) and several authors, including Burian et al. (1954) and Sugar (1965), have reported such an association. Glaucoma is also frequently seen in Rieger's anomaly[1] appearing most commonly in the 2nd and 3rd decades, and its occurrence is evidently related to the degree of abnormality present in the angle of the anterior chamber. In addition to the pectinate strands that are invariably present, mesodermal tissue may fill the angle (Fig. 603).

These cases of glaucoma should be managed in the same way as buphthalmos or simple glaucoma, depending upon the age of the patient.

DIFFUSE NEUROFIBROMATOSIS (*von Recklinghausen's Disease*)

We have already mentioned[2] the relatively common association of buphthalmos with diffuse neurofibromatosis, an association which is particularly liable to occur if a plexiform neuroma of the eyelid is present indicating intra-ocular involvement (50%, Birch-Hirschfeld, 1930). Anderson (1939) believed that buphthalmos occurred only when the upper lid was affected, but several cases have been reported of the presence of the condition at birth without any discernible involvement of the eyelid (Wheeler, 1937;

FIGS. 604 and 605.—NEUROFIBROMATOSIS (J. R. Wolter *et al.*).

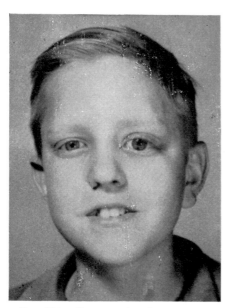 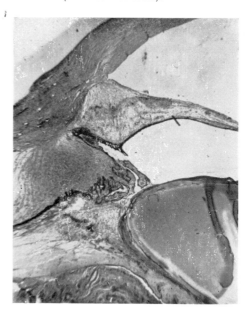

FIG. 604.—Occurring in a boy, showing a plexiform neuroma extending from the upper lid to the left temple. The left eye is buphthalmic.

FIG. 605.—To show the involvement of the iris and ciliary body with closure of the angle of the anterior chamber and a fibrous membrane over the retina and surrounding the cataractous lens.

[1] Seefelder and Wolfrum (1906), Waardenburg (1932), Gasteiger (1937), Braendstrup (1948), Falls (1949), Streiff (1949), Sakic (1952), Callahan (1956), Henkind *et al.* (1965), Rivara (1965), Pearce and Kerr (1965), Breebaart (1966), and others.
[2] Vol. IX, p. 823.

PLATE VII

DEVELOPMENTAL GLAUCOMA (A. Lister, Inst. Ophthal.)

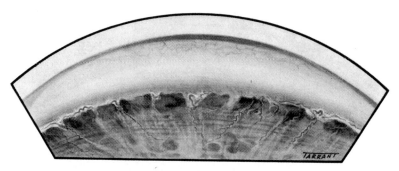

FIG. 1.—THE ANGLE OF THE ANTERIOR CHAMBER IN BUPHTHALMOS.

FIGS. 2 and 3.—DIFFUSE NEUROFIBROMATOSIS.

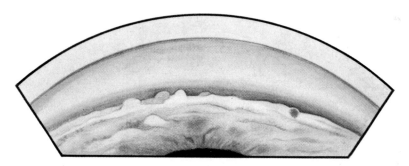

FIG. 2.—Showing nodules at the angle of the anterior chamber.

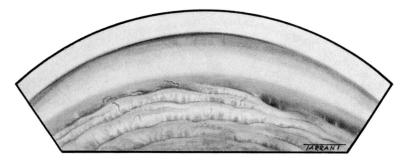

FIG. 3.—Partial closure of the angle of the anterior chamber.

PLATE VIII

The Sturge-Weber Syndrome (A. Lister, Inst. Ophthal.)

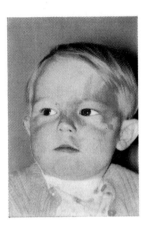

Fig. 1.—The Typical Appearance with Involvement of the Upper Lid and Buphthalmos.

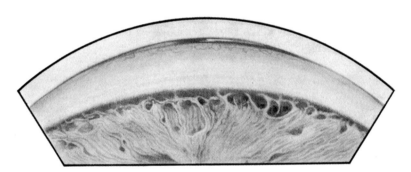

Fig. 2.—The Angle of the Anterior Chamber showing Vascularized Mesodermal Tissue.

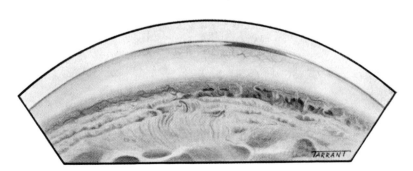

Fig. 3.—The Angle of the Anterior Chamber showing Partial Closure.

Lascu *et al.*, 1963; Grant and Walton, 1968). It is relevant to mention here the observation of François and his co-workers (1955) that the association of buphthalmos, involvement of the eyelid and facial hemi-hypertrophy is diagnostic of neurofibromatosis. In most of the reported cases that have been examined histologically the choroid has been densely infiltrated with the typical cells of Schwann (Fig. 604–5),[1] but choroidal involvement is not invariably associated with buphthalmos (Snell and Collins, 1903); in a few cases an adult glaucoma has resulted (Meeker, 1936; Noto, 1949), while occasionally a raised tension has never developed (Freeman, 1934). Glaucoma may also occur with ectropion uveæ, whether it be congenital (Hosford, 1908; Reis, 1909) or acquired (Wolter and Butler, 1963).

The aetiology of this glaucoma in most cases is ill-understood. It has been suggested that some cases result from a failure in development of the angle of the anterior chamber (Snell and Collins, 1903; Hogan and Zimmerman, 1962; Friedman and Ritchie, 1963), that others are due to infiltration of the angle itself by neurofibromatous tissue, while others appear to depend on the formation of peripheral anterior synechiæ, possibly due to the forward displacement of the uveal tract as a result of its infiltration by neoplasic cells (Davis, 1939) (Plate VII, Figs. 2 and 3). A case in which the angle in the greater part of its circumference was completely blanketed by a layer of dense abnormal tissue, presumably neurofibromatous in nature, was reported by Grant and Walton (1968).

As with other forms of buphthalmos, the treatment is surgical, but despite this many cases end in blindness and enucleation has become necessary, while intracranial extension is always a possibility that should be remembered (Bracher, 1967).

ENCEPHALO-(OCULO)-FACIAL ANGIOMATOSIS (*the Sturge-Weber Syndrome*)

An association of glaucoma with a capillary nævus affecting the skin of the face (nævus flammeus)[2] was first observed by Schirmer (1860) and since then several hundred cases have appeared in the literature; most of these have been summarized by Larmande (1948), Danis (1950) and Alexander and Norman (1960). The association occurs in about 30% of cases (73 out of 257—Alexander and Norman, 1960) and is sufficiently common to suggest a relationship of cause and effect. It occurs when the facial nævus involves the lids and usually some of the ocular structures; thus Anderson (1939) observed that glaucoma did not occur in the presence of normal adnexæ. In the vast majority of cases the condition is unilateral; bilateral cases are rare and may occur when the nævus is widespread,

---

[1] Sachsalber (1898), Snell and Collins (1903), Collins and Batten (1905), Sutherland and Mayou (1907), Weinstein (1909), Murakami (1913), Wiener (1925), Wheeler (1937), Davis (1939), Oravisto (1949), François and Katz (1961), Wolter *et al.* (1962), Friedman and Ritchey (1963), and others.
[2] Vol. III, p. 1120.

affecting also the pharynx and nasal mucosa and sometimes the limbs and trunk (Beltman, 1904; Safar, 1923; Knapp, 1928; Djacos, 1951; Pietruschka, 1960; and others) (Plate VIII).

Although the angiomatous condition is invariably congenital, buphthalmos occurs only in between half and two-thirds of the cases of glaucoma (Danis, 1950—84 cases of buphthalmos and 90 of glaucoma without enlargement of the globe; Alexander and Norman, 1960—48 cases of buphthalmos and 25 of glaucoma); the remaining cases develop a raised ocular tension in adolescence or adult life, although the onset of glaucoma late in life is uncommon.[1] Such a condition is similar to simple glaucoma in its clinical

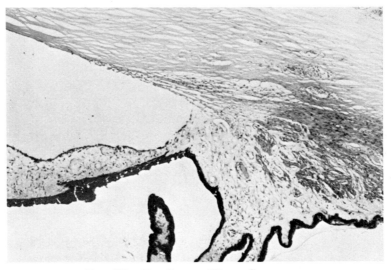

FIG. 606.—THE STURGE–WEBER SYNDROME.
The angle of the anterior chamber, showing the anomalous insertion of the root of the iris (J. W. Berkow).

features, associated with a characteristically deeply cupped and atrophic disc, inducing typical field defects and frequently progressing to complete blindness. This result, however, is by no means invariable, and the visual acuity and fields may remain normal for an indefinite period even although the tension is raised (Vogele, 1928), while in other cases the condition appears to become arrested (O'Brien and Porter, 1933). Other changes which may occur in the eye include a dilatation of the vessels of the conjunctiva, sclera and iris, heterochromia, hyperplasia of the iris, and very frequently a choroidal angioma and tortuous and dilated retinal vessels.

Pathological examinations have been reported on a number of occasions

[1] Salus (1923), Zvereva (1927), Yamanaka (1927), Vagts (1937), Pincus (1939), and others.

(Fig. 606). A choroidal angioma has been found in about 40% of the eyes which have been examined histologically even although the tumour may not have been ophthalmoscopically visible (Danis and van Bogaert, 1951), and anomalies in the angle of the anterior chamber have also been described (Safar, 1934; Anderson, 1939; Sedláček and Vrabec, 1961; and others). In a review of the literature François (1951) found that of 21 cases with glaucoma, 18 had an angioma of the choroid, 2 showed vascular abnormalities of the iris and only 1 case failed to show any vascular anomaly in the uveal tract. In 4 out of 5 of Anderson's (1939) cases with glaucoma examined histologically, anomalies of the angle were noted.

An interesting feature of these cases is a co-existent angiomatous condition of the meninges, an association suggested by Sturge (1879) and Horrocks (1883), confirmed at autopsy by Kalischer (1897) and at operation by Cushing (1906). Evidence of intracranial angiomata or tortuous or calcified diploic vessels has also been brought forward on many occasions by x-ray examination,[2] or by the occurrence of a spastic hemiplegia or epileptiform convulsions (Horrocks, 1883; von Rötth, 1928; Aynsley, 1929; Weber, 1929). This association of facial and meningeal angiomatous changes probably has an embryological explanation.[3]

The cause of the glaucoma is disputed. The very frequent occurrence of choroidal angiomata has suggested that increased permeability of the uveal vessels may be partly responsible for the raised tension (the "plethoric glaucoma" of Elschnig, 1918) (Nakamura, 1922; Tyson, 1932; Mehney, 1937; Joy, 1949), and tonographic studies (Mansheim, 1953; Miller, 1963) have seemed to support a hypersecretory aetiology. On the other hand, choroidal angiomata are frequently linked with structural anomalies in the anterior segment (Safar, 1923), and several authors have described the gonioscopic appearance of an angle containing abnormal mesodermal tissue (Barkan, 1954–57; Berkow, 1966); Lister (1966) has stressed the variable appearance of the angle in this condition. Occasionally, vascular malformations have been present in the iris (François, 1951; Ara et al., 1966) and these may be responsible for occluding the angle of the anterior chamber. In the present state of our knowledge it is impossible to say which mechanism, if there is but one, is responsible for the glaucoma, although the balance of recent evidence is in favour of a structural abnormality of the angle of the anterior chamber (Plate VIII, Figs. 2 and 3).

The treatment of the buphthalmos is surgical and, although an expulsive hæmorrhage is a possibility, such intervention may successfully control the

[1] Milles (1884), Lawford (1885), Snell (1886), Wagenmann (1900), Stoewer (1908), Quackenboss and Verhoeff (1908), Love (1914), Safar (1923), Knapp (1928), Clausen (1928), de Haas (1928), Weber (1929), Ballantyne (1930–40), Jahnke (1931), Dunphy (1935), Anderson (1939), J. J. and P. J. Evans (1939), Danis and van Bogaert (1951), Sedláček and Vrabec (1961), and many others.
[2] Brushfield and Wyatt (1927), von Rötth (1928), Aynsley (1929), Weber (1929), Hudelo (1929), Jahnke (1931), Tyson (1932), O'Brien and Porter (1933), and many others.
[3] Vol. III, p. 1122.

tension (Dunphy, 1935). Barkan (1954–57) was able to do so in 2 eyes by repeated goniotomies, although Lister (1966) has found this procedure unsuccessful. For juvenile and adult glaucomas, cyclodiathermy is probably the safest procedure (Miller, 1963).

GLAUCOMA SECONDARY TO SYSTEMIC SYNDROMES

It is convenient at this point to review the association of buphthalmos with a number of systemic syndromes, the ocular manifestations of which have been discussed in previous Volumes.

A secondary glaucoma is a frequent accompaniment of the group of syndromes characterized, among other changes, by ECTOPIA LENTIS. We

FIGS. 607 AND 608.—THE MARFAN SYNDROME (M. J. Reeh and W. L. Lehman).

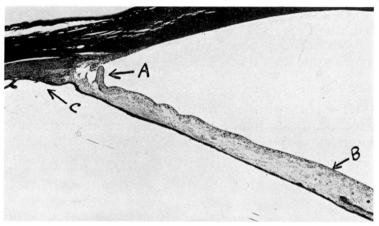

FIG. 607.—Strands of the iris crossing the filtration angle (A). The iris shows a lack of crypts and collarette with an endothelial membrane on the anterior surface (B). The ciliary body is small and flat with few circular muscle fibres (C).

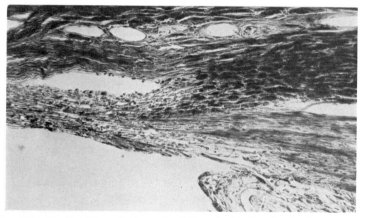

FIG. 608.—Section through the angle of the anterior chamber in the same case.

shall presently discuss the raised ocular tension consequent upon anterior dislocation and subluxation of the lens, and that resulting less frequently from a phacolytic glaucoma or a phaco-anaphylactic endophthalmitis when the lens is dislocated posteriorly. There remains a number of these cases wherein the glaucoma, sometimes buphthalmic in type, is due to a congenital malformation of the angle of the anterior chamber.

In the MARFAN SYNDROME[1] persistent mesodermal tissue in the angle of the anterior chamber and dense pectinate remnants are common findings (Figs. 607–8)[2] and there may be irregularities in the size, shape and position of the canal of Schlemm (Burian and Allen, 1961; Wachtel, 1966). Similar malformations of the angle may occur in the MARCHESANI SYNDROME[3] (Duque Estrada, 1961) (Fig. 609).

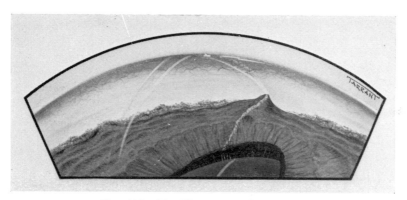

FIG. 609.—THE MARCHESANI SYNDROME.
There is a subluxated lens and the formation of peripheral anterior synechiæ, in a woman aged 21 (Inst. Ophthal.).

There remains a heterogeneous group of multiple syndromes in which buphthalmos has been reported, in some as a common finding, in others exceptionally. In the OCULO-CEREBRO-RENAL SYNDROME of Lowe[4] buphthalmos occurs in about half the cases (28 out of 55, Haut and Joannides, 1966). There are few reports of the appearance either gonioscopic or histological of the angle of the anterior chamber in this syndrome, partly because of the frequent occurrence of corneal opacities, and partly because of the paucity of histological material, but this region is usually said to be normal (Fisher et al., 1967). Curtin and his colleagues (1967), however, described the histological appearances in two patients; in both, the angles of the anterior chambers were incompletely developed with the insertion of the longitudinal part of the ciliary muscle into the trabecular meshwork

---

[1] Vol. III, p. 1102.
[2] Theobald (1941), Reeh and Lehman (1954), Burian (1958), Burian et al. (1960), Burian and Allen (1961).
[3] Vol. III, p. 1107.   [4] p. 193.

(Fig. 610). The literature has been reviewed on several occasions, notably by Chutorian and Rowland (1966, 46 cases) and by Haut and Joannides (1966, 55 cases). It is relevant to note here that in uncomplicated buphthalmos an abnormal amino-aciduria was found in 50% of males and 30% of females (Franceschetti, 1962); the significance of this observation and its possible relationship with Lowe's syndrome is unknown but has already been discussed.[1]

Buphthalmos is an occasional finding in the PIERRE-ROBIN SYNDROME[2] (Lawton Smith *et al.*, 1960–61; Saraux *et al.*, 1963; Ortlepp and Brandt,

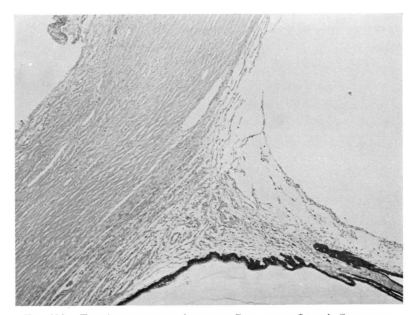

FIG. 610.—THE ANGLE OF THE ANTERIOR CHAMBER IN LOWE'S SYNDROME.

The angle is incompletely cleaved. Iris tissue is attached to the trabecular meshwork. Schlemm's canal is well defined. The longitudinal muscle of the ciliary body extends beyond the scleral spur to attach to the trabecular meshwork. The ciliary processes arise from the posterior surface of the iris and are pulled towards the lens by the zonule (H. & E.) (L. E. Zimmerman and V. T. Curtin).

1966). In the 39 cases reported by Lawton Smith and Stowe (1961), 15 of which were examined ophthalmoscopically, buphthalmos was present only in one. It also occasionally occurs in OCULO-DENTO-DIGITAL DYSPLASIA[3] (Meyer-Schwickerath *et al.*, 1957) being associated with microphthalmos and anomalies of the iris, and in MUCOPOLYSACCHARIDOSIS I (*the Hurler syndrome*)[4] (Déjean *et al.*, 1958; Stergar, 1964). The anomaly has also been reported in a few cases of the TURNER SYNDROME (Laurent *et al.*, 1961;

[1] p. 192. [2] Vol. III, p. 1025.
[3] Vol. III, p. 1115. [4] Vol. VIII, p. 1071.

Khodadoust and Paton, 1967), TRISOMY D (13–15) (Keith, 1966; Snodgrass *et al.*, 1966) (Fig. 611), and in one case of TRISOMY F (17–18) (Townes *et al.*, 1962).[1]

The treatment of these various forms of complicated buphthalmos is similar to that of the uncomplicated condition. Medical therapy is only of limited value and the surgical procedures of choice are goniotomy and gonio-puncture. Even so, the prognosis in many cases is poor, particularly

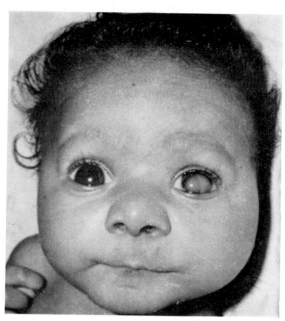

FIG. 611.—BUPHTHALMOS DUE TO TRISOMY 13–15.
With asymmetry of the face, and corneal opacities in the left eye (C. G. Keith).

if the malformation of the angle is severe. The best results appear to occur in those cases wherein the outflow of aqueous is obstructed by mesodermal remnants in the angle of the anterior chamber.

It is important, however, to appreciate the existence of buphthalmos in these various systemic syndromes, not only because an early diagnosis of the raised tension gives the best chance of successful treatment, but also because the presence of ocular malformations may shed some light on the basic ætiology of the primary condition. Unfortunately, few cases have been available for histological investigation at an early stage, but in most so far examined the typical pathological picture of buphthalmos has been found.

[1] Vol. III, p. 341.

Alexander and Norman. *The Sturge-Weber Syndrome*, Bristol (1960).

Anderson. *Hydrophthalmia or Congenital Glaucoma*, Cambridge (1939).

Ara, Sözen and Menderes. *Ankara Hast. Derg.*, **1**, 331 (1966).

Aynsley. *Brit. J. Ophthal.*, **13**, 612 (1929).

Ballantyne. *Brit. J. Ophthal.*, **14**, 481 (1930); **24**, 65 (1940).

Barkan. *Arch. Ophthal.*, **49**, 1 (1953). *Acta XVII int. Cong. Ophthal.*, Montreal-N.Y., **2**, 1101 (1954). *Amer. J. Ophthal.*, **43**, 545 (1957).

Barkan and Borley. *Amer. J. Ophthal.*, **19**, 307 (1936).

Bartolozzi, Franco and Hernández Gómez. *Arch. Soc. oftal. hisp.-amer.*, **24**, 465 (1964).

Beltman. *v. Graefes Arch. Ophthal.*, **59**, 502 (1904).

Berkow. *Arch. Ophthal.*, **75**, 72 (1966).

Birch-Hirschfeld. *Graefe-Saemisch Hb. d. ges. Augenheilk.*, 2nd ed., Berlin, **9**, (1), 491 (1930).

Bracher. *v. Graefes Arch. Ophthal.*, **173**, 351 (1967).

Braendstrup. *Acta ophthal.* (Kbh.), **26**, 495 (1948).

Breebaart. *Arch. Ophthal.*, **76**, 825 (1966).

Brushfield and Wyatt. *Brit. J. Child. Dis.*, **24**, 98, 2094 (1927).

Burian. *Missouri Med.*, **55**, 1088 (1958).

Burian and Allen. *Arch. Ophthal.*, **65**, 323 (1961).

Burian, Braley and Allen. *Trans. Amer. ophthal. Soc.*, **52**, 389 (1954).

Burian, von Noorden and Ponseti. *Arch. Ophthal.*, **64**, 671 (1960).

Callahan. *Amer. J. Ophthal.*, **32** (2), 28 (1949); **41**, 745 (1956).

Chutorian and Rowland. *Neurology* (Minneap.), **16**, 115 (1966).

Clausen. *Klin. Mbl. Augenheilk.*, **81**, 393 (1928).

Collins. *Ophthal. Rev.*, **10**, 101 (1891).

Collins and Batten. *Trans. ophthal. Soc. U.K.*, **25**, 248 (1905).

Curtin, Joyce and Ballin. *Amer. J. Ophthal.*, **64**, 533 (1967).

Cushing. *J. Amer. med. Ass.*, **47**, 178 (1906).

Danis. *Acta neurol. psychiat. belge*, **50**, 615 (1950).

Danis and van Bogaert. *Acta neurol. psychiat. belge*, **51**, 74 (1951).

Davis. *Arch. Ophthal.*, **22**, 761 (1939).

Déjean, Viallefont, Boudet and Boulad. *Rev. Oto-neuro-ophtal.*, **30**, 368 (1958).

Djacos. *Bull. Soc. hellén. Ophtal.*, **19**, 34 (1951).

Dunphy. *Amer. J. Ophthal.*, **18**, 709 (1935).

Duque Estrada. *Bull. Soc. franç. Ophtal.*, **74**, 729 (1961).

Elschnig. *Z. Augenheilk.*, **39**, 189 (1918).

Evans, J. J. and P. J. *Brit. J. Ophthal.*, **23**, 95 (1939).

Falls. *Amer. J. Ophthal.*, **32** (2), 41 (1949).

Fisher, Hallett and Carpenter. *Arch. Ophthal.*, **77**, 642 (1967).

Franceschetti. *Bull. schweiz. Akad. med. Wiss.*, **17**, 414 (1962).

François. *Acta neurol. psychiat. belge*, **51**, 521 (1951).

François, Haustrate and Philips. *Bull. Soc. belge Ophtal.*, No. 108, 625 (1955).

François and Katz. *Ophthalmologica*, **142**, 549 (1961).

François and Neetens. *Acta Genet. med.* (Roma), **4**, 217 (1955).

Freeman. *Arch. Ophthal.*, **11**, 641 (1934).

Friede. *Klin. Mbl. Augenheilk.*, **67**, 192 (1921); **79**, 464 (1927); **102**, 16 (1939).

Friedman and Ritchey. *Arch. Ophthal.*, **70**, 294 (1963).

Gasteiger. *Klin. Mbl. Augenheilk.*, **99**, 36 (1937).

Grant and Walton. *Arch. Ophthal.*, **79**, 127 (1968).

de Haas. *Ned. T. Geneesk.*, **72**, 4326 (1928).

Haut and Joannides. *Arch. Ophtal.*, **26**, 21 (1966).

Henkind, Siegel and Carr. *Arch. Ophthal.*, **73**, 810 (1965).

Hogan and Zimmerman. *Ophthalmic Pathology Atlas and Textbook*, Phila., 443 (1962).

Horrocks. *Trans. ophthal. Soc. U.K.*, **3**, 106 (1883).

Hosford. *Trans. ophthal. Soc. U.K.*, **28**, 152 (1908).

Hudelo. *Ann. Oculist.* (Paris), **166**, 889 (1929).

Jahnke. *Z. Augenheilk.*, **74**, 165 (1931).

Joy. *Trans. Amer. ophthal. Soc.*, **47**, 93 (1949).

Kalischer. *Berl. klin. Wschr.*, **34**, 1059 (1897).

Keith. *Trans. ophthal. Soc. U.K.*, **86**, 435 (1966).

Khodadoust and Paton. *Arch. Ophthal.*, **77**, 630 (1967).

Knapp. *Arch. Ophthal.*, **57**, 219 (1928).

Larmande. *La neuro-angiomatose encéphalofaciale*, Paris (1948).

Lascu, Niculescu, Oprescu and Hagiopol. *Oftalmologia* (Buc.), **7**, 15 (1963).

Laurent, Royer and Noel. *Bull. Soc. Ophtal. Fr.*, 367 (1961).

Lawford. *Trans. ophthal. Soc. U.K.*, **5**, 136 (1885).

Lister. *Trans. ophthal. Soc. U.K.*, **86**, 5 (1966).

Love. *Arch. Ophthal.*, **43**, 607 (1914).

Mansheim. *Arch. Ophthal.*, **50**, 580 (1953).

Meeker. *Arch. Ophthal.*, **16**, 152 (1936).

Mehney. *Arch. Ophthal.*, **17**, 1018 (1937).

Meyer-Schwickerath and Grüterich. *Acta genet.* (Basel), **7**, 277 (1957).

Miller. *Proc. roy. Soc. Med.*, **56**, 419 (1963).

Milles. *Trans. ophthal. Soc. U.K.*, **4**, 168 (1884).

Murakami. *Klin. Mbl. Augenheilk.*, **51** (2), 514 (1913).

Nakamura. *Klin. Mbl. Augenheilk.*, **69**, 312 (1922).

Noto. *G. ital. Oftal.*, **2**, 137 (1949).

O'Brien and Porter. *Arch. Ophthal.*, **9**, 715 (1933).

Oravisto. *Acta ophthal.* (Kbh.), **27**, 89 (1949).

Ortlepp and Brandt. *Klin. Mbl. Augenheilk.*, **148**, 46 (1966).

Pearce and Kerr. *Brit. J. Ophthal.*, **49**, 530 (1965).

Pietruschka. *Klin. Mbl. Augenheilk.*, **137**, 545 (1960).

Pincus. *Arch. Ophthal.*, **21**, 741 (1939).

Quackenboss and Verhoeff. *Trans. Amer. ophthal. Soc.*, **11**, 510 (1908).

Reeh and Lehman. *Trans. Amer. Acad. Ophthal.*, **58**, 212 (1954).

Reis. *Z. Augenheilk.*, **22**, 499 (1909).

Rivara. *Minerva oftal.*, **7**, 15 (1965).

von Rötth. *Klin. Mbl. Augenheilk.*, **80**, 405 (1928).

Sachsalber. *Beitr. Augenheilk.*, **3**, 523 (1898).

Safar. *Z. Augenheilk.*, **51**, 301 (1923).

Sakic. *Ophthalmologica*, **123**, 31 (1952).

Salus. *Klin. Mbl. Augenheilk.*, **71**, 305 (1923).

Saraux, Laplane, Delaitre and Testard. *Bull. Soc. Ophtal. Fr.*, **63**, 465 (1963).

Schirmer. *v. Graefes Arch. Ophthal.*, **7** (1), 119 (1860).

Sedlácek and Vrabec. *Cs. Oftal.*, **17**, 232 (1961).

Seefelder and Wolfrum. *v. Graefes Arch. Ophthal.*, **63**, 430 (1906).

Smith, J. L., Cavanaugh and Stowe. *Arch. Ophthal.*, **63**, 984 (1960).

Smith, J. L. and Stowe. *Pediatrics*, **27**, 128 (1961).

Snell. *Brit. med. J.*, **2**, 68 (1886).

Snell and Collins. *Trans. ophthal. Soc. U.K.*, **23**, 157 (1903).

Snodgrass, Butler, France *et al.* *Arch. Dis. Childh.*, **41**, 250 (1966).

Stergar. *Ann. Oculist.* (Paris), **197**, 1134 (1964).

Stoewer. *Klin. Mbl. Augenheilk.*, **46** (2), 323 (1908).

Streiff. *Ophthalmologica*, **118**, 815 (1949).

Sturge. *Trans. clin. Soc. Lond.*, **12**, 162 (1879).

Sugar. *Amer. J. Ophthal.*, **59**, 1012 (1965).

Sutherland and Mayou. *Trans. ophthal. Soc. U.K.*, **27**, 179 (1907).

Sweet. *Amer. J. Ophthal.*, **7**, 437 (1921).

Theobald. *Amer. J. Ophthal.*, **24**, 1132 (1941).

Townes, Manning and DeHart. *J. Pediat.*, **61**, 755 (1962).

Tyson. *Arch. Ophthal.*, **8**, 365 (1932).

Vagts. *Nævus flammeus und Glaukom* (Diss.), Kiel (1937).

Vögele. *Klin. Mbl. Augenheilk.*, **81**, 393 (1928).

Waardenburg. *Das mensch. Auge u. seine Erbanlagen*, Haag, 331 (1932).

Wachtel. *Arch. Ophthal.*, **76**, 512 (1966).

Wagenmann. *v. Graefes Arch. Ophthal.*, **51**, 532 (1900).

Weber. *Proc. roy. Soc. Med.*, **22**, 431 (1929).

Weinstein. *Klin. Mbl. Augenheilk.*, **47** (2), 577 (1909).

Wheeler. *Amer. J. Ophthal.*, **20**, 368 (1937).

Wiener. *Arch. Ophthal.*, **54**, 481 (1925).

Wolter and Butler. *Amer. J. Ophthal.*, **56**, 964 (1963).

Wolter, Gonzales-Sirit and Mankin. *Amer. J. Ophthal.*, **54**, 217 (1962).

Yamanaka. *Klin. Mbl. Augenheilk.*, **78**, 372 (1927).

Zvereva. *Trudy II Moskovsk. Univ.*, **1**, 159 (1927). See *Zbl. ges. Ophthal.*, **20**, 847 (1929).

Glaucoma Secondary to Intra-ocular Inflammations

We have already discussed at length the fact that a raised ocular tension is not an uncommon, and too frequently a formidable complication of intra-ocular inflammations of all types, most typically of an anterior uveitis,[1] less commonly of posterior uveitis, and frequently of a keratitis and a scleritis.[2] From an ætiological point of view it is convenient to divide such cases into two categories, the first in which the raised tension occurs as a complication of the inflammatory process itself (HYPERTENSIVE UVEITIS), and the second wherein the complication results from structural changes produced by the inflammation (POST-INFLAMMATORY OBSTRUCTIVE GLAU-COMA); the induction of glaucoma by the treatment of the uveitis is discussed at a later stage as IATROGENIC GLAUCOMA.[3]

[1] Vol. IX, Chap. III.   [2] Vol. VIII, Chaps. VI and VIII.
[3] p. 699.

From the clinical point of view hypertensive uveitis may be divided into two types depending on whether the tension complicates an acute anterior uveitis or a more chronic cyclitis; in the first the symptoms of inflammation dominate the picture in which the raised tension is obviously secondary, while in the second the glaucomatous symptoms may occur with evidences of inflammation so slight that their inflammatory origin frequently escapes notice.

(i) ACUTE ANTERIOR UVEITIS

In an acute anterior uveitis the ocular tension rises a few days after the onset of the illness when the picture of the inflammatory reaction, frequently characterized by a liberal outpouring of keratic precipitates and a deep

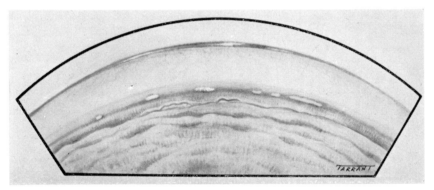

FIG. 612.—INFLAMMATORY SECONDARY GLAUCOMA.
Large precipitates are seen in the angle of the anterior chamber (Inst. Ophthal.).

anterior chamber, is suddenly intensified by increased congestion and sometimes by the development of a steamy cornea, while the pain becomes unbearable and the vision much more blurred. In some cases this rise of tension may result from the administration of a mydriatic to an eye predisposed to primary closed-angle glaucoma, in others from inflammatory œdema of the ciliary body producing peripheral anterior synechiæ and thus a secondary closed-angle glaucoma (Busacca, 1964), but in the majority of cases the anterior chamber is deep and the angle patently open. The ætiology of this secondary open-angle glaucoma is complex, resulting from the interaction of a number of conflicting factors, the important ones being an increase in the resistance to the outflow of aqueous tending to cause a rise in tension, and a diminution in the production of aqueous tending to cause a fall. Although Mansheim (1953) found tonographic evidence for excessive formation of aqueous in hypertensive uveitis, this has not been confirmed by other authors (Grant, 1951; Higgitt, 1956; Tulloh, 1960; and others). On the other hand, it has been amply demonstrated that there is an obstruction to the outflow of aqueous[1] and an increase in the resistance to outflow has been confirmed experimentally in rabbits (Auricchio and Bárány, 1958). The nature of this obstruction is more controversial. It would seem reasonable to assume that the increased viscosity of the aqueous, loaded as it is with proteins, fibrin and exudative cells, would clog the meshes of a filtration angle which may already be embarrassed by inflammatory œdema, and the presence of a secondary glaucoma without visible evidence of synechial formation has been frequently reported (Figs. 612–3).[2] Higgitt (1956), on the other hand, found a distinct correlation between the presence of peripheral anterior synechiæ and a raised tension; if 50% of the angle was open,

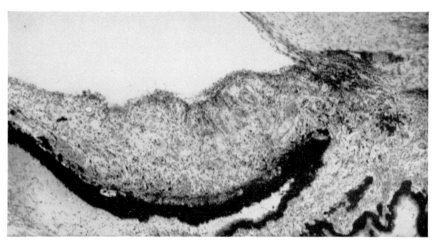

FIG. 613.—THE ANGLE OF THE ANTERIOR CHAMBER IN PANOPHTHALMITIS.

A purulent exudate infiltrates the iris, extends into the anterior chamber and is dense in the region of the trabeculæ at the filtration angle (H. & E.; × 75) (N. Ashton).

glaucoma did not occur, while it was inevitable if two-thirds of the angle was closed by synechiæ. Grant (1951) considered that the unaffected eye in unilateral hypertensive uveitis was basically normal, while Tulloh (1960) found that cases which developed secondary glaucoma had a pre-existing obstruction to outflow which predisposed to the glaucoma when the uveitis supervened.

This increase in the resistance to the outflow of aqueous is frequently overshadowed by a diminution in its production (Grant, 1951; Weekers et al., 1956–60; Auricchio and Bárány, 1958); as a result, particularly when the ciliary body is involved, hypotony is a common finding in acute anterior

[1] Thomassen (1947), Grant (1951), Weekers et al. (1953–56), Higgitt (1956), Tulloh (1960), and others.

[2] Fralick et al. (1942), Loewenstein (1948), Stankovic (1952), Weekers et al. (1956), Tulloh (1960), and others.

uveitis even when the anterior chamber is filled with an almost solid gelatinous exudate. It is probable, therefore, that the occurrence of glaucoma
depends upon the effect of obstruction to the outflow channels predominating
over the diminution in the production of aqueous, and that it is more likely
to occur in an eye wherein there is a pre-existing obstruction to the outflow
of aqueous.

Hypertensive uveitis may also occur during the course of a severe
KERATITIS, whether it be an interstitial keratitis or a corneal ulceration,
more particularly a hypopyon ulcer with which a raised tension forms a
serious complication; herpes simplex or zoster may also be associated with a
severe and recalcitrant glaucoma. In SCLERITIS, also, a secondary rise of
tension is a frequent and sometimes very persistent complication. In all
these conditions, of course, the uveal tract is involved in the inflammatory
process, so that the mechanism of the glaucoma is similar to that which
we have already considered.

(ii) CYCLITIS

The chronic inflammations of the ciliary body present a more difficult
problem both in their clinical recognition and in their treatment, so much
so that certain types do not respond to any current method of therapy. The
clinical picture of the secondary glaucoma associated with cyclitis may
resemble an acute closed-angle or a simple glaucoma, usually the latter.
Three groups of conditions, often difficult to separate, have already been
described,[1] but their salient features will be repeated.

(a) CHRONIC CYCLITIS. This condition, first described by Fuchs (1889)
as cyclitis, has been termed peripheral uveitis (Brockhurst et al., 1956–61),
pars planitis (Welch et al., 1960; Martenet, 1964), cyclitis with peripheral
chorioretinitis (Hogan and Kimura, 1961), and chronic cyclitis (Kimura
and Hogan, 1964).[2] It occurs typically in children and young adults, is
bilateral in 70% of cases, and usually has an insidious onset without ocular
congestion or discomfort; an acute onset is a rarity. The first symptom is
usually blurred vision with or without vitreous floaters. The aqueous flare
is minimal and there are a few small keratic precipitates although larger
deposits may be present on the trabeculæ leading to the formation of peripheral anterior synechiæ. The iris appears normal and posterior synechiæ
do not occur. The main changes are seen in the anterior vitreous which at
first contains a cloud of fine dust-like opacities followed at a later stage by
coarse accumulations which tend to settle on the periphery of the retina.
Perivascular sheathing may occur at the periphery of the retina, and macular
œdema which may extend to involve the optic disc may be severe, particularly in children; but glaucoma seems to be an uncommon complication
(2 out of 136 cases—Kimura and Hogan, 1964).

[1] Vol. IX.   [2] Vol. IX, p. 200.

(b) GLAUCOMATO-CYCLITIC CRISES. This condition was described in detail by Posner and Schlossman (1948) although previously reported on a number of occasions (Streiff, 1919; Terrien and Veil, 1929; Knapp, 1935; Kraupa, 1936; Kronfeld, 1944).[1] It is usually unilateral, occurs predominantly in young or middle-aged people, and is characterized by attacks of slight blurring of vision, the appearance of haloes, and ocular discomfort, but no pain. During the attack the ocular tension is raised, sometimes to a considerable degree, and there is a faint aqueous flare with the deposition on the cornea of fine well-defined non-pigmented precipitates. The attacks last from several hours to several weeks, synechiæ never form, but it is usual for the affected iris eventually to become depigmented so that heterochromia results. A striking reduction or complete disappearance of pigmentation in the angle of the anterior chamber has been described as being characteristic (Shimizu, 1965), while Hart and Wetherill (1968) observed gonioscopically in 7 patients an appearance similar to that seen in congenital glaucoma. During the attacks the angle of the anterior chamber is open, although Posner (1958) described a case wherein primary closed-angle glaucoma and glaucomato-cyclitic crises were coincident. During an attack there is an obstruction to the outflow of aqueous (Grant, 1951; Mansheim, 1953; Posner and Schlossman, 1953; Delmarcelle, 1957; Spivey and Armaly, 1963; Sugar, 1965). The rate of aqueous formation during an attack has been reported as normal (Grant, 1951; Rouher and Cantat, 1963), low normal (Mansheim, 1953), or increased (Spivey and Armaly, 1963; Sugar, 1965).

(c) HETEROCHROMIC CYCLITIS. The condition of heterochromia together with clinical evidence of cyclitis was established, as we have seen,[2] as a clinical entity by Fuchs (1906). It is usually a unilateral condition characterized by signs of a quiet anterior uveitis with little or no ciliary congestion and without discomfort or pain. The iris loses its architecture and becomes atrophic. Small non-pigmented precipitates are formed on the posterior corneal surface, posterior synechiæ never occur, the aqueous humour is sometimes clear and at other times it shows a definite haze in the beam of the slit-lamp, and the vitreous body is not uncommonly clouded with dust-like opacities. Gonioscopic examination frequently shows the presence of fine vessels on the trabeculæ (François, 1946; Franceschetti, 1955), and gross vascularization of the angle resembling that following occlusion of the central vein of the retina has been recorded (Lerman and Levy, 1964). The frequent occurrence of gonio-hæmorrhages has been reported (Begg, 1969).

The most serious complication of this form of cyclitis is the development in the hypochromic eye of an insidious glaucoma which clinically and histologically is indistinguishable from simple glaucoma (Ilday, 1956;

[1] Vol. IX, p. 202.　　　　[2] Vol. IX, p. 594.

Goldberg *et al.*, 1965; Doughman, 1966). Its incidence has varied in different series,[1] but that of Huber (1961) is representative: he found glaucoma in 5 to 13% of unilateral and in 25 to 33% of bilateral cases. In those without frank glaucoma the coefficient of aqueous outflow is often low (11 out of 65 cases, Georgiadès and Tsinopoulos, 1965; 66% of cases, Ward and Hart, 1967). Ward and Hart (1967) also noted that this coefficient is further reduced after extraction of the cataract; curiously, the uninvolved eye may also show abnormal tonographic readings (Hart and Ward, 1967; Gloster and Hartley, 1968). Coles (1964) found that glaucoma was particularly liable to occur in eyes that had developed a cataract.

The course of the condition is similar to that of simple glaucoma and pathological changes suggest that the obstruction to outflow is due to sclerosis of the trabeculæ with obliteration of the inter-trabecular spaces. An acute glaucoma is unusual; Lerman and Levy (1964) reported a case due to vascularization of the angle of the anterior chamber, while Lemke (1966) observed 8 acute out of 31 cases of glaucoma in his series.

The mechanism of the rise of tension in these various types of cyclitis appears, therefore, to be an obstruction to the outflow of aqueous. In chronic cyclitis the obstruction probably results from inflammatory cells blocking the trabecular meshwork, in glaucomato-cyclitic crises the mechanism is unknown although an allergic vasodilatation and increased permeability of the ciliary body have recently received most support, while in heterochromic cyclitis the rise of tension appears to be indistinguishable from that of simple glaucoma.

The *treatment* of hypertensive uveitis frequently presents difficult and anxious problems, some of which have already been touched upon.[2] It goes without saying, of course, that the underlying cause of the inflammation, if it is known, should receive the appropriate therapy.

With regard to the treatment of the actual complication of the raised tension the choice lies between medical and surgical measures, and it may be said at once that in general the more apparent the inflammation the less the indication for surgery, a ruling which applies even although the condition looks alarmingly acute. The best way to deal with the secondary glaucoma complicating an acute anterior uveitis is to combat the inflammation which produces it, and if structural changes have not developed to obstruct the circulation of fluid in the eye, it is surprising how frequently this can be done. The dilemma which presents itself as to whether the uveitis should

[1] 31%, Lloyd (1931); 4 to 5% unilateral, 33% bilateral, François (1954); 13% unilateral, 25% bilateral, Franceschetti (1955); 7·7%, Georgiadès (1956); 14%, de Rosa (1959); 18%, Hollwich (1963); 15 to 25%, Coles (1964); 14·5% unilateral, 22% bilateral, Velický (1964); 9·3%, Georgiadès and Tsinopoulos (1965); 9%, Sugar (1965); 21%, Lemke (1966).
[2] Vol. IX, p. 178.

be treated with mydriatics or the glaucoma with miotics has already been discussed, but it is usually more apparent than real. Certainly in those cases wherein the inflammation is acute and when the anterior chamber is deep, the urgent necessity is to establish dilatation of the pupil with the attendant decongestion of the anterior segment of the uveal tract and the breaking down of existing synechiæ, and for these atropine is generally safe to use. If the angle of the anterior chamber is narrow—and if the picture is obscured an estimate of this may be made by gonioscopy on the fellow eye—it is probably safer to employ the shorter-acting mydriatics. Here the choice is more difficult and lies between the tropine group of drugs, such as homatropine, cyclopentolate and tropicamide, which produce peripheral folding of the iris and thus tend to encourage the formation of peripheral anterior synechiæ, and the adrenergic drugs, such as adrenaline and phenylephrine, which tend to produce pupillary block (Lowe, 1966). The latter group is probably the safer since, in addition to their mydriatic effect, they inhibit the formation of aqueous. Together with the mydriatics, topical and subconjunctival steroids should be intensively administered.

The mydriatics and steroids should always be accompanied by the use of systemic hypotensive drugs, the more important of these being the carbonic anhydrase inhibitors and intravenous and oral hypertonic agents. The use of these drugs has been fully discussed in previous Volumes.[1] One or other is usually effective in controlling the glaucoma secondary to an acute anterior uveitis so long as structural changes have not occurred, and surgery need only be contemplated if the anterior chamber is so shallow as to raise the suspicion of a tendency for the development of a closed-angle glaucoma. Paracentesis—formerly a popular method of therapy—should be avoided, as any temporary benefit is counterbalanced by the resulting tendency to the development of peripheral anterior synechiæ.

In the glaucoma secondary to cyclitis the problem is sometimes more difficult and may call for more judgement. It is to be remembered that chronic cyclitis appears to be very resistant to treatment (Welch et al., 1960; Kimura and Hogan, 1964). Steroids, both topically (Brockhurst et al., 1961) and subconjunctivally (Kimura and Hogan, 1964) have been recommended, while mydriatics are necessary only in those cases with an acute onset since in most instances synechiæ do not form. Systemic hypotensive drugs are the mainstay of treatment for this type of glaucoma although cyclodiathermy has been recommended (Welch et al., 1960).

Miotics, mydriatics, steroids, carbonic anhydrase inhibitors, and many other drugs have been recommended for the treatment of glaucomato-cyclitic crises. Pilocarpine may lower the tension temporarily while stronger miotics may cause it to rise. Homatropine and atropine usually have no effect while adrenaline and phenylephrine usually reduce the tension. The best course is to administer topical or subconjunctival steroids and systemic

[1] Vol. VII, pp. 623, 629; Vol. IX, p. 179.

acetazolamide during the attack; if the tension continues to give rise to anxiety, it can usually be controlled by oral glycerol. Surgical treatment has been recommended on a number of occasions; it is effective only if a filtering bleb results (Lowe, 1953; Rouher, 1955; Sugar, 1965).

Treatment is necessary only for the complications of heterochromic cyclitis; the condition itself does not respond to steroids, and mydriatics are not indicated as synechiæ do not occur. If the tension becomes raised it may be controlled by miotics, adrenaline and acetazolamide, but a drainage operation may be required. In cases wherein glaucoma and cataract are co-existent, extraction of the lens may control the tension (Coles, 1964).

POST-INFLAMMATORY OBSTRUCTIVE GLAUCOMA

A secondary rise of tension is by no means unusual as a result of the pathological changes which may follow inflammation; these all act by obstructing the circulation of the intra-ocular fluid either in the region of the pupil or its drainage at the angle of the anterior chamber.

(i) *In the region of the pupil* adhesions between the iris and the capsule of the lens or the hyaloid surface of the vitreous in an aphakic eye may produce a seclusion of the pupil by forming annular posterior synechiæ. Such an

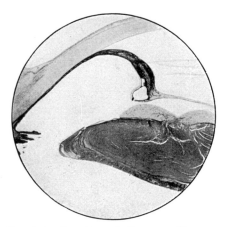

Fig. 614.—Iris Bombé: Seclusio Pupillæ.

Extensive peripheral anterior synechiæ. Posterior synechiæ with seclusio pupillæ; inflammatory pupillary membrane with occlusio pupillæ; anterior capsular cataract (J. H. Parsons).

occurrence stops the circulation of the intra-ocular fluid which is banked up under pressure behind the iris producing an iris bombé and secondary glaucoma (Fig. 614). A more serious obstruction may occur if a total posterior synechia binds the entire posterior surface of the iris to the lens so that the circumlental space is blocked with cyclitic exudate, but in such cases the more common termination is hypotony and phthisis bulbi owing to wide-spread destruction of the ciliary body by the inflammatory process.

(ii) *In the angle of the anterior chamber* obstruction may be produced by three mechanisms. The inflammatory swelling of the tissues at the root of the iris and the anterior part of the ciliary body, aided frequently by the forward bellying of the former tissue, makes this region of the uvea approach the cornea so closely that the narrowed angle becomes bridged across by strands of new-formed tissue which gradually consolidate to form peripheral anterior synechiæ which may eventually completely block the filtration angle (Figs. 615–16) (Junius, 1932; Busacca, 1964). Peripheral anterior

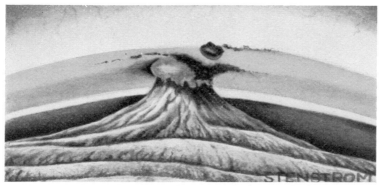

FIG. 615.—PERIPHERAL ANTERIOR SYNECHIA.

Seen gonioscopically, the exudate on the trabeculæ at the angle of the anterior chamber has led to an adhesion of the iris, the forerunner of an organized peripheral anterior synechia (R. J. Brockhurst, C. L. Schepens and I. D. Okamura).

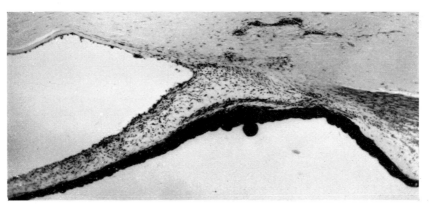

FIG. 616.—PERIPHERAL ANTERIOR SYNECHIÆ.

From a blind painful eye, in an old case of iridocyclitis, showing the consolidation of peripheral anterior synechiæ with the formation of a false angle (H. & E.; × 64) (N. Ashton).

synechiæ, which are seen gonioscopically, may also result from a shallow anterior chamber due to the presence of a pupillary block and the formation of an iris bombé. Again, obstruction to the drainage of aqueous may occur owing to post-inflammatory changes in the tissues of the angle itself. Here the trabecular meshwork is at first clogged with fibrin and inflammatory cells and then by granulation tissue which may eventually consolidate into fibrous tissue, so that ultimately, as pathological investigations have demonstrated (Parsons, 1904 ; Greeves, 1928 ; and others), the trabecular meshwork may be converted into a solid mass, sometimes associated with the formation of new hyaline membranes lined by endothelium and with proliferation of the endothelium forming the wall of the canal of Schlemm (Fig. 617). In all

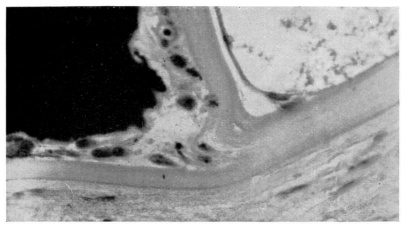

Fig. 617.—The Formation of a Hyaline Membrane in Iridocyclitis.

In a case of old iridocyclitis. Descemet's membrane appears to split and the new hyaline layer passes over the anterior surface of the iris blocking the filtration angle (N. Ashton).

these cases the ætiology of the glaucoma is primarily mechanical, the tension rising because of obstruction to the circulation and blockage of the outflow channels.

It is interesting that in cases of glaucoma secondary to inflammation, pathological changes of this nature may be seen not only in the pupillary region and the angle of the anterior chamber but also at the optic nerve-head. Here the glaucomatous cup may be partially or completely filled with organizing exudate of inflammatory origin which may consolidate to form loose connective tissue supplied by new vessels (Fig. 618) and even bone (Moretti, 1928). It may happen, indeed, that the subsequent contraction of this tissue pulls upon the retina and drags it as a folded and degenerated mass into the concavity of the excavation (Parsons, 1905).

The *treatment* of such a mechanical condition must be essentially surgical—the opening up of the channels of circulation. The best treatment is, of course, prophylactic and lies in the prevention of the formation of organized adhesions by the establishment of opportune mydriasis and by the reduction of the uveitis with steroids from the earliest stages of the inflammation, but once they have become consolidated sufficiently to cause hypertension, it is rare for even the strongest available mydriatics to be effective in breaking them down. In the case of an iris bombé, communication between the posterior and anterior chambers can be re-established by an iridectomy and, so long as peripheral anterior synechiæ have not formed, the glaucoma will be relieved. The operation of choice is an iridectomy *ab externo* wherein, under a conjunctival flap, an incision at the corneo-scleral junction parallel to the limbus is deepened with a Bard-Parker knife until the root of the iris is reached. A peripheral iridectomy or, in the presence of total posterior

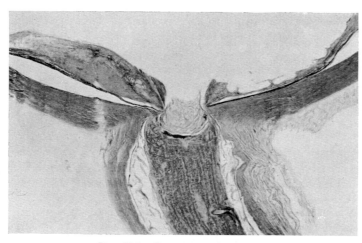

FIG. 618.—SECONDARY GLAUCOMA.

Showing cupping and optic atrophy in a man of 75 with glaucoma following a hypopyon ulcer. Note the thickening and degeneration of the retina and the organized exudate filling the cup. The subarachnoid space is widely dilated ($\times$ 10) (after J. H. Parsons).

synechiæ, a sector iridectomy, is then performed. Sometimes, however, in the presence of total posterior synechiæ and an atrophic iris, an attempted iridectomy results in a splitting of the iris so that its posterior ectodermal layer is left adhering to the capsule of the lens; indeed, any operation upon a fragile and atrophic iris may be most unsatisfactory, and when its tissues tear so that an adequate basal iridectomy is impossible, a greater chance of success may lie in abandoning the idea of an iridectomy and performing an iris-inclusion operation instead.

In a congested eye during the acute inflammatory phase, where an iridectomy is thought to be too hazardous, a transfixation of the iris may be performed. In Fuchs's four-point iridotomy a narrow Graefe knife is passed through the cornea in the horizontal meridian to pierce the iris, pass beneath it and emerge from it near the pupillary aperture, and then to transfix the iris again in a similar manner on the opposite side of the pupil before it finally re-emerges through the cornea at the opposite point in the limbus. In this way the iris is transfixed four times.

Once peripheral anterior synechiæ have formed and are sufficiently extensive to cause glaucoma an iridectomy will not relieve the condition. If the tension is not too high it may be controlled (if the uveitis has settled) by miotics, adrenaline and carbonic anhydrase inhibitors, but any coincident pupillary block must be treated separately. If the tension is uncontrolled in spite of medical therapy, a drainage operation must be considered.[1] Considerable judgement is necessary in deciding when this step has to be taken, for although an otherwise normal eye can tolerate a moderate increase in tension for some considerable time, the operation should be performed before the increased tension has caused irreparable damage to the eye.

NEONATAL RUBELLA, caused by maternal infection usually in the first trimester of pregnancy,[2] is frequently associated with a raised ocular tension. Since the first record of this complication by Swan and his colleagues (1943) in Australia, some 20 reports have appeared in the literature. It will be remembered[3] that the ocular tension in normal infants often shows an ephemeral rise up to 40 or even 60 mm. Hg; but a frank and lasting condition of secondary congenital glaucoma has been recorded in large series of cases of infected infants occurring with an incidence varying between 2 and 15% (Geltzer et al., 1967; Sears, 1967) and even reaching a figure of 25% (Alfano, 1966). The cause of the raised tension seems to differ and is not always clear, for the full investigation of the eyes of very young children presents considerable difficulties; many such eyes have a small cornea sometimes associated with opacities, others have anomalies at the drainage angle, but in others this angle has been anatomically normal and in these it is probable that the decreased facility of outflow of the aqueous is the result of inflammatory changes (Sears, 1967; Zimmerman, 1968). In some cases the rise of tension is temporary and spontaneous recovery may ensue (Long and Danielson, 1945; Waardenburg et al., 1961), or it may be controlled by medical measures such as topical adrenaline and carbonic anhydrase inhibitors; in others surgical relief may be necessary by such measures as goniotomy, a filtering operation or cyclodiathermy.

Alfano. *Trans. Amer. Acad. Ophthal.*, **70**, 235 (1966).

Auricchio and Bárány. *Ophthalmologica*, **136**, 249 (1958).

Begg. *Brit. J. Ophthal.*, **53**, 1 (1969).

Brockhurst, Schepens and Okamura. *Amer. J. Ophthal.*, **42**, 545 (1956); **49**, 1257 (1960); **51**, 19 (1961).

Busacca. *Amer. J. Ophthal.*, **57**, 383 (1964).

Coles. Sorsby's *Modern Ophthalmology*, London, **4**, 636 (1964).

Delmarcelle. *Bull. Soc. belge Ophtal.*, No. 114, 566 (1957).

Doughman. *Surv. Ophthal.*, **11**, 297 (1966).

Fralick, Cooper and Armstrong. *Trans. Amer. Acad. Ophthal.*, **47**, 92 (1942).

Franceschetti. *Amer. J. Ophthal.*, **39** (2), 50 (1955).

François. *Ann. Oculist.* (Paris), **179**, 559 (1946); **187**, 255 (1954).

Fuchs. *Lhb. d. Augenheilk.*, Leipzig (1889). *Z. Augenheilk.*, **15**, 191 (1906).

[1] p. 534. [2] p. 220; Vol. III, p. 392. [3] Vol. IV, p. 240.

Geltzer, Guber and Sears. *Amer. J. Ophthal.*, **63**, 221 (1967).
Georgiadès. *Bull. Soc. franç. Ophtal.*, **69**, 470 (1956).
Georgiadès and Tsinopoulos. *Arch. ophthal. Hetair. borei. hellad.*, **13**, 200 (1965).
Gloster and Hartley. *Brit. J. Ophthal.*, **52**, 912 (1968).
Goldberg, Erozan, Duke and Frost. *Arch. Ophthal.*, **74**, 604 (1965).
Grant. *Arch. Ophthal.*, **46**, 113 (1951).
Greeves. *Trans. ophthal. Soc. U.K.*, **48**, 45 (1928).
Hart and Ward. *Brit. J. Ophthal.*, **51**, 739 (1967).
Hart and Wetherill. *Brit. J. Ophthal.*, **52**, 682 (1968).
Higgitt. *Trans. ophthal. Soc. U.K.*, **76**, 73 (1956).
Hogan and Kimura. *Arch. Ophthal.*, **66**, 667 (1961).
Hollwich. *Klin. Mbl. Augenheilk.*, **142**, 129 (1963).
Huber. *Ophthalmologica*, **141**, 122 (1961).
Ilday. *Oto-Nörö-Oftal.*, **11**, 35 (1956).
Junius. *Arch. Augenheilk.*, **106**, 475 (1932).
Kimura and Hogan. *Arch. Ophthal.*, **71**, 193 (1964).
Knapp. *Klin. Mbl. Augenheilk.*, **94**, 748 (1935).
Kraupa. *Arch. Augenheilk.*, **109**, 416 (1936).
Kronfeld. *Arch. Ophthal.*, **32**, 447 (1944).
Lemke. *Ophthalmologica*, **151**, 457 (1966).
Lerman and Levy. *Amer. J. Ophthal.*, **57**, 479 (1964).
Lloyd. *Amer. J. Ophthal.*, **15**, 287 (1931).
Loewenstein. *Trans. ophthal. Soc. U.K.*, **68**, 485 (1948).
Long and Danielson. *Arch. Ophthal.*, **34**, 24 (1945).
Lowe. *Trans. ophthal. Soc. Aust.*, **13**, 168 (1953).
Med. J. Aust., **2**, 1037 (1966).
Mansheim. *Arch. Ophthal.*, **50**, 580 (1953).
Martenet. *Ophthalmologica*, **147**, 282 (1964).

Moretti. *Z. Augenheilk.*, **66**, 239 (1928).
Parsons. *Pathology of the Eye*, London, **1**, 304 (1904).
Trans. ophthal. Soc. U.K., **25**, 99 (1905).
Posner. *Eye, Ear, Nose, Thr. Monthly*, **37**, 402 (1958).
Posner and Schlossman. *Arch. Ophthal.*, **39**, 517 (1948).
Trans. Amer. Acad. Ophthal., **57**, 531 (1953).
de Rosa. *Arch. Ottal.*, **63**, 437 (1959).
Rouher. *Bull. Soc. Ophtal. Fr.*, 534 (1955).
Rouher and Cantat. *Arch. Ophtal.*, **16**, 798 (1956).
Sears. *Brit. J. Ophthal.*, **51**, 744 (1967).
Shimizu. *Rinsho Ganka*, **19**, 297 (1965).
Spivey and Armaly. *Amer. J. Ophthal.*, **55**, 47 (1963).
Stankovic. *Bull. Soc. Ophtal. Fr.*, 493 (1952).
Streiff. *Klin. Mbl. Augenheilk.*, **62**, 353 (1919).
Sugar. *Amer. J. Ophthal.*, **60**, 1 (1965).
Swan, Tostevin, Moore et al. *Med. J. Aust.*, **2**, 201 (1943).
Terrien and Veil. *Bull. Soc. franç. Ophtal.*, **42**, 349 (1929).
Thomassen. *Acta ophthal.* (Kbh.), **25**, 243 (1947).
Tulloh. *Trans. ophthal. Soc. U.K.*, **80**, 187 (1960).
Velický. *Csl. Ofthal.*, **20**, 298 (1964).
Waardenburg, Franceschetti and Klein. *Genetics and Ophthalmology*, Oxford, **1**, 142, 580, 601 (1961).
Ward and Hart. *Brit. J. Ophthal.*, **51**, 530 (1967).
Weekers, Delmarcelle and Prijot. *Bull. Soc. belge Ophtal.*, No. 104, 235 (1953).
Bull. Soc. Ophtal. Fr., 208 (1956).
Weekers, Lavergne, Feron and Vermer. *Klin. Mbl. Augenheilk.*, **137**, 1 (1960).
Welch, Maumenee and Wahlen. *Arch. Ophthal.*, **64**, 540 (1960).
Zimmerman. *Amer. J. Ophthal.*, **65**, 837 (1968).

EXTRA-OCULAR INFLAMMATIONS

The occurrence of glaucoma secondary to extra-ocular inflammations is rare but raises the question of the development of this disease in *trachoma* owing to the obstruction of the outflow of aqueous by the infiltration of the limbal region. The question is difficult to decide but depends upon the relative incidence of glaucoma in populations free from trachoma and in those heavily infected with the disease. Conflicting reports have appeared in the literature. Thus many writers[1] have found a higher frequency of raised tension among trachomatous people, a view corroborated by Nema and his colleagues (1964) in India. On the other hand, an equal number has

[1] Müller (1900), de Wecker (1900), Cuénod and Nataf (1930), MacCallan (1936), Adamantiadis (1937), Bietti (1947), Boles Carenini and Cambiaggi (1957).

concluded that raised tension is no more frequent among these people and therefore that the two diseases are independent,[1] a view corroborated by Aouchiche and his co-workers (1966) in Northern Africa. At present the problem must remain undecided.

Adamantiadis. *Rev. int. Trachome*, **14**, 241 (1937).

Aouchiche, Boyer, Djennas and Landeiro. *Rev. int. Trachome*, **43**, 275 (1966).

Bailliart. *Bull. Soc. franç. Ophtal.*, **41**, 323 (1928).

Bietti. *Il tracoma*, Rome (1947).

Boles Carenini and Cambiaggi. *Rev. int. Trachome*, **34**, 62 (1957).

Cuénod and Nataf. *Le trachome*, Paris (1930).

Guarino. *Studio critico sull'evoluzione tracomatosa*, Cairo (1914).

Lagrange. *Du glaucome et de l'hypotonie*, Paris (1922).

MacCallan. *Trachoma*, London, 53 (1936).

Müller. *Arch. Augenheilk.*, **40**, 13 (1900).

Nema, Saiduzzafar, Nath and Shukla. *Brit. J. Ophthal.*, **48**, 563 (1964).

Pasino. *Studi sassaresi*, **35**, 25 (1957).

Terson. *Bull. Soc. franç. Ophtal.*, **41**, 329 (1928).

Trantas. *Rev. int. Trachome*, **14**, 131 (1937).

de Wecker. *Ann. Oculist.* (Paris), **124**, 45 (1900).

Glaucoma Secondary to Changes in the Lens

DEFORMITIES OF THE LENS

MICROPHAKIA (or SPHEROPHAKIA), a congenital and bilateral condition frequently associated with skeletal changes (the *Marfan* and the *Marchesani* syndromes),[2] may be complicated by glaucoma, a circumstance remarked by Bowman (1865) and studied by several subsequent writers.[3] The glaucoma is usually due to the spherical lens blocking the pupillary aperture, thus obstructing the flow of aqueous from the posterior to the anterior chamber (pupillary-block glaucoma). As in other forms of this type of glaucoma, mydriatics will usually relieve the condition so long as peripheral anterior synechiæ have not developed, while miotics may precipitate an acute attack of raised tension (*inverse glaucoma*—Urbanek, 1930; Probert, 1953).

When the symptoms come on in early life there may be coincident anomalies at the angle of the anterior chamber and buphthalmos may result, but more usually the onset is delayed until youth, when acute attacks of raised tension are liable to occur. These repeated self-limiting attacks of glaucoma may ultimately result in the formation of extensive peripheral anterior synechiæ and a permanent rise in pressure (Gärtner, 1958; Zoldan, 1959; Levy and Anderson, 1961). Before this occurs the attacks of raised tension can be controlled by mydriatics but permanent relief from the recurrent episodes usually follows a peripheral iridectomy (Rosenthal and Kloepfer, 1956; Levy and Anderson, 1961). Once the angle of the anterior chamber has been permanently closed some form of drainage operation is necessary (iridencleisis or cyclodialysis—Zoldan, 1959). Removal of the lens is far from

---

[1] Guarino (1914), Lagrange (1922), Bailliart (1928), Terson (1928), Trantas (1937), Pasino (1957), and others.

[2] Vol. III, p. 1107.

[3] Wessely (1910), Fleischer (1916), Urbanek (1930), Gnad (1931), Shapira (1934), Serr (1940), Rosenthal and Kloepfer (1956), Dodo (1957), Zabriskie and Reisman (1958), Nirankari and Maudgal (1959), Tjanidis *et al.* (1962), Nirankari and Chaddah (1963), Chandler (1964), Magnasco and Zingirian (1965), Janotka (1966), McGavic (1966).

satisfactory, particularly in its long-term results, and should be considered only if the lens is cataractous.

A complication which may occur is subluxation or luxation of the lens owing to the congenitally weak zonule. If the subluxated lens becomes incarcerated in the pupil, an attempt should be made to replace it with the use of mydriatics. If this fails, the glaucoma can be relieved by a peripheral iridectomy, after which the lens can usually be replaced when the pupil is dilated, with or without massage. The management of luxation of the lens into the anterior or posterior chambers is discussed elsewhere.[1]

DISPLACEMENTS OF THE LENS

A subluxation or luxation of the lens,[2] whether it be congenital, traumatic or secondary to intra-ocular disease, is frequently but by no means invariably followed by the development of secondary glaucoma.[3] Glaucoma is not uncommonly associated with congenital *subluxation* as an isolated finding (Bowman, 1865) or as part of the Marfan or Marchesani syndrome, or less frequently in homocystinuria.[4] In traumatic cases this complication is even more common (Fig. 619) (36 out of 70 cases, Hegner, 1915; 15 out of 38, H. McDonald and Purnell, 1951; 6 out of 11, Calhoun and Hagler, 1960). In subluxations secondary to intra-ocular disease a rise of tension is also common, but here the condition is usually overshadowed by more serious events.

A complete *dislocation* of the lens is more frequently followed by the complication of raised tension. In anterior dislocations, whether spontaneous or traumatic, an immediate secondary glaucoma is very common (Fig. 620); thus in 15 cases of dislocations into the anterior chamber (7 traumatic and 7 spontaneous) Hegner (1915) found glaucoma in 14, while Rodman (1963) found that 34 out of 44 cases of traumatic anterior dislocation of the lens had a clinical history or pathological evidence of glaucoma. Chandler (1964) has commented on the frequent occurrence of glaucoma in spontaneous anterior dislocation of the lens in ectopia lentis, the Marfan syndrome and the Marchesani syndrome, and a similar glaucoma has been described in homocystinuria.[5] In posterior dislocations of traumatic origin glaucoma is not so frequent an occurrence (2 out of 11 cases, Hegner, 1915; 4 out of 15, H. McDonald and Purnell, 1951; 5 out of 9, Calhoun and Hagler, 1960) and when it does occur the rise in tension is usually the result of the trauma, not of the dislocated lens (Rodman, 1963). A spontaneous posteriorly dislocated lens may be tolerated without complications for many years, and in those instances in which glaucoma has been reported, it is probable that in most cases it was not caused by the dislocated lens itself (Chandler, 1964).

[1] p. 307.   [2] p. 298.
[3] p. 307.   [4] Vol. IX, p. 646
[5] Gibson *et al.* (1964), Carson *et al.* (1965), Henkind and Ashton (1965), Schimke *et al.* (1965), Lieberman *et al.* (1966), Johnston (1968).

Ætiologically there are many factors concerned in the development of this type of glaucoma and these are best discussed by dividing cases of subluxated and luxated lenses into those of spontaneous and those of traumatic origin. In a spontaneous subluxation, the lens is often smaller and more spherical than normal and because of a coincident congenitally

FIGS. 619 and 620.—SECONDARY GLAUCOMA AFTER SUBLUXATION OF THE LENS (H. I. Rodman).

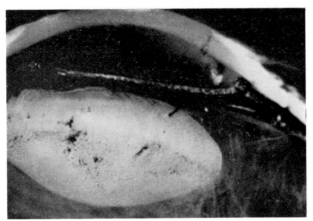

FIG. 619.—The eye was enucleated 4 months after a traumatic subluxation of the lens. The vitreous is prolapsed through the aphakic portion of the pupil (to the right) and is adherent to the posterior surface of the iris. As a result of this vitreous-pupillary block, the angle of the anterior chamber is completely closed.

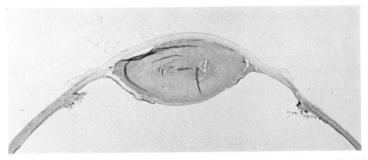

FIG. 620.—The result of an anterior dislocation of the lens. The pupil is blocked by the posterior surface of the lens so that the anterior chamber is completely closed by peripheral anterior synechiæ.

weak zonule it is liable to block the pupillary aperture, resulting in pupillary-block glaucoma. A similar mechanism obtains in some of these cases from a herniation of the vitreous blocking the pupillary aperture. Moreover, congenital ectopia lentis is often associated with other congenital anomalies which may involve the angle of the anterior chamber and be factors in the development of glaucoma. This applies particularly to the syndromes of

Marfan and Marchesani,[1] and also to ectopia lentis unassociated with systemic anomalies (Smeral, 1962; Segal, 1962).

In spontaneous anterior dislocations the lens is sometimes incarcerated in the pupil resulting in pupillary-block glaucoma, while if it lies completely in the anterior chamber the pupil may be blocked by the iris coming forward against the posterior surface of the lens, and as pressure increases in the posterior chamber the iris is pressed more and more tightly against it. If the lens is repeatedly incarcerated in the pupil or has remained for a long period in the anterior chamber, the formation of extensive peripheral anterior synechiæ and permanent glaucoma may result (Rodman, 1963; Chandler, 1964) (Fig. 620).

A spontaneous posteriorly dislocated lens, as we have already seen,[2] is usually well tolerated by the eye, causing no serious complications and may be associated for many years with the preservation of useful vision. In those cases wherein hypertension occurs it is due to vitreo-pupillary block, rubeosis secondary to a retinal detachment (Rodman, 1963), phaco-anaphylactic or phacolytic glaucoma (Chandler, 1959) or a coincident primary glaucoma (Chandler, 1964).

In subluxated and luxated lenses of traumatic origin there are several possible causes for any associated glaucoma. The pupillary aperture may be blocked by the vitreous or lens; if not relieved this may lead to the formation of peripheral anterior synechiæ. Recession of the angle of the anterior chamber[3] is frequently seen in such patients (Rodman, 1963); this deformity of the angle is sometimes associated with a chronic open-angle glaucoma which develops several years after the injury. In traumatic cases of a posteriorly subluxated or luxated lens, glaucoma in the presence of an open angle is almost always due to recession of the angle (30 out of 31 cases, Rodman, 1963), a post-concussive event not primarily associated with the lens; glaucoma in the presence of a closed angle is the result of rubeosis secondary to retinal detachment or extensive chorioretinal scarring, vitreo-pupillary block, or the organization of exudates and hæmorrhages into the anterior chamber. On the other hand, phacolytic glaucoma appears to be a rare cause of the development of hypertension in eyes with a posteriorly dislocated lens (Rodman, 1963; Chandler, 1964).

The *treatment* of glaucoma in the presence of a subluxated or luxated lens depends upon the cause of the hypertension. Although extraction of the lens has been recommended as the treatment of choice in all cases of luxated lenses, with or without glaucoma (Barraquer, 1958; Dryden *et al.*, 1961), or as the immediate treatment of all lenses luxated into the anterior chamber (Rodman, 1963), this is usually a hazardous procedure and should not be undertaken without very careful consideration (Chandler, 1964).[4] With the development of glaucoma, however, treatment becomes urgent

[1] Vol. III, p. 1107. [2] p. 304. [3] p. 707. [4] p. 309.

and should be undertaken, particularly in cases of pupillary blockage, before repeated attacks result in the formation of permanent peripheral synechiæ. If the lens is incarcerated in the pupil or dislocated anteriorly, relief of the acute glaucoma may be obtained by the vigorous use of mydriatics when it may slip back to its original position (Axenfeld, 1914; Hegner, 1915; Zeeman, 1942; Harshman, 1948; and others), a process which may be aided by massage of the cornea (Rampoldi, 1886; Boggi, 1896; Kravitz, 1959); in such cases miotics tend to increase the hypertension. The lens has even been pushed backwards by a spatula inserted through a keratome incision (Bickerton, 1897). Once back in its normal position, it may be temporarily retained by the use of miotics; if the tension remains high a much safer and usually effective procedure is to relieve the condition by a peripheral iridectomy whereafter replacement of the lens can often be effected (Wessely, 1919; Harshman, 1948; Rosenthal and Kloepfer, 1956). This is probably a safer procedure than an immediate attempt to extract the lens (Chandler, 1964); and in bilateral cases of subluxation wherein a rise of tension has occurred in one eye, a prophylactic peripheral iridectomy is advisable in the other if the rise had been due to a dislocation of the lens into the anterior chamber. In pupillary blockage by the vitreous, mydriasis may also relieve the tension; alternatively and more safely, a peripheral iridectomy frequently does. When recurrent attacks of tension have resulted in the formation of peripheral anterior synechiæ, the glaucoma should be treated by a cyclodialysis or a drainage operation. Cases wherein the angle is wide should be treated as for simple glaucoma, by medical measures or by surgery in which cyclodialysis is often a suitable procedure. Whether or not the lens is then removed is a matter of assessment in each particular case, except that in phacolytic glaucoma this is a necessity if the eye is to remain useful.[1]

INTUMESCENCE OF THE LENS

A rapid swelling of the lens frequently excites a secondary rise in tension, a sequence first clearly recognized by von Graefe (1869). This may occur in two conditions: (a) with a rapidly developing intumescent cataract of the senile type[2] and (b) in traumatic cataract, caused either by a perforating injury or an operation of discission. It is generally accepted that the mechanism is similar to that in primary acute closed-angle glaucoma: the swollen lens pushes the iris forwards making the anterior chamber sufficiently shallow to block its angle or to permit other factors, such as mydriasis, to do so (Priestley Smith, 1879). Although it is widely agreed that acute glaucoma with an intumescent lens usually occurs in an otherwise normal eye, the fellow eye having an anterior chamber of normal depth, it occurs more readily when the angle is narrow (Diotallevi, 1961). Indeed,

[1] p. 663.
[2] Priestley Smith (1879), Ischreyt (1909), Salus (1910), Wright (1910), Morax (1922), Gonzales (1922), Sugar (1941), Nemetz (1956).

Nemetz (1956) considered that it should be regarded as a true primary glaucoma since he commonly found a shallow anterior chamber and a narrow angle present in both eyes, and that a closed-angle glaucoma frequently occurred in the other eye of patients who had experienced this complication with an intumescent cataract. When the capsule is ruptured, the process may be further intensified by soft lens matter blocking the angle, by a phacolytic glaucoma, or by a phaco-anaphylactic endophthalmitis.

Treatment, in the first instance, is the same as that for primary acute closed-angle glaucoma. The tension should be reduced by medical means, and miotics, carbonic anhydrase inhibitors, and oral and intravenous hypertonic solutions may all have to be used. Once the tension has been reduced to a normal level, medical treatment should be followed by removal of the lens by extraction in the case of an intumescent cataract, or curette evacuation or aspiration in a traumatic cataract.

MORGAGNIAN CATARACT

A morgagnian cataract is frequently associated with the development of a secondary glaucoma which is usually acute and stormy in its incidence, but may develop slowly and insidiously so that all perception of light has been lost before any damage to the eye apart from the cataract has been noted. Occasionally the glaucoma is associated with various degrees of dislocation of a shrunken hypermature cataract, a phenomenon usually followed by a severe reaction and a serious secondary glaucoma (Szili, 1884; Mitvalsky, 1892; Harms, 1905; and others). A raised tension may accompany the spontaneous absorption of a cataract (v. Reuss, 1900; H. Gifford, 1900–27; Verrey, 1916; Verhoeff and Lemoine, 1922), and it will be remembered that this event is usually associated with a spontaneous rupture of the capsule which has become thin and frail. In the case of a hypermature cataract this is often marked by the sudden appearance of a milky fluid in the anterior chamber and the development of glaucoma is usually accompanied by pain and circumcorneal injection. This condition and the appropriate literature have been noted elsewhere.[1]

PHACOLYTIC GLAUCOMA

We have already discussed elsewhere the various forms of lens-induced uveitis[2] and have remarked upon the frequent occurrence of a secondary glaucoma during the course of a phaco-anaphylactic endophthalmitis, a phacotoxic uveitis, or a lens-induced uveitis in the second eye; the mechanism of the rise of tension is similar to that in other intra-ocular inflammations. One particular form of lens-induced reaction, phacolytic glaucoma, is worthy of further mention.

Phacolytic glaucoma, so called by Flocks and his colleagues (1955), is a

[1] p. 138.   [2] Vol. IX, p. 500.

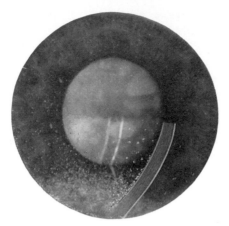

Fig. 621.—Phacolytic Glaucoma.
Note the hypermature lens and the mass of large keratic precipitates (Inst. Ophthal.).

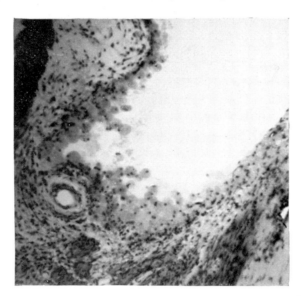

Fig. 622.—The Angle of the Anterior Chamber in Phacolytic Glaucoma.
Note the enlarged macrophages with ingested cortical material filling the angle, the trabeculæ and the anterior chamber and invading the iris (P. Henkind and B. Jay).

condition long recognized[1] but only recently clarified; it occurs in an eye with a hypermature cataract wherein the capsule may be thinned or ruptured posteriorly (16% in 138 cases, Flocks et al., 1955; 4 out of 4 cases, Schofield, 1957) but may have remained intact. Large mononuclear phagocytes accumulate in masses around the capsule and, laden with lenticular material, these clog the trabecular spaces at the angle of the

[1] Gifford (1900), von Reuss (1900), and many others.

anterior chamber and thus induce a rise of ocular tension usually mani-
festing itself as an acute or subacute glaucoma which, indeed, may be so
intractable as to lead to the excision of the eye (Fig. 622). In the classical
case there is no other type of cellular response; this contrasts with the
pathology of the various forms of lens-induced uveitis. The affected eye
is often acutely congested and may show corneal œdema, although there is
usually no disturbance of the corneal endothelium and therefore no keratic
precipitates; a flare may be present in the anterior chamber which is sometimes deeper than in the other eye owing to shrinkage of the affected lens
(Weekers and Grieten, 1965). The turbid aqueous may show a cloud
of punctate iridescent opacities (Fig. 621); the earlier authors usually

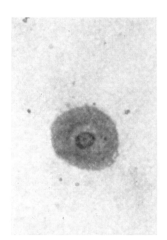 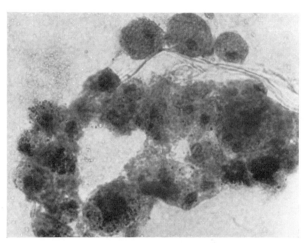

FIG. 623.   FIG. 624.

FIGS. 623 and 624.—PHACOLYTIC GLAUCOMA.

Macrophages demonstrated by the Papanicolau stain after filtration of the
aqueous through a millipore sheet (M. F. Goldberg).

described them as cholesterol crystals[1] but they may well be mononuclear
macrophages swollen with protein granules (Goldberg, 1967). In 25% of
enucleated eyes, recession of the angle of the anterior chamber has been
found (Smith and Zimmerman, 1965); this suggests that trauma may play a
significant pathogenic role in certain cases and may influence the prognosis.
Essentially, however, phacolytic glaucoma results from the leakage of lens
substance into the chambers of the eye (S. R. and A. R. Irvine, 1952;
Schofield, 1957; Fenton and de Buen, 1964).

The most effective treatment of such a secondary glaucoma in the
presence of a hypermature lens is to reduce the pressure by acetazolamide
or intravenous hypertonic solutions, followed immediately by extraction of

[1] Safar (1928), Kaufman (1933), Hubbersty and Gourlay (1953).

the lens.[1] An intracapsular extraction should, if possible, be performed, although the thinned and delicate capsule may make this difficult without the use of cryosurgery. The decision to perform a major operation on an acutely inflamed eye with a high tension may cause anxiety, particularly since phacolytic glaucoma may present bizarre clinical signs. By the relatively simple procedure of a paracentesis, however, the diagnosis may be made by the demonstration of the typical macrophages in the aqueous; these are difficult to find in the ordinary course of events but can usually be demonstrated if the fluid is passed through a millipore filter (Goldberg, 1967) (Figs. 623–4); if these are found extraction of the cataract can be performed without hesitation and, in fact, offers the only hope of saving the eye.

Axenfeld. *Klin. Mbl. Augenheilk.*, **52**, 195 (1914).

Ballen and Hughes. *Amer. J. Ophthal.*, **39**, 403 (1955).

Barraquer. *Arch. Soc. Amer. Oftal. Opt.*, **1**, 30 (1958).

Bickerton. *Trans. ophthal. Soc. U.K.*, **17**, 34 (1897).

Boggi. *Ann. Ottal.*, **25**, 7 (1896).

Bowman. *Roy. Lond. ophthal. Hosp. Rep.*, **5**, 1 (1865).

Calhoun and Hagler. *Amer. J. Ophthal.*, **50**, 701 (1960).

Carson, Dent, Field and Gaull. *J. Pediat.*, **66**, 565 (1965).

Chandler. *Arch. Ophthal.*, **60**, 828 (1958); **71**, 765 (1964).
Trans. Amer. ophthal. Soc., **57**, 242 (1959).

Diotallevi. *Boll. Oculist.*, **40**, 901 (1961).

Dodo. *Acta Soc. ophthal. jap.*, **61**, 795 (1957).

Dryden, Perraut and Seward. *Amer. J. Ophthal.*, **52**, 468 (1961).

Fenton and de Buen. *Arch. Ophthal.*, **72**, 227 (1964).

Fleischer. *Arch. Augenheilk.*, **80**, 248 (1916).

Flocks, Littwin and Zimmerman. *Arch. Ophthal.*, **54**, 37 (1955).

Gärtner. *Klin. Mbl. Augenheilk.*, **133**, 31 (1958).

Gibson, Carson and Neill. *J. clin. Path.*, **17**, 427 (1964).

Gifford. *Amer. J. Ophthal.*, **17**, 289 (1900); **1**, 83 (1918).
Arch. Ophthal., **56**, 457 (1927).

Gnad. *Klin. Mbl. Augenheilk.*, **87**, 33 (1931).

Goldberg. *Brit. J. Ophthal.*, **51**, 847 (1967).

Gonzales. *Rev. cub. Oftal.*, **4**, 100 (1922).

von Graefe. *v. Graefes Arch. Ophthal.*, **15** (2), 153 (1869).

Harms. *Klin. Mbl. Augenheilk.*, **43** (1), 147 (1905).

Harshman. *Amer. J. Ophthal.*, **31**, 833 (1948).

Heath. *Arch. Ophthal.*, **25**, 424 (1941).

Hegner. *Beitr. Augenheilk.*, **9** (90), 707 (1915).

Henkind and Ashton. *Trans. ophthal. Soc. U.K.*, **85**, 21 (1965).

Hubbersty and Gourlay. *Brit. J. Ophthal.*, **37**, 432 (1953).

Irvine, S. R. and A. R. *Amer. J. Ophthal.*, **35**, 177, 370, 489 (1952).

Ischreyt. *Arch. Augenheilk.*, **62**, 272 (1909).

Janotka. *Klin. oczna*, **36**, 619 (1966).

Johnston. *Brit. J. Ophthal.*, **52**, 251 (1968).

Kaufman. *Arch. Ophthal.*, **9**, 56 (1933).

Knapp. *Amer. J. Ophthal.*, **20**, 820 (1937).

Kravitz. *Arch. Ophthal.*, **62**, 764 (1959).

Levy and Anderson. *Brit. J. Ophthal.*, **45**, 223 (1961).

Lieberman, Podos and Hartstein. *Amer. J. Ophthal.*, **61**, 252 (1966).

Magnasco and Zingirian. *Ann. Ottal.*, **91**, 489 (1965).

McDonald and Purnell. *J. Amer. med. Ass.*, **145**, 220 (1951).

McGavic. *Amer. J. Ophthal.*, **62**, 820 (1966).

Mitvalsky. *Zbl. prakt. Augenheilk.*, **16**, 289 (1892).

Morax. *Ann. Oculist.* (Paris), **159**, 185 (1922).

Nemetz. *Klin. Mbl. Augenheilk.*, **128**, 483 (1956).

Nirankari and Chaddah. *J. All-India ophthal. Soc.*, **11**, 104 (1963).

Nirankari and Maudgal. *Brit. J. Ophthal.*, **43**, 314 (1959).

Probert. *Amer. J. Ophthal.*, **36**, 1571 (1953).

Rampoldi. *Ann. Ottal.*, **15**, 179 (1886).

von Reuss. *Zbl. prakt. Augenheilk.*, **24**, 33 (1900).

Rodman. *Arch. Ophthal.*, **69**, 445 (1963).

Rosenthal and Kloepfer. *Arch. Ophthal.*, **55**, 28 (1956).

Safar. *Z. Augenheilk.*, **64**, 46 (1928).

Salus. *Klin. Mbl. Augenheilk.*, **48** (2), 167 (1910).

Schimke, McKusick, Huang and Pollack. *J. Amer. med. Ass.*, **193**, 711 (1965).

Schofield. *Trans. ophthal. Soc. U.K.*, **77**, 193 (1957).

Scott. *Brit. J. Ophthal.*, **37**, 58 (1953).

[1] Gifford (1900–27), Safar (1928), Knapp (1937), Heath (1941), S. R. and A. R. Irvine (1952), Verhoeff (1952), Scott (1953), Ballen and Hughes (1955), Chandler (1958), and others.

Segal. *Oftalmologia* (Buc.), **6**, 207 (1962).
Serr. *Ber. dtsch. ophthal. Ges.*, **53**, 306 (1940).
Shapira. *Amer. J. Ophthal.*, **17**, 726 (1934).
Smeral. *Sborn. věd. Praci lék. Fak. Hradci Králové*, **5**, 93 (1962).
Smith, M. E. and Zimmerman. *Arch. Ophthal.*, **74**, 799 (1965).
Smith, Priestley. *Glaucoma*, London (1879).
Sugar. *Amer. J. Ophthal.*, **24**, 851 (1941).
Szili. *Zbl. prakt. Augenheilk.*, **8**, 17 (1884).
Tjanidis, Georgiades, Chilas and Bessas. *Arch. Soc. Ophtal. Grèce Nord*, **11**, 67 (1962).
Urbanek. *Z. Augenheilk.*, **71**, 171 (1930).

Verhoeff. *Amer. J. Ophthal.*, **35**, 498 (1952).
Verhoeff and Lemoine. *Amer. J. Ophthal.*, **5**, 700 (1922).
Verrey. *Amer. J. Ophthal.*, **33**, 230 (1916).
Weekers and Grieten. *Ophthalmologica*, **150**, 36 (1965).
Wessely. *Arch. Augenheilk.*, **65**, 295 (1910); **85**, 63 (1919).
Wright. *Ophthal. Rec.*, **19**, 303 (1910).
Zabriskie and Reisman. *J. Pediat.*, **52**, 158 (1958).
Zeeman. *Acta ophthal.* (Kbh.), **20**, 1 (1942).
Zoldan. *Boll. Oculist.*, **38**, 753 (1959).

Glaucoma Secondary to Vascular Diseases

HÆMORRHAGIC GLAUCOMA

A severe and intractable secondary glaucoma may occur during the course of or following a number of apparently dissimilar affections which have in common a widespread hypoxia of the retina. The acute rise of tension characterized by the development of new vessels covering the iris and lining the angle of the anterior chamber has been termed HÆMORRHAGIC GLAUCOMA.

OCCLUSION OF THE CENTRAL VEIN OF THE RETINA

The frequent occurrence of secondary glaucoma after occlusion of the central vein of the retina (but not of a tributary vein) has already been fully discussed.[1] At the time of the vascular occlusion the tension in the affected eye may be normal or lower than that of its fellow (Foster Moore, 1922; Wessely, 1935; Bianchi and Barrenechea, 1966), but in some 20% of cases of complete occlusion, hypertension becomes evident as a rule within 3 months after the start of the illness. The resultant *hæmorrhagic* or *thrombotic glaucoma* is usually a disastrous condition, severe and extremely painful (Fig. 625): the cornea is hazy and may become vascularized, the anterior chamber is typically of normal depth and may contain some blood, the pupil is small and the iris and trabeculæ show new vessels on their surface, the vitreous is usually clouded with red cells often precluding any view of the fundus, the tension is stony-hard, all perception of light is lost, and the associated pain is sometimes sufficient to demand excision of the globe. Any attempt at operative reduction of the ocular tension merely makes matters more acutely worse by inducing profuse and recurrent hæmorrhages, and the only practical method of treatment, if a retrobulbar injection of alcohol or cyclodiathermy fails to relieve the pain, is enucleation.

The ætiology of this type of glaucoma has given rise to much speculation. Pathological examinations[2] have shown that, besides an intense inflammatory reaction in the anterior segment of the globe, a highly vascularized

[1] Vol. X, p. 112.   [2] Vol. X, p. 114.

membrane finally covers the entire anterior surface of the iris and the angle of the anterior chamber (Figs. 626–30) (Verhoeff, 1907; Inouye, 1910; Samuels, 1935; Smith, 1955; Auricchio and Diotallevi, 1959). The presence of this vascularized membrane and the occurrence of extensive peripheral anterior synechiæ are responsible for the acute rise of tension which in the past has been attributed to other causes—the effect of a highly albuminous aqueous (Coats, 1904), a perivascular sclerosis (Fisher, 1925), a turgescence

Figs. 625 and 626.—Thrombotic Glaucoma.

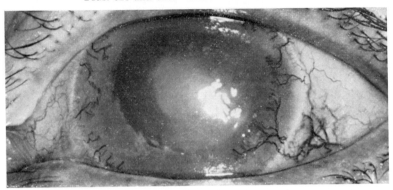

Fig. 625.—In a woman aged 62 (J. H. Dobree).

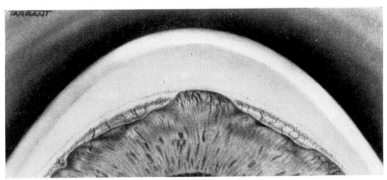

Fig. 626.—Rubeosis of the base of the iris and of the corneo-scleral trabeculæ following occlusion of the central retinal vein (R. Smith).

of the vitreous owing to the absorption of hæmorrhagic products (Wood, 1932; Vannas, 1960), or of other tissue metabolites (Weinstein, 1939).

At this point it must be emphasized once again that retinal venous occlusion frequently occurs in eyes with well-established simple glaucoma, a relationship which, although first described by Verhoeff (1913),[1] has until recently received little confirmation. Dryden (1965), in a clinical and histological study of 31 eyes enucleated for secondary glaucoma following

[1] Vol. X, p. 101.

Figs. 627 and 628.—Thrombotic Glaucoma (N. Ashton).

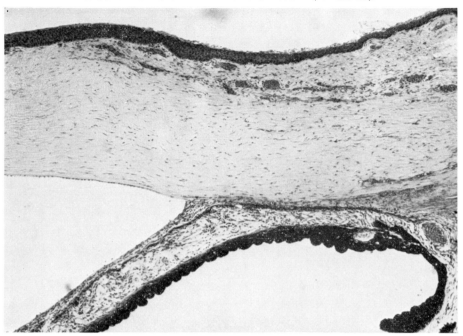

Fig. 627.—Peripheral anterior synechiæ associated with a vascular membrane of new vessels on the anterior face of the iris obliterating the drainage channels.

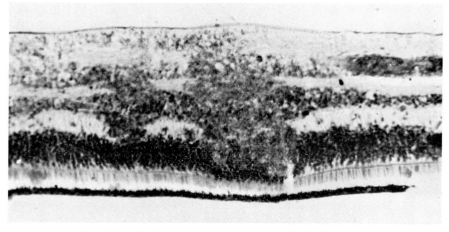

Fig. 628.—Retinal hæmorrhages in thrombotic glaucoma.

Figs. 629 and 630.—The Optic Nerve-head in Thrombotic Glaucoma (N. Ashton).

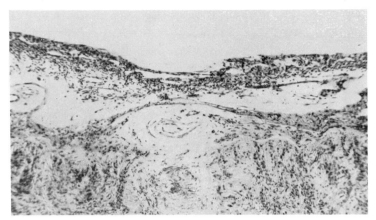

Fig. 629.—There is slight cupping and a large number of new vessels on the optic disc.

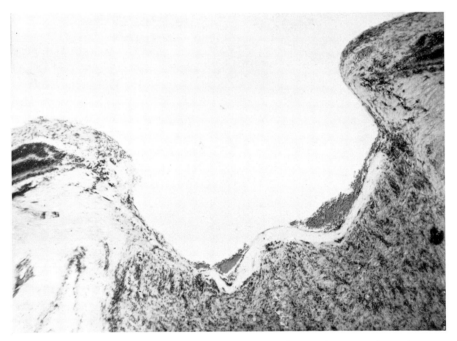

Fig. 630.—In a more advanced case. There are hæmorrhages on the optic disc and much fibrous organization.

venous occlusion, found that simple glaucoma was present in one eye prior to the occlusion and was discovered in the contralateral eye of 9 patients following enucleation. In the same study he examined clinically 26 patients with venous occlusion, 7 of whom had been seen prior to the occlusion and of whom 5 had bilateral simple glaucoma. In the remaining 19 patients first seen after the occlusion, 13 were found with simple glaucoma in the contralateral eye. These observations confirm those of several other authors[1]; although the incidence of simple glaucoma has been found to show wide variations, the discrepancy is probably due to the different criteria used in making the diagnosis.

There is thus no doubt that the presence of simple glaucoma plays an important role in the production of occlusion of the central retinal vein but the mechanism of this association is ill-understood. Verhoeff (1913) suggested that the glaucoma produced proliferative degenerative changes in the vein, while Behrman (1962) believed that it acted by producing a backward bulging of the lamina cribrosa with a resulting mechanical stenosis of the vein. Either factor would aggravate the effect of any concurrent venous sclerosis.

OCCLUSION OF THE CENTRAL ARTERY OF THE RETINA

In contrast to the relatively common occurrence of secondary glaucoma following occlusion of the central vein, that following occlusion of the central artery of the retina[2] is distinctly uncommon, occurring in about 1% of cases. Although a number of isolated reports appeared in the earlier literature[3] it is only more recently that attention has been drawn to this association.[4] Smith (1962) reported a case of hæmorrhagic glaucoma following occlusion of the central artery of the retina subsequent to occlusion of the carotid artery on the same side. In the majority of cases the rise in tension has occurred between 5 and 9 weeks after the arterial occlusion (Perraut and Zimmerman, 1959), a considerably shorter interval than that of the glaucoma which follows occlusion of the central vein, although the clinical picture in the two circumstances is otherwise similar.

The ætiology is as ill-understood as that of the secondary glaucoma following occlusion of the central vein. Pathological examinations have shown that a fibro-vascular membrane lines the angle of the anterior chamber

[1] Braendstrup (1950–52), Larsson and Nord (1950), Becker and Post 1951), Higgitt (1956), Vannas et al. (1957–61), Waubke (1960), Bertelsen (1961), Raitta (1965), Bianchi and Barrenechea (1966), Trux (1966), and others.

[2] Vol. X, p. 77.

[3] Loring (1874), Nettleship (1874), Watson and Nettleship (1875), Knapp (1881), Manz (1891), Marple (1895), Ridley (1895), Galinowsky (1901), Coats (1905–13), Harms (1905), Schwitzer (1906), Opin (1927), Villard and Dejean (1928), Bussola (1930).

[4] Ross (1950), Holt (1951), Benton (1953), Winter (1957), Wolter and Liddicoat (1958), Wolter and Lubeck (1958), Davenport (1959), Perraut and Zimmerman (1959), Wolter and Phillips (1959), Gupta (1960), Wagener (1960), Weiss and Leopold (1961), Liversedge and Smith (1962), Haye et al. (1964), Etienne et al. (1965), Ibrahim (1965), Lebas (1965), Madsen (1965), Tota (1965), Paufique and Ravault (1968), and others.

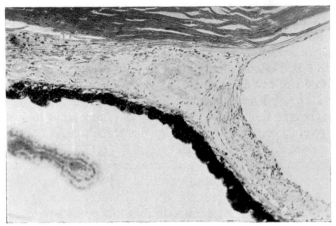

Fig. 631.—Secondary Glaucoma after Occlusion of the Central
Retinal Artery.

The entire angle is occluded by peripheral anterior synechiæ and a layer of
delicate capillaries extends onto the anterior surface of the atrophic iris (L. E. Perraut
and L. E. Zimmerman).

and covers the surface of the iris (Fig. 631),[1] and this membrane is believed
to cause the initial impairment of the outflow of aqueous; subsequently the
formation of peripheral anterior synechiæ aggravates the obstruction.

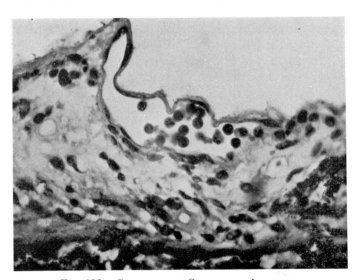

Fig. 632.—Glaucoma in Giant-cell Arteritis.

Thin-walled new formed vessels on the surface of the iris (J. R. Wolter and
R. L. Phillips).

[1] Perraut and Zimmerman (1959), Wolter and Liddicoat (1958), Wolter and Phillips
(1959), Wagener (1960).

A similar ætiological mechanism probably exists in the rare cases of hæmorrhagic glaucoma following LIGATION OF THE INTERNAL CAROTID ARTERY in the treatment of a carotico-cavernous aneurysm (Henderson and Schneider, 1958; Weiss et al., 1963). In the case described by Weiss and his colleagues (1963) an ocular tension of 32 mm. Hg was noted following the development of a traumatic carotico-cavernous aneurysm; there was no apparent neovascularization of the iris. Eight weeks after ligation of the internal carotid artery, a secondary glaucoma developed with many new vessels on the iris, rubeosis of the angle of the anterior chamber, and peripheral anterior synechiæ. Although no frank occlusion of the central artery or vein of the retina had occurred, there was diminished arterial input and venous stasis, indicating the probable presence of retinal hypoxia.

Also comparable is the case of hæmorrhagic glaucoma reported by Wolter and Phillips (1965) in a patient with giant-cell arteritis[1] (Fig. 632).

DIABETIC RUBEOSIS OF THE IRIS

A diabetic rubeosis of the iris often causes a hæmorrhagic glaucoma, an association that has already been remarked upon.[2] In this condition the surface of the iris is festooned with new-formed vessels, often concentrated near the pupillary margin. On gonioscopic examination the circumferential vessel frequently seen at the root of the iris in normal eyes becomes congested in the early stages (Ohrt, 1958), and large new vessels may be formed running peripherally into the angle where they break up again into innumerable branches forming extensive peripheral anterior synechiæ. Hæmorrhagic glaucoma occurs in about 2/3 of cases of rubeosis[3] and is almost always associated with a diabetic retinopathy, usually proliferative in type (Gasteiger, 1949; Ohrt, 1964; Cristiansson, 1965) but not invariably (van Beuningen, 1960); it also appears to be more common in patients with vascular hypertension (Waldman and Naidoff, 1948; François, 1951). The ætiology of the neovascularization is probably similar to that in other types of hæmorrhagic glaucoma, the stimulus being again associated with retinal hypoxia (Smith, 1954).

Treatment in most cases is ineffective. It is generally assumed that the condition is unrelated to the control of the diabetes although Cristiansson (1965) found that this was inadequate in the majority of his patients. Drainage operations are generally contra-indicated because of the risk of recurrent hyphæmata, but some success has been reported with cyclo-diathermy.[4]

[1] Vol. X, p. 238.
[2] Malbrán and Rebay (1948), Waldman and Naidoff (1948), Gasteiger (1949), Bonnet (1949), Pietruschka (1958), Ohrt (1961–64), Cristiansson (1965). Vol. IX, p. 651.
[3] Five out of 9 cases, Gasteiger (1949); 25 out of 30, Pietruschka (1958); 24 out of 41, Ohrt (1961); 15 out of 33, Ohrt (1964).
[4] Scobee (1944), Meyer and Sternberg (1944), deRoetth (1946), François and Neetens (1955), Cristini (1959), Calmettes et al. (1964).

SICKLE-CELL DISEASE

A secondary glaucoma may occasionally occur in sickle-cell disease.[1] Boniuk and Burton (1964) reported 2 cases with sickle-cell retinopathy wherein a unilateral hæmorrhagic glaucoma developed; one patient had hæmoglobin S-C disease and the other hæmoglobin S-A disease. The glaucoma was considered to be due to neovascularization of the angle of the anterior chamber and the formation of peripheral anterior synechiæ resulting from multiple areas of intravascular sickling and arteriolar obstruction (Fig. 633). Another case of hæmoglobin S-A disease reported by Shapiro and Baum (1964) developed uveitis and a secondary glaucoma. The canal of Schlemm was filled with blood for 18 days and it was believed that sickling within the canal resulted in the increase in tension.

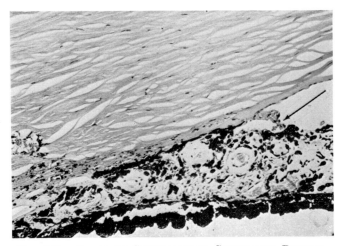

FIG. 633.—GLAUCOMA SECONDARY TO SICKLE-CELL DISEASE.

The angle of the anterior chamber is closed by anterior synechiæ with a fine vascular membrane (arrowed) which covers the anterior surface of the peripheral part of the iris (M. Boniuk and G. L. Burton).

RHEGMATOGENOUS AND EXUDATIVE RETINAL DETACHMENTS

A secondary glaucoma complicating a simple detachment of the retina is rare, but it occurs in a small proportion of cases in which the detachment is of some duration. Thus Nordenson (1887) found no rise of tension in 62 recent cases but in 4 of 58 long-standing cases it was raised; Kümmell (1921) reported a raised tension in 2 out of 52 cases, and Thomas (1925) in 1 out of 247. Such a rise of tension is usually preceded by inflammatory lesions accompanying the detachment suggesting a toxic origin (Fuchs. 1920; Morax, 1920; Maggiore, 1923; Wilder, 1931), but it has also been associated with recurrent hæmorrhages (Bergmeister, 1919; Stanka, 1923)

[1] Vol. X, p. 393.

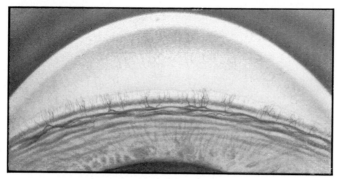

FIG. 634.—RUBEOSIS IN EALES'S DISEASE.
In a male aged 27 (Inst. Ophthal.).

suggesting that in some cases it is hæmorrhagic in nature, as indicated by Zollinger (1951).

A similar hæmorrhagic glaucoma may also occur in COATS'S SYNDROME (Coats, 1912; Böhringer, 1952) and in EALES'S DISEASE (Smith, 1955) (Fig. 634).

FOLLOWING IRRADIATION

Glaucoma occurs extremely rarely after intensive radiotherapy which has produced a general telangiectatic condition of the skin and conjunctiva (Birch-Hirschfeld, 1921; Gifford, 1940; Goulden, 1942; Bedford, 1966). A secondary open-angle glaucoma may occur in such cases (Bedford, 1966). Bothman (1940) described a case wherein, following irradiation, the ciliary processes had become atrophic and depigmented and the angle of the anterior chamber and the canal of Schlemm were filled with pigment which had apparently blocked the outflow channels to produce the hypertension. Similar changes were produced in guinea-pigs by Cecio and Menna (1960). Fry (1952) described a 5-year-old child who developed peripheral anterior synechiæ and a secondary glaucoma, Jones (1958) found vascularization of the angle of the anterior chamber following radiotherapy, while Haye and his co-workers (1965) reported a case of hypertensive uveitis which developed 18 months after intensive irradiation to the eyelids.

Auricchio and Diotallevi. *Rass. ital. Ottal.*, **28**, 321 (1959).
Becker and Post. *Amer. J. Ophthal.*, **34**, 677 (1951).
Bedford. *Proc. roy. Soc. Med.*, **59**, 529 (1966).
Behrman. *Brit. J. Ophthal.*, **46**, 336 (1962).
Benton. *Arch. Ophthal.*, **49**, 280 (1953).
Bergmeister. *Z. Augenheilk.*, **42**, 254 (1919).
Bertelsen. *Acta ophthal.* (Kbh.), **39**, 603 (1961).
van Beuningen. *Ber. dtsch. ophthal. Ges.*, **63**, 91 (1960).

Bianchi and Barrenechea. *Arch. chil. Oftal.*, **23**, 21 (1966).
Birch-Hirschfeld. *Z. Augenheilk.*, **45**, 199 (1921).
Böhringer. *Ophthalmologica*, **123**, 211 (1952).
Boniuk and Burton. *Trans. Amer. Acad. Ophthal.*, **68**, 316 (1964).
Bonnet. *Ophthalmologica*, **118**, 575 (1949).
Bothman. *Arch. Ophthal.*, **23**, 1198 (1940).
Braendstrup. *Acta ophthal.* (Kbh.), Suppl. 35 (1950).
  Nord. Med., **48**, 1668 (1952).

Bussola. *Boll. Oculist.*, **9**, 495 (1930).
Calmettes, Déodati and Bec. *Bull. Soc. Ophtal. Fr.*, **64**, 1040 (1964).
Cecio and Menna. *Arch. Ottal.*, **64**, 359 (1960).
Coats. *Roy. Lond. ophthal. Hosp. Rep.*, **16**, 62 (1904); 262 (1905); 516 (1906); **19**, 45, 71, 78 (1913).
  Trans. ophthal. Soc. U.K., **24**, 161 (1904); **33**, 30 (1913).
  v. Graefes Arch. Ophthal., **81**, 275 (1912); **86**, 341 (1913).
Cristiansson. *Acta ophthal.* (Kbh.), **43**, 224 (1965).
Cristini. *Rass. ital. Ottal.*, **28**, 401 (1959).
Davenport. *Trans. ophthal. Soc. U.K.*, **79**, 3 (1959).
Dryden. *Arch. Ophthal.*, **73**, 659 (1965).
Etienne, Barut and Ravault. *Ann. Oculist.* (Paris), **198**, 991 (1965).
Fisher. *Trans. ophthal. Soc. U.K.*, **45**, 288 (1925).
François. *Ophthalmologica*, **121**, 313 (1951).
François and Neetens. *Bull. Soc. belge Ophtal.*, No. 111, 318 (1955).
Fry. *Trans. Amer. Acad. Ophthal.*, **56**, 888 (1952).
Fuchs. *v. Graefes Arch. Ophthal.*, **101**, 265 (1920).
Galinowsky. *Arch. Augenheilk.*, **43**, 183 (1901).
Gasteiger. *Ber. dtsch. ophthal. Ges.*, **55**, 181 (1949).
Gifford. *Arch. Ophthal.*, **23**, 301 (1940).
Goulden. *Trans. ophthal. Soc. U.K.*, **62**, 112 (1942).
Gupta. *Brit. J. Ophthal.*, **44**, 52 (1960).
Harms. *v. Graefes Arch. Ophthal.*, **61**, 1, 245 (1905).
Haye, Demailly and Reca. *Bull. Soc. Ophtal. Fr.*, **64**, 269 (1964).
Haye, Jammet and Dollfus. *L'oeil et les radiations ionisantes*, Paris, 335 (1965).
Henderson and Schneider. *Trans. Amer. ophthal. Soc.*, **56**, 123 (1958).
Higgitt. *Trans. ophthal. Soc. U.K.*, **76**, 73 (1956).
Holt. *Amer. J. Ophthal.*, **34**, 1758 (1951).
Ibrahim. *Bull. ophthal. Soc. Egypt*, **58**, 367 (1965).
Inouye. *Roy. Lond. ophthal. Hosp. Rep.*, **18**, 24 (1910).
Jones. *Brit. J. Ophthal.*, **42**, 636 (1958).
Knapp. *Arch. Augenheilk.*, **10**, 96 (1881).
Kümmell. *Klin. Mbl. Augenheilk.*, **67**, 180 (1921).
Larsson and Nord. *Acta ophthal.* (Kbh.), **28**, 187 (1950).
Lebas. *J. All-India ophthal. Soc.*, **13**, 130 (1965).
Liversedge and Smith. *Trans. ophthal. Soc. U.K.*, **82**, 571 (1962).
Loring. *Amer. J. med. Sci.*, **67**, 313 (1874).
Madsen. *Acta ophthal.* (Kbh.), **43**, 350 (1965).
Maggiore. *Ann. Ottal.*, **51**, 1 (1923).

Malbrán and Rebay. *Arch. Oftal. B. Aires*, **23**, 276 (1948).
Manz. *Festschr. z. Feier d. 70 Geburtstages v. H. von Helmholtz*, Stuttgart, 9 (1891).
Marple. *N.Y. Ear and Eye Inf. Rep.*, **3**, 1 (1895).
Meyer and Sternberg. *Trans. Amer. Acad. Ophthal.*, **49**, 147 (1944).
Moore, Foster. *Trans. ophthal. Soc. U.K.*, **42**, 115 (1922).
Morax. *Bull. Soc. franç. Ophtal.*, **33**, 160 (1920).
Nettleship. *Roy. Lond. ophthal. Hosp. Rep.*, **8**, 9 (1874).
Nordenson. *Die Netzhautablösung*, Wiesbaden (1887).
Ohrt. *Acta ophthal.* (Kbh.), **36**, 556 (1958).
  Ophthalmologica, **142**, 356 (1961).
  Dan. med. Bull., **11**, 17 (1964).
Opin. *Arch. Ophtal.*, **44**, 321 (1927).
Paufique and Ravault. *Bibl. ophthal.*, No. 76, 54 (1968).
Perraut and Zimmerman. *Arch. Ophthal.*, **61**, 845 (1959).
Pietruschka. *Dtsch. Gesundh.-Wes.*, **13**, 1182 (1958).
Raitta. *Der Zentralvenen- u. Netzhautvenenverschluss*, Helsinki (1965).
Ridley. *Roy. Lond. ophthal. Hosp. Rep.*, **14**, 264 (1895).
deRoetth. *Arch. Ophthal.*, **35**, 20 (1946).
Ross. *Eye, Ear, Nose, Thr. Monthly*, **29**, 561 (1950).
Samuels. *Arch. Ophthal.*, **13**, 404 (1935).
Schwitzer. *Z. Augenheilk.*, **16**, 61 (1906).
Scobee. *Tex. St. J. Med.*, **40**, 432 (1944).
Shapiro and Baum. *Amer. J. Ophthal.*, **58**, 292 (1964).
Smith, J. L. *J. Amer. med. Ass.*, **182**, 683 (1962).
Smith, R. *Acta XVII int. Cong. Ophthal.*, Montreal-N.Y., **2**, 1164 (1954).
  Trans. ophthal. Soc. U.K., **75**, 265 (1955).
Stanka. *Klin. Mbl. Augenheilk.*, **70**, 707 (1923).
Thomas. *Z. Augenheilk.*, **54**, 333 (1925).
Tota. *Boll. Oculist.*, **44**, 186 (1965).
Trux. *Bull. Soc. franç. Ophtal.*, **79**, 540 (1966).
Vannas. *Acta ophthal.* (Kbh.), **38**, 254 (1960).
  Ophthalmologica, **142**, 266 (1961).
Vannas and Orma. *Arch. Ophthal.*, **58**, 812 (1957).
Vannas and Tarkkanen. *Brit. J. Ophthal.*, **44**, 583 (1960).
  Acta ophthal. (Kbh.), **38**, 50 (1960).
Verhoeff. *Arch. Ophthal.*, **36**, 1 (1907); **42**, 145 (1913).
Villard and Dejean. *Ann. Oculist.* (Paris), **165**, 241 (1928).
Wagener. *Amer. J. med. Sci.*, **240**, 253 (1960).
Waldman and Naidoff. *Amer. J. Ophthal.*, **31**, 468 (1948).
Watson and Nettleship. *Roy. Lond. ophthal. Hosp. Rep.*, **8**, 251 (1875).

Waubke. *Klin. Mbl. Augenheilk.*, **136,** 224 (1960).

Weinstein. *Brit. J. Ophthal.*, **23,** 392 (1939).

Weiss and Leopold. *Amer. J. Ophthal.*, **51,** 793 (1961).

Weiss, Shaffer and Nehrenberg. *Arch. Ophthal.*, **69,** 304 (1963).

Wessely. *Klin. Mbl. Augenheilk.*, **95,** 398 (1935).

Wilder. *Arch. Ophthal.*, **5,** 55 (1931).

Winter. *Trans. Pac. Cst. oto-ophthal. Soc.*, **38,** 9 (1957).

Wolter and Liddicoat. *Amer. J. Ophthal.*, **46,** 182 (1958).

Wolter and Lubeck. *Klin. Mbl. Augenheilk.*, **133,** 179 (1958).

Wolter and Phillips. *Amer. J. Ophthal.*, **47,** 335 (1959); **59,** 625 (1965).

Wood. *Brit. J. Ophthal.*, **16,** 423 (1932).

Zollinger. *Ophthalmologica*, **121,** 168 (1951).

GLAUCOMA SECONDARY TO INTRA-OCULAR HÆMORRHAGE

INTRA-OCULAR ARTERIAL HÆMORRHAGES, if at all profuse, are always followed by an extremely acute rise of tension wherein the intra-ocular pressure is suddenly raised to approximately the level of the blood-pressure in the arteries. We have already seen that the most typical instance of this distressing accident is in the case of an expulsive hæmorrhage during or after an intra-ocular operation, that the hæmorrhage is usually choroidal from one of the posterior ciliary arteries, and that the only treatment usually effective in relieving the excruciating pain is excision of the globe.[1]

CAPILLARY AND VENOUS HÆMORRHAGES are not usually followed by secondary glaucoma unless they are recurrent, although occasional cases of

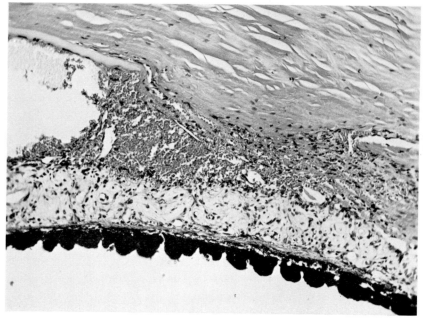

FIG. 635.—GLAUCOMA SECONDARY TO INTRA-OCULAR HÆMORRHAGE.

In a case of occlusion of the central retinal artery. A blood clot in the anterior chamber is becoming organized, pulling the iris forward against the cornea (L. E. Perraut and L. E. Zimmerman).

[1] Vol. IX, p. 27.

acute secondary glaucoma following a vitreous hæmorrhage have been
reported (Fenton and Zimmerman, 1963; Fenton and Hunter, 1965). In
the cases on which histological examination has been carried out, the
angle of the anterior chamber was found to be filled with hæmorrhagic debris
and pigment-laden macrophages which were considered responsible for the
rise in intra-ocular pressure (Fig. 635). As the ætiological mechanism is
similar to that operative in phacolytic glaucoma, the term *hæmolytic glaucoma*
has been suggested for this condition (Fenton and Zimmerman, 1963).

GLAUCOMA SECONDARY TO OBSTRUCTION OF VENOUS DRAINAGE FROM THE EYE

Any condition which causes an obstruction of the venous drainage from
the eye is liable to produce a secondary glaucoma. This may arise from

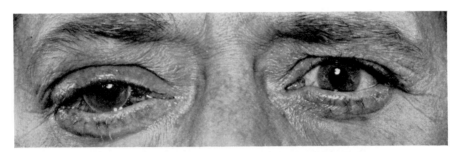

FIG. 636.

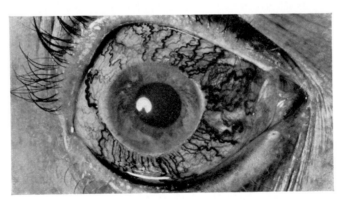

FIG. 637.

FIGS. 636 and 637.—CAROTICO-CAVERNOUS ANEURYSM.
On the right side, in a male aged 34. (Inst. Ophthal.)

various orbital conditions including idiopathic THROMBOSIS of the orbital
veins (Morax, 1967), INFLAMMATIONS (Guist, 1925; inflammatory œdema—
Davis, 1928; abscess—Magitot, 1918; tenonitis—Seefelder, 1924; Larsson,
1926), HÆMORRHAGES (Magitot, 1918; Magitot and Tillé, 1932; Terrien,
1932), TUMOURS (van Duyse, 1896; Cory, 1947; Plamondon and Lacerte,

1954; Orlowski and Korobowicz, 1958; Bayard, 1963; vom Hofe and Schmidt, 1965; and others), PSEUDO-TUMOURS (Aten, 1948; Rosselet, 1960), and PAGET'S DISEASE involving the orbit (Moro and Bello, 1951; Olaru and Diaconu, 1959). It also occurs in about 10% of cases of PULSATING EXOPHTHALMOS determined by carotico-cavernous aneurysm (Figs. 636–7)[1]. The rise of tension in these cases is generally thought to be due to an increased venous back-pressure[2] since the resistance to the outflow of aqueor is normal; Auricchio and Diotallevi (1961), however, found a decrease in the production of aqueous and an increased resistance to outflow, while Weekers and Grieten (1965) later observed that there may be a superadded increase in the resistance to outflow in long-standing and severe cases. In many instances of glaucoma complicating a carotico-cavernous aneurysm, ligation of the internal carotid artery reduces the tension to a normal level, but, as we have seen,[3] on a few occasions a typical hæmorrhagic glaucoma has been reported to follow this procedure.

Glaucoma associated with an idiopathic elevation of the episcleral venous pressure affecting both eyes in a mother and one eye in a daughter was reported by Minas and Podos (1968). In the affected eyes the episcleral veins were engorged for no discoverable reason with a blood pressure of about 20 mm. Hg. The drainage angles were open but there was blood in Schlemm's canal, the ocular tensions were raised, the discs were cupped and there were typical glaucomatous defects in the visual fields.

The venous drainage from the eye may also be impaired by OBSTRUCTION OF THE SUPERIOR VENA CAVA by a mediastinal tumour or other lesions (Fig. 638).[4] An interesting case was reported by J. E. Alfano (1965) wherein the superior vena cava was occluded for less than one minute during cardiac surgery; the 5-year-old girl suffered an acute glaucoma associated with œdema of the lids and retina. In such a case the intra-ocular pressure is frequently within normal limits when the patient is upright but raised when the recumbent position is assumed. Pilocarpine usually reduces this type of raised tension.

At this point it is relevant to discuss the possible relationship between ENDOCRINE EXOPHTHALMOS and raised intra-ocular pressure. Although Brailey and Eyre described 5 cases of thyrotoxicosis in young women with glaucoma as long ago as 1900, it is only recently that many reports of the association between glaucoma and endocrine exophthalmos have appeared in the literature.[5] The position, however, is complicated by the observations

[1] H. Sattler (1880), C. H. Sattler (1920), Hudelo (1928), Hanford and Wheeler (1930), Terry and Fred (1938), Sugar and Meyer (1940), Crawford (1942), Gazepis (1951), Swan and Raaf (1951), Weekers et al. (1954–65), Henderson and Schneider (1958), Lobstein and Lévy (1958), Auricchio and Diotallevi (1961), Weiss et al. (1963), and others.
[2] Weekers and Delmarcelle (1952–56), Henderson and Schneider (1958), vom Hofe and Schmidt (1965), and others.
[3] p. 673.
[4] Brolin (1949), Bedrossian (1952), J. E. and P. A. Alfano (1956), Lévy and Lobstein (1958).
[5] Pesme (1947), Beierwaltes (1951), Vanni (1958), Vanni and Vozza (1960), Rosselet (1960), Gördüren (1962), Sandston (1963), Rogova (1964), Rose (1965), Vasilieva (1965), Haddad (1967).

of Weekers and his colleagues (1959–60), which have been confirmed by Draeger (1960), Böck and Stepanik (1961) and Strazhdina (1968), that the ocular tension increases on elevation of the eyes.   In addition, there have been conflicting reports on the effect of thyroid disease on the ocular rigidity. Weekers and his colleagues (1957–58) at first thought that the coefficient of ocular rigidity was reduced in thyrotropic exophthalmos although normal in

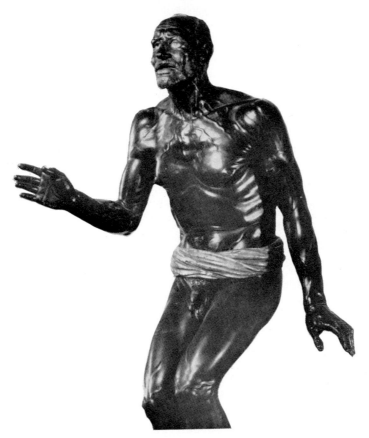

Fig. 638.—Le Vieux Pêcheur.

The statue in the Louvre, Paris, probably represents the syndrome of compression of the superior vena cava resulting in glaucoma in the left eye due to elevation of the episcleral venous pressure.

thyrotoxic exophthalmos, but in later papers (1959–60) they found it to be normal in both forms of endocrine disturbance, findings confirmed by Böck and Stepanik (1961); on the other hand, Vanni (1958), Draeger (1960) and Ytteborg (1961) found a low coefficient in these cases, while Haddad (1967) found that it showed wide variations.   In view of these reports on the increased ocular tension on elevation of the eyes and on the variability of the coefficient of ocular rigidity, it is difficult to assess the significance of glaucoma occurring in endocrine exophthalmos. To complicate the situation further, there have recently been reports that the function of the thyroid is abnormal in many cases of simple glaucoma (McLenachan and Davies, 1965; Becker *et al.*, 1966).

In spite of reports to the contrary it appears probable that the ocular tension is normal in thyrotoxic exophthalmos (Vanni and Vozza, 1960; Cheng and Perkins, 1967), while in thyrotropic exophthalmos there is an increased incidence of secondary glaucoma possibly caused by obstruction of the venous drainage from the eye.

GLAUCOMA SECONDARY TO SCAR-TISSUE ASSOCIATED WITH VASCULAR ANOMALIES

In RETROLENTAL FIBROPLASIA (the RETINOPATHY OF PREMATURITY)[1] a secondary glaucoma is not an uncommon event; it is always associated with a shallow anterior chamber and is therefore of the closed-angle type. In the

FIGS. 639 and 640.—RETROLENTAL FIBROPLASIA (F. C. Blodi).

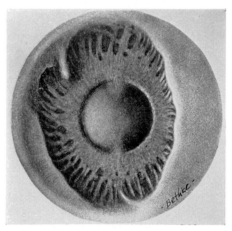 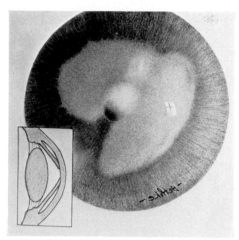

FIG. 639.—Peripheral anterior synechiæ causing glaucoma, associated with extensive peripheral corneal opacities.

FIG. 640.—Gross peripheral anterior synechiæ causing glaucoma and central corneal opacities.

early stages of the disease this may be caused by a pushing forward of the vitreous by the œdema and other changes in the retina, and the raised tension thus caused may be controlled by miotics. The more serious type of glaucoma, however, arises in the later stages when the fibrous tissue consolidates, forcing the lens–iris diaphragm forward and progressively narrowing the anterior chamber until it may become completely obliterated and permanent peripheral synechiæ develop (King, 1950; Blodi, 1955)

[1] Vol. X, p. 197.

(Figs. 639–40). In a considerable number of cases further contraction of the fibrous tissue may deepen the anterior chamber and open the angle to some extent; in this event the ultimate fate of the eye may be softening and atrophy.

In such an eye at a varying period after birth, the glaucoma tends to develop acutely, with pain and vomiting. At this stage miotics are valueless, but relief may be obtained by such hypotensive measures as acetazolamide; an alternative is cyclodiathermy (Reese and Blodi, 1951). These expedients may tide the child over the crisis until the globe begins to shrink but otherwise the useless eye should be enucleated.

A CONGENITAL PERSISTENCE OF THE VASCULAR SHEATH OF THE LENS is a second condition wherein the prolific formation of vascularized fibroblastic tissue behind the lens, often complicated by hæmorrhages, may result in a similar type of secondary glaucoma.[1] In addition to the displacement of the lens–iris diaphragm, the ciliary body is usually distorted and the retina detached in this malformation, of which the usual culmination is necessarily enucleation of the eye.

Alfano, J. E. *Amer. J. Ophthal.*, **60**, 412 (1965).

Alfano, J. E. and P. A. *Amer. J. Ophthal.*, **42**, 685 (1956).

Aten. *Ophthalmologica*, **115**, 121 (1948).

Auricchio and Diotallevi. *Ann. Ottal.*, **87**, 59 (1961).

Bayard. *Arch. Ophthal.*, **70**, 647 (1963).

Becker, Kolker and Ballin. *Amer. J. Ophthal.*, **61**, 997 (1966).

Bedrossian. *Arch. Ophthal.*, **47**, 641 (1952).

Beierwaltes. *J. clin. Endocrinol.*, **11**, 512 (1951).

Blodi. *Trans. Amer. ophthal. Soc.*, **59**, 35 (1955).

Böck and Stepanik. *Ophthalmologica*, **142**, 365 (1961).

Brailey and Eyre. *Guy's Hosp. Rep.*, **54**, 65 (1900).

Brolin. *Acta ophthal.* (Kbh.), **27**, 393 (1949).

Cheng and Perkins. *Brit. J. Ophthal.*, **51**, 547 (1967).

Cory. *Brit. J. Ophthal.*, **31**, 731 (1947).

Crawford. *Arch. Ophthal.*, **27**, 539 (1942).

Davis. *Trans. ophthal. Soc. U.K.*, **48**, 34 (1928).

Draeger. *Ber. dtsch. ophthal. Ges.*, **63**, 148 (1960).

van Duyse. *Arch. Ophtal.*, **16**, 604 (1896).

Fenton and Hunter. *Surv. Ophthal.*, **10**, 335 (1965).

Fenton and Zimmerman. *Arch. Ophthal.*, **70**, 236 (1963).

Gazepis. *Trans. Greek ophthal. Soc.*, **19**, 1 (1951).

Gördüren. *Brit. J. Ophthal.*, **46**, 491 (1962).

Guist. *Z. Augenheilk.*, **55**, 308 (1925).

Haddad. *Amer. J. Ophthal.*, **64**, 63 (1967).

Hanford and Wheeler. *Ann. Surg.*, **92**, 8 (1930).

vom Hofe and Schmidt. *Klin. Mbl. Augenheilk.*, **147**, 375 (1965).

Hudelo. *Le glaucome dans l'exophtalmos pulsatile* (Thèse), Paris (1928).

King. *Arch. Ophthal.*, **43**, 694 (1950).

Larsson. *Acta ophthal.* (Kbh.), **3**, 207 (1926).

Lavergne, Weekers and Prijot. *Bull. Soc. belge Ophtal.*, No. 116, 298 (1957).

Lévy and Lobstein. *Bull. Soc. Ophtal. Fr.*, 602 (1958).

Lobstein and Lévy. *Bull. Soc. Ophtal. Fr.*, 609 (1958).

McLenachan and Davies. *Brit. J. Ophthal.*, **49**, 441 (1965).

Magitot. *Ann. Oculist.* (Paris), **155**, 1 (1918).

Magitot and Tillé. *Bull. Soc. Ophtal. Paris*, 170 (1932).

Minas and Podos. *Arch. Ophthal.*, **80**, 202 (1968).

Morax. *Ann. Oculist.* (Paris), **200**, 23 (1967).

Moro and Bello. *Rass. ital. Ottal.*, **20**, 340 (1951).

Olaru and Diaconu. *Neurol. Psihiat. Neurochir.* (Buc.), **4**, 165 (1959).

Orlowski and Korobowicz. *Klin. oczna*, **28**, 307 (1958).

Pesme. *Bull. Soc. franç. Ophtal.*, **60**, 32 (1947).

Plamondon and Lacerte. *Acta XVII int. Cong. Ophthal.*, Montreal-N.Y., **1**, 31 (1954).

Reese and Blodi. *Amer. J. Ophthal.*, **34**, 1 (1951).

Rogova. *Vestn. Oftal.*, **77**, 38 (1964).

[1] Vol. III, p. 770.

Rose. *Amer. J. Ophthal.*, **59,** 1 (1965).

Rosselet. *Ophthalmologica*, **139,** 275 (1960).

Sandston. *Trans. ophthal. Soc. N.Z.*, **16,** 61 (1963).

Sattler, C. H. *Graefe-Saemisch Hb. d. ges. Augenheilk.*, 2nd ed., Berlin, **9** (1), Kap. XIII (2) (1920).

Sattler, H. *Graefe-Saemisch Hb. d. ges. Augenheilk.*, 1st ed., Leipzig, **6,** 745 (1880).

Seefelder. *Wien. med. Wschr.*, **74,** 2053 (1924).

Strazhdina. *Vestn. Oftal.*, **81,** 54 (1968).

Sugar and Meyer. *Arch. Ophthal.*, **23,** 1288 (1940).

Swan and Raaf. *Trans. Amer. ophthal. Soc.*, **49,** 435 (1951).

Terrien. *Bull. Soc. Ophtal. Paris*, 173 (1932).

Terry and Fred. *Arch. Ophthal.*, **19,** 90 (1938).

Vanni. *Boll. Oculist.*, **37,** 636 (1958).

Vanni and Vozza. *Boll. Oculist.*, **39,** 189 (1960).

Vasilieva. *Vestn. Oftal.*, **78,** 70 (1965).

Weekers and Delmarcelle. *Arch. Ophthal.*, **48,** 338 (1952).

Arch. Ophtal., **16,** 380 (1956).

Weekers and Grieten. *Arch. Ophtal.*, **25,** 531 (1965).

Weekers and Lavergne. *Ophthalmologica*, **134,** 276 (1957).

Brit. J. Ophthal., **42,** 680 (1958).

Weekers, Prijot and Lavergne. *Bull. Soc. belge Ophtal.*, No. 123, 564 (1959).

Ophthalmological, **139,** 382 (1960).

Ytteborg. *Acta ophthal.* (Kbh.), **39,** 540 (1961).

Glaucoma Secondary to Hæmopoietic Diseases

We have already seen[1] that the uveal tract is involved in about half the cases of leucæmia, when the choroid is implicated most commonly and the iris only exceptionally. In the ACUTE LEUCÆMIAS the infiltration of the uvea is frequently complicated by a rise in the ocular tension.[2] The iris may be intensely hyperæmic with an associated ciliary injection and if it is diffusely involved there is a loss of its architecture with neovascularization of its surface and intensive leucæmic infiltration of the tissues (Fig. 641).

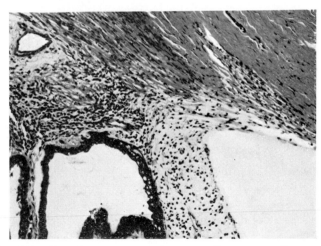

FIG. 641.—THE ANGLE OF THE ANTERIOR CHAMBER IN LEUCÆMIA.

In a 6½-year-old girl, showing dense infiltration of the root of the iris, the trabecular meshwork, Schlemm's canal and the ciliary body with leucæmic cells (H. A. Fonken and P. P. Ellis).

[1] Vol. IX, p. 634.

[2] Meller (1906–7), Triebenstein (1920), Weve (1932), McGavic (1943), Sommers (1949), Weekers and Prijot (1950), Cooper and Riker (1951), Thomas *et al.* (1954), Deitch and Wilson (1963), Marcus (1963), Fonken and Ellis (1966).

The consequent heterochromia is often associated with a hypopyon or a hyphæma and keratic precipitates may be deposited on the cornea. A perilimbal conjunctival infiltration has also been reported (Weekers and Prijot, 1950). The ocular condition responds to radiotherapy (Plate IX, Figs. 1 and 2).

In the CHRONIC LEUCÆMIAS, on the other hand, glaucoma is exceptional. Glaser and Smith (1966) reported a case of chronic lymphatic leucæmia wherein the presenting sign was a raised ocular tension associated with open drainage angles and the glaucoma was thought to be due to a blockage of the outflow channels by the infiltration of the limbus, while Martin (1968) described a case of chronic lymphatic leucæmia wherein bilateral acute glaucoma developed due to leucæmic infiltration of the angles of the anterior chamber (Plate IX, Figs. 3 and 4). Both cases responded to radiotherapy. Scholtyssek (1949) described a patient who developed a hæmorrhagic glaucoma following occlusion of his central retinal vein; 18 months later he presented the picture of myeloid leucæmia. It is possible that at the time of the occlusion leucæmia was already present and resulted in an increase in the viscosity of the blood which precipitated the condition.

Other diseases which cause an increase in the viscosity of the blood, such as POLYCYTHÆMIA and the DYSPROTEINÆMIAS, may also precipitate an occlusion of the central vein of the retina and thus result in a hæmorrhagic glaucoma. The cases reported by Goldzieher (1904), Baquis (1908) and Ginzburg (1928) may fall into this group.

Baquis. *v. Graefes Arch. Ophthal.*, **68,** 177 (1908).
Cooper and Riker. *Amer. J. Ophthal.*, **34,** 1153 (1951).
Deitch and Wilson. *Arch. Ophthal.*, **69,** 560 (1963).
Fonken and Ellis. *Arch. Ophthal.*, **76,** 32 (1966).
Ginzburg. *Klin. Mbl. Augenheilk.*, **81,** 591 (1928).
Glaser and Smith. *Brit. J. Ophthal.*, **50,** 92 (1966).
Goldzieher. *Zbl. prakt. Augenheilk.*, **28,** 257 (1904).
Marcus. *Arch. Ophthal.*, **69,** 251 (1963).
Martin. *Brit. J. Ophthal.*, **52,** 781 (1968).

McGavic. *Arch. Ophthal.*, **30,** 179 (1943).
Meller. *Z. Augenheilk.*, **15,** 538 (1906).
    v. Graefes Arch. Ophthal., **62,** 130 (1906).
    Klin. Mbl. Augenheilk., **45,** 491 (1907).
Scholtyssek. *Klin. Mbl. Augenheilk.*, **115,** 251 (1949).
Sommers. *Histology and Histopathology of the Eye and its Adnexa*, N.Y., 240 (1949).
Thomas, Vitte and Guidat. *Bull. Soc. Ophtal. Fr.*, 75 (1954).
Triebenstein. *Klin. Mbl. Augenheilk.*, **64,** 825 (1920).
Weekers and Prijot. *Bull. Soc. belge Ophtal.*, No. 96, 623 (1950).
Weve. *Arch. Augenheilk.*, **105,** 710 (1932).

Glaucoma Secondary to Epidemic Dropsy

Epidemic dropsy is a disease commonly seen in India; it is characterized by œdema of the extremities, gastro-intestinal disturbances, hypertrophy and dilatation of the heart, changes in the skin and, rarely, peripheral neuritis. It is a toxic condition caused by the contamination of cooking oil with seeds of the herb, *Argemone mexicana* (S. L. Sarker, 1926; Kamath, 1928; Lal and Roy, 1937); an alkaloid, sanguinarine, isolated from samples of argemone oil, has been shown to be the responsible agent (S. N. Sarkar, 1948).

PLATE IX

LEUCÆMIC INFILTRATES IN THE IRIS

FIGS. 1 and 2.—ACUTE LYMPHATIC LEUCÆMIA IN A GIRL AGED 6½ YEARS
(H. A. Fonken and P. P. Ellis).

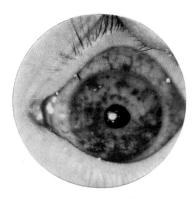 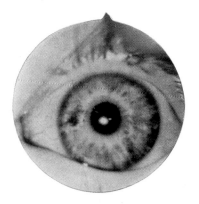

FIG. 1.—Showing the iris covered with vascularized tissue.

FIG. 2.—The same eye two weeks after radiation treatment, showing a minimal amount of infiltration of the iris.

FIGS. 3 and 4.—CHRONIC LYMPHATIC LEUCÆMIA IN A MAN AGED 59
(B. Martin).

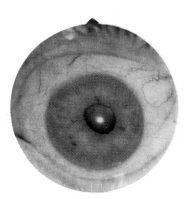 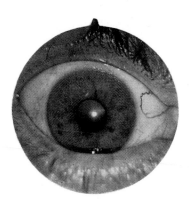

FIG. 3.—The eye before treatment, showing loss of the pattern of the iris and the deformed pupil.

FIG. 4.—The same eye after radiation treatment.

The most interesting pathological feature is a generalized telangiectatic dilatation of the capillaries, without an inflammatory reaction or a hæmorrhagic tendency, a phenomenon seen throughout the body and in all the blood vessels of the uveal tract even in cases which have shown no clinical signs and symptoms of glaucoma before death.

Glaucoma was first noted in association with epidemic dropsy by Maynard (1909) who reported a series of 100 cases in an epidemic in 1908–9; Mukerjee (1927) observed another series of 253 cases in Bengal, and Kirwan (1934) 325 cases between 1929 and 1933. The condition may occur in youth from 8 years of age upwards, and is most common between the ages of 20 and 35. It is bilateral and chronic in type, for the eye remains white even when the tension is extremely high; it is rarely accompanied by pain, and the two essential symptoms are the appearance of haloes due to corneal œdema and a gradual deterioration of vision. The anterior chamber is usually deep, although Mathur (1951) found it shallow in 52·6% of cases, and the pupil normal, while cupping and atrophy of the optic disc are late in appearance. The visual fields show the defects typical of simple glaucoma but the outstanding feature is the height of the tension which is rarely below 50 mm. Hg and may readily reach 100.

Pathologically an enormous dilatation of the small vessels of the uveal tract is a constant feature (Figs. 642–3); but there is no evidence of any inflammatory process and the filtration angle is open and shows no abnormality (Kirwan, 1936), although Leach (1955) found that sanguinarine produced a proliferation of the endothelial lining of the trabeculæ in monkeys. The aqueous humour shows a marked increase of albumin, a raised osmotic pressure due to its presence (Kirwan and Mukerjee, 1938), and contains a histamine-like substance in considerable quantity.

Hakim (1954) found experimentally that sanguinarine produced ocular changes similar to those seen in simple glaucoma in rabbits, guinea-pigs and rats, and that it could cause a marked and prolonged increase in the intra-ocular pressure. Similar increases in tension have been observed by Lieb and Scherf (1956) in rabbits, by Leach and Lloyd (1956) in monkeys, and by Shevalev (1957) in cats. The mode of action of this substance is not clearly understood although Hakim (1954–62) and Lieb and Scherf (1956) considered that the hypertensive reaction was due to the action of the alkaloid on the central nervous system; on the other hand, Kabelík (1966) suggested that the carbohydrate metabolism was deranged with a predominantly rice diet.

In *treatment* the first step ought to be the elimination of the seeds of *Argemone mexicana* completely from the diet. There are conflicting reports as to the value of miotics in this type of glaucoma, although Leach and Lloyd (1956) found that pilocarpine, eserine and DFP reduced the intra-ocular pressure to a normal level. As sanguinarine appears to have an anti-adrenaline action (Hakim, 1954), there is a theoretical reason for using

Figs. 642 and 643.—Glaucoma in Epidemic Dropsy (E. O'G. Kirwan).

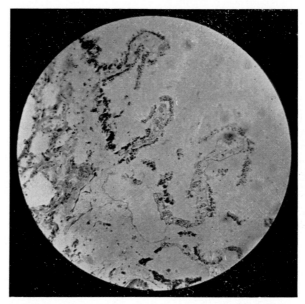

Fig. 642.—The ciliary body, showing vascular dilatation and œdema of the tissues without abnormality of the epithelium.

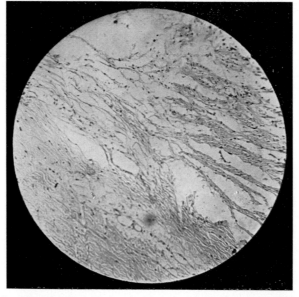

Fig. 643.—The filtration angle, showing complete absence of abnormality.

adrenaline in the treatment; cysteine has also been found to prevent the experimental glaucoma produced by sanguinarine (Hakim, 1954) and its use has been recommended by Leach and Lloyd (1956). Fuchs (1959) found that 31 out of 43 patients required surgery which should be undertaken if the ocular tension remains high and the deterioration of the visual fields is progressive in spite of medical therapy; various operations have been recommended but an anterior sclerectomy or a trephining operation appears to be effective.

Fuchs. *J. Ophtal. soc.*, Nos. 27 and 28, 14 (1959).

Hakim. *Brit. J. Ophthal.*, **38**, 193 (1954).
J. All-India ophthal. Soc., **10**, 83 (1962).

Kabelík. *Cs. Oftal.*, **22**, 49 (1966).

Kamath. *Indian med. Gaz.*, **63**, 555 (1928).

Kirwan. *Arch. Ophthal.*, **12**, 1 (1934).
Brit. J. Ophthal., **20**, 321 (1936).

Kirwan and Mukerjee. *Brit. J. Ophthal.*, **22**, 329 (1938).

Lal and Roy. *Indian J. med. Res.*, **25**, 163, 177, 233, 239 (1937).

Leach. *Trans. ophthal. Soc. U.K.*, **75**, 425 (1955).

Leach and Lloyd. *Trans. ophthal. Soc. U.K.*, **76**, 453 (1956).

Lieb and Scherf. *Klin. Mbl. Augenheilk.*, **128**, 686 (1956).

Mathur. *Proc. All-India ophthal. Soc.*, **12**, 145 (1951).

Maynard. *Indian med. Gaz.*, **44**, 373 (1909).

Mukerjee. *Trans. VII Cong. Far Eastern Ass. trop. Med.*, Calcutta, **1**, 272 (1927).

Sarkar, S. L. *Indian med. Gaz.*, **61**, 62 (1926).

Sarkar, S. N. *Nature* (Lond.), **162**, 265 (1948).

Shevalev. *Bengal Glaucoma* (in Russian), Odessa (1957).

Glaucoma Secondary to Ocular Dystrophies and Degenerations

ESSENTIAL (PROGRESSIVE) ATROPHY OF THE IRIS

We have already described in detail the features of this disease of unknown ætiology characterized by slowly progressive atrophic changes in the iris which ultimately lead to blindness from absolute glaucoma.[1] It is usually unilateral, developing most commonly in females in the 3rd decade, although bilateral cases are more common in males in whom the condition occurs at an earlier age and advances more rapidly and disastrously. It presents initially as a displacement of the pupil, followed by progressive atrophy of the iris resulting in the formation of holes in this tissue which enlarge and coalesce until only a few strands of stroma remain with immense apertures between them (Fig. 644). Eventually the ocular tension rises and the glaucoma which develops is very recalcitrant to any form of treatment, so that the usual end-result is blindness.

In the majority of cases glaucoma develops within 8 years of the onset of the disease (Henderson and Benedict, 1940) and results from the formation of peripheral anterior synechiæ which may be demonstrated gonioscopically (Fig. 645)[2] and histologically.[3] On a number of occasions a hyaline membrane has been described extending over the angle,[4] which may contribute to the occurrence of the raised tension (Fig. 646).

[1] Vol. IX, p. 686.

[2] Post (1939), Scharf (1941), Sugar (1945), Chang and Ojers (1949), Pau *et al.* (1962), Sokolić (1963), Koyama *et al.* (1965).

[3] Bentzen and Leber (1895), Wood (1910), Feingold (1918), Lisckó (1923), Rochat and Mulder (1924), Ellett (1928), Rones (1940), Heath (1953).

[4] Feingold (1918), Licskó (1923), Rochat and Mulder (1924), Rones (1940), Amsler and Landolt (1958), Pau *et al.* (1962).

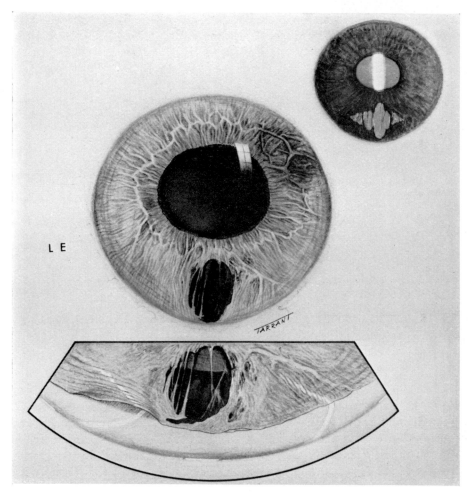

Fig. 644.—Essential Atrophy of the Iris.
Showing the changes in the iris and the occurrence of peripheral anterior
synechiæ (J. Winstanley).

Treatment is difficult and often ineffective. Miotics and acetazolamide may control the tension for some time but eventually recourse has to be made to surgery. A prophylactic peripheral iridectomy was recommended by L. and R. K. Daily (1957) and Tarkkanen and Forsius (1963), but was found ineffective by Clarke (1960) who suggested that complete removal of the atrophic iris might prevent the onset of glaucoma. A cyclodialysis has successfully controlled the tension in a number of cases[1] while several other procedures have been occasionally successful: sclerectomy (Waite, 1928),

[1] von Grósz (1937), Sugar (1945), Thorne-Thorne (1949), Eliezer and Carvalho (1960), Vancea (1960), Forsius and Tarkkanen (1961), Sokolić (1963).

FIGS. 645 and 646.—ESSENTIAL ATROPHY OF THE IRIS (P. Heath).

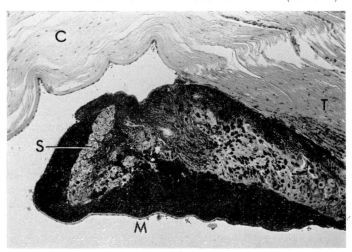

FIG. 645.—At a late stage, to show the collapsed folded iris with the heavy ectropion of the uveal pigment and an extensive peripheral anterior synechia; note the membrane, M, on the posterior surface of the iris. C, cornea; S, sphincter; T, trabeculæ.

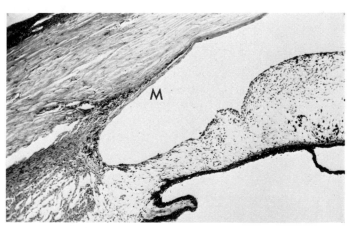

FIG. 646.—Endothelialized cuticular membrane, M, lying over the corneo-scleral trabeculæ.

sclero-iridectomy (de Ferrari, 1954), Scheie's operation (Weseley, 1961), Preziosi's operation (Papierbuch and Kurz, 1960), trephining (Paufique *et al.*, 1966), trephine with beta-radiation (Friedenwald, 1950), cyclodiathermy (Castroviejo, 1953), cyclodiathermy and goniotomy (Redi, 1957) and iridencleisis (Forsius and Tarkkanen, 1961; Mehra, 1963).

CHANDLER'S SYNDROME (1956) is a variant of this condition wherein the atrophy of the iris is patchy and incomplete without the formation of holes in this tissue, but irregular attachments of the superficial leaf of the iris to the trabeculæ are present associated with a corneal endothelial dystrophy. When the ocular tension increases above a certain level (such as 25 mm. Hg), œdema of the corneal epithelium develops with the formation of haloes. Such cases are uniocular and the glaucoma is rarely severe with little involvement of the optic disc; but as time passes the corneal œdema appears at lower levels of tension until it may become permanent in which case it is probably caused by the endothelial dystrophy. The ocular tension should be kept as low as possible with miotics, adrenaline and carbonic anhydrase inhibitors, but if the glaucoma cannot be adequately controlled a filtration operation becomes advisable.

IRIDOSCHISIS

In a previous volume[1] we have described in detail this rare condition characterized by a localized cleavage of the mesodermal stroma of the iris into two layers so that the anterior leaf separates from the posterior and

FIGS. 647 to 649.—IRIDOSCHISIS (Inst. Ophthal.).

FIGS. 647 and 648.—In a male aged 61.

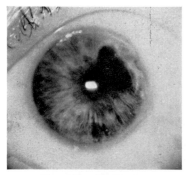 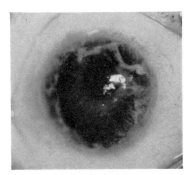

FIG. 647.—Right eye.   FIG. 648.—Left eye.

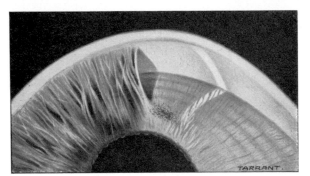

FIG. 649.—To show gross peripheral anterior synechiæ.

[1] Vol. IX, p. 694.

disintegrates into fibrils, the distal ends of which float freely in the anterior chamber (Figs. 647–8). Most cases seemed to have occurred spontaneously in aged eyes, a few have been associated with other ocular defects of a congenital nature, while others have followed a concussional trauma. There are several reports in the literature of the association of iridoschisis and glaucoma, but in some instances the description is inadequate to confirm the diagnosis, in some the condition may have been a progressive atrophy of the iris, while in others the atrophy is apparently secondary to primary closed-angle glaucoma. There appears to be little doubt that senile iridoschisis may occur in the presence of either a normal or a raised ocular tension, but in the present state of our knowledge it is impossible to be certain whether the occurrence of glaucoma is fortuitous or is the result of the formation of peripheral anterior synechiæ[1] (Fig. 649).

PSEUDO-EXFOLIATION OF THE LENS CAPSULE

We have already discussed at length the condition usually termed pseudo-exfoliation of the lens capsule,[2] essentially a degenerative state affecting not only the lens capsule but also the entire anterior uveal tract,

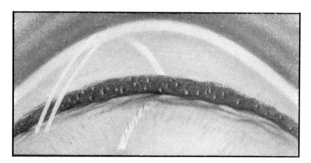

FIG. 650.—EXFOLIATIVE GLAUCOMA.
In a woman aged 57 with exfoliation of the lens capsule, showing heavy pigmentation and the deposition of exudative material on the trabeculæ (Inst. Ophthal.).

wherein a characteristic exudative material accumulates in association with the limiting membranes of the iris and ciliary body, around their vessels and upon their surfaces, as well as on the capsule of the lens, the zonule and in the angle of the anterior chamber (Fig. 650). We have also noted its frequent association with simple glaucoma and described the difference of opinion still existing regarding the ætiology of this complication—whether the rise in ocular tension should be ascribed to a mechanical blockage of the drainage channels by the exudative material (the *glaucoma capsulare* of

---

[1] Schoenberg (1927), Loewenstein *et al.* (1945–48), Garden and Wear (1949), Linn and Linn (1949), McCulloch (1950), Haik *et al.* (1952), Carter (1953), Törnquist and Swegmark (1961), Morales Ledesma (1964), Goetz (1966), Sódan (1966), Mills (1967), and others.
[2] p. 45.

Vogt) or develops as a part of the same degenerative changes which cause the pseudo-exfoliation. We have also seen that the glaucoma should be treated as the primary simple type by medical means if possible or, if this is ineffective, by a drainage operation.

PIGMENTARY RETINAL DYSTROPHY

The association between pigmentary retinal dystrophy[1] and glaucoma, although uncommon, has been noted by many observers, and while most of the reported cases have been of simple (or presumably simple) glaucoma,[2] a few examples of the acute (or closed-angle) type can be found in the literature.[3] In view of the rarity of closed-angle glaucoma in retinal dystrophies the association may well be fortuitous, but this does not appear to be true of simple glaucoma which occurs in about 3% of cases of this condition. Schmidthauser (1904), for example, found glaucoma in 2·78% of 180 such patients, Ciotola (1950) in 3·1% of 194 patients, and Raimondo and Gennaro (1955) also in 3·1% of 160 patients. It is significant that if the retinal dystrophy is unilateral the glaucoma is limited to the affected eye (de Carvalho et al., 1962).

Few cases have been examined histologically and these have all been at an advanced stage of glaucoma; the presence of peripheral anterior synechiæ in these cases is therefore not surprising, and has not helped to elucidate the ætiology of the rise in tension. Gartner and Schlossman (1949) examined three such eyes and indicated that pigment was not deposited in the trabecular meshwork, thus exonerating pigmentary dispersion as the cause.

The glaucoma associated with retinal dystrophy, whether simple or closed-angle, should be treated as a primary glaucoma.

PRIMARY FAMILIAL AMYLOIDOSIS

In a case of this rare disease of unknown ætiology characterized by an accumulation of amyloid material throughout many tissues of the body including the eye, a secondary glaucoma became one of the major complications leading to the necessity for enucleation[4] (Kaufman, 1958; Paton and Duke, 1966). In such an eye the latter authors found on the anterior surface of the iris a marked proliferative fibroblastic reaction forming a membrane containing giant cells of the foreign-body type with empty vacuoles and without inflammatory evidences (Fig. 651).

[1] Vol. X, p. 608.
[2] Bellarminoff (1893), Heinersdorff (1897), Goldzieher (1897), Filatov (1903), Weiss (1903), Wainstein (1911), Müller (1916), Bradburne (1916), Kotliarevsky (1931), Attiah (1941), Gartner and Schlossman (1949), Ciotola (1950), Panepinto and Lo Cascio (1951), Jayle and Ourgaud (1951), Cartasegna (1952), Salvi (1953), Raimondo and Gennaro (1955), Pacurariu and Radian (1959), Scialfa (1964), and others.
[3] Galezowski (1862), Schnabel (1878), Ayres (1886), Bradburne (1916), Krill and Iser (1959).
[4] p. 330.

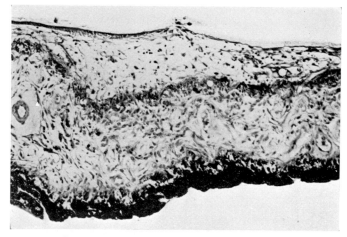

FIG. 651.—PRIMARY FAMILIAL AMYLOIDOSIS.
A fibrous membrane covers the anterior surface of the iris with giant cells
containing empty vacuoles (D. Paton and J. R. Duke).

Amsler and Landolt. *Ophthalmologica*, **135**, 584 (1958).

Attiah. *Bull. ophthal. Soc. Egypt*, **34**, 21 (1941).

Ayres. *Amer. J. Ophthal.*, **3**, 81 (1886).

Bellarminoff. *Arch. Augenheilk.*, **27**, 53 (1893).

Bentzen and Leber. *v. Graefes Arch. Ophthal.*, **41** (3), 208 (1895).

Bradburne. *Ophthal. Rev.*, **35**, 65 (1916).

Cartasegna. *Atti Soc. oftal. Lombarda*, **7**, 244 (1952).

Carter. *Amer. J. Ophthal.*, **36**, 967 (1953).

de Carvalho, de Magalhães Castro and Braga de Magalhães. *Rev. bras. Oftal.*, **21**, 339 (1962).

Castroviejo. *Trans. Amer. ophthal. Soc.*, **51**, 189 (1953).

Chandler. *Amer. J. Ophthal.*, **41**, 607 (1956).

Chang and Ojers. *Amer. J. Ophthal.*, **32**, 369 (1949).

Ciotola. *Boll. Oculist.*, **29**, 489 (1950).

Clarke. *Amer. J. Ophthal.*, **49**, 147 (1960).

Daily, L. and R. K. *Amer. J. Ophthal.*, **44**, 487 (1957).

Eliezer and de Carvalho. *Rev. bras. Oftal.*, **19**, 55 (1960).

Ellett. *Trans. Amer. ophthal. Soc.*, **26**, 306 (1928).

Feingold. *Amer. J. Ophthal.*, **1**, 1 (1918).

de Ferrari. *Boll. Oculist.*, **33**, 290 (1954).

Filatov. *Vestn. Oftal.*, **20**, 108 (1903).

Forsius and Tarkkanen. *Acta ophthal.* (Kbh.), **39**, 356 (1961).

Friedenwald. *Amer. J. Ophthal.*, **33**, 1523 (1950).

Galezowski. *Ann. Oculist.* (Paris), **48**, 265 (1862).

Garden and Wear. *Brit. J. Ophthal.*, **33**, 509 (1949).

Gartner and Schlossman. *Amer. J. Ophthal.*, **32**, 1337 (1949).

Goetz. *Klin. oczna*, **36**, 229 (1966).

Goldzieher. *Zbl. prakt. Augenheilk.*, **21**, 116 (1897).

von Grósz. *Arch. Augenheilk.*, **110**, 111 (1937).

Haik, Lyda and Waugh. *Arch. Ophthal.*, **48**, 40 (1952).

Heath. *Trans. Amer. ophthal. Soc.*, **51**, 167 (1953).

Heinersdorff. *Arch. Augenheilk.*, **34**, 230 (1897).

Henderson and Benedict. *Amer. J. Ophthal.*, **23**, 644 (1940).

Jayle and Ourgaud. *Bull. Soc. Ophtal. Fr.*, 590 (1951).

Kaufman. *Arch. Ophthal.*, **60**, 1036 (1958).

Kotliarevsky. *Russ. Arch. Oftal.*, **8**, 159 (1931).

Koyama, Sarai and Hirokawa. *Folia ophthal. jap.*, **16**, 498 (1965).

Krill and Iser. *Arch. Ophthal.*, **61**, 626 (1959).

Licskó. *Klin. Mbl. Augenheilk.*, **71**, 456 (1923).

Linn, J. G. and J. G. Jr. *Amer. J. Ophthal.*, **32**, 1700 (1949).

Loewenstein and Foster. *Brit. J. Ophthal.*, **29**, 277 (1945).

Loewenstein, Foster and Sledge. *Brit. J. Ophthal.*, **32**, 129 (1948).

McCulloch. *Amer. J. Ophthal.*, **33**, 1398 (1950).

Mehra. *Acta ophthal.* (Kbh.), **41**, 9 (1963).

Mills. *Brit. J. Ophthal.*, **51**, 158 (1967).

Morales Ledesma. *Arch. Asoc. Ceguera Méx.*, **6**, 51 (1964).

Müller. *Retinitis pigmentosa und Glaukom* (Diss.), Giessen (1916).

Pacurariu and Radian. *Ruman. med. Rev.*, **3**, 75 (1959).

Panepinto and Lo Cascio. *G. ital. Oftal.*, **4**, 209 (1951).

Papierbuch and Kurz. *Israel med. J.*, **19**, 260 (1960).

Paton and Duke. *Amer. J. Ophthal.*, **61**, 736 (1966).

Pau, Graeber and Holtermann. *Klin. Mbl. Augenheilk.*, **141**, 568 (1962).

Paufique, Ravault and Malterre. *Bull. Soc. Ophtal. Fr.*, **66**, 757 (1966).

Post. *Amer. J. Ophthal.*, **22**, 755 (1939).

Raimondo and Gennaro. *Atti Soc. oftal. Lombarda*, **10**, 278 (1955).

Redi. *Boll. Oculist.*, **36**, 65 (1957).

Rochat and Mulder. *Brit. J. Ophthal.*, **8**, 362 (1924).

Rones. *Amer. J. Ophthal.*, **23**, 163 (1940).

Salvi. *Boll. Oculist.*, **32**, 36 (1953).

Scharf. *Klin. Mbl. Augenheilk.*, **106**, 411 (1941).

Schmidthäuser. *Retinitis pigmentosa und Glaukom* (Diss.), Tübingen (1904).

Schnabel. *Arch. Ophthal.*, **7**, 12 (1878).

Schoenberg. *Arch. Ophthal.*, **56**, 538 (1927).

Scialfa. *Atti Soc. oftal. ital.*, **22**, 283 (1964).

Sédan. *Ann. Oculist.* (Paris), **199**, 699 (1966).

Sokolić. *Jugoslav. oftal. Arh.*, **1**, 65 (1963).

Sugar. *Amer. J. Ophthal.*, **28**, 744 (1945).

Tarkkanen and Forsius. *Acta ophthal.* (Kbh.), **41**, 473 (1963).

Thorne-Thorne. *Trans. ophthal. Soc. U.K.*, **69**, 311 (1949).

Törnquist and Swegmark. *Acta ophthal.* (Kbh.), **39**, 940 (1961).

Vancea. *Arch. Ophtal.*, **20**, 490 (1960).

Wainstein. *Vestn. Oftal.*, **28**, 149 (1911).

Waite. *Amer. J. Ophthal.*, **11**, 187 (1928).

Weiss. *Samml. zwangl. Abhandl. Geb. Augenheilk.*, **5** (5) (1903).

Weseley. *Arch. Ophthal.*, **65**, 779 (1961).

Wood. *Ophthalmoscope*, **8**, 858 (1910).

Glaucoma Secondary to Intra-ocular Cysts and Tumours

It is well known that although intra-ocular cysts and neoplasms may frequently be associated with a secondary glaucoma, the sequence is by no means inevitable, and that the development of glaucoma depends little upon the size of the tumour or the degree of exudation as evinced, for example, by the presence of a secondary serous detachment of the retina; even with very large tumours the tension may remain normal or low (Heymans-May, 1921). It was suggested by Priestley Smith (1879) that the anatomical displacement forwards of the lens–iris diaphragm accounted for the rise of tension, a view supported by Fuchs (1917) and Nakayama (1927), but it has now been established that the factors responsible are not those of size and volume, but rather those of site (Figs. 652–6). In the early stages of the development of a tumour the tension is usually normal or subnormal (Dunnington, 1938), and the frequency of raised tension varies in the anterior and posterior segments of the globe. Although a raised tension due to embarrassment of the angle of the anterior chamber may occasionally occur in cysts of the iris, it is infiltrative tumours of the anterior uvea that are particularly prone to cause a secondary glaucoma, the mechanism of which is usually the direct invasion of the trabecular meshwork by neoplasic cells; in other cases the hypertension may be the result of the organization of the recurrent hyphæmata that frequently accompany certain of these tumours. Infiltration of the angle of the anterior chamber by such tumours as dictyomata, leiomyomata, and malignant melanomata of the uvea have been discussed at length elsewhere (Fig. 657),[1] but it is worth stressing that simple melanomata of the uvea do not give rise to glaucoma (Fig. 653); the occur-

[1] Vol. IX, p. 863.

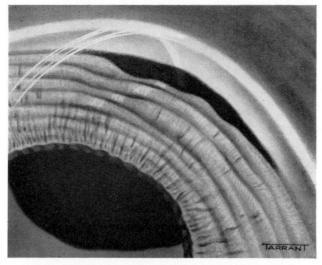

FIG. 652.—MALIGNANT MELANOMA OF THE CILIARY BODY.
In a man aged 46 with 6/6 vision, seen gonioscopically (Inst. Ophthal.).

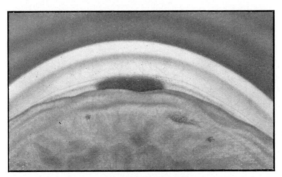

FIG. 653.—SIMPLE MELANOMA OF THE CILIARY BODY.
In a male aged 67.   This type of melanoma does not give rise to glaucoma
(Inst. Ophthal.).

rence of a raised tension in an eye with such a melanoma should always be looked upon with suspicion since it indicates that the tumour is infiltrative and has invaded the trabecular meshwork.

Glaucoma is a feature in about 33% of the cases of choroidal melanomata,[1] being more frequent when they involve the anterior uvea and particularly when they are of the infiltrating type.   In most cases this is probably due to obstruction of the circulation of the intra-ocular fluid at the trabeculæ, in some cases by actual infiltration of the angle, in others by accumulations of malignant cells at the angle of the anterior chamber which

[1] Vol. IX, p. 859.

FIGS. 654 to 656.—NEOPLASIC SECONDARY GLAUCOMA.

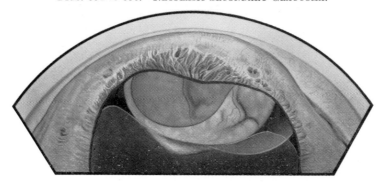

FIG. 654.—Blockage of the angle due to a medullo-epithelioma, in a female aged 22 (Inst. Ophthal.).

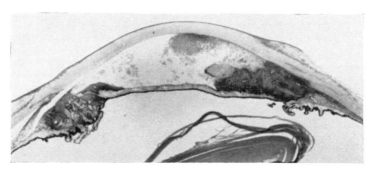

FIG. 655.—In a woman aged 82, a limbal epithelioma had infiltrated intra-ocularly to the ciliary body, the iris and the trabecular meshwork (C. H. Greer).

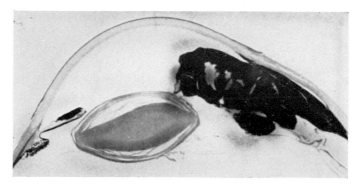

FIG. 656.—Malignant melanoma of the iris and ciliary body (on the right) (W. B. Doherty).

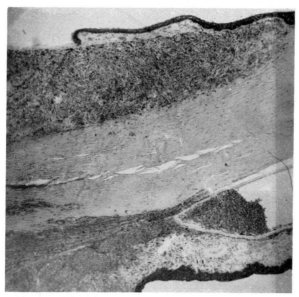

FIG. 657.—MALIGNANT RING MELANOMA OF THE IRIS.

The tumour invades the structures of the angle and forms an extra-ocular
subconjunctival mass (N. Ashton).

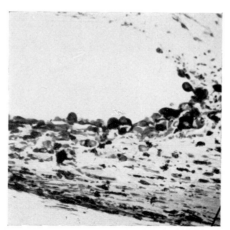

FIG. 658.—THE EXFOLIATION OF NEOPLASIC CELLS.

From a malignant melanoma of the ciliary body; the cells are carried by the
aqueous to be deposited on the trabeculæ (R. E. Hopkins and F. R. Carriker).

have been carried thither in the aqueous stream (Coats, 1912; Hopkins and
Carriker, 1958) (Fig. 658); in other cases it may be due to the formation of a
vascularized membrane on the iris, in others to recurrent hæmorrhages, in
others to necrosis and uveitis, but the concept advocated by Evans (1939)
that the rise of tension may be due to circulatory congestion and stasis causing

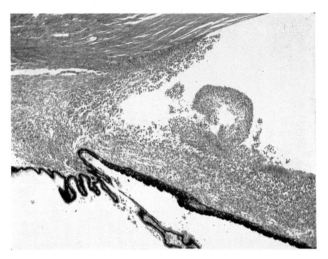

FIG. 659.—JUVENILE XANTHOGRANULOMA.

The infiltration of the angle of the anterior chamber with histiocytes and a
nodule on the surface of the iris (T. E. Sanders).

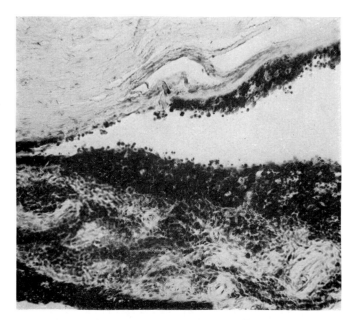

FIG. 660.—INTRA-OCULAR EXTENSION OF A RETINOBLASTOMA.

Retinoblastoma cells within the iris stroma and lining the occluded filtration
angle (P. B. Schofield).

an obstruction of the venous return from the ciliary body and choroid is probably rarely operative. This type of glaucoma is therefore primarily obstructive but in the later stages, when irritative products of necrosis are liberated and inflammatory symptoms appear, these may intensify the process. In all such cases, of course, the only adequate treatment is excision of the globe, a method usually advisable in all cases of blind painful eyes with raised tension in view of the likelihood of the presence of a neoplasm.

A secondary glaucoma is a common accompaniment of a juvenile xanthogranuloma.[1] The glaucoma is obstructive for the angle of the anterior chamber and the trabeculæ become clogged with large, pale-staining mononuclear histiocytes accompanied by variable numbers of Touton giant cells (Fig. 659). Eventually peripheral synechiæ may form. The treatment of such cases is difficult. Some respond to radiotherapy, but when a raised tension occurs enucleation is usually the only expedient although a successful filtration operation was reported by Newell (1957).

A similar secondary glaucoma is an almost constant feature of a retinoblastoma[2] which has been allowed to progress to an advanced stage (Fig. 660). In this event the globe enlarges owing to the stretching of its coats accompanied by much pain, a process which is intensified until relief is obtained when the sclera is eventually ruptured.

Coats. *Roy. Lond. ophthal. Hosp. Rep.*, **18**, 284 (1912).
 Trans. ophthal. Soc. U.K., **32**, 165 (1912).
Dunnington. *Arch. Ophthal.*, **20**, 359 (1938).
Evans. *Brit. J. Ophthal.*, **23**, 745 (1939).
Fuchs. *v. Graefes Arch. Ophthal.*, **94**, 43 (1917).

Heymans-May. *Arch. Ophtal.*, **38**, 479 (1921).
Hopkins and Carriker. *Amer. J. Ophthal.*, **45**, 835 (1958).
Nakayama. *v. Graefes Arch. Ophthal.*, **118**, 311 (1927).
Newell. *Arch. Ophthal.*, **58**, 321 (1957).
Smith, Priestley. *Glaucoma*, London (1879).

Iatrogenic Glaucoma

A secondary glaucoma may follow the use of certain drugs, particularly mydriatics and the corticosteroids, sometimes the miotics, and (very occasionally) certain vasomotor drugs and the sulphonamides.

MYDRIATIC GLAUCOMA

That glaucoma could follow the instillation of atropine was known to von Graefe (1858) and its occurrence has been amply attested[3]; the sequence has also been reported following the subcutaneous injection of atropine (Myashita, 1914; Larmande, 1949), its use as a suppository, or has arisen during the prolonged treatment of gastric conditions by belladonna given by mouth (Ullman and Mossman, 1950; Larmande and Toulant, 1951). Less frequently, cases have been reported following the topical instillation of less

---

[1] Vol. IX, p. 656.   [2] Vol. X, p. 688.
[3] See among others, Derby (1867), Laqueur (1877), Gifford (1916), Gradle (1935), Beach and Holt (1941), Sugar (1941).

potent and more transient mydriatics: homatropine,[1] scopolamine (Walter, 1898), euphthalmine (Ring, 1903; Breuil, 1909), cocaine,[2] and even holo-caine.[3] The most common occurrence is after the use of atropine in the treat-ment of iridocyclitis, but this unfortunate sequel has also followed the use of mydriatics in the routine testing of the refraction or examining the fundus.

Such a secondary glaucoma is of the closed-angle type and occurs only in eyes with a shallow anterior chamber and a narrow drainage angle or a moderately deep anterior chamber and a plateau iris, in both of which cases the dilatation of the pupil closes the angle sufficiently to embarrass drainage; if the angle is wide mydriasis is a perfectly safe procedure, even in cases of simple glaucoma.[4] When it does occur the rise in tension may be acute and recalcitrant to treatment until miosis is achieved by powerful miotics such as eserine combined if necessary with hypotensive measures such as osmotic therapy or acetazolamide. Particularly in cases of iritis, if the anterior chamber of the involved eye cannot be adequately examined, the angle of the fellow eye should be examined gonioscopically. In the presence of a narrow angle the use of atropine for the treatment of uveitis is contra-indicated, and one of the shorter-acting mydriatics, such as adrenaline or phenylephrine, should be substituted. If during the course of a hypertensive uveitis the tendency for the development of a primary closed-angle glaucoma is suspected, a prophylactic peripheral iridectomy should be contemplated.

MIOTIC GLAUCOMA

A PARADOXICAL (INVERSE) GLAUCOMA may result from the adminis-tration of miotics owing to the occurrence of a pupillary blockage when the iris is strongly apposed to the lens. Such an accident may arise after the instillation of pilocarpine in spherophakia or in the Marfan syndrome[5] (Urbanek, 1930; Probert, 1953), or when the lens is dislocated into the anterior chamber.[6] The same reaction may occur in an apparently normal eye or in cases of iritis when miotics (or reading) may bring on a glauco-matous attack and mydriatics may relieve the tension (Leydhecker, 1953–54; Higgitt and Smith, 1955; Gorin, 1966). This paradoxical reaction is asso-ciated with closure of the angle of the anterior chamber and may be due to an increased convexity of the lens blocking the pupil and ballooning the root of the iris forwards. A similar reaction has been seen in a case of iritis with

[1] Hodges (1885), Rogers (1895), Shears (1900), Gifford (1900–16), Pyle (1903), Friedmann (1908), Stevenson (1913), Levitt (1917), Levinsohn (1918), Desai (1919), Linhart (1950).

[2] Manz (1885), Javal (1886), Hinshelwood (1900), Snell (1901), Sergiewski (1903), Hamilton (1916), Ganguly (1923), and others.

[3] Plastinin (1914), Gjessing (1914), Hughes (1917).

[4] It may be noted here that although it is usually stated that a mydriatic does not cause a rise in the ocular tension in patients with simple glaucoma, in an appreciable number of such cases a small rise of some 6 mm. Hg or more may occur on the instillation of a cycloplegic (not a mydriatic) drug (Kronfeld et al., 1943; Harris, 1968).

[5] Vol. III, p. 1107.   [6] p. 658.

iris bombé wherein pilocarpine caused an accentuation of the bellying of the iris and a consequent increase in tension (Penn, 1948). Finally, the strong miotics in the group of organic phosphates (DFP, TEPP and others) which produce a ciliary œdema with increased capillary permeability may accentuate a congestive attack of hypertension in an eye with a narrow angle (Zekman and Snydacker, 1953) or induce such an attack in a non-congested eye (Stone, 1950; Andreani, 1954). Thus a bilateral attack of closed-angle glaucoma has been reported in a child aged 7 years after treatment by Phospholine iodide for accommodative esotropia (Jones and Watson, 1967); the reaction was associated with a marked decrease in the depth of the anterior chamber and the ocular tension was lowered by atropine.

CORTICOSTEROID GLAUCOMA

Since the introduction of corticosteroids into ophthalmic therapeutics their long-continued use has been found to give rise in a significant number of cases to the development of a secondary glaucoma of the simple (open-angle) type occasionally associated with a posterior cortical cataract.[1] We have already seen[2] that its occurrence probably depends on the susceptibility of the individual, a factor genetically determined. Armaly (1963–65) has shown that in normal eyes the topical application of a 0·1% solution of dexamethasone can produce an increase in ocular tension from 5 to 16 mm. Hg and a reduction in the facility of the outflow of aqueous in the treated eye, that the hypertensive response increases with the duration of treatment and is completely reversible on its cessation, and that the magnitude of this dexamethasone-induced hypertension increases with age. He also found that in cases of simple glaucoma, whether with low-tension or medically-controlled tension, the dexamethasone-induced response is greater than in normal individuals, an observation amply confirmed (Nicholas, 1964; Pasmanik and Miranda, 1965; Spiers, 1965; Weekers et al., 1967; and others). Similar results have been reported with topical betamethasone (Becker et al., 1963–65). It has now been established that a secondary glaucoma may also develop during the prolonged systemic treatment of patients with such conditions as rheumatoid arthritis or disseminated lupus erythematosus, and after its long topical use in cases of uveitis or even allergic conjunctivitis or spring catarrh. This steroid-induced glaucoma may be difficult to differentiate from hypertensive uveitis, but in unilateral conditions a steroid provocative test in the fellow eye may permit such a differentiation. It is possible that there is no close relationship between the magnitude of the hypertensive response and the previous presence of glaucoma since Levene and his associates (1967) found that the effect after topical administration was similar in normal eyes and glaucomatous suspects.

Although the steroid-induced rise of ocular tension is most marked with dexamethasone and betamethasone, it also occurs with other glucocorticoids. Becker and

[1] p. 230.   [2] p. 400.

Hahn (1964) found that the effect with 0·1% prednisolone or 0·1% triamcinolone used four times a day was similar to betamethasone once a day, and Ramsell and his co-workers (1967) produced a rise in ocular tension of 6 mm. Hg or more in 5 out of 20 normal volunteers on 0·5% prednisolone.

Such a simple glaucoma has been reported after the systemic use of the corticosteroids, usually for two years or more, on several occasions,[1] while following the observation by François (1954) reports of a similar increase in the ocular tension have been more numerous following its topical application.[2] The rise of tension may be slight but, particularly after its topical instillation in susceptible individuals, it may be severe, up to 60 mm. Hg or more, with cupping and atrophy of the optic disc and typical glaucomatous defects in the visual fields; but in all cases the symptoms are slight and the angle of the anterior chamber is gonioscopically open. The curious feature of the condition is that it is frequently reversible, for on the cessation of treatment with the drug the tension tends to fall, sometimes rapidly and sometimes after one or two months. If, however, the rise in tension is allowed to persist for a considerable time, irreversible damage may be caused to the eye (Miller, 1965; Spiers, 1965; François et al., 1966). Moreover, the cupping of the disc and the defects in the visual fields may develop with remarkable rapidity (within a few months with topical applications, Roberts, 1968), an occurrence which emphasizes the need for the repeated examination of patients treated with these drugs.

It is now generally believed that the glucocorticoids cause the increase in the ocular tension owing to a decrease in the facility of outflow of the aqueous,[3] although several workers have demonstrated an increased production of aqueous, either with no change in the facility of outflow (Linnér, 1959; Draeger, 1965; Kitazawa, 1966) or with a reduced facility (Frandsen, 1964).

The intimate mode of action of these drugs, however, is unknown but tentative hypotheses have been advanced. Armaly (1963) suggested that the action of dexamethasone was to increase the mucopolysaccharide content of the trabecular meshwork and thus reduce the pore-size and therefore the facility of the outflow of aqueous; he also postulated a greater accumulation of mucopolysaccharides in the degenerated trabecular meshwork of glaucomatous when compared with normal eyes. Weekers and his co-workers (1966) postulated a similar mechanism for the steroid-induced rise in tension without specifying the steroid-sensitive substance in the

[1] Stern (1953), Covell (1958), Harris (1960), Bernstein and Schwartz (1962), Bernstein et al. (1963), Lerman (1963), Hofmann and Hauser (1964), and others.

[2] François (1961), Goldmann (1962), Valerio et al. (1962), Armaly (1963), Becker and Mills (1963), Briggs (1963), Quaranta and Serafini (1963), Bouzas (1964–67), Lerner et al. (1964), Ljungström (1964), Nicholas (1964), Weekers et al. (1964–66), Cantat (1965), Draeger (1965), Grieten and Collignon-Brach (1965), Kojima et al. (1965), Miller (1965), Spiers (1965), Cucco (1966), Kitazawa (1966), Spaeth (1966), Drance and Scott (1968), and many others.

[3] François (1961), Goldmann (1962), Armaly (1963), Becker and Mills (1963), Quaranta and Serafini (1963), Miller et al. (1965), and others.

outflow channels. Becker (1964), however, showed that the response of patients with secondary glaucoma to betamethasone was similar to that of normal individuals and different from that of patients with simple glaucoma, thus tending to contradict Armaly's hypothesis. Kern (1967), experimenting on monkeys, found that the ciliary muscle showed a decreased tonus in response to acetylcholine and suggested that steroids promoted glaucoma by their adrenergic and anticholinergic action, a hypothesis which might be said to explain the failure of miotics to control the tension in these cases.

In many cases considerable judgment is necessary both in the diagnosis and in the management of this steroid-induced hypertension. In some instances, topical adrenaline and systemic carbonic anhydrase inhibitors will maintain the intra-ocular pressure within normal limits, but in others it may be necessary to reduce the frequency of administration of the steroids, or to substitute less potent hypertension-inducing compounds, such as hydrocortisone or prednisolone, for the more potent betamethasone or dexamethasone; miotics have little effect on the ocular tension. In particularly recalcitrant cases the systemic administration of steroids instead of the more potent topical method may suppress the inflammatory process without precipitating a damaging rise of ocular tension. The occurrence of this complication should suggest care, certainly in patients with a hereditary history of simple glaucoma, in the use of corticosteroids for mild and unimportant ocular inflammations, such as an allergic conjunctivitis; while patients who develop corticosteroid glaucoma should be subsequently observed as potential candidates for the development of simple glaucoma.

VASOMOTOR DRUGS have occasionally caused an acute rise in ocular tension. After a subconjunctival injection of *adrenaline* in a patient with a vasomotor disturbance of the Raynaud type, Schiff-Wertheimer and Jonquères (1947) reported such an incident which required an iridectomy for its control. Similarly, after a parenteral injection of adrenaline in a patient with bronchial asthma Saubermann (1948) recorded an ocular tension of over 100 mm. Hg which, however, was controlled by pilocarpine.

The administration of *Priscol* has also been reported to have given rise to an acute glaucomatous attack (Gallois, 1951).

SULPHONAMIDE GLAUCOMA

The few cases which have been reported wherein a secondary glaucoma has developed after the systemic administration of sulphonamides in comparison with the large number who have been treated with these drugs suggest that any relationship may perhaps be incidental rather than causal. Such cases have been reported by Fritz and Kesert (1947) and Pavisic (1949); both were in patients susceptible to sulphonamides and both developed an acute closed-angle glaucoma. If this sequence does occur, the mechanism is not clear; it has been suggested that a swelling of the lens with an associated myopia which can complicate the absorption of these drugs may be sufficient to obstruct the drainage of the aqueous in an eye with a narrow angle.

TRANQUILLIZING DRUGS have been said to give rise exceptionally to a secondary glaucoma. Thus Isayama and Yasui (1967) found an increase in the intra-ocular pressure combined with a diminution of accommodation in 22 out of 69 schizophrenic patients receiving massive oral doses of phenothiazine derivatives.

As an addendum, the effect of TETRA-ETHYL LEAD may be mentioned, a substance added to petrol (gasoline) to decrease engine knocking. Largely on the evidence of experiments on rabbits and rats, it has been claimed to alter the ocular elasticity, to change the diurnal rhythm of the intra-ocular pressure, and to induce a transient increase in tension (Skripnitschenko, 1956–62; Posner, 1961–62). The most prominent features of poisoning are disturbances of the central nervous system, particularly excitement, insomnia and headache, but the evidence so far available for this effect on the intra-ocular pressure is still unconvincing.

Andreani. *Ann. Ottal.*, **80**, 341 (1954).
Armaly. *Arch. Ophthal.*, **70**, 482, 492 (1963).
  Invest. Ophthal., **4**, 187 (1965).
Beach and Holt. *Amer. J. Ophthal.*, **24**, 668 (1941).
Becker. *Arch. Ophthal.*, **72**, 769 (1964).
Becker and Ballin. *Arch. Ophthal.*, **74**, 621 (1965).
Becker and Hahn. *Amer. J. Ophthal.*, **57**, 543 (1964).
Becker and Mills. *Arch. Ophthal.*, **70**, 500 (1963).
Bernstein, Mills and Becker. *Arch. Ophthal.*, **70**, 15 (1963).
Bernstein and Schwartz. *Arch. Ophthal.*, **68**, 742 (1962).
Bouzas. *Bull. Soc. hellén. Ophtal.*, **32**, 226 (1964).
  Bull. Soc. franç. Ophtal., **80**, 652 (1967).
Breuil. *Clin. Ophtal.*, **15**, 146 (1909).
Briggs. *Arch. Ophthal.*, **70**, 312 (1963).
Cantat. *Bull. Soc. Ophtal. Fr.*, **65**, 1130 (1965).
Covell. *Amer. J. Ophthal.*, **45**, 108 (1958).
Cucco. *Ann. Ottal.*, **92**, 686 (1966).
Derby. *Trans. Amer. ophthal. Soc.*, **1** (4), 35 (1867).
Desai. *Brit. J. Ophthal.*, **3**, 251 (1919).
Draeger. *Klin. Mbl. Augenheilk.*, **147**, 386 (1965).
Drance and Scott. *Canad. J. Ophthal.*, **3**, 159 (1968).
François. *Ann. Oculist.* (Paris), **187**, 805 (1954).
  Ophthalmologica, **142**, 517 (1961).
François, Heintz-de Bree and Tripathi. *Amer. J. Ophthal.*, **62**, 844 (1966).
Frandsen. *Acta ophthal.* (Kbh.), **42**, 108 (1964).
Friedmann. *Ophthal. Rec.*, **17**, 92 (1908).
Fritz and Kesert. *Amer. J. Ophthal.*, **30**, 197 (1947).
Gallois. *Bull. Soc. Ophtal. Fr.*, 131 (1951).
Ganguly. *Indian med. Gaz.*, **58**, 379 (1923).
Gifford. *Ophthal. Rec.*, **9**, 328 (1900).
  J. Amer. med. Ass., **67**, 112 (1916).
Gjessing. *Klin. Mbl. Augenheilk.*, **53**, 379 (1914).
Goldmann. *Arch. Ophthal.*, **68**, 621 (1962).

Gorin. *Amer. J. Ophthal.*, **62**, 1063 (1966).
Gradle. *Trans. Amer. ophthal. Soc.*, **33**, 175 (1935).
von Graefe. *v. Graefes Arch. Ophthal.*, **4** (2), 127 (1858).
Grieten and Collignon-Brach. *Bull. Soc. belge Ophtal.*, No. 141, 564 (1965).
Hamilton. *Liverpool med. chir. J.*, **36**, 156 (1916).
Harris. *Amer. J. Ophthal.*, **49**, 351 (1960).
  Arch. Ophthal., **79**, 242 (1968).
Higgitt and Smith. *Brit. J. Ophthal.*, **39**, 103 (1955).
Hinshelwood. *Ophthal. Rev.*, **19**, 305 (1900).
Hodges. *Arch. Ophthal.*, **14**, 42 (1885).
Hofmann and Hauser. *Amer. J. Ophthal.* **57**, 1043 (1964).
Hughes. *Amer. J. Ophthal.*, **34**, 140 (1917).
Isayama and Yasui. *Rinsho Ganka*, **21**, 635 (1967).
Javal. *Progr. méd.*, **17**, 355 (1886).
Jones and Watson. *Brit. J. Ophthal.*, **51**, 783 (1967).
Kern. *Ophthalmologica*, **154**, 341 (1967).
Kitazawa. *Acta Soc. ophthal. jap.*, **70**, 292 (1966).
Kojima *et al. Rinsho Ganka*, **19**, 551 (1965).
Kronfeld, McGarry and Smith. *Amer. J. Ophthal.*, **26**, 245 (1943).
Laqueur. *v. Graefes Arch. Ophthal.*, **23** (3), 149 (1877).
Larmande. *Algérie Méd.*, **52**, 113 (1949).
Larmande and Toulant. *Presse Med.*, **59**, 1611 (1951).
Lerman. *Amer. J. Ophthal.*, **56**, 31 (1963).
Lerner, Stocker and Gans. *J. Mich. med. Soc.*, **63**, 349 (1964).
Levene, Wigdor, Edelstein and Baum. *Arch. Ophthal.*, **77**, 593 (1967).
Levinsohn. *Klin. Mbl. Augenheilk.*, **61**, 174 (1918).
Levitt. *N.Y. med. J.*, **106**, 362 (1917).
Leydhecker. *Ber. dtsch. ophthal. Ges.*, **58**, 326 (1953).
  v. Graefes Arch. Ophthal., **155**, 255 (1954).
Linhart. *Amer. J. Ophthal.*, **33**, 448 (1950).
Linnér. *Docum. ophthal.*, **13**, 191 (1959).
Ljungström. *Opusc. med.* (Stockh.), **9**, 132 (1964).

Manz. *Ber. dtsch. ophthal. Ges.*, **17**, 118 (1885).

Miller. *Trans. ophthal. Soc. U.K.*, **85**, 289 (1965).

Miller, Peczon and Whitworth. *Amer. J. Ophthal.*, **59**, 31 (1965).

Myashita. *Klin. Mbl. Augenheilk.*, **52**, 561 (1914).

Nicholas. *Arch. Ophthal.*, **72**, 189 (1964).

Pasmanik and Miranda. *Arch. chil. Oftal.*, **22**, 30 (1965).

Pavisic. *Med. Arh. Sarajevo*, **3**, 81 (1949).

Penn. *Amer. J. Ophthal.*, **31**, 228 (1948).

Plastinin. *Klin. Mbl. Augenheilk.*, **52**, 896 (1914).

Posner. *Eye, Ear, Nose, Thr. Monthly*, **40**, 853 (1961); **41**, 57, 129 (1962).

Probert. *Amer. J. Ophthal.*, **36**, 1571 (1953).

Pyle. *J. Amer. med. Ass.*, **40**, 1725 (1903).

Quaranta and Serafini. *Boll. Oculist.*, **42**, 525 (1963).

Atti Cong. Soc. oftal. ital., **21**, 294 (1963).

Ramsell, Trillwood and Draper. *Brit. J. Ophthal.*, **51**, 398 (1967).

Ring. *Trans. Amer. ophthal. Soc.*, **10**, 109 (1903).

Roberts. *Amer. J. Ophthal.*, **66**, 520 (1968).

Rogers. *Ophthal. Rec.*, **5**, 421 (1895).

Saubermann. *Ophthalmologica*, **115**, 246 (1948).

Schiff-Wertheimer and Jonquères. *Bull. Soc. Ophtal. Paris*, 470 (1947).

Sergiewski. *Klin. Mbl. Augenheilk.*, **41** (1), 554 (1903).

Shears. *Trans. ophthal. Soc. U.K.*, **20**, 254 (1900).

Skripnitschenko. *Oftal. Z.*, **11**, 143 (1956); **12**, 372 (1957).

Acta XIX int. Cong. Ophthal., New Delhi, **2**, 1284 (1962).

Snell. *Ophthal. Rev.*, **20**, 31 (1901).

Spaeth. *Arch. Ophthal.*, **76**, 772 (1966).

Spiers. *Acta ophthal.* (Kbh.), **43**, 419 (1965).

Stern. *Amer. J. Ophthal.*, **36**, 389 (1953).

Stevenson. *Ophthalmoscope*, **11**, 73 (1913).

Stone. *Arch. Ophthal.*, **43**, 36 (1950).

Sugar. *Amer. J. Ophthal.*, **24**, 851 (1941).

Ullman and Mossman. *Amer. J. Ophthal.*, **33**, 757 (1950).

Urbanek. *Z. Augenheilk.*, **71**, 171 (1930).

Valerio, Carones and de Poli. *G. ital. Oftal.*, **15**, 143 (1962).

Walter. *Clin. Ophtal.*, **4**, 265 (1898).

Weekers, Grieten and Collignon-Brach. *Ophthalmologica*, **152**, 81 (1966).

Weekers, Grieten, Watillon and Prijot. *Ophthalmologica*, **148**, 81 (1964).

Weekers, Lennes, Demailly and Grieten. *Arch. Ophtal.*, **27**, 457 (1967).

Zekman and Snydacker. *Amer. J. Ophthal.*, **36**, 1709 (1953).

Traumatic Glaucoma

A rise of tension following trauma to the eye may occur after contusions whether they be uncomplicated or involve gross intra-ocular lesions, or may develop after a perforating injury, either traumatic or operative. The rise of tension may occur shortly after the injury, or may develop some considerable time later.

CONCUSSION GLAUCOMA

The behaviour of the tension of the eye after a simple contusion is very variable. In animals there is usually a short initial period (lasting some 30 minutes) of hypertension followed by a longer period of hypotony (lasting some 3 to 7 days), a reaction which may be evident also in the fellow eye even although it had not been injured (Magitot, 1920; Leplat, 1922–25; Schmidt and de Decker, 1930; Larsson, 1930; Chuistova, 1965). In man it is usually impossible to take tonometric readings so frequently, but the evidence suggests that in general terms a somewhat similar reaction takes place although any short period of hypertension is usually overshadowed by the following hypotony.[1]

The occurrence of concussion glaucoma of early onset is uncommon. The condition was first adequately noted by Priestley Smith (1882); the literature has been annotated by Schindhelm (1917) and Tillema (1937), and

[1] p. 733.

now well over 100 cases have been reported. These have occurred at all ages (6 years, Villard, 1905; 75, Agnello, 1931). The rise in tension usually develops immediately or shortly after the injury; less frequently (some 20% of cases) its onset is delayed beyond a week. An analysis of 74 recorded cases, in which the time interval between the concussion and the onset of

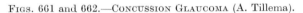

FIGS. 661 and 662.—CONCUSSION GLAUCOMA (A. Tillema).

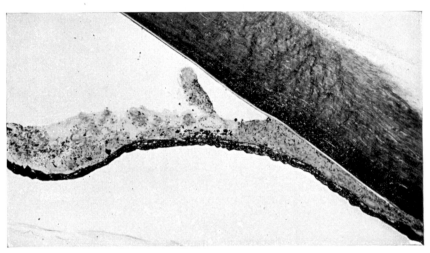

FIG. 661.—Acute concussion necrosis of the iris. The stroma shows advanced necrosis with a tear of the anterior lamella. There is considerable scattering of pigment and a peripheral anterior synechia closes the angle of the anterior chamber.

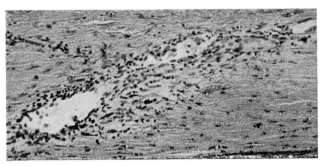

FIG. 662.—A ciliary artery showing a partially disorganized wall. The surrounding sclera is infiltrated and contains both uveal and hæmatogenous pigment.

glaucoma is given, shows that in 32 the raised tension came on immediately, in 21 from 3 to 5 days, in 6 from 5 to 7, in 6 in the 2nd week, in 2 in the 3rd week, and in the remaining 7 at longer intervals up to 7 weeks. The rise of tension may be relatively mild, or alternatively the glaucoma may be acute with much pain, an immobile pupil, vomiting and prostration, symptoms which may subside rapidly on miotic treatment or may require more energetic measures.

Pathological examinations of such eyes have been rare—von Garnier (1891), Morax (1921), and Tillema (1937). These have shown the usual changes following concussion, essentially a generalized œdema of the uveal tract which may be associated with tearing of the ciliary muscle accompanied by widespread vasodilatation and necrosis of the tissues, sometimes with the formation of peripheral anterior synechiæ (Figs. 661–2). François and his associates (1956) described a case wherein abundant new vessels had developed on the iris constituting a rubeosis and percolating the trabecular tissue.

The cause of the glaucoma may be complex, for several events may have occurred in the eye each sufficient to determine a rise of tension, the most important of which are damage to the angle of the anterior chamber, intra-ocular hæmorrhages and subluxation or dislocation of the lens. These, however, are by no means invariable occurrences; nor does their presence always lead to glaucoma. Thus Hegner (1915) found only 15 cases of glaucoma in 48 traumatic dislocations of the lens, although Rodman (1963) found 63 cases in 76 wherein the lens was posteriorly dislocated or subluxated after injury. Similarly, in the presence of a primary traumatic hyphæma early glaucoma is uncommon, but after a secondary hyphæma it occurs more frequently (25%, Shea, 1957; 33%, Leone, 1966). It is important that in all recently reported cases of concussion glaucoma, whether uncomplicated or complicated, wherein adequate gonioscopic examination has been performed, recession of the angle of the anterior chamber has been a very common finding.

TRAUMATIC RECESSION OF THE ANGLE OF THE ANTERIOR CHAMBER

It is only recently that the significance of tears into the face of the ciliary body after blunt trauma and their relationship to the occurrence of glaucoma has been realized, although the pathological appearance of such tears was pointed out many years ago (Collins, 1892; Stoewer, 1904–7; Lister, 1924; Lamb, 1927) (Fig. 665). Wolff and Zimmerman (1962) described a chronic secondary glaucoma which develops insidiously as a late complication of ocular injuries. Histologically there are longitudinal tears in the face of the ciliary body which split the circular from the radial fibres; similar changes were described by Rodman (1963). These changes result in a prolongation backward of the angle of the anterior chamber with a retroplacement of the lens–iris diaphragm and a consequent deepening of the anterior chamber (Figs. 663–4). Wolff and Zimmerman suggested that glaucoma was the result of subtle ultramicroscopic damage to the inner wall of Schlemm's canal, a suggestion confirmed by the electron-microscopic studies of Yamashita and Rosen (1965) of two angles from patients with traumatic glaucoma secondary to hyphæma; these showed an

FIGS. 663 and 664.—RECESSION OF THE ANGLE OF THE ANTERIOR CHAMBER
(T. H. Pettit and E. U. Keates).

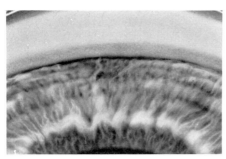

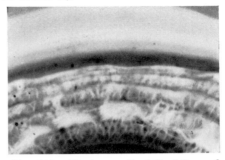

FIG. 663.—Gonioscopic view of the anterior
chamber of the right (normal) eye.

FIG. 664.—The traumatic cleft of the angle
of the anterior chamber with a tear into the
face of the ciliary body. Note the clumps of
pigment scattered in the angle.

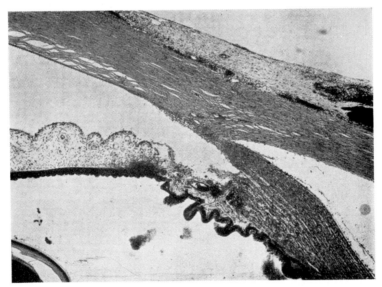

FIG. 665.—TEARING OF THE CILIARY BODY IN A CONCUSSION INJURY.

The rent runs deeply into the ciliary body from the angle of the anterior chamber,
separating the circular from the longitudinal muscle fibres (W. Lister).

obliteration of the pores in the inner aspect of Schlemm's canal, an increase
in the size and number of the endothelial cells and an accumulation of an
amorphous material between them.

Following this description of the histological appearance of traumatic recession
of the angle, it has become apparent that when eyes are examined gonioscopically this
condition is a common sequel of concussion injuries. Rodman (1963) found recession
of the angle in 30 of 31 cases of open-angle glaucoma associated with traumatic posterior
dislocation or subluxation of the lens, and Blanton (1964) observed a similar change in

the angle of 130 out of 182 cases of hyphæma following non-penetrating injuries. Howard and his colleagues (1965) found a recessed angle in 47 out of 50 consecutive patients with traumatic hyphæma examined 2 to 3 weeks after injury, Kitazawa and Takeuchi (1966) in 18 out of 22 eyes with traumatic hyphæma or iritis, and Bitrán (1965) in 55% of patients with traumatic hyphæma. Tönjum (1966) examined gonio-scopically 53 patients with traumatic hyphæma: 35 had deep clefts and 15 had super-ficial tears in the ciliary body and the root of the iris; Smith and Zimmerman (1965) found that it was commonly associated with phacolytic glaucoma (Figs. 666–8).

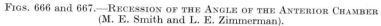

FIGS. 666 and 667.—RECESSION OF THE ANGLE OF THE ANTERIOR CHAMBER
(M. E. Smith and L. E. Zimmerman).

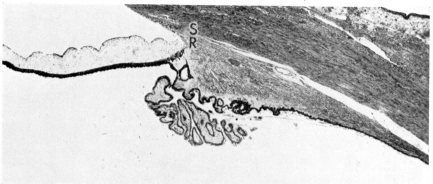

FIG. 666.—The normal angle of the anterior chamber.

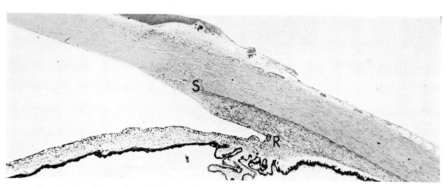

FIG. 667.—Recession of the angle of the anterior chamber. The root of the iris (R) is retroplaced with reference to the scleral spur (S) and the contour of the ciliary body is fusiform instead of the normal wedge shape seen in Fig. 666.

Although recession of the angle is a common finding after concussion injuries, glaucoma occurs far less frequently. In Blanton's (1964) series of 182 cases of traumatic hyphæma following non-penetrating injury, 130 had recession of the angle and 15 of these patients developed glaucoma. Six patients developed a transient glaucoma 2 months to 2 years after the injury and once the intra-ocular pressure became reduced the coefficient of aqueous outflow was found to be normal; nine patients developed glaucoma

10 years or more after the injury. In those patients in whom the angle of the anterior chamber appeared undamaged, the coefficient of aqueous outflow was normal, while in those with recession of the angle there was a positive correlation between the amount of recession of the angle and a low coefficient of outflow. Pettit and Keates (1963) described 8 cases of traumatic recession of the angle; two developed transient episodes of acute glaucoma 9 days and several weeks respectively after the injury, two had a reduced coefficient of outflow, and one developed glaucoma 8 years after the injury. Alper (1963) described 27 cases of traumatic recession of which 16 developed glaucoma in the injured eye; 15 of these 16 cases showed recession of two-thirds or more

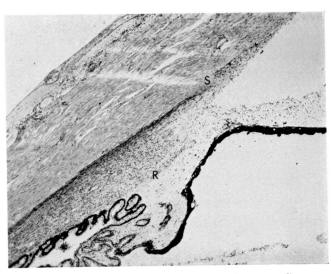

Fig. 668.—Recession of the Angle of the Anterior Chamber.

The recessed iris has become adherent to the longitudinal ciliary muscle giving the illusion that the angle is not recessed. R, root of the iris; S, scleral spur. (M. E. Smith and L. E. Zimmerman.)

of the angle. In two cases glaucoma was diagnosed the day after injury (both had subluxated lenses and one had, in addition, pupillary block); in the remaining 13 cases glaucoma occurred as a late event. Similarly, Howard and his colleagues (1965) found that the coefficient of outflow was reduced in 13 out of 25 cases of traumatic recession.

Although, as has already been stated, recession of the angle of the anterior chamber is an almost invariable gonioscopic finding in traumatic glaucoma, there is still some doubt as to whether it is the cause of the glaucoma, or only an indication that the eye has sustained severe trauma. Miles and Boniuk (1966) reported on 26 eyes enucleated for glaucoma following concussion and considered that the primary cause of the raised tension was deformity of the angle in 11 cases, hyphæma in 7, scarring and vascularization of the anterior chamber in 4, phacolytic glaucoma in 2, and iritis and hæmorrhagic glaucoma each in 1 case. That various ætiological factors may be responsible for traumatic glaucoma was also stressed by Rodman (1963) who reported on 76 eyes with traumatic posteriorly dislocated or subluxated lenses: 63 eyes developed glaucoma, in 32 of which the angle was closed while in 31 it was open. In the cases with closed angles the glaucoma was due to rubeosis and peripheral anterior synechiæ in 14 (12 of these patients had a retinal detachment), while in other cases in this group the glaucoma was due either to pupillary block or to the formation of peripheral anterior synechiæ by the organization of hæmorrhages and exudates. In the 31 cases with open angles there was a demonstrable deformity of the angle in 30. Similarly, in traumatic glaucoma associated with hyphæma, although recession of the angle is usually found[1] this may not be the primary cause of the rise in tension.

It is apparent, therefore, that several ætiological factors are responsible for this type of traumatic glaucoma. The traumatic hypertension that has been reported to occur in a few cases within the first 30 minutes after injury is probably due to the release of a histamine-like substance from damaged cells and the associated vasodilatation in the uveal tract. This vascular reaction together with the increased permeability of the capillaries associated with it was demonstrated by Amsler (1946–48) who found after a concussion to one eye a bilateral increase in the transference of fluorescein into the anterior chamber after its intravenous injection; and the involvement of the second eye by reflex action[2] explains the occasional instability in the fellow eye after one has been concussed. The early glaucoma that occurs within the first few weeks of an injury is due to trabecular damage, the glaucoma often being masked by the hyposecretion of aqueous that commonly occurs at this time (Blanton, 1964). This damage may be the direct result of the injury, or may be secondary to a hyphæma or uveitis. The late glaucoma that occurs 10 years or more after an injury is almost invariably associated with a severe degree of recession of the angle of the anterior chamber and damage to the drainage channels, notably an atrophy and compression of the trabecular meshwork or an actual growth of corneal endothelium and Descemet's membrane over the trabecular area (Rodman, 1963).

The interesting observation of Spaeth (1967) that traumatized eyes show a marked hypertensive response to the topical administration of dexamethasone may indicate that this type of glaucoma occurs more readily when an inherent susceptibility is present.

Of historical interest are the various causes that have been invoked to explain traumatic glaucoma in the past. Lagrange (1922) concluded that such an entity did

---

[1] Blanton (1964), Howard *et al.* (1965), Bitrán (1965), Kitazawa and Takeuchi (1966), Tönjum (1966).
[2] Vol. IV, p. 308.

not exist, but considered that hypertension occurred in traumatized eyes only of persons who were already predisposed to glaucoma. Granting the occurrence of the condition, a large number of hypotheses has been put forward to explain its rationale —œdema of the uvea due to blockage of the perivascular lymphatics with loose cells (von Garnier, 1891); the increased protein content of the aqueous caused by vaso-dilatation owing to vascular paralysis blocking the filtration angle (Sala, 1904; Peters, 1904); sympathetic irritation causing hypersecretion (C. and H. Fromaget, 1913); thrombosis of the ciliary vessels (von Garnier, 1891); the presence of intra-ocular hæmorrhages (Morax, 1921); the development of an orbital hæmatoma obstructing the venous outflow from the eye (Magitot, 1917–18); or an upset of the local nervous control of the circulation (Duke-Elder, 1931).

The *prognosis* of a traumatic glaucoma depends largely on the serious-ness of the associated lesions. In uncomplicated cases at an early stage the tension usually returns to normal in the course of a few weeks; but when serious intra-ocular lesions are present the outlook is more doubtful. Par-ticularly is this the case when a dislocation of the lens is present or a hæmor-rhage into the vitreous has occurred. The late traumatic glaucoma, occurring 10 years or more after the injury, appears to behave like simple glaucoma.

Treatment. In cases of early simple hypertension without evidence of acute glaucoma no special treatment is required, for the tension almost always returns to normal. In more serious cases characterized by a rise of tension sufficient to produce symptoms, carbonic anhydrase inhibitors are the most valuable drugs available. There has been some controversy as to whether to use mydriatics or miotics in these cases; it is usually wisest to use neither, but if the tension is uncontrolled on carbonic anhydrase inhibitors, topical adrenaline, so long as the angle is open, is probably the safest drug (R. Weekers *et al.*, 1954). A retrobulbar injection of alcohol sometimes serves as a hypotensive agent and also has a local anæsthetizing effect (L. Weekers, 1939). Total hyphæmata with secondary glaucoma are best treated by irrigation of the anterior chamber, preferably with urokinase,[1] and pupillary-block glaucoma by iridotomy or iridectomy. Glaucoma in the presence of a subluxated or dislocated lens is discussed elsewhere.[2] In the more acute cases when drugs fail to control the condition, surgical treatment (except that outlined above) is frequently exceedingly difficult and dis-appointing; every anti-glaucomatous technique has been recommended and the choice of procedure depends upon the particular surgeon; but it is not unusual, especially in grossly injured eyes, for excision to become necessary for the relief of pain.

GLAUCOMA AFTER PERFORATION

Post-traumatic glaucoma after a perforating injury is usually due to the incarceration of some of the intra-ocular tissues in the wound, the most common example being a corneal perforation with anterior synechiæ; a similar result may follow a perforated corneal ulcer. The pathological picture

[1] Vol. IX, p. 23.   [2] p. 659.

may vary from a simple incarceration of the iris to the formation of an anterior staphyloma, wherein the cornea, the iris and the lens are fused into one mass of cicatricial tissue. In such cases the rise of tension is due to obliteration of the filtration angle which, indeed, may be abolished. The treatment of such a condition is entirely surgical—a freeing of the tied-up iris, an extensive sector iridectomy or, at the least, an isolation of the adherent part of the iris by an iridectomy on either side of it.[1] Operations undertaken purely for the relief of tension are frequently disappointing, and if the glaucoma remains uncontrolled, enucleation may be necessary. It frequently happens, however, even if the tension is apparently controlled, that such cases tend slowly and gradually to suffer a decline in vision.

TRAUMATIC GLAUCOMA COMPLICATED BY A RETAINED FOREIGN BODY

The presence of a minute foreign body is sometimes responsible for the development of a delayed secondary glaucoma. Almost all intra-ocular foreign bodies excite an inflammatory reaction of some degree which can give rise to a secondary glaucoma. In addition, the trauma accompanying the entrance of the foreign body into the eye can of itself be responsible for the development of a concussion or post-traumatic glaucoma. Iron and steel foreign bodies, however, excite the peculiarly characteristic changes of *siderosis* which may result in a chronic secondary glaucoma coming on at a period varying from 18 months to 19 years after the injury (Clegg, 1915). This condition produces alterations in the structure of the trabecular meshwork which closely resemble those of simple glaucoma and decrease the facility of aqueous outflow. The trabecular meshwork is usually heavily stained by the Prussian blue reaction, but even in cases of glaucoma the angle is usually open (Mayou, 1926; Loewenstein and Foster, 1947). This secondary open-angle glaucoma is difficult to treat. If possible the foreign body should be removed even if siderosis has developed (Sédan-Bauby *et al.*, 1952; Pontal, 1955; Borioni, 1957), and the case managed as one of simple glaucoma. A drainage operation is frequently necessary although often unsuccessful, in which case enucleation of an irritable eye must be considered (Morax, 1917–21; Greeves, 1937; and others). This subject will be discussed more fully in a subsequent Volume.[2]

Cases of *chalcosis* due to the retention of a copper foreign body have been said to develop secondary glaucoma. Those reported, however, have been few and are confined to the literature before post-concussive recession of the angle of the anterior chamber was described; it may be, therefore, that they were due to the trauma and do not specifically depend on chalcosis (Jess, 1926; Clausen, 1930; Colrat, 1931; Belthle, 1938; Metzger, 1939).

[1] Vol. VIII, p. 644.
[2] Vol. XIV.

Agnello. *Lettura Oftal.*, **8**, 520 (1931).
Alper. *Arch. Ophthal.*, **69**, 455 (1963).
Amsler. *Bull. Soc. franç. Ophtal.*, **59**, 304 (1946).
  Trans. ophthal. Soc. U.K., **68**, 45 (1948).
Belthle. *Ueber intraokulare Kupfersplitter* (Diss.), Tübingen (1938).
Bitrán. *Arch. chil. Oftal.*, **22**, 59 (1965).
Blanton. *Arch. Ophthal.*, **72**, 39 (1964).
Borioni. *Minerva med.*, **48**, 3991 (1957).
Chuistova. *Oftal. Zh.*, No. 3, 167 (1965).
Clausen. *Klin. Mbl. Augenheilk.*, **85**, 584 (1930).
Clegg. *Ophthalmoscope*, **13**, 501 (1915).
Colrat. *Ann. Oculist.* (Paris), **168**, 935 (1931).
Collins. *Trans. ophthal. Soc. U.K.*, **12**, 180 (1892).
Duke-Elder. *Proc. roy. Soc. B*, **109**, 19 (1931).
François, Rabaey and Neetens. *Arch. Ophthal.*, **55**, 193 (1956).
Fromaget, C. and H. *Ann. Oculist.* (Paris), **149**, 1 (1913).
von Garnier. *Wratsch*, **12**, 636 (1891).
Greeves. *Brit. med. J.*, **2**, 1107 (1937).
Hegner. *Beitr. Augenheilk.*, **9**, 707 (1915).
Howard, Hutchinson and Frederick. *Trans. Amer. Acad. Ophthal.*, **69**, 295 (1965).
Jess. *Klin. Mbl. Augenheilk.*, **76**, 464 (1926).
Kitazawa and Takeuchi. *Acta Soc. ophthal. jap.*, **70**, 92 (1966).
Lagrange. *Du glaucome et de l'hypotonie*, Paris (1922).
Lamb. *Arch. Ophthal.*, **56**, 332 (1927).
Larsson. *Acta ophthal.* (Kbh.), **8**, 261 (1930).
Leone. *J. pediat. Ophthal.*, **3**, 7 (1966).
Leplat. *C.R. Soc. Biol.* (Paris), **87**, 982 (1922).
  Ann. Oculist. (Paris), **162**, 81 (1925).
Lister. *Brit. J. Ophthal.*, **8**, 305 (1924).
Loewenstein and Foster. *Amer. J. Ophthal.*, **30**, 275 (1947).
Magitot. *Ann. Oculist.* (Paris), **154**, 667 (1917); **155**, 1, 66 (1918); **157**, 680 (1920).

Mayou. *Trans. ophthal. Soc. U.K.*, **46**, 167 (1926).
Metzger. *Klin. Mbl. Augenheilk.*, **102**, 720 (1939).
Miles and Boniuk. *Amer. J. Ophthal.*, **62**, 493 (1966).
Morax. *Ann. Oculist.* (Paris), **154**, 11 (1917).
  Glaucome et glaucomateux, Paris (1921).
Peters. *Klin. Mbl. Augenheilk.*, **42** (2), 545 (1904).
Pettit and Keates. *Arch. Ophthal.*, **69**, 438 (1963).
Pontal. *Bull. Soc. Ophtal. Fr.*, 438 (1955).
Rodman. *Arch. Ophthal.*, **69**, 445 (1963).
Sala. *Klin. Mbl. Augenheilk.*, **42** (1), 316 (1904).
Schindhelm. *Klin. Mbl. Augenheilk.*, **58**, 195 (1917).
Schmidt and de Decker. *Arch. Augenheilk.*, **102**, 700 (1930).
Sédan-Bauby, Sédan and Farnarier. *Atti Soc. oftal. Lombarda*, **7**, 19 (1952).
Shea. *Canad. med. Ass. J.*, **76**, 466 (1957).
Smith, M. E. and Zimmerman. *Arch. Ophthal.*, **74**, 799 (1965).
Smith, Priestley. *Ophthal. Rev.*, **1**, 273 (1882).
Spaeth. *Arch. Ophthal.*, **78**, 714 (1967).
Stoewer. *Klin. Mbl. Augenheilk.*, **42** (1), 143 (1904); **45** (1), 347 (1907).
Tillema. *Arch. Ophthal.*, **17**, 586 (1937).
Tönjum. *Acta ophthal.* (Kbh.), **44**, 650 (1966).
Villard. *Ann. Oculist.* (Paris), **134**, 241 (1905).
Weekers, L. *Ann. Oculist.* (Paris), **176**, 81 (1939).
Weekers, R., Prijot and Gustin. *Ophthalmologica*, **128**, 213 (1954).
Wolff and Zimmerman. *Amer. J. Ophthal.*, **54**, 547 (1962).
Yamashita and Rosen. *Amer. J. Ophthal.*, **60**, 427 (1965).

POST-OPERATIVE GLAUCOMA

A peculiar and important type of post-traumatic hypertension sometimes occurs after glaucoma surgery, but more usually after one of the various operations for cataract. Thus of 27 cases studied by Lehrfeld and Rebre (1937), 3 followed iridectomy, 1 capsulotomy, 1 discission, and 22 cataract extraction. The ætiology of this sequel varies, the most important factors being pupillary blockage, malignant glaucoma, the formation of peripheral anterior synechiæ and phacogenic glaucoma.

AFTER GLAUCOMA SURGERY

A secondary glaucoma after glaucoma surgery is not particularly common, and when it does occur, apart from accidental wounding of the lens, it is associated with conditions which embarrass the filtration angle. These especially concern the formation of peripheral anterior synechiæ and the peculiar condition called malignant glaucoma wherein there is a forward displacement of the lens–iris diaphragm.

MALIGNANT GLAUCOMA. von Graefe (1869) first described the relentless elevation of the ocular tension associated with a flat anterior chamber which sometimes followed glaucoma surgery (Fig. 669). Chandler (1950) described 6 cases, 4 following iridencleisis and 2 following trephinings, and ascribed this complication to an abnormal slackness of the zonule and a forward displacement of the lens–iris diaphragm completely closing the angle of the anterior chamber and blocking the wound. This disastrous event usually occurs shortly after the operation but its onset may occasionally

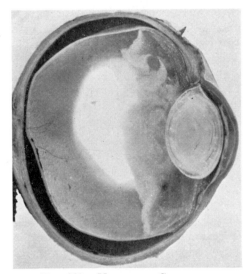

FIG. 669.—MALIGNANT GLAUCOMA.
After corneo-scleral trephining (H. E. Hobbs and R. J. H. Smith).

be delayed for some weeks or months. Moreover, it may be assumed that if malignant glaucoma occurs in one eye it invariably follows an operation on the second (Chandler, 1950; Hobbs and Smith, 1954; Birge, 1956; Cross, 1959; Posner, 1961; Hoshiwara, 1964; and others).

The *treatment* of malignant glaucoma is difficult. In some cases the tension may be controlled by the instillation of mydriatic and cycloplegic drugs into the affected eye as was first successfully practised by Heuser (1877) (Chandler and Grant, 1962), a measure which may be supplemented by osmotic therapy[1] (Weiss *et al.*, 1963; Lippas, 1964; Hoshiwara, 1964; Frezzotti and Gentili, 1964; Etienne, 1966; Chandler *et al.*, 1968). Should these expedients not be rapidly successful, surgical relief must be attempted. The classical method, originally proposed by Pagenstecher (1877), was removal of the lens, a difficult procedure which, however, may be dramati-

[1] p. 610.

cally successful (Chandler, 1950; Birge, 1956). If the tension still remains high thereafter owing to pupillary blockage by the vitreous, treatment should be on the lines to be presently indicated.[1] An alternative and less drastic procedure than removal of the lens, first recommended by Weber (1877), is a posterior sclerotomy, preferably through the pars plana which may well be supplemented by the injection of air into the anterior chamber (Chandler, 1950; Cross, 1959; Scott and Smith, 1961; and others). It was suggested by Sugar (1966) and Christensen and Irvine (1966) that the aqueous, denied its normal exit, tended to accumulate at the posterior pole of the globe where it collects and the vitreous is displaced and liquefied, and that this region should therefore be aspirated. Should all these measures fail, enucleation is the only course available; but if malignant glaucoma occurs in one eye a prophylactic peripheral iridectomy should be undertaken on the other.

AFTER CATARACT EXTRACTION: APHAKIC GLAUCOMA

The occurrence of glaucoma after the extraction or discission of a cataract is a complication recognized since the time of Bowman (1865) and von Graefe (1869), the very considerable literature on which has been discussed at length by Natanson (1889), Dalén (1901), Chance (1910), Fox (1936), and Legrand and Hervouët (1964). In the early literature its incidence after extracapsular extractions was said to vary from 0·6 to 3·0% (0·64%—Collins, 1905; 1·2%—Fox, 1936; 2%—da Gama Pinto, 1897; 3%—A. Knapp, 1928), while after intracapsular extractions its incidence was said to be less (0%—Fox, 1936; Davis, 1938; Gifford, 1940; 0·4%—Sinclair, 1932; 0·8%—A. Knapp, 1936; 2·5%—A. Knapp, 1926–33). These early figures are certainly artificially low, and in more recent series the incidence after all cataract extractions has been found to vary between 2 and 7%.

Thus Owens (1948) encountered 4·2% in all cataract extractions, but only 1·6% in intracapsular extractions, Meyer and Sternberg (1950) found 5·5% in their series but the incidence declined to 3·5% in those cases wherein corneo-scleral sutures were used, Cinotti and Jacobson (1953) experienced 7·5% in extracapsular and 5·4% in intracapsular extractions but in their diabetic patients the incidence increased to 10%, Post and Harper (1953) found an incidence of 7%, Barraquer (1962) encountered 2·1% in those cases in which alpha-chymotrypsin was used and 0·94% in those in which it was not. Legrand and Hervouet (1964) quote incidences of between 2 and 4% in various recent series, while in their own series of 600 cases operated upon since 1961 the incidence was 5·8%, a relatively high figure accounted for by their routine of systematically measuring the intra-ocular pressure of all their post-operative patients.

In the majority of cases of glaucoma following cataract extraction the tension rises during the first few days or weeks after the operation; glaucoma which develops months or years after an extraction is probably primary and unrelated to the surgery. Most cases of secondary glaucoma are the result of closure of the angle of the anterior chamber, usually by peripheral anterior synechiæ (Fig. 670). These were described histologically by Czermak (1897)

[1] p. 718.

but gonioscopic evidence of their existence and their importance in aphakic glaucoma was presented by Sugar (1940). Kronfeld (1955) and Miller and his colleagues (1957) have shown tonographically that the resistance to the outflow of aqueous is related to the extent of the peripheral anterior synechiæ, although occasional cases have been reported wherein a completely closed angle following cataract extraction has occurred in the presence of a normal intra-ocular pressure. The probable explanation for this is the existence of a filtering bleb or cicatrix (Sugar, 1941).

There are several causes for closure of the angle of the anterior chamber, the more important of which are as follows:

1. DELAYED RE-FORMATION OF THE ANTERIOR CHAMBER. This is probably the most important factor in the ætiology of secondary aphakic glaucoma, although until fairly recently its significance was not fully appreciated.[1] The more obvious causes of a leaking wound have been

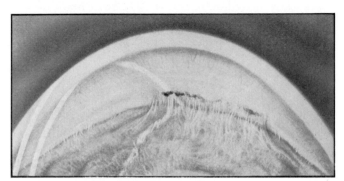

FIG. 670.—APHAKIC GLAUCOMA.
Showing the presence of peripheral anterior synechiæ (Inst. Ophthal.).

known for some considerable time. Incarceration of the iris has been verified by many pathological examinations (Stölting, 1887; Collins, 1888–1914; Dalén, 1901; Fox, 1936; and others), entanglement of the capsule of the lens in the wound has been described on many occasions (Collins, 1888–1914; Natanson, 1889; A. Knapp, 1910–28; Stölting, 1912; Gros, 1925; and others), while a prolapse of the vitreous into the wound and a blocking of the angle of the anterior chamber is known to have caused glaucoma (H. Knapp, 1895; Risley, 1910; Weill, 1920; Stieren, 1921; Urbanek, 1924). In the majority of cases of delayed re-formation of the anterior chamber, however, these florid complications have not occurred and the leak is due to insecure or inaccurate apposition of the lips of the wound. The duration of the delay in the re-formation of the anterior chamber influences the incidence of secondary glaucoma, and although this varies in different series of cases, a delay in re-formation of more than 5 days carries an appreciable risk of the

[1] Sugar (1940), Meyer and Sternberg (1950), Weekers and Delmarcelle (1952), Ross (1953), Kronfeld (1954), Giardini (1956–62), McLean (1957), Simpson (1959–66), Huber (1962), and others.

formation of extensive peripheral anterior synechiæ and therefore of secondary glaucoma.

If the anterior chamber remained shallow for more than 5 days Meyer and Stern-berg (1950) found the incidence of secondary glaucoma to be 22% while Weekers and Delmarcelle (1952) found it to be 43%. Kronfeld (1954) experienced a 12% incidence of glaucoma if the anterior chamber were flat for 5 to 8 days and of 44% if it were flat for 9 to 12 days. Bernard (1963) encountered glaucoma in 22% of cases wherein the anterior had been flat for 8 to 15 days, in 44% of cases between 15 and 20 days, in 72% of cases between 20 and 45 days, and in 100% of cases if the anterior chamber were flat for more than 45 days. Huber (1962) observed glaucoma in 50% of cases wherein the anterior chamber remained flat for more than 9 days.

The presence of a cilio-choroidal detachment has been considered to cause a delay in the re-formation of the anterior chamber by a number of authors (Weekers and Delmarcelle, 1952; McLean, 1957; Simpson, 1959; Bernard, 1963). The detachment is associated with a shallow anterior chamber which predisposes to the formation of peripheral anterior synechiæ and hence to closed-angle glaucoma.

2. PUPILLARY BLOCK. Dupuy-Dutemps (1904) and Hudson (1911) both believed that the vitreous could block the pupillary aperture and cause a secondary glaucoma, but it was Chandler and Johnson (1947) who fully established the concept of pupillary block as a cause of secondary glaucoma in aphakia and in eyes with dislocated lenses. This concept has been con-firmed by subsequent authors.[1] Chandler (1954) described four types of pupillary block: (1) ring synechiæ of the pupil to an intact vitreous face, (2) a plug of vitreous occluding the pupillary aperture and any iridectomy that may be present, (3) the formation of a pupillary membrane, and (4) the blocking by vitreous of a gap in a pupillary membrane following an extra-capsular extraction. In each of these instances there is an obstruction to the flow of aqueous from the posterior to the anterior chamber, and the vitreous–iris diaphragm is pushed forward so that the peripheral iris comes into contact with the cornea and peripheral anterior synechiæ are liable to form (Shaffer, 1954). Pupillary block may occur in many conditions: (1) after an otherwise uneventful extracapsular extraction, (2) after an otherwise uneventful intracapsular extraction, (3) after any type of lens extraction which is followed by delayed re-formation or late shallowing of the anterior chamber, (4) after the discission of a cataract or of an after-cataract, and (5) in air-blockage after a cataract extraction (Sugar, 1966). Pupillary block is more common after extracapsular than after intracapsular extrac-tions owing to the greater post-operative inflammation resulting from the presence of lens material in the anterior chamber (Chandler, 1962).

Pupillary block characteristically presents as a shallow or a flat anterior chamber, usually without evidence of a leakage from the wound, associated

[1] Reese (1948), Chandler (1954–62), Shaffer (1954), Sugar (1960–66), Swan (1963), Etienne (1967), and others.

with an elevated intra-ocular pressure and with herniation of the hyaloid face of the vitreous into the anterior chamber.[1] If the pupillary block is unrelieved, peripheral anterior synechiæ develop and the intra-ocular pressure, if not already raised, then becomes so. If the condition is diagnosed before glaucoma has occurred, an attempt should be made to break the adhesions between the iris and the vitreous or the remnants of the lens by the use of mydriatics. If these are unsuccessful, iridotomy or iridectomy may relieve the block. Should these measures not be successful, more dramatic steps must be taken. If the pupillary block persists there is evidence that it may be due to an increased pressure in the vitreous itself, conditioned by the accumulation of aqueous formed by the ciliary body which cannot find an exit into the anterior chamber owing to the impermeability of the hyaloid face of the gel and its fusion with the iris (Christensen and Irvine, 1966; Sugar, 1966). In this event the aqueous percolates into the vitreous, often accumulating in the posterior region where the gel is displaced and liquefied. To relieve the tension thus caused Chandler (1951) advised cutting the hyaloid face of the vitreous, Shaffer (1954) practised cutting deeply into the vitreous itself, while Sugar (1966) and Meisekothen and Allen (1968) aspirated the vitreous through a small incision in the region of the pars plana, whereupon as much as 1 ml. of clear fluid could be removed before any formed gel appeared. Once peripheral anterior synechiæ have formed, however, both the pupillary block and the closed-angle glaucoma must be treated by a combined iridectomy and cyclodialysis.

3. EPITHELIAL INGROWTH. An ingrowth of epithelium through the surgical wound into the anterior chamber, the whole of which may eventually be lined by the proliferating cells, occasionally produces a most recalcitrant type of glaucoma.[2] Although an uncommon complication of cataract extraction, it is responsible for about 20% of the eyes that are enucleated after this operation. Theobald and Haas (1948) reported 14 eyes with epithelial ingrowths out of 75 eyes enucleated after cataract extraction; in 9 there was a history of post-operative gaping of the wound or delayed reformation of the anterior chamber. Blodi (1954) studied 150 enucleated eyes following extraction: about 20% had epithelial ingrowths which were twice as common after intracapsular as after extracapsular extraction. Payne and his colleagues (1955) found that 60 out of 333 eyes enucleated after cataract extraction had epithelial ingrowths; 36 of these eyes had developed secondary glaucoma. The treatment of this condition has already been discussed.[3]

4. A POST-OPERATIVE ANTERIOR UVEITIS may determine the onset of an inflammatory glaucoma, to which may be added the mechanical effect of

[1] p. 368.
[2] Meller (1901), Elschnig (1903), Collins (1914), Salus (1927), Corrado (1931), Levine (1933), Vail (1936), Terry et al. (1939), Theobald and Haas (1948), Blodi (1954), Payne et al. (1955), Maumenee (1957–64), Payne (1958), Paufique and Hervouët (1964), and others.
[3] p. 281.

pupillary block due to an adhesion of the iris to the capsule (Priestley Smith, 1891).

5. A POST-OPERATIVE HYPHÆMA, if it becomes organized, may obstruct the outflow of aqueous at the angle of the anterior chamber. In the series of cases of secondary glaucoma reported by Post and Harper (1953) a hyphæma occurred in 14·3%.

6. Massive quantities of SOFT LENS MATTER in the anterior chamber may clog the filtration angle and also excite an inflammatory reaction (Fox, 1936). This is particularly liable to occur following discission of a congenital cataract. As a rule such a secondary glaucoma is readily controlled by evacuation of the lenticular material.

7. THE INJECTION OF AIR INTO THE ANTERIOR CHAMBER, a procedure often employed at the end of an operation for cataract extraction to separate the face of the vitreous and the iris from the cornea and thus re-form the anterior chamber,[1] may give rise to a secondary glaucoma in two circumstances. If too much air is injected the pupillary aperture may be blocked by a valve-like action between the posterior surface of the bubble of air and the anterior surface of the iris, thus obstructing the flow of aqueous out of the posterior chamber and causing an iris bombé which may embarrass the drainage angle (Sallmann, 1931; Barkan, 1947–51; Scheie and Frayer, 1950; Brognoli, 1955). Alternatively, if the bubble of air gets behind the iris, this tissue may be pushed forward to occlude the angle, an accident likely to happen if the pupil is dilated and the patient inadvertently bends his head forward (Wyman, 1954).

THE DISPLACEMENT OF A POST-IRIDIC LENTICULUS inserted after an extraction of the lens may induce a secondary glaucoma necessitating the very difficult procedure of its removal. This subject has previously been discussed.[2]

At this stage it is worth mentioning the transient, often severe, rise of intra-ocular pressure following the use of *alpha-chymotrypsin* in cataract surgery. This was described by Kirsch (1964) who noted it in 72·5% of extractions when this enzyme was used. A similar rise of tension was noted in only 23·6% of extractions when the enzyme was not used. The peak in the rise of intra-ocular pressure occurs between the 2nd and 5th post-operative days, and in most cases the pressure has returned to normal levels by the 7th day, in all cases by the 19th day. The rise is due to a low coefficient of facility of outflow with no evidence of hypersecretion, and it was suggested that this transient glaucoma was an important factor in the production of complications in wound-healing after cataract extraction when this enzyme was employed (Kirsch, 1965). These findings have been confirmed by Acers (1965) and Galin and his colleagues (1966) although the latter workers found a lower incidence of this form of glaucoma. Fanta (1963) showed histologically that in eyes in which alpha-chymotrypsin had been used there was an inflammatory reaction in the angle of the anterior chamber with swelling and degeneration of cells of the trabecular meshwork. Kirsch (1965) demonstrated that these changes were probably not the result of a hypersensitivity reaction, and that the most likely ætiological mechanism for this rise of pressure was a toxic or possibly a mechanical interference with outflow. These complications, however, are usually avoided if the enzyme is carefully washed out of the anterior chamber

[1] p. 276.   [2] p. 289.

within 2 or 3 minutes after its use, but their incidence does not appear to be reduced by the post-operative use of pilocarpine, acetazolamide or subconjunctival steroids (Bloomfield, 1968).

The *prognosis* in such cases of post-operative glaucoma following cataract surgery is on the whole poor, although recently since the ætiology of many types has become better understood the prognosis has improved. The best treatment is prophylactic—the elimination of the factors which pre-dispose to operative and post-operative complications, for it is when these occur that a secondary glaucoma is particularly liable to develop (Post and Harper, 1953). In particular, accurate and adequate closure of the wound and the prevention of vitreous loss will reduce the incidence of this compli-cation. If pupillary block develops, this should be relieved before peripheral anterior synechiæ have formed. Once glaucoma has developed, medical measures should be tried; miotics, and particularly the long-acting anti-cholinesterase drugs, may produce a dramatic fall in tension, and these topical drugs may be combined with the systemic carbonic anhydrase inhibitors. If the tension remains uncontrolled, however, surgery should not be too long delayed if vision is to be retained, for the prognosis depends largely on the promptness of the relief of tension before irreversible damage to the optic nerve has occurred. Although a number of surgical techniques has been recommended at different times for the treatment of aphakic glaucoma, cyclodialysis is probably the most widely useful operation, particularly when the glaucoma is of the closed-angle variety; it is a procedure unaffected by the condition of aphakia and does not entail the presentation of vitreous. Cases of epithelial ingrowth are particularly difficult and unrewarding to treat. Radiotherapy relieves the tension in some cases (Vail, 1936; Wolff and Naquin, 1955; Anton, 1967), while in others relief has been obtained by wide iridectomy and removal of the epithelial tissues from the cornea by curettage (Maumenee, 1957–64) or cryosurgery.[1]

After penetrating KERATOPLASTY a secondary glaucoma may be due to the presence of anterior synechiæ usually as a result of a delay in the re-formation of the anterior chamber (see Leahey, 1957; and others); occasionally hypertension results from an associated iridocyclitis and after a lamellar keratoplasty a pupillary block may be the causal factor sometimes due to synechiæ involving the pupillary margin (Bushmitch and Kalfa, 1960).

SCLERAL BUCKLING AND ENCIRCLING OPERATIONS FOR RETINAL DETACHMENT[2] may be followed by the development of a secondary glaucoma, due sometimes to a blockage of the venous return and sometimes to narrowing of the anterior chamber and the formation of anterior synechiæ (Sebestyn et al., 1962).

LIGHT-COAGULATION OF THE IRIS may be followed by the development of a secondary glaucoma caused possibly by the inflammatory reaction of the tissues; a gross accumulation of pigmentary deposits in the trabeculæ sometimes suggests the occurrence of a pigmentary type of glaucoma.

[1] p. 283.   [2] Vol. X, p. 835.

Acers. *Trans. Amer. Acad. Ophthal.*, **69**, 1022 (1965).
Anton. *Klin. Mbl. Augenheilk.*, **150**, 675 (1967).
Barkan. *Amer. J. Ophthal.*, **30**, 1063 (1947); **34**, 567 (1951).
Barraquer. *La extracción intracapsular del cristalino*, Madrid (1962).
Bernard. *Bull. Soc. Ophtal. Fr.*, Suppl. (1963).
Birge. *Trans. Amer. ophthal. Soc.*, **54**, 311 (1956).
Blodi. *J. Iowa St. med. Soc.*, **44**, 514 (1954).
Bloomfield. *Amer. J. Ophthal.*, **65**, 405 (1968).
Bowman. *Roy. Lond. ophthal. Hosp. Rep.*, **4**, 332, 365 (1865).
Brognoli. *Ann. Ottal.*, **81**, 411 (1955).
Bushmitch and Kalfa. *Oftal. Zh.*, No. 4, 195 (1960).
Chance. *Ophthalmology*, **6**, 565 (1910).
Chandler. *Trans. Amer. ophthal. Soc.*, **48**, 128 (1950).
　Amer. J. Ophthal., **34**, 993 (1951).
　Trans. Amer. Acad. Ophthal., **58**, 382 (1954).
　Arch. Ophthal., **67**, 14 (1962).
Chandler and Grant. *Arch. Ophthal.*, **68**, 353 (1962).
Chandler and Johnson. *Arch. Ophthal.*, **37**, 740 (1947).
Chandler, Simmons and Grant. *Amer. J. Ophthal.*, **66**, 495 (1968).
Christensen and Irvine. *Arch. Ophthal.*, **75**, 490 (1966).
Cinotti and Jacobson. *Amer. J. Ophthal.*, **36**, 929 (1953).
Collins. *Roy. Lond. ophthal. Hosp. Rep.*, **12**, 19 (1888); **16**, 247 (1905).
　Trans. ophthal. Soc. U.K., **34**, 18 (1914).
Corrado. *Ann. Ottal.*, **59**, 706 (1931).
Cross. *Brit. J. Ophthal.*, **43**, 57 (1959).
Czermak. *Prag. med. Wschr.*, **22**, 1, 15, 38 (1897).
Dalén. *Mitt. Augenklin. Carol. med.-chir. Inst.*, Stockholm, **3**, 75 (1901).
Davis. *Arch. Ophthal.*, **19**, 867 (1938).
Dupuy-Dutemps. *Ann. Oculist.* (Paris), **132**, 93 (1904).
Elschnig. *Klin. Mbl. Augenheilk.*, **41** (1), 247 (1903).
Etienne. *Ann. Oculist.* (Paris), **199**, 1121 (1966); **200**, 729 (1967).
Fanta. *Klin. Mbl. Augenheilk.*, **142**, 1011 (1963).
Fox. *Arch. Ophthal.*, **16**, 585 (1936).
Frezzotti and Gentili. *Amer. J. Ophthal.*, **57**, 402 (1964).
Galin, Barasch and Harris. *Amer. J. Ophthal.*, **61**, 690 (1966).
Giardini. *Boll. Oculist.*, **35**, 275 (1956). *Docum. ophthal.*, **16**, 338 (1962).
Gifford. *Arch. Ophthal.*, **23**, 301 (1940).
von Graefe. *v. Graefes Arch. Ophthal.*, **15** (3), 108 (1869).
Gros. *Clin. Ophtal.*, **29**, 691 (1925).
Heuser. *Zbl. prakt. Augenheilk.*, **1**, 256 (1877).

Hobbs and Smith. *Brit. J. Ophthal.*, **38**, 279 (1954).
Hoshiwara. *Arch. Ophthal.*, **72**, 601 (1964).
Huber. *An. Inst. Barraquer*, **3**, 399 (1962).
Hudson. *Roy. Lond. ophthal. Hosp. Rep.*, **18**, 203 (1911).
Kirsch. *Arch. Ophthal.*, **72**, 612 (1964).
　Trans. Amer. Acad. Ophthal., **69**, 1011 (1965).
Knapp, A. *Trans. Amer. ophthal. Soc.*, **12**, 472 (1910).
　Arch. Ophthal., **55**, 257 (1926); **10**, 6 (1933); **16**, 770 (1936).
　J. Amer. med. Ass., **91**, 1794 (1928).
Knapp, H. *Arch. Augenheilk.*, **30**, 1 (1895).
Kronfeld. *Amer. J. Ophthal.*, **38**, 453 (1954); **39**, 147 (1955).
Leahey. *Trans. Amer. ophthal. Soc.*, **55**, 575 (1957).
Legrand and Hervouët. *Bull. Soc. Ophtal. Fr.*, Annual Report (1964).
Lehrfeld and Reber. *Arch. Ophthal.*, **18**, 712 (1937).
Levine. *Amer. J. Ophthal.*, **16**, 796 (1933).
Lippas. *Amer. J. Ophthal.*, **57**, 620 (1964).
McLean. *Trans. Amer. Acad. Ophthal.*, **61**, 20 (1957).
Maumenee. *Trans. Amer. Acad. Ophthal.*, **61**, 51 (1957).
　Trans. Amer. ophthal. Soc., **62**, 153 (1964).
Meisekothen and Allen. *Amer. J. Ophthal.*, **65**, 877 (1968).
Meller. *v. Graefes Arch. Ophthal.*, **52**, 436 (1901).
Meyer and Sternberg. *Trans. Amer. Acad. Ophthal.*, **54**, 326 (1950).
Miller, Keskey and Becker. *Arch. Ophthal.*, **58**, 401 (1957).
Natanson. *Ueber Glaukom in aphakischen Augen* (Diss.), Dorpat (1889).
Owens. *South. med. J.*, **41**, 357 (1948).
Pagenstecher. *Ber. dtsch. ophthal. Ges.*, **10**, 7 (1877).
Paufique and Hervouët. *Ann. Oculist.* (Paris), **197**, 1, 105 (1964).
Payne. *Amer. J. Ophthal.*, **45**, 182 (1958).
Payne, Simonton and Cury. *Trans. Amer. ophthal. Soc.*, **53**, 231 (1955).
Pinto, da Gama. *Ann. Oculist.* (Paris), **117**, 22 (1897).
Posner. *Eye, Ear, Nose Thr. Monthly*, **40**, 203 (1961).
Post and Harper. *Amer. J. Ophthal.*, **36**, 103 (1953).
Reese. *Trans. Amer. ophthal. Soc.*, **46**, 73 (1948).
Risley. *Ophthalmology*, **6**, 572 (1910).
Ross. *Acta ophthal.* (Kbh.), **31**, 43 (1953).
Sallmann. *Nat. med. J. China*, **17**, 6 (1931).
Salus. *Klin. Mbl. Augenheilk.*, **78**, 368 (1927).
Scheie and Frayer. *Arch. Ophthal.*, **44**, 691 (1950).
Scott and Smith. *Brit. J. Ophthal.*, **45**, 654 (1961).
Sebestyn, Schepens and Rosenthal. *Arch. Ophthal.*, **67**, 736 (1962).

Shaffer. *Trans. Amer. Acad. Ophthal.*, **58**, 217 (1954).

Simpson. *Trans. Canad. ophthal. Soc.*, **21** and **22**, 56 (1959).
Canad. J. Ophthal., **1**, 67 (1966).

Sinclair. *Trans. ophthal. Soc. U.K.*, **52**, lvii (1932).

Smith, Priestley. *Glaucoma*, London (1891).

Stieren. *Amer. J. Ophthal.*, **4**, 424 (1921).

Stölting. *v. Graefes Arch. Ophthal.*, **33** (2), 177 (1887); **81**, 518 (1912).

Sugar. *Amer. J. Ophthal.*, **23**, 853 (1940); **61**, 435 (1966).
Arch. Ophthal., **25**, 674 (1941).
J. int. Coll. Surg., **33**, 312 (1960).

Swan. *Arch. Ophthal.*, **69**, 191 (1963).

Terry, Chisholm and Schonberg. *Amer. J. Ophthal.*, **22**, 1083 (1939).

Theobald and Haas. *Trans. Amer. Acad. Ophthal.*, **53**, 470 (1948).

Urbanek. *Z. Augenheilk.*, **54**, 164 (1924).

Vail. *Arch. Ophthal.*, **15**, 270 (1936).

Weber. *v. Graefes Arch. Ophthal.*, **23** (1), 1 (1877).

Weekers, R. and Delmarcelle. *Bull. Soc. belge Ophtal.*, No. 102, 668 (1952).

Weekers, R., Prijot and Gustin. *Brit. J. Ophthal.*, **38**, 742 (1954).

Weill. *Arch. Ophthal.*, **37**, 716 (1920).

Weiss, Shaffer and Harrington. *Arch. Ophthal.*, **69**, 154 (1963).

Wolff and Naquin (1955). Quoted in Sugar, *The Glaucomas*, 2nd ed., N.Y., 339 (1957).

Wyman. *Amer. J. Ophthal.*, **37**, 424 (1954).

CHAPTER X

OCULAR HYPOTONY

THE subject of ocular hypotension has excited much less interest and speculation than that of hypertension, partly because its effects are less dramatic and partly because it is usually a consequential and incidental event in a clinical picture dominated by other more compelling factors; nevertheless, it is of considerable theoretical and practical importance. In general, if the tension is below the average the condition is called HYPO-TONY if the fall is considerable and persistent and is sufficient to cause structural and functional changes it is known as OPHTHALMOMALACIA ($\mu\alpha\lambda\alpha\kappa\iota\alpha$, softness). The latter condition is important since in its acute and dramatic forms the damage caused to the eye can be as great as that caused by acute hypertension.

Historically, the first writer to devote particular attention to states of markedly low tension was von Graefe (1866), who termed the condition *essential phthisis bulbi*. Then followed the work of Nagel (1867), Swanzy (1869–70), Landesberg (1871) and others, the general opinion being that whereas glaucoma represented an increased secretion of the intra-ocular fluid, ophthalmomalacia was the result of a diminution of secretion which could be caused by vascular or nervous disorders. Among the most comprehensive studies on the pathology of the condition are those of Treacher Collins (1916–18) who induced it experimentally by repeated paracenteses in rabbits, investigations repeated by Meesmann (1922), and by creating a fistula by Orzalesi (1947) and Capper and Leopold (1956), while more recently the clinical pathology was extensively detailed by Frazzetto and his associates (1967). From the physiological and aetiological points of view, the work of Magitot (1917–33) of Paris was outstanding, and the clinical studies of Lagrange (1922), Parker Heath (1947) and Poos (1952) embrace much of the subject.

SIR HENRY ROSBOROUGH SWANZY [1844–1913] (Fig. 671) of Dublin, following Arthur Jacob [1790–1874], famous for his researches on anatomy, and Sir William R. W. Wilde [1815–76], more notorious for his indiscretions than famous for his professional contributions, succeeded in giving Irish ophthalmology an international prestige just as did William Mackenzie for Scotland and Sir William Bowman for England. After an assistantship to von Graefe in Berlin and serving as a surgeon in the Prussian Army in 1866, Swanzy returned to his native Dublin where he spent the remainder of his professional life, eventually becoming senior surgeon to the Royal Victoria Eye and Ear Hospital and the leading figure in ophthalmology in his country, universally popular because of his clinical ability, charming personality and humour. He delivered the Bowman Lecture in 1888 on the localization of cerebral disease, was President of the Ophthalmological Society of the United Kingdom (1897–99) and President of the Royal College of Surgeons of Ireland (1906–8). He contributed to many aspects of our specialty, his first paper being written from von Graefe's clinic on " Essential Phthisis Bulbi " (1869).

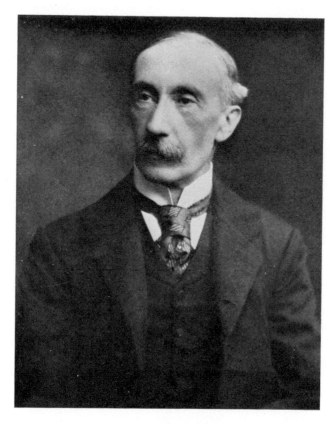

FIG. 671.—HENRY ROSBOROUGH SWANZY
[1844–1913].

Essential Hypotension

Just as it is impossible to establish an upper limit to the "normal" range of the intra-ocular pressure, so is it difficult to define a lower level. As we have seen, the height of the ocular tension in any population follows an asymmetrical curve of distribution around a mean of 14 to 16 mm. Hg. Measuring the tension of 10,000 apparently normal eyes, Leydhecker (1959–60) found that in 95·5% the pressure lay between 10·5 and 20·5 mm. Hg; it was below 10·0 mm. Hg in about 2% of the population and below 9·0 in 0·6%; and in his view a pressure below 6·5 mm. Hg should be considered as abnormal. These figures have been corroborated by other investigators using less extensive populations (Bertelsen et al., 1965; Davanger and Holter, 1965; and others). The condition of essential hypotension is bilateral and a suggestion that heredity may be a determining factor is shown by the findings of Forsius and Eriksson (1961) in the Åland Islands that the inhabitants had a remarkably low average level of intra-ocular pressure and a low incidence of glaucoma. Such an eye, provided it shows no signs of ocular pathology, is not associated with a systemic disease causing a low tension, and shows no deterioration in structure or function, may be considered to belong to the category of essential hypotension and requires no treatment.

Secondary Hypotony

ÆTIOLOGY

In the Volume of this *System* devoted to Physiology[1] we have seen that prolonged changes in the intra-ocular pressure may be produced by one of three factors—changes in the rate of the formation of the aqueous humour, changes in the resistance to its outflow, or changes in the pressure in the episcleral veins; a fall in this venous pressure is probably of little clinical significance in the production of hypotony, but the first two factors are important. A multitude of other conditions such as a fall in blood pressure or a ligation of the carotid artery may cause a fall in the intra-ocular pressure, but in such cases the decrease is slight and transitory and of little clinical significance. Only when the arterial pressure in the eye is dramatically lowered over a long period does it become important, as is seen in pulseless disease and carotid occlusion[2] (Hollenhorst, 1959; and others), or widespread giant-cell arteritis[3] (Haimböck, 1961). It is to be remembered, however, that in a number of cases of hypotony no obvious ætiology can be detected.

A diminution in the production of the aqueous may therefore produce hypotony and, in fact, is the most common factor in its ætiology. Pharmacologically this can be brought about by the carbonic anhydrase inhibitors such as acetazolamide which probably decrease the secretory element in the formation of aqueous up to some 50% (B. Becker, 1954; and many

[1] Vol. IV, p. 243.   [2] Vol. X, p. 356.   [3] Vol. X, p. 238.

others)[1]; the cardiac glycosides (such as ouabain) act similarly but to a less extent, probably by inhibiting the sodium–potassium activated adenosine triphosphatase (NA-K-ATPase) which participates in the secretion of the aqueous (Simon *et al.*, 1962; and others).[2] Similarly, a slight degree of hypotony may follow irradiation either by x-rays (1,300 r, B. Becker *et al.*, 1956) or beta-rays (strontium-90, Schiff, 1959). In so far as the intra-ocular fluid is formed by ultrafiltration, a lowering of the ocular tension may occur if the osmotic pressure of the serum is raised; if the increased osmolarity is due to diffusible substances, the lowering of the intra-ocular pressure is transient, but if the colloid content of the serum is raised a slight hypotony of some duration results.[3] A similar condition may occur in states of systemic dehydration.

A considerable number of pathological conditions may produce the same effect, such as the accumulation of fluid in the suprachoroidal lamellæ sufficient to detach the ciliary body from the sclera, or degenerative or inflammatory processes in which the ciliary body is involved. A dramatic hypotensive effect may also occur in diseases which cause widespread metabolic disturbances.

A diminution of the resistance to the outflow of the aqueous may also result in ocular hypotony which persists as long as the cause is effective. The most dramatic example of this is seen in perforating wounds or fistulous scars such as constitute the rationale of the surgical treatment of glaucoma. By tearing the ciliary muscle, a concussion of the globe may similarly be responsible for a prolonged period of hypotony.

Nervous influences have frequently been cited as an ætiological factor in the development of hypotony, the usual explanations being that the fall in intra-ocular pressure is due to a diminution of the secretion of aqueous owing to vasoconstriction of the vessels in the ciliary body or, alternatively, a lowering of the resistance to outflow owing to the release of sympatho-mimetic amines from degenerating nerve-endings (Langham and Taylor, 1960). Our knowledge of these effects in man, however, is fragmentary and the clinically observed changes in the intra-ocular pressure are small and transient. It has been said that a slight hypotony occurs in patients who have undergone a leucotomy (Weinstein, 1954; Cavka, 1956) or on the paralysed side in cases of cerebral hemiplegia (Kahler and Sallmann, 1923), in the post-encephalitic syndrome (Ludwig and Vurdelja, 1951; Brand, 1956), in states of deep coma (Restivo-Manfridi and Serafini, 1966), following severe cerebral trauma (Casari, 1951), in deep anæsthesia (Kornblueth *et al.*, 1959; Müller-Jensen, 1964) or barbiturate poisoning (Magitot and Offret, 1936). Finally, in zoster an acute hypotony may develop (Juler, 1928; Sédan, 1933; and others), an effect possibly due to the disturbance of local axon reflexes.

[1] Vol. IV, p. 316.
[2] Vol. IV, p. 188.
[3] Vol. IV, p. 292.

Hormonal factors are also said to be capable of producing hypotony—hyperpituitarism (Imre, 1921), hyperthyroidism (Terrien, 1922; von Csapody, 1923), castration (Radnót, 1944–49), ovariectomy (Sédan, 1965), or Addison's disease, independently of the blood pressure (Cervino *et al.*, 1960). These effects, however, are small and incidental.

On this basis we shall now shortly discuss the various clinical conditions characterized by a persistent lowering of tension. The most common of these are:

1. Cilio-choroidal detachment.
2. Retinal detachment.
3. Cyclitis.
4. Systemic disturbances.
5. Myotonic dystrophy.
6. Myopia.
7. Congenital anomalies.
8. Trauma.

1. CILIO-CHOROIDAL DETACHMENT

In a previous Volume[1] we have already seen that a cilio-choroidal detachment or, more exactly, a cilio-choroidal œdema resulting from a vasodilatation of the uvea, is a common feature of hypotonic eyes; indeed, by many authorities it is considered to be much the most common cause (Leber, 1916; Kümmell, 1925; Baurmann, 1929; Gonin, 1934; Hertz, 1954; and many others). The lesion accompanies a variety of ocular conditions including chorioretinal inflammations, severe vascular disturbances, vascular congestion due to ocular neoplasms, and all types of trauma including many surgical procedures. The detachment is due to the effusion of fluid into the suprachoroidal lamellæ as the result of vascular dilatation in the uveal tract.[2] The fluid is usually serous but may be albuminous, hæmorrhagic or occasionally purulent, depending on the causal lesion. It is difficult to define a specific reason why its presence in this region should determine the development of a fall in the ocular tension and its persistence until the exudate is absorbed; Chandler and Maumenee (1961), however, reasoning that the intra-ocular pressure tended to return to a normal level on the disappearance of the cilio-choroidal detachment, suggested that its presence inhibited the formation of the aqueous humour and they found that in order to be an effective cause the entire ciliary region from the scleral spur to the ora serrata had to be undermined with fluid, which in some cases was merely a thin film not more than 0·5 mm. thick (Fig. 672). In such cases the ocular tension may be 5·0 mm. Hg or less. Moreover, after allowing the release of fluid from beneath the ciliary body, a normal tension may dramatically return (Miller, 1963). A hypotony was induced experimentally in rabbits by

[1] Vol. IX, p. 939.
[2] Marshall (1896), Hudson (1914), Hagen (1921), Fuchs (1921), O'Brien (1935), Klien (1937), Hertz (1954), Dobree (1961), Bernard (1963), and others.

Dellaporta and Obear (1964) by injecting citrated blood between the ciliary body and the sclera.

In this connection, the occurrence of hypotony after trauma, particularly contusions and perforating wounds, is interesting; in the former, tears in the ciliary muscle are common and in the latter there is sudden vaso-dilatation. To the latter class also belong the hypotonic conditions which follow intra-ocular surgery, particularly cyclodialysis, filtering operations for glaucoma, operations for cataract and, more rarely, keratoplasty and surgical procedures for retinal detachment. These are discussed at length elsewhere.[1]

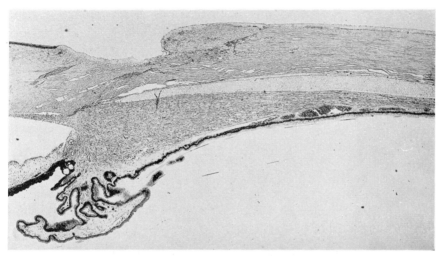

Fig. 672.—Cilio-choroidal Detachment.
In a case of marked hypotony. There is a flat detachment of the ciliary body (P. A. Chandler and A. E. Maumenee).

2. RETINAL DETACHMENT

We have already seen[2] that although a retinal detachment is popularly associated with a low tension, this is by no means the rule; while statistics vary considerably, some authors finding hypotension almost invariably (Lauber, 1908; Kummell, 1920), some in equal proportions with a normal tension (Horstmann, 1891), and others rarely (Deutschmann, 1910; Thomas, 1925), it is probable that in the majority of cases the tension is normal at first, or may even on occasion be raised, but tends to fall to a subnormal level as the age of the detachment increases (Nordenson, 1887; Leber, 1916; Kleiner, 1933). The duration of the hypotony in such cases averages from 4 to 5 weeks (Porsaa, 1942). The cause of this phenomenon probably varies. It has been suggested that drainage of the intra-ocular fluid is

[1] Vol. IX, p. 951.   [2] Vol. X, p. 808.

facilitated by escape through the tear in the retina into the subretinal space, a route found by Arruga (1934) to be preferentially taken in the rabbit if Indian ink is injected into the vitreous. On the other hand, using the fluorescein technique, Dobbie (1963) found that the formation of aqueous was diminished, a factor which may participate in lowering the tension, while an imbalance between the formation and drainage of the intra-ocular fluid was established by Rousseau and Regan (1965) and Regan and Rousseau (1966) using the suction-cup technique. The disorganization of the dynamics of the aqueous humour is seen in a lessening of the influence of the general blood pressure upon the intra-ocular pressure, the loss of the diurnal pressure variation, and in the failure of the ophthalmotonic response after paracentesis (Magitot and Hallard-Alibert, 1931). On the other hand, many cases are complicated by the presence of a cilio-choroidal detachment in addition[1] so that both these ætiological factors come into play.

The fall in tension in retinal detachments is usually not very great; but occasionally an *acute phase of hypotony* occurs suddenly when the tension of the eye falls so that the globe can hardly be palpated through the closed lids, a phenomenon first noted by Schnabel (1876) and fully authenticated by Leber (1916). In some cases the malacia may be so acute that on opening the lids the cornea appears cupped (Khosla *et al.*, 1967). In investigating this manifestation, Beigelman (1929) concluded that it was due to the passage of fluid from a liquefied vitreous in quantity through the retinal hole to the subretinal space and its absorption into the choroidal circulation; but an alternative explanation is that the fall is due to an irritative cyclitis caused by the detachment.

3. CYCLITIS

Any prolonged inflammation of the inner eye is liable to be followed by a condition of lowered tension, a result most frequently seen when the ciliary body is seriously involved, in which case the eyeball shrinks and may become completely disorganized.[2] It will be remembered that such a condition of ophthalmomalacia is particularly common in cases of interstitial keratitis[3] with which, of course, some degree of uveitis is almost always combined. It can also be brought about experimentally; for, as shown by L. Weekers (1932), scleral cauterization over the ciliary region in animals leads to a short-lived phase of hypertension followed by a prolonged hypotonic phase. It is also noteworthy that in these cases a cilio-choroidal detachment is by no means uncommon (Procksch, 1933). An interesting observation was made by Paufique and his associates (1950) that a permanently lowered tension could occur in the degenerative condition of siderosis; detecting hypotony in the other eye of a case of this kind which

---

[1] Nordenson (1887), Deutschmann (1890), Ginsberg and Simon (1898), Bret (1907), von Hippel (1908), Kümmell (1925), Baurmann (1929), Procksch (1933), Gonin (1934), Klien (1937).
[2] Vol. IX, p. 103. [3] Vol. VIII, p. 827.

rectified itself after excision of the siderotic eye, they suggested that the fall in tension was the initial sign in the development of sympathetic ophthalmitis.

4. SYSTEMIC DISTURBANCES

A hypotony, sometimes acute and usually bilateral, may be associated with a considerable number of systemic diseases, particularly those involving dehydration, acidosis, and gross metabolic disturbances.

DIABETIC COMA ranks as the most dramatic of these. The occurrence of acute bilateral hypotony in this condition was first noted by Krause (1904) and Heine (1906), and has since received a considerable amount of attention.[1] It is a phenomenon, however, which has become much more rare since the more modern and efficient treatment of diabetes has become universal. Abnormally low pressures in this condition used to be relatively common, but with replenishment of the body-fluids these are usually rapidly made good (Waite and Beetham, 1935); occasionally, however, in the most severe cases, especially in patients who do not survive, the loss of tension may be extremely profound, the cornea at times collapsing as if a negative pressure existed. The hypotony is independent of the height of the blood pressure and the blood-sugar.

The cause of the hypotony is not clear. Hertel (1913) assumed that it was due to changes in the molar concentration of the blood; a second hypothesis attributed it to a condition of acidosis (Ehrmann and Esser, 1911; Elschnig, 1929); it has been said to be due to diminution in the volume of the vitreous with a lowered pH, but the degree of acidosis which could cause this is incompatible with life.[2] It is significant, however, that hypotony does not occur in acidosis without coma and it attains its maximum with the development of coma and disappears with it. Moreover, Pellicciotta (1933) produced profound acidosis in rabbits with ammonium chloride and no hypotony developed, while Böck and Moro (1951) found that the ocular tension varied with the degree of dehydration and not with the acidosis.

Poos (1932), on the other hand, suggested that the hypotony was caused by some unknown substance toxic to the capillaries. In this connection it is interesting that Rønne (1913) and Kochmann and Römer (1914) produced a prolonged hypotony in rabbits by the injection of a small quantity of serum from comatose diabetics, while de Jongh and Wolff (1924–25) produced a comparable diminution of tension associated with convulsions in the hypoglycæmia induced by insulin and suggested that a substance which they called *antitonin* found in the serum of patients in diabetic coma was responsible. For these suggestions, however, there is no concrete evidence.

[1] Gallus (1924), Elschnig (1929), Patek (1929), Poos (1932), Giesmann (1959), Haimböck (1961), Moreau *et al.* (1963), and others.
[2] Vol. IV, p. 205.

Hypotonia, sometimes of an acute nature, may develop in other severe systemic disturbances. It has been observed in *uræmic coma* (Bietti, 1932), in *cardiac œdema* (Pietruschka, 1958; Giessmann, 1959; Keitel and Giessmann, 1959), in extreme *dehydration* due to malnutrition (Moreau *et al.*, 1963), after severe *abdominal disturbances* such as intestinal perforation or obstruction (Bietti, 1967), in a case of cardiac disease complicated by jaundice due to hepatic metastases from an intestinal reticulosarcoma (Frazzetto *et al.*, 1967), or after a violent diarrhœa which had persisted for 7 years (Verhoeff and Waite, 1925). Hypotony is also said to occur in the stage of shock which sometimes follows an intravenous injection of typhoid vaccine (Kotania, 1957; Kapuściński and Hańczyc, 1963; Kapuściński and Prestowska, 1967); the cause of this is unknown.

The primary *anæmias*, particularly agranulocytosis and pernicious anæmia, are said to be associated with a slight degree of hypotonia (Suker, 1934).

Bettelheim (1968) reported 2 cases of *giant-cell arteritis* associated with acute hypotony and suggested that these resulted from a transient impairment of the blood supply to the ciliary body.

5. MYOTONIC DYSTROPHY

Hypotony was first observed in the usual form of myotonic dystrophy by Granström (1934) and was incidentally noted by Vos (1936); since these early observations this has been amply confirmed in the majority of such patients by many clinicians.[1] Junge (1966) found that the average ocular tension measured by applanation tonometry was 8·8 mm. Hg, while levels of 2 to 6 mm. Hg were frequently encountered. The hypotony seems to be unrelated to the blood pressure although it is frequently low in this disease; it shows no correlation with age or the degree of myotonia and the diurnal variations in tension may be considerable. The cause of the hypotension, as is the case with the myotonia, is not clear, but tonography suggests that the facility of the outflow of aqueous is often increased (Junge, 1966).

It is interesting that this clinical feature does not occur in congenital myotonia, but hypotony is seen in some abortive cases of myotonia in relatives of patients with the disease (Junge, 1966).

6. MYOPIA

It has long been held that a connection existed between hypotension and high myopia, a combination usually associated with chorioretinal degeneration and a fluid and degenerated vitreous (Caso, 1931; Kraupa, 1931; Poos, 1952; and others). Thus Lagrange (1922) held that about 1/3 of myopic eyes over −8 or −10 D had a subnormal tension, a tendency

---

[1] Herner (1940), Ladekarl and Stürup (1940), Brand (1950–63), Boersner (1952), de Jong (1955), Kuhn and Piesbergen (1957), Bégaux and Decock (1957), Collier (1959), Paganoni (1961), Simon (1962), Adriaenssens (1963), Zucchini (1963), Pendefunda *et al.* (1964), Junge (1966), and others.

confirmed by Urio (1933) who found over a series of 35 markedly aniso-
metropic cases with unilateral myopia that in 80% the eye with high myopia
had a tension lower than its fellow. This relation between the two was
known to be by no means invariable; indeed, as we have already seen,
myopia is often associated with simple glaucoma. It is to be remembered,
however, that these measurements were taken by indentation tonometry,
and since the ocular rigidity of such eyes is usually low, false values are
frequently given by this technique; using applanation tonometry, Blach and
Jay (1965) found a normal distribution of the ocular tension in the eyes of
77 high myopes. This relationship cannot therefore be considered as established.

7. CONGENITAL LESIONS

The occurrence of marked hypotony in association with congenital anomalies of
the eye is a rare and incidental phenomenon. Thus Knapová (1929) reported a case of
an enophthalmic hypermetropic eye the tension of which never rose above 8 mm. Hg
(Schiøtz), and Mazal (1933) a family in which the three siblings showed hypotension
with aniridia or colobomata.

8. TRAUMA

Trauma is one of the commonest causes of ocular hypotension. It is,
of course, understandable that in PERFORATING WOUNDS wherein a loss
of aqueous or vitreous occurs, a profound hypotony follows immediately,
but the same result may be seen after a minimal perforating wound, as by a
minute foreign body which has not allowed the escape of any of the contents
of the globe, a clinical phenomenon which has been verified experimentally
in animals (L. Weekers, 1932). If the wound heals incompletely and remains
fistulous, the hypotony may be profound and prolonged.

The effects of a CONCUSSION INJURY in lowering the ocular tension may
be dramatic and, indeed, may be the dominant factor in determining the
fate of the eye. A disturbance of the normal equilibrium is usual and may
occur in the absence of any observable intra-ocular lesion; a similar reaction
may result from an indirect contusion which has primarily affected the
facial bones. Prolonged pressure on the globe by bandaging or massage
has the same effect, as well as orbital pressure as by a hæmatoma. As a
rule after such an injury the tension is unstable, sometimes being raised,
sometimes lowered, and occasionally alternating between the two extremes.
This instability may be shared to some extent by the other (uninjured) eye,
both varying within considerable limits for a number of days, periods of
mild and transient hypertension alternating with periods of hypotony until
stability is again attained (Fig. 673). Usually the instability passes away
without serious effects, but occasionally, on the one hand, a traumatic
glaucoma may develop,[1] so severe and intractable as to involve rapid loss of
sight or to necessitate excision of the eye owing to pain; on the other, a

[1] p. 705.

persistent hypotony may as surely lead to changes which eventually render the eye useless.

The variation in the ocular tension is probably due to several factors. An initial transient period of hypotony may be caused by an inhibition of secretion of the aqueous humour by the trauma (Goldmann, 1951) and this is associated with a stage of vascular instability—an irritative vasocon-striction and a vasodilatation resulting from the liberation of histamine-like substances following the period of ischæmia, an effect which may be aug-mented on occasion by a paresis of the vasomotor nerves aided perhaps by direct concussion damage to the capillary endothelium.   Both of these effects may be relayed all over the affected eye and to the fellow eye by axon reflexes, and the resultant behaviour of the ocular tension depends

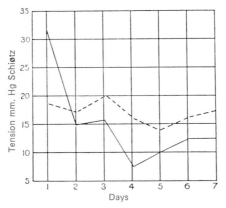

FIG. 673.—TRAUMATIC HYPOTONY.

After an ocular concussion.   The continuous line represents the pressure in the injured eye.   Note the consensual reaction in the sound eye (broken line).

largely on the relative importance of either at any particular time.   A simple hypertony or a transient hypotony is the physiological response to trauma, a traumatic glaucoma or a profound and prolonged hypotony the pathological effect; in the first case, a healthy vascular system readjusts itself rapidly, but in the second it cannot, perhaps because the vessels and nerves have themselves suffered structural damage by the injury, perhaps because the reaction is accentuated and prolonged by other lesions already present or newly created in the eye.

Experimental work on animals has considerably clarified these problems.[1] On the receipt of a concussion to the globe the tension may show considerable variations, but the usual response is a period of relatively acute hyper-tension lasting some 30 to 40 minutes, which is followed by a period of hypotony which may last a variable time from 3 to 7 days, but usually

[1] Magitot (1917–33), G. Leplat (1922–25), L. Weekers (1924–32), Schmidt and de Decker (1930), Larsson (1930), and others.

shows periods when the tension rises temporarily or falls more profoundly—reactions which may be shared by the other eye even although it has not been injured.[1] These effects are obviously vasomotor in their origin and are associated with an increased capillary permeability, as shown by the ease with which fluorescein injected intravenously finds its way into the aqueous humour, an effect which also occurs bilaterally although one eye only has suffered a contusion (Amsler, 1946–48) (Fig. 674). In other cases the drainage of the aqueous is facilitated by a rupture of the pectinate ligament and the ciliary muscle (Collins, 1892–1916), a circumstance which also may result in a cilio-choroidal detachment. It is interesting that the hypotony which occasionally follows an acute attack of glaucoma was said

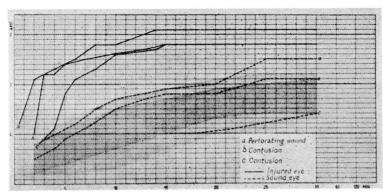

FIG. 674.—THE FLUORESCEIN TEST AFTER OCULAR INJURY.

a. The curve after a perforating wound (continuous line) and in the sound eye (dotted line).

b and c. The increased permeability after a contusion (continuous lines) and in the sound eye (dotted lines).

The limits of normal are indicated in the shaded area. It is seen that the permeability in the sound fellow eye in a is abnormally high and in b is in the upper limits of normal (M. Amsler and A. Huber).

by vom Hofe (1959) to be due to leakage of aqueous through tears in Descemet's membrane and the endothelium allowing its seepage through the cornea.

A fall in tension is a common sequel of an ocular contusion but, as we have just seen, it is usually slight in degree and lasts only a few days, the tension slowly attaining its normal height after some variations; again, it is to be noted that this instability is frequently shared by the fellow eye. Occasionally, however, the ophthalmomalacia is profound and lasts so long as to appear permanent[2]; indeed, after a relatively severe contusion a common development is the triad of hypotony, myopia and mydriasis.[3]

[1] p. 705.
[2] L. Leplat (1890), Collins and Hinnell (1901), Collins (1916–17), Magitot (1917–33), L. Weekers (1932), Bonnet and Chavanne (1948), and many others.
[3] Knapp (1883), Fromaget (1911), Brøns (1930), Morgan (1940), Fox (1942), L. Weekers et al. (1949), Luntz (1959).

One interesting result occasionally seen is the appearance of œdema at the optic disc and of the retina, due presumably to a disturbance of the normal relationship between the intra-ocular and intracranial pressures (Collins and Hinnell, 1901 ; Collins, 1917 ; Arkle, 1944 ; Bonnet and Chavanne, 1948), a phenomenon which can be induced experimentally (Parker, 1916). A persistently soft cyc of this type may retain good vision indefinitely, but its function is liable to deteriorate slowly and progressively, occasionally with the development of degenerative changes such as rucking and opacity of the cornea, cataract, or a quiet irritative iritis, and sometimes without apparent cause.

POST-OPERATIVE HYPOTONY comes into this category and, apart from the immediate effect of trauma, is usually caused either by a cilio-choroidal detachment or an increased facility of drainage. As occurs after most types of trauma to the anterior segment of the uvea, most surgical operations involving this segment of the globe are followed by a period of hypotony due to a partial or almost complete inhibition of the formation of the aqueous humour (Goldmann, 1951) ; this reaction, however, is transitory.

After an operation for *cataract* the development of hypotony may also be due to leakage from a wound which becomes fistulous.[1] If this is uncomplicated the hypotony may be intermittent and attacks of vague discomfort and congestion may persist for weeks. If, however, it is complicated by a cilio-choroidal detachment of any size the anterior chamber becomes shallow, the vitreous balloons through the pupil, sometimes to come into contact with the cornea which tends to become somewhat hazy, and eventually peripheral anterior synechiæ may form and lead to the development of a secondary glaucoma if the anterior chamber is lost for more than 4 to 6 days.[2]

Filtering operations for glaucoma may lead to hypotony if the drainage is too free owing to fistulization of the scar or to the development of a cilio-choroidal detachment, whether the technique has been sclerectomy, trephining or iridencleisis (Chandler and Maumenee, 1961 ; Paufique *et al.*, 1965 ; Cristiansson, 1967). When the anterior chamber has been lost after such an operation, small discrete subcapsular opacities have been seen on the anterior surface of the lens resembling those seen after an acute attack of hypertension (Lowe, 1964), while if the condition persists the subsequent development of a cataract is common. An interesting feature of these operations for glaucoma is the consensual hypotonic reaction which may occur in the fellow eye so that its tension may fall, sometimes to the normal level or even below this (Blatt and Regenbogen, 1960) ; such a reaction must depend on the nervous regulation of the intra-ocular pressure.

In the operation of *cyclodialysis* the resulting cilio-choroidal detachment

---

[1] p. 279.

[2] Chandler (1947–54), Kronfeld (1953–54), Post and Harper (1953), R. Weekers and Delmarcelle (1953), Dunnington (1956), Gormaz (1962), Simpson (1966), and others.

may occasionally lead to profound and acute hypotony (Fanta, 1949; Vannas and Björkheim, 1952; Viikari and Tuovinen, 1957; Miller, 1963; Sédan, 1966).

In *destructive techniques* on the ciliary body to reduce the intra-ocular pressure in glaucoma, such as cyclodiathermy, partial atrophy of the ciliary body has been found histologically sufficient in degree to lower the formation of the aqueous (Scheie *et al.*, 1955).

After operations for *retinal detachment* a condition of hypotony may develop, frequently associated with a choroidal detachment[1]; this may assume dangerous proportions and even result in phthisis bulbi when a scleral fistula develops and is not effectively closed (Heydenreich, 1966). After diathermocoagulation or buckling or encircling operations the unpleasant syndrome of necrosis of the anterior segment is characterized by an acute hypotony due to constriction of the long ciliary arteries supplying the ciliary body.[2]

CLINICAL FEATURES

Unless the hypotony is acute, an eye with low tension may present no dramatic clinical features and retain its function indefinitely, although after some weeks it may become vaguely uncomfortable and signs of irritation with ciliary congestion may be evident associated with an irritative iridocyclitis which may result in pigmentary degeneration and occlusion of the pupil (Juler, 1939); in such cases there may be a varying amount of pain, frequently intermittent in its incidence. In phthisical eyes resulting from a uveitis, this pain may be considerable. In the presence of a cilio-choroidal detachment of some size the anterior chamber is usually shallow, the iridocyclitic signs are more marked and a secondary cataract may develop as well as a secondary glaucoma if extensive peripheral anterior synechiæ develop. Fine vitreous opacities are the rule. A further complication in the case of fistulous scars is the development of an exogenous infection (Kraus and Myska, 1965). It is interesting that Stepanik (1956–57) found that the intra-ocular pressure may be lower than the episcleral venous pressure so that the outflow of aqueous would appear to be by the posterior uveal route.

In acute cases, however, ocular signs and visual disabilities may be dramatic. The cornea may show signs of keratopathy or may become obviously rucked or may even collapse into a saucer-shape when the lids are opened (Figs. 675–6); the sclera may be deeply grooved by the rectus muscles. The œdematous condition of the fundus may be evident in the formation of retinal folds (Kyrieleis, 1929; Dellaporta, 1948–55; Pau, 1950; Miller, 1963), macular œdema and papillœdema (Toselli, 1959; Zamorani,

---

[1] Lauber (1908), Leber (1916), Vogt (1924), Kümmell (1925), Lindner (1931), Arruga (1933), Gonin (1934), Ladekarl (1935), Porsaa (1942), Schiff-Wertheimer and Frileux (1946), and many others.
[2] Vol. X, p. 840.

Figs. 675 and 676.—The Eye in Acute Hypotony (F. Frazzetto *et al.*).

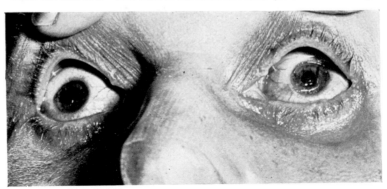

Fig. 675.—In a patient aged 57 with heart failure and jaundice due to hepatic metastases from an intestinal reticulosarcoma after Longmire's cholangio-jejunostomy followed by acidosis. The illustration shows flattening and folding of the right cornea.

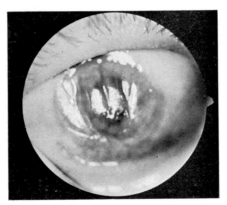

Fig. 676.—The right eye of the same case, one hour after death, showing marked folds in the cornea.

1961; Paufique *et al.*, 1965; and others) (Fig. 677). In the most acute cases the pain may be so severe as to demand excision of the globe for its relief. So dramatic may the destruction be that the onset of an acute hypotony may lead to the spontaneous necrosis of a melanoma in the eye (Samuels, 1934; Wolter, 1968).

PATHOLOGY

The pathological changes which result from an acute fall in the intra-ocular pressure are first seen in the vascular circulation and the composition of the intra-ocular fluid which escapes from dilated and freely permeable capillaries. The universal vasodilatation which occurs throughout the uveal tract is essentially a pressure-effect, for the walls of the small vessels, deprived of the outer support of the normal intra-ocular pressure, give way before

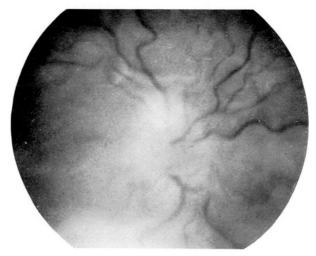

FIG. 677.—THE FUNDUS IN HYPOTONY.

The œdema of the optic disc and the macular region and surrounding retina seen in acute hypotony following an operation of cyclodialysis in a patient aged 50 who had subacute attacks of closed-angle glaucoma unrelieved by pilocarpine and an initial broad iridectomy (S. J. H. Miller).

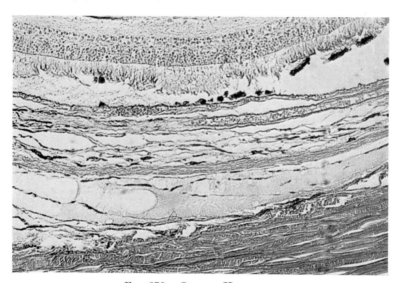

FIG. 678.—OCULAR HYPOTONY.

To show the intense vasodilatation and œdema of the choriocapillaris with the presence of lacunæ filled with an amorphous PAS-positive exudate (F. Frazzetto et al.).

the blood pressure. A plasmoid fluid therefore escapes from them in all directions, into the tissues of the iris, the ciliary body and the choroid, causing an œdema throughout (Fig. 678). This becomes most evident in the richly vascularized regions, such as the ciliary body, where large vesicles

FIGS. 679 and 680.—OCULAR HYPOTONY (F. Frazzetto *et al.*).

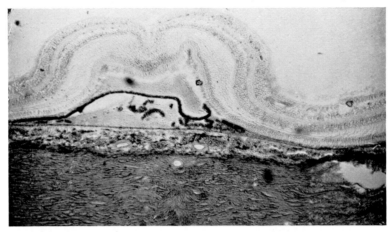

FIG. 679.—From the same case as Fig. 675. The retina shows gross folding, the pigmentary epithelium also lies in folds and is reduced to a clump of granules. A PAS-positive exudate raises the retina and infiltrates the choriocapillaris.

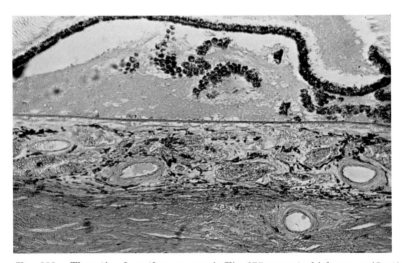

FIG. 680.—The retina from the case seen in Fig. 675, seen at a higher magnification to show the intense vasodilatation of the choriocapillaris and the granular appearance of the PAS-positive material.

of œdematous fluid may form under the ciliary epithelium (the vesicles of Greeff, 1894) (Bauer, 1896; Henderson and Lane-Claypon, 1907; Rados, 1922; Klien, 1937) or in the iris, on the posterior surface of which similar collections of fluid may become evident under the epithelium (Carlini, 1910; Rados, 1922; Carrère, 1923; Samojloff, 1925–27). Escaping out from the tissues, this protein-rich fluid reaches all the available spaces in the eye, filling the anterior and posterior chambers with a plasmoid aqueous, percolating the vitreous causing liquefaction and opacification, distending the suprachoroidal space and thus causing a detachment of the choroid and sometimes of the ciliary body from the sclera, and occasionally accumulating in mass between the retina and the pigmentary epithelium and causing a detachment of the former tissue or raising it in œdematous folds (Della-porta, 1954; Frazzetto *et al.*, 1967) (Figs. 679–80). A final œdematous

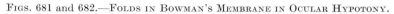

FIGS. 681 and 682.—FOLDS IN BOWMAN'S MEMBRANE IN OCULAR HYPOTONY.

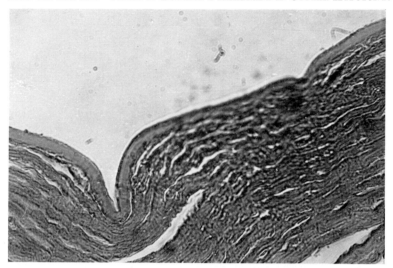

FIG. 681.—From the same case as Fig. 675. Deep folds in Bowman's membrane and the anterior layers of the stroma. The epithelium is absent (F. Frazzetto *et al.*).

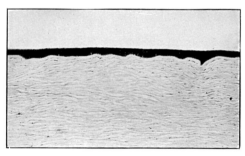

FIG. 682.—A common histological feature of shrunken globes. The depressions are filled in with epithelium, which maintains the surface level (J. H. Parsons).

manifestation is the development of papillœdema from the uncompensated intracranial pressure, a phenomenon which may be fleeting but may last so long as to appear to be permanent.

In marked degrees of ophthalmomalacia, particularly when the condition is of long standing, the pathological picture is dominated by a relaxation of the tissues usually kept taut. The cornea becomes wrinkled, and the two elastic laminæ show folds, those in Bowman's membrane producing superficial double contour lines and those in Descemet's membrane giving rise to the clinical picture of striate keratopathy.[1] Pathologically the folds in Bowman's membrane were first noted by Schirmer (1896) in a shrunken globe in which the cornea was much diminished in size, and they have repeatedly been described in conditions of ophthalmomalacia from any cause[2]; the membrane itself shows pronounced waves, a configuration in which the anterior lamellæ of the substantia propria participate, but in mild cases the epithelium may fill in the troughs of the waves anteriorly so that the surface of the cornea is smooth and regular (Figs. 681–2). The folds in Descemet's membrane were first noted in phthisical eyes by von Graefe (1866) and were studied experimentally by Hess (1892–96), Schirmer

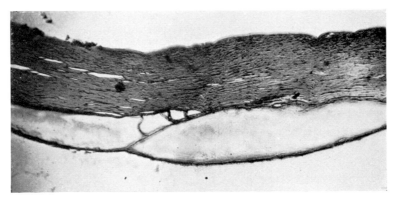

FIG. 683.—THE CORNEA IN HYPOTONY.

From the same case as Fig. 675. The deep layers of the cornea. Descemet's membrane is separated from the stroma, the space being filled by fluid and an amorphous substance (F. Frazzetto *et al.*).

(1896) and Vogt (1919), and pathologically by O. Becker (1875), Fuchs (1902), Parsons (1904) and others. They may represent a purely mechanical deformation in which the deeper layers of the substantia propria also take part, and the changes may be complicated by œdema (Fig. 683). In the most severe cases the entire cornea may collapse in folds.

The sclera, too, becomes thickened and puckered, large furrows being found behind the insertions of the rectus muscles, while a wrinkling and spacing-out of the fibres throughout, particularly in the deeper layers, result in a thickening of the whole membrane. A similar wrinkling of the elastic lamina of the choroid occurs, a process associated as a rule with a heaping up of the pigmentary epithelium on the inner surface where the folds are deep (Collins, 1917). Finally, the loss of tension in the coats of the eye leads

[1] Vol. VIII, p. 662.
[2] Caspar (1903–16), Weche (1905), Haab (1916), Spicer and Greeves (1916), Collins (1917), Fuchs (1918), Reis (1921). Frazzetto *et al.* (1967).

to a relaxation of the zonule and a forward displacement of the lens with a resulting myopia.

TREATMENT

In mild cases of hypotony the structure and function of the eye remain unimpaired and symptoms are absent, for an eye may tolerate a tension considerably lower than 8 mm. Hg for a long period without any significant harm. In acute cases, however, more active steps must be taken if the eye is to be saved and these should be directed towards the causal lesion although topical corticosteroids may control any inflammatory reaction. The old procedure of cauterization around the limbus (colmatage) (Kümmell, 1912; Lagrange, 1922) is usually ineffective or illegitimate. If there is a fistulous wound or a leaking surgical scar this should be reinforced and covered by a conjunctival flap. Sometimes an excessive leak from a filtering operation can be controlled by light diathermocoagulation (Fornes, 1962). If the leak is due to a necrotic area of sclera, closure of the fistula by a suture is rarely successful; a scleral graft (Hervouët, 1961) or lyophilized dura mater (Heydenreich, 1966) has been usefully employed to reinforce and cover the defect. If a cilio-choroidal detachment is present a dramatic result may be obtained by releasing the fluid through a barrage of perforating diathermic punctures through the ciliary region of the sclera (Chandler and Maumenee, 1961; Miller, 1963); and in the case of a surgical cyclodialysis this may be supplemented by an attempt to close the cleft by surface diathermy of the overlying sclera (Vannas and Björkheim, 1952) or by electro-coagulation (Viikari and Tuovinen, 1957).

A hypertensive effect has been observed after the subconjunctival injection of phosphorylcholine chloride, particularly in traumatic cases and after ocular surgery (Hupsel and Henkes, 1954; Boet, 1956; Aguilar Bartolomé, 1958), but this technique has not been consistently successful (R. Weekers and Delmarcelle, 1958) and has not been widely used.

When these measures fail or when the cause of the condition is unknown, excision of the eye may be the only practical procedure to relieve distressing pain in a useless eye.

Adriaenssens. *Ann. Oculist.* (Paris), **196,** 1140 (1963).

Aguilar Bartolomé. *Arch. Soc. oftal hisp.-amer.*, **18,** 451 (1958).

Amsler. *Bull. Soc. franç. Ophtal.*, **59,** 304 (1946).
  Trans. ophthal. Soc. U.K., **68,** 45 (1948).

Amsler and Huber. *Ophthalmologica*, **111,** 155 (1946).

Arkle. *Trans. ophthal. Soc. U.K.*, **64,** 233 (1944).

Arruga. *XIV int. Cong. Ophthal.*, Madrid, **2** (1), 5, 86 (1933).
  Klin. Mbl. Augenheilk., **93,** 52 (1934).

Bauer. *v. Graefes Arch. Ophthal.*, **42** (3), 193 (1896).

Baurmann. *v. Graefes Arch. Ophthal.*, **122,** 415 (1929).

Becker, B. *Amer. J. Ophthal.*, **37,** 13 (1954).

Becker, B., Constant, Cibis and Ter-Pogossian *Amer. J. Ophthal.*, **42,** 51 (1956).

Becker, O. *Atlas d. pathologischen Topographie d. Auges*, Wien (1875).

Bégaux and Decock. *Mod. Probl. Ophthal.*, **1,** 551 (1957).

Beigelman. *Arch. Ophthal.*, **1,** 463 (1929).

Bernard. *Bull. Soc. Ophtal. Fr.*, Suppl. (1963).

Bertelsen, Davanger, Kolstad *et al.* *T. norske Lægeforen.*, **85,** 449 (1965).

Bettelheim. *v. Graefes Arch. Ophthal.*, **174,** 359 (1968).

Bietti. *Atti Cong. Soc. oftal. ital.*, **10**, 240 (1932).
Bull. Soc. franç. Ophtal., **80**, 684 (1967).
Blach and Jay. *Trans. ophthal. Soc. U.K.*, **85**, 161 (1965).
Blatt and Regenbogen. *Klin. Mbl. Augenheilk.*, **136**, 761 (1960).
Böck and Moro. *Ber. dtsch. ophthal. Ges.*, **57**, 217 (1951).
Boersner. *Confin. neurol.* (Basel), **12**, 1 (1952).
Boet. *Ophthalmologica*, **132**, 150 (1956).
Bonnet and Chavanne. *Bull. Soc. Ophtal. Paris*, 792 (1948).
Brand. *Ophthalmologica*, **119**, 157 (1950); **129**, 81 (1955).
Orv. Hetil., **97**, 461 (1956).
Klin. Mbl. Augenheilk., **136**, 241 (1960).
Szemészet, **100**, 193 (1963).
Bret. *Arch. Ophtal.*, **27**, 544 (1907).
Brøns. *Danish ophthal. Soc.*, 1930. *See* *Zbl. ges. Ophthal.*, **25**, 534 (1931).
Capper and Leopold. *Arch. Ophthal.*, **55**, 101 (1956).
Carlini. *v. Graefes Arch. Ophthal.*, **77**, 96 (1910).
Carrère. *C.R. Soc. Biol.* (Paris), **88**, 475 (1923).
Casari. *Boll. Oculist.*, **30**, 649 (1951).
Caso. *Lettura oftal.*, **8**, 287 (1931).
Caspar. *Klin. Mbl. Augenheilk.*, **41** (2), 289 (1903); **57**, 385 (1916).
Cavka. *Ophthalmologica*, **132**, 76 (1956).
Cervino, Garbino, Maggiolo *et al.* *An. Fac. Med. Montevideo*, **45**, 223 (1960).
Chandler. *Amer. J. Ophthal.*, **30**, 484 (1947).
Trans. Amer. Acad. Ophthal., **58**, 382 (1954).
Chandler and Maumenee. *Amer. J. Ophthal.*, **52**, 609 (1961).
Collier. *Arch. Ophtal.*, **19**, 850 (1959).
Collins. *Trans. ophthal. Soc. U.K.*, **12**, 180 (1892); **36**, 204 (1916); **37**, 281 (1917); **38**, 217 (1918).
Ophthalmoscope, **14**, 348 (1916).
Collins and Hinnell. *Trans. ophthal. Soc. U.K.*, **21**, 100 (1901).
Cristiansson. *Acta ophthal.* (Kbh.), **45**, 837 (1967).
von Csapody. *Klin. Mbl. Augenheilk.*, **70**, 111 (1923).
Davanger and Holter. *Acta ophthal.* (Kbh.), **43**, 314 (1965).
Dellaporta. *Ophthalmologica*, **116**, 51 (1948).
Klin. Mbl. Augenheilk., **125**, 672 (1954).
Amer. J. Ophthal., **40**, 781 (1955).
Dellaporta and Obear. *Amer. J. Ophthal.*, **58**, 785 (1964).
Deutschmann. *Beitr. Augenheilk.*, **1** (1), 41 (1890).
v. Graefes Arch. Ophthal., **74**, 206 (1910).
Dobbie. *Arch. Ophthal.*, **69**, 159 (1963).
Dobree. *Trans. ophthal. Soc. U.K.*, **81**, 113 (1961).
Dunnington. *Brit. J. Ophthal.*, **40**, 30 (1956).

Ehrmann and Esser. *Z. klin. Med.*, **72**, 496 (1911).
Elschnig. *Med. Klin.*, **25**, 49 (1929).
Fanta. *Ophthalmologica*, **118**, 205 (1949).
Fornes. *Arch. Soc. oftal. hisp.-amer.*, **22**, 691 (1962).
Forsius and Eriksson. *Acta ophthal.* (Kbh.), **39**, 318 (1961).
Fox. *Arch. Ophthal.*, **28**, 218 (1942).
Frazzetto, Faggioni, Rebagliati and Esposito. *Bull. Soc. franç. Ophtal.*, **80**, 670 (1967).
Fromaget. *Bull. Soc. franç. Ophtal.*, **28**, 346 (1911).
Fuchs. *Trans. ophthal. Soc. U.K.*, **22**, 15 (1902).
v. Graefes Arch. Ophthal., **79**, 53 (1911); **96**, 315 (1918); **104**, 247 (1921).
Gallus. *Klin. Mbl. Augenheilk.*, **73**, 491 (1924).
Giessmann. *Klin. Mbl. Augenheilk.*, **134**, 890 (1959).
Ginsberg and Simon. *Zbl. prakt. Augenheilk.*, **22**, 161 (1898).
Goldmann. *Ophthalmologica*, **121**, 94 (1951).
Gonin. *Arch. Ophtal.*, **51**, 426, 428 (1934).
Gormaz. *Amer. J. Ophthal.*, **53**, 832 (1962).
von Graefe. *v. Graefes Arch. Ophthal.*, **12** (2), 256 (1866).
Granström. *Acta ophthal.* (Kbh.), **12**, 165 (1934).
Greeff. *Arch. Augenheilk.*, **28**, 178 (1894).
Haab. *Beitr. Augenheilk.*, **10**, 1 (1916).
Hagen. *Klin. Mbl. Augenheilk.*, **66**, 161 (1921).
Haimböck. *Wien. klin. Wschr.*, **73**, 378 (1961).
Klin. Mbl. Augenheilk., **138**, 596 (1961).
Heath. *Trans. Amer. Acad. Ophthal.*, **52**, 613 (1947).
Heine. *Klin. Mbl. Augenheilk.*, **44** (2), 451 (1906).
Henderson and Lane-Claypon. *Roy. Lond. ophthal. Hosp. Rep.*, **17**, 97 (1907).
Herner. *Acta med. scand.*, **105**, 17 (1940).
Hertel. *Klin. Mbl. Augenheilk.*, **51**, 351 (1913).
Münch. med. Wschr., **60**, 1191 (1913).
Hertz. *Brit. J. Ophthal.*, **38**, 364 (1954).
Acta ophthal. (Kbh.), Suppl. 41 (1954).
Hervouët. *Bull. Soc. Ophtal. Fr.*, 583 (1961).
Hess. *v. Graefes Arch. Ophthal.*, **38** (4), 1 (1892).
Arch. Augenheilk., **33**, 204 (1896).
Heydenreich. *Klin. Mbl. Augenheilk.*, **148**, 413 (1966).
von Hippel. *v. Graefes Arch. Ophthal.*, **68**, 38, 58 (1908).
vom Hofe. *Öst. ophthal. Ges.*, **4**, 36 (1959).
Hollenhorst. *Amer. J. Ophthal.*, **47**, 753 (1959).
Horstmann. *Ber. dtsch. ophthal. Ges.*, **21**, 140 (1891).
Hudson. *Roy. Lond. ophthal. Hosp. Rep.*, **19**, 301 (1914).
Hupsel and Henkes. *Acta XVII int. Cong. Ophthal.*, Montreal-N.Y., **1**, 143 (1954).

Imre. *Arch. Augenheilk.*, **88**, 155 (1921).

de Jong. *Dystrophia myotonica, Paramyotonia and Myotonia congenita* (Thesis), Utrecht (1955).

de Jongh and Wolff. *Ned. T. Geneesk.*, **68**, 2703 (1924); **69**, 2665 (1925).

Juler. *Trans. ophthal. Soc. U.K.*, **48**, 179 (1928); **59**, 253 (1939).

Junge. *Ocular Changes in Dystrophia myotonica, Paramyotonia and Myotonia congenita* (Thesis), Amsterdam (1966).

Kahler and Sallmann. *Wien. klin. Wschr.*, **36**, 883 (1923).

Kapuściński and Hańczyc. *Bull. Soc. franç. Ophtal.*, **76**, 501 (1963).

Kapuściński and Prestowska. *Bull. Soc. franç. Ophtal.*, **80**, 688 (1967).

Keitel and Giessmann. *Dtsch. Gesundh.-Wes.*, **14**, 854 (1959).

Khosla, Angra and Agarwal. *Orient. Arch. Ophthal.*, **5**, 184 (1967).

Kleiner. *v. Graefes Arch. Ophthal.*, **129**, 485 (1933).

Klien. *Amer. J. Ophthal.*, **20**, 812, 817 (1937).

Knapová. *Cas. lék. cesk.*, **68**, 348 (1929).

Knapp, H. *Arch. Augenheilk.*, **12**, 85 (1883).

Kochmann and Römer. *v. Graefes Arch. ophthal.*, **88**, 528 (1914).

Kornblueth, Aladjemoff, Magora and Gabbay. *Arch. Ophthal.*, **61**, 84 (1959).

Kotania. *Klin. oczna*, **27**, 239 (1957).

Kraupa. *Klin. Mbl. Augenheilk.*, **87**, 837 (1931).

Kraus and Myska. *Sborn. lék.*, **67**, 199 (1965).

Krause, P. *XXI Cong. inn. Med.*, Wiesbaden, 439 (1904).

Kronfeld. *Amer. J. Ophthal.*, **36**, 1271 (1953); **38**, 453 (1954).

Kümmell. *Arch. Augenheilk.*, **72**, 261 (1912); **95**, 214 (1925).
Ber. dtsch. ophthal. Ges., **42**, 231 (1920).

Kuhn and Piesbergen. *Klin. Mbl. Augenheilk.*, **130**, 329 (1957).

Kyrieleis. *v. Graefes Arch. Ophthal.*, **121**, 560 (1929).

Ladekarl. *Acta ophthal.* (Kbh.), **13**, 301 (1935).

Ladekarl and Stürup. *Nord. Med.*, **7**, 1376 (1940).

Lagrange. *Du glaucome et de l'hypotonie*, Paris (1922).

Landesberg. *v. Graefes Arch. Ophthal.*, **17** (1), 292 (1871).

Langham and Taylor. *J. Physiol.*, **152**, 437, 447 (1960).

Larsson. *Acta ophthal.* (Kbh.), **8**, 261 (1930).

Lauber. *Z. Augenheilk.*, **20**, 118, 208 (1908).

Leber. *Graefe-Saemisch Hb. d. ges. Augenheilk.*, 2nd ed., Leipzig, **7A** (2), 1422 (1916).

Leplat, G. *C.R. Soc. Biol.* (Paris), **87**, 982 (1922).
Ann. Oculist. (Paris), **160**, 348 (1923); **161**, 87 (1924); **162**, 81 (1925).

Leplat, L. *Ann. Oculist.* (Paris), **103**, 209 (1890).

Leydhecker. *Docum. ophthal.*, **13**, 359 (1959).
Glaukom – ein Handbuch, Berlin (1960).

Lindner. *v. Graefes Arch. Ophthal.*, **127**, 177 (1931).

Lowe. *Orient. Arch. Ophthal.*, **2**, 267 (1964).

Ludwig and Vurdelja. *Ophthalmologica*, **122**, 295 (1951).

Luntz. *Brit. J. Ophthal.*, **43**, 566 (1959).

Magitot. *Ann. Oculist.* (Paris), **154**, 667 (1917); **155**, 1, 66 (1918); **157**, 680 (1920); **170**, 465 (1933).

Magitot and Hallard-Alibert. *Bull. Soc. Ophtal. Paris*, 100 (1931).

Magitot and Offret. *Bull. Soc. Ophtal. Paris*, 163 (1936).

Marshall. *Trans. ophthal. Soc. U.K.*, **16**, 98 (1896).

Mazal. *Cs. Oftal.*, **1**, 185 (1933).

Meesmann. *Arch. Augenheilk.*, **90**, 69 (1922).

Miller. *Brit. J. Ophthal.*, **47**, 211 (1963).

Moreau, Cornibert and Mugneret. *Bull. Soc. Ophtal. Fr.*, **63**, 243 (1963).

Morgan. *Brit. J. Ophthal.*, **24**, 403 (1940).

Müller-Jensen. *Klin. Mbl. Augenheilk.*, **145**, 526 (1964).

Nagel. *v. Graefes Arch. Ophthal.*, **13** (1), 407 (1867).

Nordenson. *Die Netzhautablösung*, Wiesbaden (1887).

O'Brien. *Arch. Ophthal.*, **14**, 527 (1935).

Orzalesi. *Ann. Ottal.*, **73**, 129 (1947).

Paganoni. *Riv. oto-neuro-oftal.*, **36**, 28 (1961).

Parker. *J. Amer. med. Ass.*, **67**, 1053 (1916).

Parsons. *The Pathology of the Eye*, London, **1**, 181 (1904).

Patek. *J. Amer. med. Ass.*, **92**, 438 (1929).

Pau. *Klin. Mbl. Augenheilk.*, **117**, 591 (1950).

Paufique, Étienne, Bonnet and Lequin. *Bull. Soc. Ophtal. Fr.*, **65**, 477 (1965).

Paufique, Grange and Barut. *Bull. Soc. Ophtal. Fr.*, 124 (1950).

Pellicciotta. *Rass. Ter. Pat. clin.*, **5**, 776 (1933).

Pendefunda, Cernea and Dobrescu. *Oftalmologia* (Buc.), **8**, 219 (1964).

Pietruschka. *Klin. Mbl. Augenheilk.*, **132**, 839 (1958).

Poos. *Klin. Mbl. Augenheilk.*, **89**, 145 (1932).
Ber. dtsch. ophthal. Ges., **49**, 319 (1932).
Arch. Augenheilk., **109**, 162 (1935).
v. Graefes Arch. Ophthal., **152**, 609 (1952).

Porsaa. *Acta ophthal.* (Kbh.), **20**, 379 (1942).

Post and Harper. *Amer. J. Ophthal.*, **36**, 103 (1953).

Procksch. *Z. Augenheilk.*, **81**, 224 (1933).

Radnót. *Ophthalmologica*, **107**, 282 (1944).
Klin. Mbl. Augenheilk., **110**, 595 (1944); **115**, 524 (1949).

Rados. *v. Graefes Arch. Ophthal.*, **109**, 342 (1922).

Regan and Rousseau. *Amer. J. Ophthal.*, **61**, 696 (1966).

Reis. *v. Graefes Arch. Ophthal.*, **105**, 617 (1921).

Restivo-Manfridi and Serafini. *Ann. Ottal.*, **92**, 84 (1966).

Rønne. *v. Graefes Arch. Ophthal.*, **85**, 489 (1913).

Rousseau and Regan. *Arch. Ophthal.*, **73**, 803 (1965).

Samojloff. *Klin. Mbl. Augenheilk.*, **75**, 382 (1925).

v. Graefes Arch. Ophthal., **118**, 391 (1927).

Samuels. *Arch. Ophthal.*, **11**, 998 (1934).

Scheie, Frayer and Spencer. *Arch. Ophthal.*, **53**, 839 (1955).

Schiff. *Amer. J. Ophthal.*, **47** (2), 553 (1959).

Schiff-Wertheimer and Frileux. *Bull. Soc. franç. Ophtal.*, **59**, 265 (1946).

Schirmer. *v. Graefes Arch. Ophthal.*, **42** (3), 1 (1896).

Schmidt and de Decker. *Arch. Augenheilk.*, **102**, 700 (1930).

Schnabel. *Arch. Augenheilk.*, **5**, 50, 69, 71 (1876).

Sédan. *Rev. oto-neuro-ophtal.*, **11**, 601 (1933).
Bull. Soc. Ophtal. Fr., **65**, 1095 (1965); **66**, 959 (1966).

Simon. *Arch. Ophthal.*, **67**, 312 (1962).

Simon, Bonting and Hawkins. *Exp. Eye Res.*, **1**, 253 (1962).

Simpson. *Canad. J. Ophthal.*, **1**, 67 (1966).

Spicer and Greeves. *Ophthalmoscope*, **14**, 116 (1916).

Stepanik. *Wien. klin. Wschr.*, **68**, 490 (1956).
Ophthalmologica, **133**, 397 (1957).

Suker. *Amer. J. Ophthal.*, **17**, 125 (1934).

Swanzy. *Dubl. quart. J.*, **48**, 531 (1869).

Swanzy. *Ann. Oculist.* (Paris), **64**, 212 (1870).

Terrien. *Arch. Ophtal.*, **39**, 716 (1922).

Thomas. *Z. Augenheilk.*, **54**, 333 (1925).

Toselli. *Ann. Ottal.*, **85**, 98 (1959).

Urio. *v. Graefes Arch. Ophthal.*, **131**, 377 (1933).

Vannas and Bjorkheim. *Acta ophthal.* (Kbh.), **30**, 63 (1952).

Verhoeff and Waite. *Trans. Amer. ophthal. Soc.*, **23**, 120 (1925).

Viikari and Tuovinen. *Acta ophthal.* (Kbh.), **35**, 543 (1957).

Vogt. *v. Graefes Arch. Ophthal.*, **99**, 296 (1919).
Klin. Mbl. Augenheilk., **72**, 335 (1924).

Vos. *Cataracta myotonica* (Diss.), Groningen (1936).
Ned. T. Geneesk., **80**, 2399 (1936).

Waite and Beetham. *New Engl. J. Med.*, **212**, 367, 429 (1935).

Weche. *Hornhauttrübungen durch Faltungen d. Bowman'schen Membran* (Diss.), Greifswald (1905).

Weekers, L. *Arch. Ophtal.*, **41**, 641 (1924); **48**, 321, 593 (1931); **49**, 24 (1932).

Weekers, L. and R., and Dedoyard. *Bull. Soc. belge Ophtal.*, No. 93, 366 (1949).

Weekers, R. and Delmarcelle. *Ann. Oculist.* (Paris), **186**, 415 (1953).
Actualites latines d'ophtalmologie, Paris, 176 (1958).

Weinstein. *Ophthalmologica*, **127**, 164 (1954).

Wolter. *Eye, Ear, Nose, Thr. Mthly.*, **47**, 31 (1968).

Zamorani. *G. ital. Oftal.*, **14**, 202 (1961).

Zucchini. *Ann. Ottal.*, **89**, 617 (1963).

APPENDICES

APPENDIX I

THE OCULAR RIGIDITY

FRIEDENWALD'S (1955) (*Trans. Amer. Acad. Ophthal.*, **61**, 108, 1957) calibration for readings with the Schiøtz tonometer using different plunger-loads (5·5 G., 7·5 G., 10 G., and 15 G.).*

TABLE IV

Scale reading	Plunger-weight											
	5·5 G			7·5 G			10 G			15 G		
	P_0 mm.Hg	v_c cu. mm.	P_t mm. Hg	P_0 mm. Hg	v_c cu. mm.	P_t mm. Hg	P_0 mm.Hg	v_0 cu. mm.	P_t mm. Hg	P_0 mm. Hg	v_c cu. mm.	P_t mm. Hg
0	41·4	4·4	51·4	59·1	3·4	70·1	81·7	2·7	93·5	127·5	1·9	140·2
0·5	37·8	5·0	48·3	54·2	3·9	65·9	75·1	3·2	87·8	117·9	2·2	131·7
1	34·5	5·6	45·5	49·8	4·5	62·1	69·3	3·6	82·8	109·3	2·6	124·2
1·5	31·6	6·3	43·1	45·8	5·0	58·7	64·0	4·1	78·3	101·4	3·0	117·5
2	29·0	7·0	40·9	42·1	5·7	55·7	59·1	4·6	74·3	94·3	3·4	111·4
2·5	26·6	7·7	38·9	38·8	6·3	53·0	54·7	5·2	70·7	88·0	3·8	106·0
3	24·4	8·5	37·1	35·8	7·0	50·5	50·6	5·8	67·4	81·8	4·3	101·1
3·5	22·4	9·3	35·4	33·0	7·7	48·3	46·9	6·4	64·4	76·2	4·8	96·6
4	20·6	10·1	33·9	30·4	8·5	46·2	43·4	7·1	61·7	71·0	5·3	92·5
4·5	18·9	11·0	32·5	28·0	9·3	44·4	40·2	7·8	59·1	66·2	5·9	88·7
5	17·3	11·9	31·3	25·8	10·1	42·6	37·2	8·6	56·8	61·8	6·5	85·2
5·5	15·9	12·9	30·1	23·8	11·0	41·0	34·4	9·4	54·7	57·6	7·2	82·0
6	14·6	13·9	29·0	21·9	11·9	39·5	31·8	10·2	52·7	53·6	7·8	79·0
6·5	13·4	14·9	28·0	20·1	12·9	38·1	29·4	11·1	50·8	49·9	8·6	76·3
7	12·2	16·0	27·0	18·5	13·9	36·8	27·2	12·0	49·1	46·5	9·3	73·7
7·5	11·2	17·1	26·1	17·0	14·9	35·6	25·1	12·9	47·5	43·2	10·1	71·3
8	10·2	18·3	25·3	15·6	16·0	34·5	23·1	13·9	46·0	40·2	10·9	69·0
8·5	9·4	19·5	24·5	14·3	17·2	33·4	21·3	15·0	44·6	38·1	11·8	66·9
9	8·5	20·7	23·8	13·1	18·3	32·4	19·6	16·0	43·3	34·6	12·7	64·9
9·5	7·8	22·0	23·1	12·0	19·5	31·5	18·0	17·2	42·0	32·0	13·7	63·0
10	7·1	23·3	22·5	10·9	20·8	30·6	16·5	18·3	40·8	29·6	14·7	61·2
10·5	6·5	24·6	21·8	10·0	22·1	29·8	15·1	19·5	39·7	27·4	15·7	59·6
11	5·9	26·0	21·3	9·1	23·4	29·0	13·8	20·8	38·6	25·3	16·8	58·0
11·5	5·3	27·4	20·7	8·3	24·8	28·2	12·6	22·1	37·6	23·3	17·9	56·5
12	4·9	28·8	20·2	7·5	26·2	27·5	11·5	23·4	36·7	21·4	19·1	55·0
12·5	4·4	30·3	19·7	6·8	27·7	26·8	10·5	24·8	35·8	19·7	20·3	53·7
13	4·0	31·9	19·2	6·2	29·2	26·2	9·5	26·2	34·9	18·1	21·5	52·4
13·5		33·4	18·8	5·6	30·7	25·6	8·6	27·7	34·1	16·5	22·8	51·1
14		35·0	18·3	5·0	32·3	25·0	7·8	29·3	33·3	15·1	24·2	50·0
14·5		36·7	17·9	4·5	34·0	24·4	7·1	30·8	32·6	13·7	25·5	48·8
15		38·3	17·5	4·1	35·6	23·9	6·4	32·4	31·9	12·6	27·0	47·8
15·5		40·1	17·1		37·4	23·4	5·8	34·1	31·2	11·4	28·5	46·7
16		41·8	16·8		39·1	22·9	5·2	35·8	30·5	10·4	30·0	45·8
16·5		43·6	16·4		40·9	22·4	4·7	37·6	29·9	9·4	31·5	44·8
17		45·5	16·1		42·8	22·0	4·2	39·4	29·3	8·5	33·2	43·9
17·5		47·3	15·8		44·7	21·5		41·2	28·7	7·7	34·8	43·0
18		49·2	15·5		46·7	21·1		43·1	28·1	6·9	36·5	42·2
18·5		51·2	15·2		48·7	20·7		45·1	27·6	6·2	38·3	41·4
19		53·1	14·9		50·7	20·3		47·1	27·1	5·6	40·1	40·6
19·5		55·2	14·6		52·8	19·9		49·1	26·6	4·9	42·0	39·9
20		57·2	14·4		54·9	19·6		51·2	26·1	4·5	43·9	39·2

* Values are given here to one decimal.

P_0 = pressure in the undisturbed eye.

v_c = volume of corneal indentation.

P_t = intra-ocular pressure with tonometer resting on the eye.

FRIEDENWALD'S (1957) NOMOGRAM FOR OCULAR RIGIDITY

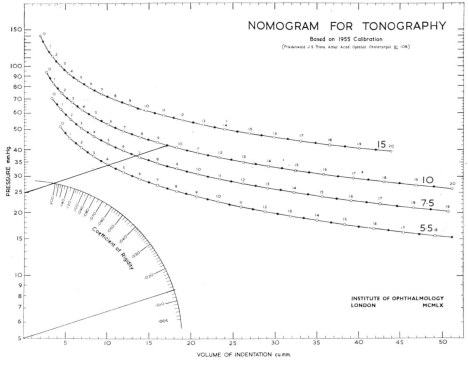

Fig. 684.

The ordinate represents the intra-ocular pressure in mm. Hg on a logarithmic scale, the abscissa the volume of corneal indentation in cu. mm. Tonometric readings are taken with two different plunger-loads and the line joining these two points has a specific slope intersecting the ordinate at a pressure-reading corresponding to the initial intra-ocular pressure (P_0). If a line parallel to this is drawn from the lower left-hand corner of the chart, it will meet the quadrant-scale at a point corresponding to the ocular rigidity.

In the example illustrated in Fig. 684, the reading with the 5·5 G. plunger-load was 4, and with the 10 G. load 9·5, the initial intra-ocular pressure was 25, and the coefficient of rigidity 0·013.

It will be seen that a small error of 0·5 unit in either reading results in a wide range of uncertainty in the level of the initial intra-ocular pressure and in the coefficient of rigidity.

APPENDIX II

TONOGRAPHIC TABLES

For eyes of average rigidity (Moses and Becker, *Amer. J. Ophthal.*, **45**, 196, 1958). The values for the coefficient of aqueous outflow (C) corresponding to all possible scale-readings have been calculated in accordance with the equation

$$C = \frac{(V_{c4} - V_{c0}) + \dfrac{1}{K}(\log P_{t0} - \log P_{t4})}{\left(\dfrac{P_{t0} + P_{t4}}{2} - P_0 - \Delta P_v\right)t}$$

For the explanation of terms, see p. 462.

KEY TO THE USE OF THE TABLES

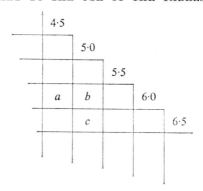

FIG. 685.—USE OF TABLES V, VI AND VII.

The value of C is given at the intersection of the vertical column indicated by the initial scale-reading, and the horizontal column indicated by the scale-reading after 4 minutes of tonography.

Thus (a) if the scale-reading changed from 4·5 to 6·0, the value of C would be as shown at a;

(b) if the scale-reading changed from 4·75 to 6·0, the value of C would be the average of a and b;

(c) if the scale-reading changed from 4·75 to 6·25, the value of C would be the average of a and c.

TABLE V

TONOGRAPHY WITH 5·5 G. WT.

2·0	2·5	3·0	3·5	4·0	4·5	5·0	5·5	6·0	6·5	7·0	7·5	8·0	8·5	9·0	9·5	10·0	10·5	11·0	11·5	12·0	12·5	13·0
0·05	**2·5**																					
0·10	0·04	**3·0**																				
0·16	0·09	0·04	**3·5**																			
0·24	0·15	0·09	0·04	**4·0**																		
0·33	0·22	0·14	0·08	0·04	**4·5**																	
0·44	0·30	0·20	0·13	0·08	0·04	**5·0**																
0·58	0·39	0·27	0·19	0·13	0·08	0·04	**5·5**															
0·74	0·49	0·35	0·25	0·18	0·12	0·08	0·04	**6·0**														
0·93	0·62	0·44	0·32	0·24	0·17	0·12	0·08	0·03	**6·5**													
	0·76	0·54	0·40	0·30	0·23	0·17	0·12	0·07	0·03	**7·0**												
	0·92	0·65	0·49	0·37	0·29	0·22	0·16	0·11	0·07	0·03	**7·5**											
		0·78	0·59	0·45	0·35	0·27	0·21	0·15	0·11	0·07	0·03	**8·0**										
			0·70	0·54	0·42	0·33	0·26	0·20	0·15	0·11	0·07	0·03	**8·5**									
				0·63	0·50	0·40	0·32	0·25	0·20	0·15	0·11	0·07	0·03	**9·0**								
					0·58	0·47	0·38	0·31	0·25	0·20	0·15	0·11	0·07		**9·5**							
						0·54	0·45	0·37	0·30	0·24	0·19	0·15	0·11			**10·0**						
							0·52	0·43	0·36	0·29	0·24	0·19	0·15				**10·5**					
								0·49	0·42	0·35	0·29	0·24	0·19					**11·0**				
									0·48	0·40	0·34	0·29	0·23						**11·5**			
										0·46	0·39	0·34	0·28							**12·0**		
											0·45	0·39	0·33								**12·5**	
												0·45	0·39									**13·0**

TABLE VI

TONOGRAPHY WITH 7·5 G. WT.

2·0	2·5	3·0	3·5	4·0	4·5	5·0	5·5	6·0	6·5	7·0	7·5	8·0	8·5	9·0	9·5	10·0	10·5	11·0	11·5	12·0	12·5	13·0
0·04																						
0·09	0·04																					
0·14	0·08	0·03																				
0·22	0·13	0·07	0·03																			
0·31	0·19	0·12	0·07	0·03																		
0·43	0·27	0·17	0·11	0·06	0·03																	
0·58	0·36	0·23	0·16	0·10	0·06	0·03																
0·78	0·47	0·31	0·21	0·15	0·10	0·06	0·03															
	0·60	0·40	0·28	0·20	0·14	0·10	0·06	0·03														
	0·77	0·50	0·35	0·25	0·18	0·13	0·09	0·06	0·03													
		0·62	0·43	0·32	0·24	0·17	0·13	0·09	0·05	0·03												
		0·76	0·53	0·39	0·29	0·22	0·16	0·12	0·09	0·05	0·03											
			0·63	0·46	0·35	0·27	0·21	0·16	0·12	0·08	0·05	0·03										
				0·55	0·42	0·33	0·26	0·20	0·15	0·12	0·08	0·05	0·03									
						0·50	0·39	0·31	0·25	0·19	0·15	0·12	0·08	0·05								
								0·45	0·37	0·30	0·24	0·19	0·15	0·11	0·08							
										0·42	0·35	0·28	0·23	0·19	0·15	0·11						
												0·40	0·33	0·27	0·23	0·18	0·15					
														0·38	0·32	0·27	0·22	0·18				
																0·37	0·31	0·26	0·22			
																		0·36	0·30	0·26		
																				0·35	0·30	

TABLE VII

TONOGRAPHY WITH 10 G. WT.

2·0	2·5	3·0	3·5	4·0	4·5	5·0	5·5	6·0	6·5	7·0	7·5	8·0	8·5	9·0	9·5	10·0	10·5	11·0	11·5	12·0	12·5	13·0	13·5
2·0																							
0·03	**2·5**																						
0·08	0·03	**3·0**																					
0·13	0·07	0·03	**3·5**																				
0·20	0·11	0·06	0·03	**4·0**																			
0·31	0·17	0·10	0·06	0·02	**4·5**																		
0·45	0·25	0·15	0·09	0·05	0·02	**5·0**																	
0·66	0·35	0·21	0·13	0·08	0·05	0·02	**5·5**																
	0·47	0·29	0·19	0·12	0·07	0·05	0·02	**6·0**															
		0·38	0·25	0·17	0·11	0·07	0·05	0·02	**6·5**														
		0·49	0·32	0·22	0·16	0·10	0·07	0·04	0·02	**7·0**													
			0·40	0·28	0·20	0·15	0·10	0·07	0·04	0·02	**7·5**												
			0·50	0·35	0·25	0·19	0·14	0·10	0·07	0·04	0·02	**8·0**											
				0·43	0·31	0·23	0·18	0·13	0·10	0·07	0·04	0·02	**8·5**										
				0·52	0·38	0·28	0·22	0·17	0·13	0·09	0·07	0·04	0·02	**9·0**									
						0·44	0·34	0·26	0·21	0·16	0·12	0·09	0·06	0·04	**9·5**								
								0·40	0·31	0·24	0·20	0·15	0·12	0·09	0·06	**10·0**							
										0·36	0·29	0·23	0·19	0·15	0·12	0·09	**10·5**						
												0·33	0·27	0·22	0·18	0·14	0·11	**11·0**					
														0·31	0·26	0·21	0·18	0·14	**11·5**				
																0·30	0·25	0·21	0·18	**12·0**			
																		0·29	0·24	0·20	**12·5**		
																				0·28	0·23	**13·0**	
																					0·27	**13·5**

FRIEDENWALD'S NOMOGRAM IN TONOGRAPHY

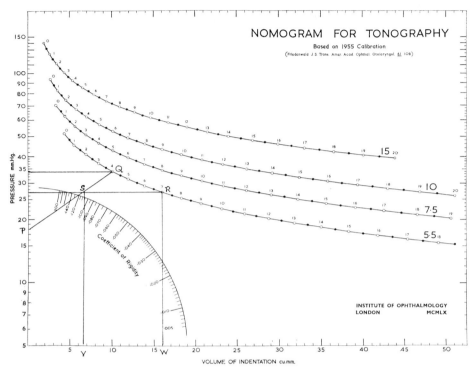

FIG. 686.

The ordinate represents the intra-ocular pressure on a logarithmic scale, the abscissa the volume of indentation. The initial applanation reading is indicated at P and the scale-readings at the beginning and end of the tonography at Q and R with an interval of 4 mins. Horizontal lines through two points give the value of the two readings as 34 and 27 mm. Hg. The slope of the line joining P and Q represents the ocular rigidity and it cuts the horizontal line from R at S. Vertical lines from R and S meet the abscissa at W and V. The total amount of fluid lost (ΔV) is represented by VW which can be read from the nomogram as 9·5 cu. mm. This evaluates the entire numeral of the equation on p. 750. The facility of outflow (C) is therefore calculated from the simplified equation.

$$\frac{\Delta V}{\left(\dfrac{P_{t0} + P_{t4}}{2} - P_0 - 1\cdot25\right) \times 4}.$$

INDEX

A

Abscess, of lens, 5
  orbital, glaucoma and, 678
Accommodation, cataract and, 123, 151, 246
  glaucoma and, 574
Aceclydine, for glaucoma, 511
Acetazolamide, for cataract, 246
  for glaucoma, acute, 619
    simple, 520
  See also Carbonic anhydrase inhibitors.
Acidification, cataract due to, 81
Acromegaly, glaucoma and, 409
  vitreous changes, senile, and, 356
Adamük, Ämilian, 628, 629
Adaptometry, in glaucoma, 480
Addison's disease, hypotony in, 728
Adrenaline, cataract due to, 104
  causing glaucoma, 703
  for glaucoma, closed-angle, 609
    simple, 517, 551
Adrenergic drugs, for glaucoma, 516
After-cataract, 233
  capsular remains causing, 234
  cyclitic exudates causing, 234, 238
  hæmorrhages causing, 234, 238
  lentoid bodies causing, 234, 238
  pigmentary remains causing, 234, 238
  prevention of, 241
  treatment of, 241
Age changes, in lens capsule, 14
  in lens, chemical, 13
    morphological, 10
  in vitreous, 355
Agnew, Cornelius Rea, 295, 296
Akinesia, for cataract surgery, 261, 269
Albright's syndrome, 176
Albuminoid in lens, in age, 13
  in cataract, 68
Alcohol, for glaucoma, closed-angle, 612
  simple, 523
Alloxan cataract, 92
Alopœcia areata, cataract and, 203
  total, cataract and, 203

Alpha-chymotrypsin with cataract extraction. *See* Zonulysis.
  injection into eye, glaucoma and, 584, 631
Alport's syndrome, cataract in, 208
  lenticonus in, 61
Aludrine. *See* Isoprenaline.
Amino acids, crystals of, in cataract, 134
  deficiency of, cataract and, 96
  excess of. *See* Aminoaciduria.
Aminoaciduria, cataract and, 192
  glaucoma and, 642
Amyl nitrite test, in glaucoma, 501
Amyloid deposits, in vitreous, 330
Amyloidosis, primary familial, glaucoma in, 692
  vitreous opacities in, 330
Anæmia, Cooley's, cataract in, 229
  hæmolytic, cataract in, 208
  pernicious, cataract in, 229
    hypotony in, 732
Anæsthesia, hypotony in, 727
Analgesia, for cataract surgery, 261, 269
Andogsky's syndrome, 197
Angiodiathermy, 548
Angiokeratoma corporis diffusum, cataract in, 194
Angioscotometry, 469, 471
Aniridia, buphthalmos and, 633
Ankylostomiasis, cataract in, 229
Anorexia nervosa, cataract in, 190
Anoxic cataract, 228
  experimental, 83
Anterior chamber, angle of, in glaucoma, closed-angle, 569, 571, 577, 596
    simple, 412, 448
  obstruction of, experimental, 630
  post-inflammatory, 653
  recession of, 661, 665, 707
  delayed re-formation of, after cataract extraction, 279, 717
    after keratoplasty, 721
  depth of, in glaucoma, closed-angle, 570, 595
    simple, 448
  dislocation of lens into, 302

Bone diseases, cataract and, 204
formation, in lens, 135, 213
Bowman's membrane, folds in, in
hypotony, 742
Brain, anomalies of, cataract and, 207
Bretylium, for glaucoma, 520
Buerger's disease. *See* Thrombo-
angiitis obliterans.
Bulbar pressure tests, in glaucoma, 499
Buphthalmos, 632
displacement of lens in, 298
Busulphan cataract, 112

C

Cachexia, cataract in, 229
Caffeine test, in glaucoma, 500
Calcareous degeneration, in lens, 134
Calcium, in blood, in glaucoma, 406
crystals, in cataract, 131, 132, 134
iodide, for cataract, 245
in lens, in age, 13
in cataract, 70
/phosphate ratio, low, cataract and,
101, 175
soaps, in vitreous, 325
Capillary system, disturbances of, in
glaucoma, 406
Capsule, lens, changes in, with age, 14
in cataract, 25, 27, 125
colloid bodies on, 26
cysts of, causing after-cataract, 237
duplication of, 32
exfoliation of, 42
pseudo-, 45
glaucoma and, 54, 691
senile, 14, 43
folding of, 57
glycolytic enzymes in, in age, 15
iridescence of, in age, 14
non-lenticular structures on, 62
permeability of, in age, 71
in cataract, 83, 123
remains of, causing after-cataract, 235
rupture of, 58
spontaneous, 59
hereditary, in mice, 61
traumatic, 58
thickening of, 62
wounds of, healing of, 16
wrinkling of, 24
See also Subcapsular epithelium.

Capsulectomy, 273
Capsulo-iridectomy, Elschnig's, 242
Capsulotomy, 272
vitreous prolapse after, 369
Caput medusæ, in glaucoma, closed-
angle, 591
simple, 445
Carbachol, for glaucoma, 511
Carbamates. *See* Physostigmine, *etc.*
Carbohydrate metabolism, in
cataractous lens, 73
anomalies of, cataract and, 194
Carbonic anhydrase inhibitors, for
glaucoma, closed-angle, 609
simple, 520, 552
hypotony due to, 726
Carbromal cataract, 230
Cardiac glycosides, for glaucoma, 522
hypotony due to, 727
Cardrase. *See* Ethoxzolamide.
Carotene deficiency, cataract and, 190
experimental, 100
excess, maternal, experimental cataract
and, 100
Carotico-cavernous aneurysm, glaucoma
and, 679
Carotid artery, ligation of, cataract and,
83
glaucoma and, 673
Cataract, 63
absorption of, spontaneous, 59, 138
accommodation and, 123
acidification, 81
adrenaline, 104
ætiology of, 67
theories of, 121
after-. *See* After-cataract.
aminoaciduria and, 192
angiokeratoma corporis diffusum and,
194
anorexia nervosa and, 190
anoxic, 228
experimental, 83
antibodies and, 122
antihistamines and, 119
anti-mitotics and, 112
arthrogryposis multiplex and, 206
asphyxia and, 84
astigmatism in, 143
atopic dermatitis and, 196
black, 127, 160
blood, chemical changes in, 74
blue-dot, 149

PRINTED IN GREAT BRITAIN BY THE WHITEFRIARS PRESS LTD.
LONDON AND TONBRIDGE